SUBMICRON EMULSIONS IN DRUG TARGETING AND DELIVERY

Drug Targeting and Delivery
A series of books discussing all aspects of the targeting and delivery of drugs.
Edited by A.T. Florence and G. Gregoriadis, The School of Pharmacy, University of London, UK

Volume 1
Microencapsulation of Drugs
edited by T.L. Whateley

Volume 2
Liposomes in Drug Delivery
edited by G. Gregoriadis, A.T. Florence and H.M. Patel

Volume 3
Drug Absorption Enhancement: Concepts, Possibilities, Limitations and Trends
edited by A.G. de Boer

Volume 4
Trends and Future Perspectives in Peptide and Protein Drug Delivery
edited by V.H.L. Lee, M. Hashida and Y. Mizushima

Volume 5
Interfacial Phenomena in Drug Delivery and Targeting
G. Buckton

Volume 6
Liposomes in Biomedical Applications
edited by P.N. Shek

Volume 7
Handbook of Biodegradable Polymers
edited by A.J. Domb, J. Kost and D.M. Wiseman

Volume 8
Antigen Delivery Systems: Immunological and Technological Issues
edited by B. Gander, H.P. Merkle and G. Corradin

Volume 9
Submicron Emulsions in Drug Targeting and Delivery
edited by S. Benita

Other volumes in preparation

Advanced Gene Delivery
edited by A. Rolland

An Introduction to Niosomes and Other Non-Phospholipid Systems
edited by I. Uchegbu

This book is part of a series. The publisher will accept continuation orders which may be cancelled at any time and which provide for automatic billing and shipping of each title in the series upon publication. Please write for details.

SUBMICRON EMULSIONS IN DRUG TARGETING AND DELIVERY

Edited by

Simon Benita

School of Pharmacy, Hebrew University of Jerusalem, Israel

harwood academic publishers
Australia • Canada • China • France • Germany • India • Japan
Luxembourg • Malaysia • The Netherlands • Russia • Singapore
Switzerland

Copyright © 1998 OPA (Overseas Publishers Association) N.V. Published by license under the Harwood Academic Publishers imprint, part of The Gordon and Breach Publishing Group.

All rights reserved.

No part of this book may be reproduced or utilized in any form or by any means, electronic or mechanical, including photocopying and recording, or by any information storage or retrieval system, without permission in writing from the publisher. Printed in Singapore.

Amsteldijk 166
1st Floor
1079 LH Amsterdam
The Netherlands

British Library Cataloguing in Publication Data

A catalogue record for this book is available from the British Library.

ISBN: 90-5702-349-0

To my wife, Esther

CONTENTS

Preface to the Series — ix

Preface — xi

Contributors — xiii

1 Introduction and Overview — 1
   S. Benita

INTRAVENOUS FAT EMULSIONS

2 Perspectives on the Use of Intravenous Lipid Emulsions in Man — 7
   A. Hyltander, R. Sandström and K. Lundholm

3 Particle-Sizing Technologies for Submicron Emulsions — 21
   R.J. Haskell, J.R. Shifflett and P.A. Elzinga

4 Biofate of Fat Emulsions — 99
   M. Nishikawa, Y. Takakura and M. Hashida

SUBMICRON EMULSIONS AS THERAPEUTIC DELIVERY SYSTEMS

5 Design and Evaluation of Submicron Emulsions as Colloidal Drug Carriers for Intravenous Administration — 119
   S. Klang and S. Benita

6 Submicron Emulsions as Drug Carriers for Topical Administration — 153
   S. Amselem and D. Friedman

7 Emulsions of Supercooled Melts — A Novel Drug Delivery System — 175
   H. Bunjes, B. Siekmann and K. Westesen

8 Submicron Lipid Suspensions (Solid Lipid Nanoparticles) versus Lipid Nanoemulsions: Similarities and Differences — 205
   B. Siekmann and K. Westesen

9 Solid Lipid Nanoparticles (SLN®) for Controlled Drug Delivery — 219
   R.H. Müller and S.A. Runge

PERFLUOROCHEMICAL SUBMICRON EMULSIONS

10 The Design and Engineering of Oxygen-Delivering Fluorocarbon Emulsions — 235
    M.P. Krafft, J.G. Riess and J.G. Weers

Index — 335

PREFACE TO THE SERIES

The current volume is the ninth in the series which aims to provide comprehensive surveys of topics in drug delivery and targeting for senior undergraduates, graduates and those carrying out research in the many facets of the field. Drug delivery technologies and targeting strategies grow in scope and potential, as well as complexity, almost daily. New opportunities arise through the development of new materials for the design and fabrication of drug delivery vehicles and carriers; new challenges are posed by the discovery and development of new therapeutic agents, which include not only small organic and inorganic molecules but oligomers and macromolecules usually with no natural propensity for transport across biological barriers. The book series has, to date, covered delivery technologies in microencapsulation[1] and liposomal delivery[2,3], the promotion of drug absorption[4], the important issues surrounding peptide and protein delivery[5], interfacial phenomena in drug delivery and targeting[6] and biodegradable polymers of natural, synthetic or semi-synthetic origin[7]. The technology of drug delivery can rarely be dealt with simply as a materials science topic, for systems have to be evaluated in the context of the biological environment in which they operate *in vivo*.

Professor Benita has edited the current volume dealing with an aspect of lipid nanotechnology — submicron emulsions in targeting and delivery. The field evolved from developments with intravenous fat emulsions, which are covered in Chapters 2–4 of the book. A variety of submicron systems — emulsions and lipid suspensions (solid lipid particles) have been investigated. The next part of the book addresses these topics. The final chapter covers perfluorochemical emulsions as blood substitutes, an intriguing area of research. Lipidic systems have great scope once we understand fully their physical chemistry and the manner in which they interact with the body.

Drexler[8] writes of conventional drug delivery: "Drugs are dumped into the body, tumble and bump around in solution haphazardly until they bump a target molecule, fit and stick ...". He proposed that the future of therapy will consist of nanomachines which will gain access to diseased sites, recognize the target, disassemble damaged parts, rebuild and reassemble. Many lipidic systems are, indeed, self-assembling. We are perhaps still some way from that vision, but the progress that is made step by step is the stuff of research in drug delivery and targeting. It is the role of a book series to record and analyze that progress, and we hope that this series will achieve those aims and provide some stimulus for further discovery.

Alexander T. Florence and Gregory Gregoriadis
Series Editors

REFERENCES

1. T.L. Whateley (Ed.) (1992) *Microencapsulation of Drugs*, Harwood Academic Publishers, Chur.
2. G. Gregoriadis, A.T. Florence and H.M. Patel (Eds) (1993) *Liposomes in Drug Delivery*, Harwood Academic Publishers, Chur,.
3. P.N. Shek (Ed.) (1996) *Liposomes in Biomedical Applications*, Harwood Academic Publishers, Chur.

4. A.(Bert) G. de Boer (Ed) (1994) *Drug Absorption Enhancement: Concepts, Possibilities, Limitations and Trends*, Harwood Academic Publishers, Chur.
5. V.H.L. Lee, M. Hashida, Y. Mizushima (Eds) (1995) *Trends and Future Perspectives in Peptide and Protein Drug Delivery*, Harwood Academic Publishers, Chur.
6. G. Buckton (1995) *Interfacial Phenomena in Drug Delivery and Targeting*, Harwood Academic Publishers, Chur.
7. A.J. Domb, J. Kost and D.M. Wiseman (Eds) (1997) *Handbook of Biodegradable Polymers*, Harwood Academic Publishers, Amsterdam.
8. K.E. Drexler (1990) *Engines of Creation*, Fourth Estate, London.

PREFACE

The general theme and purpose of this multi-authored book is to provide the reader with a current, updated and general overview of submicron emulsion and lipid suspensions (solid lipid nanoparticles). This book covers all the aspects of submicron emulsion outlining their therapeutic potential in a wide range of diseases. It contains the different methods of preparations, physicochemical characterization and *in vitro* drug release evaluation. Practical approaches to the various formulation problems are presented. The latest advances in the production, technology and therapeutic applications including drug targeting are discussed by the most authoritative contributors in the field of submicron emulsions and lipid suspensions. To the best of my knowledge, despite the fact that some reviews have been published on the subject, there is currently no book in the scientific community which deals only with submicron emulsions and lipid suspensions.

I believe, there is a need for such a comprehensive book since lipid submicron emulsions are receiving increasing attention as colloidal drug carriers for various potential therapeutic applications including drug targeting. They are well accepted as intravenous delivery systems for their ability to incorporate water non-soluble drugs to stabilize drug that easily undergo hydrolysis and to reduce side-effects of various potent drugs. Submicron emulsions are also used to increase bioavailability and prolong pharmacological effects of drug with poor absorption or short biological half life provided they are not administered intravenously.

Scientists in the pharmaceutical, biotechnological and medical research fields are aware that such a dosage form, although difficult to formulate adequately, might exhibit potential advantages that would result in new and improved therapeutic uses of drugs and would eliminate many disadvantages present in current therapies. Innovative submicron dosage forms such as Diazemuls (diazepam emulsion), Diprivan® (propofol submicron emulsion), Fluosol®, Etomidat Lipuro® (etomidate emulsion), Liple® (alprostadil emulsion) and Limethason® (dexamethasone palmitate emulsion) are examples of successfully marketed emulsions.

Thus, in a logical sense after an overview chapter, the book focuses in its first part on the perspectives on the use of intravenous lipid emulsion in man followed by a comprehensive chapter on particle sizing technologies. The chapter on biofate of fat emulsion completes this first part of the book. The second part of the book concentrates on the potential of submicron emulsions to function as efficient colloidal drug carriers for various route of administration. Despite their promising applications emulsions also exhibit some limitations. They are fragile, sensitive, dispersed systems. To overcome some of these inconveniences emulsions of super-cooled melts and solid lipid nanoparticles were developed as novel drug delivery systems and are covered in two chapters.

The use of a systematic approach in presenting the various applications of these lipid delivery systems should facilitate the comprehension of this increasingly complex field and clarify the differences existing between submicron emulsions and lipid suspensions (solid lipid nanoparticles). Furthermore, to avoid any confusion between the different lipid delivery system definitions, an entire chapter of the book is devoted to similarities and differences between these systems. Finally, a comprehensive and exhaustive chapter is dedicated to the designed engineering of oxygen-delivery fluorocarbon emulsions.

In all the different areas of submicron emulsions, leading authors have been approached and invited to write appropriate chapters in their field. All of the authors are scientists working in research centers of institutions or pharmaceutical research companies. Undoubtedly the readers of this book will benefit immensely from the experiences and input of the authors who have included within their chapters reports on their own scientific achievements in this field.

It is anticipated that submicron emulsion and lipid suspension delivery systems will find numerous and novel medical applications in the near future. The extensive recent results of animal studies published in the literature, using different routes of administration underline the promising properties of these lipid drug carriers as therapeutic delivery systems for a variety of drugs. I hope that the lecture of this book will improve the comprehension and knowledge of the readers in the entire field of colloidal lipid drug carriers.

CONTRIBUTORS

Shimon Amselem
Pharmos Ltd.
Kiryat Weizmann
76326 Rehovot
Israel

Simon Benita
Department of Pharmaceutics
School of Pharmacy
Faculty of Medicine
Hebrew University of Jerusalem
P.O. Box 12056
Jerusalem 91120
Israel

Heike Bunjes
Institute of Pharmaceutical Technology
Friedrich Schiller University Jena
07743 Jena
Germany

P.A. Elzinga
Pharmaceutical Development
Pharmacia and Upjohn, Inc.
7000 Portage Road
Kalamazoo, Michigan 49001
USA

Doron Friedman
Farmo-Nat Ltd.
P.O. Box 7284
78172 Ashkelon
Israel

Mitsuru Hashida
Department of Drug Delivery Research
Faculty of Pharmaceutical Sciences
Kyoto University
Sakyo-ku, Kyoto 606-01
Japan

R.J. Haskell
Pharmaceutical Development
Pharmacia and Upjohn, Inc.
7000 Portage Road
Kalamazoo, Michigan 49001
USA

Anders Hyltander
Department of Surgery
Sahlgrenska University Hospital
413 45 Göteborg
Sweden

Shmuel Klang
Department of Pharmaceutics
School of Pharmacy
Faculty of Medicine
Hebrew University of Jerusalem
P.O. Box 12056
Jerusalem 91120
Israel

Marie Pierre Krafft
Unité de Chimie Moléculaire
Université de Nice
France

Kent Lundholm
Department of Surgery
Sahlgrenska University Hospital
413 45 Göteborg
Sweden

R.H. Müller
Free University of Berlin
Department of Pharmaceutics,
  Biopharmaceutics and
  Biotechnology
Kelchstrasse 31
D-12169 Berlin
Germany

Makiya Nishikawa
Department of Drug Delivery Research
Faculty of Pharmaceutical Sciences
Kyoto University
Sakyo-ku, Kyoto 606-01
Japan

Jean G. Riess
School of Medicine
University of Calfornia
San Diego
USA
and
Alliance Pharmaceutical Corp.
San Diego
USA

S.A. Runge
Free University of Berlin
Department of Pharmaceutics,
 Biopharmaceutics and
 Biotechnology
Kelchstrasse 31
D-12169 Berlin
Germany

Rolf Sandström
Department of Surgery
Sahlgrenska University Hospital
413 45 Göteborg
Sweden

J.R. Shifflett
Pharmaceutical Development
Pharmacia and Upjohn, Inc.
7000 Portage Road
Kalamazoo, Michigan 49001
USA

Britta Siekmann
Astra Arcus AB
Department of Pharmaceutics
151 85 Södertälje
Sweden

Yoshinobu Takakura
Department of Drug Delivery Research
Faculty of Pharmaceutical Sciences
Kyoto University
Sakyo-ku, Kyoto 606-01
Japan

Jeffry G. Weers
Alliance Pharmaceutical Corp.
San Diego
USA

Kirsten Westesen
Institute of Pharmaceutical Technology
Friedrich Schiller University Jena
07743 Jena
Germany

1. INTRODUCTION AND OVERVIEW

SIMON BENITA

Department of Pharmaceutics, The School of Pharmacy,
The Hebrew University of Jerusalem, P.O.B. 12065, Jerusalem 91120, Israel

There is no doubt that intensive research efforts have been concentrated on the design of injectable emulsion formulations that led to successful marketed products such as the emulsion of 1% Propofol (Diprivan®, Zeneca, UK). Intravenously administered emulsions are excellent carriers for lipophilic drugs which are often difficult to deliver, they are biodegradable, biocompatible, physically stable and relatively easy to produce on large scale. Fat emulsion drug delivery systems seem to offer a wide variety of possibilities for preparing better tolerated intravenous formulations of selected poorly water soluble drugs while either maintaining the same characteristics concerning pharmacokinetic and tissue distribution or enhancing the site-specific delivery in targeted organs. The past decade has seen enormous activity in drug delivery and targeting research using submicron emulsions as carriers of poorly water soluble drugs.[1-3]

The first approved iv. emulsion, Intralipid® more than 30 years ago was developed for parenteral nutrition. It consists of an o/w emulsion of 10 or 20% soybean oil droplets (70–400 nm in size) stabilized by a monolayer of egg yolk mixed phospholipids (1.2%) and glycerol (2.25%) as an osmotic agent. Overall, Intralipid® exhibits a high negative zeta potential value at the physiological pH range.

The wide and clinically well-accepted usage of emulsions for parenteral nutrition has raised the possibility of using the internal oil core of this o/w emulsion for solubilizing water-insoluble drugs. However, in most cases the introduction of a drug within such an emulsion introduced a marked physical instability resulting in phase separation of the emulsion in a relatively short period of time. Another important drawback of emulsions is their fragile physical stability and sensitivity to marked and rapid environmental changes such as heat, shaking, light and storage conditions fluctuations. They must be sufficiently stable to be easily manufactured, sterilized (preferably by terminal autoclaving) and have a shelf life of at least 1–2 years or even more.

Thus, there is a need to design innovative lipid emulsions stabilized by various combinations of surface active agents able to prolong extensively the shelf life of the emulsion formulations resulting in viable commercial emulsion preparations. This is particularly well illustrated by the Fluosol-DA case which was the first commercially available fluorocarbon emulsion intended for intravenous use in man and was developed by Green Cross Corp. (Osaka, Japan). The advent of Fluosol was an extremely important milestone in the history of fluorocarbon-based injectable oxygen carriers. Fluosol-DA contains 20% by weight (~11% by volume) of a mixture of two fluorocarbons, perfluordecalin and perfluorotripropylamine in a 7:3 ratio in a frozen formulation which was dictated by the need to find a compromise between insufficient emulsion stability and excessive fluorocarbon retention in the organs.[4]

The lack of stability and consequent lack of practicality was a major cause of the commercial failure of Fluosol. Nevertheless, numerous papers confirmed the efficacy of fluorocarbon emulsions in delivering oxygen.[5] Moreover, the understanding and analysis of the drawbacks and shortcomings of Fluosol-DA have set the stage for future research, improvements and developments of stable innovative fluorocarbon emulsion formulations based on efficient but short organ retention time fluorocarbons such a perfluorooctylbromide .This is widely discussed in the last chapter of the book.

The oil droplets of a conventional o/w emulsion are rapidly captured after iv. injection by the reticuloendothelial system (RES) — organs such as the liver and spleen.[6,7] This may be advantageous for delivery of drugs to macrophages or to treat diseases involving the RES, but it is certainly problematic for drug delivery to non-RES tissues. In addition, rapid removal of the oil droplets to a large extent prevents the use of emulsions for controlled release of the drug within the vasculature. Because of this problem, the potential of emulsions as drug delivery systems for parenteral administration have not been fully explored. Thus, it is sometimes necessary to develop o/w emulsion formulations capable of escaping from the RES uptake and showing prolonged circulation in the blood. Different approaches are being tested to change the distribution pattern of emulsion in the body to yield high concentration of the drug in the plasma and tissues other than RES-rich organs.[8-13]

It was reported that a reduction in size and coating with hydrophilic poloxamer 338 or sphingomyelin on the surface of oil droplets resulted in avoidance of the RES.[12] It was found that inclusion of PEG derivatives such as dioleoyl N-(monomethoxypolyethyleneglycol succinyl)phosphatidylethanolamine (PEG-PE) into emulsions composed of Castor oil and phosphatidylcholine decreases the RES uptake and increase blood residence time of the emulsions.[13] Another approach to alter the biodistribution pattern of lipid emulsion is by conferring to the oil droplets a positive charge as suggested by our group (submitted data).

A major limitation of the emulsion delivery systems is that they cannot be adapted to the delivery of water-soluble drugs as no advantage over a simple aqueous solution could be foreseen. Furthermore, the kinetic results of a study on the *in vitro* release kinetic examination and comparative evaluation between submicron emulsions and polylactic acid nanocapsules of clofibride, a lipophilic drug used in the treatment of hypercholesterolaemia and hypertriglyceridaemia clearly exclude the use of submicron emulsions as colloidal controlled release delivery systems for any administration route where perfect sink conditions should prevail.[14] These deductions are valid for drugs which are water soluble or lipophilic drugs with log $P_{octanol/water}$ less than 8 like miconazole base.[15]

Therefore, the only viable approach to the delivery of a hydrophilic or poorly lipophilic drug is to synthesize a lipophilic prodrug or drug derivative that can be located in the oil phase of the emulsion and that can be transformed into the active drug after administration within a reasonable period of time. This approach has been used for example to formulate emulsions containing lipophilic drug derivatives such as dexamethasone palmitate[16-19], flurbiprofen axetil[20], isocarbacyclin methyl ester[21-23], Δ^8-9-0-butyril prostaglandin E_1 butyl ester[24,25], palmitoyl rhizoxin.[8,9,26] It should be emphasized that in order to alter the pharmacokinetic profile of a lipophilic drug and confer to it the intrinsic pharmacokinetic properties of the colloidal carrier, the value of the partition coefficient n-octanol-water should be above 10^8 as previously reported.[10] Thus, despite complex formulation problems exhibited by submicron emulsion delivery systems, it is possible to overcome the technical obstacles and to propose satisfactory solutions.

The main therapeutic applications of submicron emulsions should be sought in emulsion formulations designed for parenteral administration of poorly water soluble drugs as outlined above. However, there is still a marked potential for the use of submicron emulsions in non-parenteral delivery systems.

Submicron emulsions have also been investigated for the past decade as carriers for ocular, oral and transdermal drug delivery. Muchtar and Coll[27] and Naveh and Coll[28] demonstrated that submicron emulsions can also be used as an ocular delivery system for the lipophilic antiglaucoma drugs, tetrahydrocannabinol (THC), and pilocarpine base respectively. They showed that the emulsion was able to elicit a long-lasting antidepressant effect on the intraocular pressure of rabbits following a single instillation. Rubinstein and Coll[29]; Myers & Stella[30]; Kleinstern and Coll[31], and Ilan and Coll[32] used submicron emulsion delivery systems to prolong the pharmacological effect of drugs with short biological half-lives or poor bioavailability following oral administration. Finally, Friedman and Coll[33] and Schwarz and Coll.[34] clearly showed the potential of submicron emulsions to enhance transdermal delivery of diazepam and non-steroidal anti-inflammatory drugs whereas the results reported by Ezra and Coll.[35] suggested that a positively-charged submicron emulsion exhibited a more prolonged residence time in the uppermost layers of the skin than a negatively charged submicron emulsion. These overall results underline the promising properties of emulsion drug carriers as therapeutic delivery systems for a variety of drugs.

The number of references in the literature reporting on preliminary data regarding the potential of submicron emulsions as drug carriers is enormous and cannot be covered comprehensively in a single review or even in one book. Some of the drugs incorporated in lipid emulsions and currently under investigation are discussed in the actual book.

REFERENCES

1. Washinton, C. (1996) Stability of lipid emulsions for drug delivery. *Adv. Drug Del. Rev.*, **20**, 131–145.
2. Lovell, M.W., Johnson, H.W., Hui, H.W., Cannon, J.B., Gupta, P.K., Hsu, C.C. (1994) Less painful emulsion formulations for intravenous administration of clarithromycin. *Int. J. Pharm.*, **109**, 45–57.
3. Tibell, A., Lindholm, A., Sawe, J., Chen, G., Norrlind, B. (1995) Cyclosporin A in fat emulsion carriers: experimental studies on pharmacokinetics and tissue distribution. *Pharmacol. Toxicol.*, **76**, 115–121.
4. Riess, J.G. (1991) Synthetic fluorocarbon-based oxygen-transport fluids. *Vox Sang.*, **61**, 225–239.
5. Riess, J.G., Weers, J. (1996) Emulsions for biomedical uses. *Current Opinion in Colloid. Interface Sci.*, **1**, 652–659.
6. Singh, M., Ravin, L.J. (1986) Parenteral emulsions as drug carrier system. *J. Parenteral. Sci. Technol.*, **40**, 34–41.
7. Koga, Y., Swanson, V.L., Hayes, D.M. (1975) Hepatic 'intravenous fat pigment' in infants and children receiving lipid emulsion. *J. Pediatr. Surg.*, **10**, 641–648.
8. Kurihara, A., Shibayama, Y., Mizota, A., Yasuno, A., Ikeda, M., Sasagawa, K., Kobayashi, T., Hisaoka, M. (1996) Enhanced tumor delivery and antitumor activity of palmitoyl rhizoxin using stable lipid emulsions in mice. *Pharm. Res.*, **13**, 11305–11320.

9. Kurihara, A., Shibayama, Mizota, A., Y., Yasuno, A., Ikeda, M., Hisaoka, M. (1996) Pharmacokinetics of highly lipophilic antitumor agent palmitoyl rhizoxin incorporated in lipid emulsions in rats. *Biol. Pharm. Bull.*, **19**, 252–258.
10. Takino, T., Nakajima, C., Takakura, Y., Sezaki, H., Hashida, M. (1993) Controlled biodistribution of highly lipophilc drugs with various parenteral formulations. *J. Drug Targeting*, **1**, 117–124.
11. Takino, T., Konishi, K., Takakura, Y., Hashida, M. (1994) Long circulating emulsion carrier systems for highly lipophilic drugs. *Biol. Pharm. Bull.*, **17**, 121–125.
12. Lee, M.-J., Lee, M.-H., Shim, C.-K. (1995) Inverse targeting of drugs to reticuloendothelial system-rich organs by lipid microemulsion emulsified with poloxamer 338. *Int. J. Pharm.*, **113**, 175–187.
13. Liu, F., Liu, D. (1995) Long-circulating emulsions (oil-in-water) as carriers for lipophilic drugs. *Pharm. Res.*, **12**, 1060–1064.
14. Santos Magalhaes, N.S., Fessi, H., Puisieux, F., Benita, S., Seiller, M. (1995) An *in vitro* release kinetic examination and comparative evaluation between submicron emulsion and polylactic acid nanocapsules of clofibride. *J. Microcap.*, **12**, 195–205.
15. Kakutani, T., Nishihara, Y., Takahashi, K., Hirano, K. (1991) o/w lipid microemulsion for parenteral drug delivery. *Proc. Int. Symp. Controlled Release of Bioactive Materials*, **18**, 359–360.
16. Japan pharmaceutical reference. Administration and products in Japan, Japan Medical Products International Trade Association, Ed. Tanaka Printing Co., Tokyo, 3rd edition, 286–292 (1993).
17. Yokoyama, K., Watanabe, M. (1996) Limethason as a lipid microsphere preparation: An overview. *Adv. Drug Del. Rev.*, **20**, 195–201.
18. Yokoyama, K., Okamoto, H., Watanabe, M. (1985) Development of a corticosteroid incorporated in lipid microsphers (liposteroid). *Drugs Exp. Clin. Res.*, **11**, 611–620.
19. Hoshi, K., Mizushima, Y., Shiokawa, Y. (1985) Double-blind study with liposteroid in rheumatoid arthritis. *Drugs Exp. Clin. Res.*, **11**, 621–626.
20. Ohmukai, O. (1996) Lipo-NSAID preparation. *Adv. Drug Del. Rev.*, **20**, 203–207.
21. Shibasaki, M., Torisawa, Y., Ikegarni, S. (1983) Synthesis of 9(0)-methano-$\Delta(6(9\alpha)$-PGI$_1$: The highly potent carbon analog of prostacyclin. *Tetrahedron Lett.*, **24**, 3493–3496.
22. Hoshi, K., Mizushima, Y. (1990) A preliminary double-blind cross-over trial of lipo-PGI$_2$, a prostacyclin derivative incorporated in lipid microspheres, in cerebral infarction. *Prostaglandins*, **40**, 155–164.
23. Kurozumi, S., Araki, H., Tanabe, H., Kiyoki, M. (1996) Lipid microsphere preparation of a prostacyclin analogue. *Adv. Drug Del. Rev.*, **20**, 181–187.
24. Igarashi, R., Mizushima, Y., Takenaga, M., Matsumoto, K., Morizawa, Y., Yasuda, A. (1992) A stable PGE1 pro-drug for targeting therapy. *J. Control. Rel.*, **20**, 37–46.
25. Igarashi, R., Mizushima, Y. (1996) New lipo-PGE$_1$ using a stable prodrug of prostaglandin E$_1$ (PGE$_1$). *Adv. Drug Del. Rev.*, **20**, 189–194.
26. Kurihara, A., Shibayama, Y., Yasuno, A., Ikeda, M., Hisaoka, M. (1996) Lipid emulsions of palmitoylrhizoxin: Effects of particle size on blood dispositions of emulsion lipid and incorporated compound in rats. *Biopharm. Drug Disposit.*, **17**, 343–353.
27. Muchtar, S., Almog, S., Torracca, M.T., Saettone, M.F., Benita, S. (1992) A submicron emulsion as ocular vehicle for δ8-tetrahydro-cannabinol: Effect on intraocular pressure in rabbits. *Ophthalm. Res.*, **24**, 142–149.
28. Naveh, N., Muchtar, S., Benita, S. (1994) Pilocarpine incorporated into a submicron emulsion vehicle causes an unexpectedly prolonged ocular hypotensive effect in rabbits. *J. Ocular Pharmacol.*, **10**(3), 509–520.
29. Rubinstein, A., Pathak, Y.V., Kleinstern, J., Reches, A., Benita, S. (1991) *In vitro* release and intestinal absorption of physostigmine salicylate from submicron emulsion. *J. Pharm. Sci.*, **80**, 643–647.
30. Myers, R.A., Stella, V.J. (1992) Systemic bioavailability of penclomedine (NSC-338720) from oil-in-water emulsion administered intraduodenally to rats. *Int. J. Pharm.*, **78**, 217–226.
31. Kleinstern, J., Markowitz, E., Benita, S. (1993) The effect of oil nature in o/w submicron emulsions on the oral absorption profile of physostigmine salicylate in rats. *S.T.P. Pharma Sci.*, **3**(2), 163–169.
32. Ilan, E., Amselem, S., Weisspapir, M., Schwarz, J., Yogev, A., Zawoznik, E., Friedman D. (1996) Improved oral delivery of desmopressin via a novel vehicle: Mucoadhessive submicron emulsion. *Pharm. Res.*, **13**(7), 1083–1087.
33. Friedman, D.I., Schwarz, J.S., Weisspapir, M. (1995) Submicron emulsion vehicle for enhanced transdermal delivery of steroidal and nonsteroidal antiinflammatory drugs. *J. Pharm. Sci.*, **84**(3), 324–329.

34. Schwarz, J.S., Weisspapir, M.R., Friedman, D.I. (1995) Enhanced transdermal delivery of diazepam by submicron emulsion (SME) creams. *Pharm. Res.*, **12**(5), 687–692.
35. Ezra, R., Benita, S., Ginsburg, I., Kohen, R. (1996) Prevention of oxidative damage in fibroblast cells cultures and rat skin by positively charged submicron emulsion of α-tocopherol. *Eur. J. Pharm. Biopharm.*, **42**(4), 291–298.

2. PERSPECTIVES ON THE USE OF INTRAVENOUS LIPID EMULSIONS IN MAN

A. HYLTANDER, R. SANDSTRÖM and K. LUNDHOLM

Department of Surgery, Sahlgrenska University Hospital, Göteborg, Sweden

INTRODUCTION

The development and introduction of lipid emulsions for intravenous use in humans has offered possibilities for supply of energy-rich substrates within small infusion volumes and has significantly contributed to the practical application of total parenteral nutrition, TPN. Continued research within the field of lipid emulsions has revealed other indications exemplified as the use of lipids for drug delivery, for reduction of drug toxicity and for radiographic purposes, all of which are topics that will be discussed in other chapters of this book. This review will focus on aspects of the use of lipid emulsions for nutritional and pharmacological purposes in man.

BACKGROUND

TPN, which has been in clinical use for more than three decades, represents a life-saving treatment modality. Any patient can via intravenous infusion receive all substrates necessary for maintenance of nutritional status, i.e. carbohydrate, fat and amino acids, irrespective of the functional status of the gastro-intestinal tract. Carbohydrate overfeeding have since long been demonstrated in association with significant side effects such as hepatic lipogenesis, excessive CO_2 production and increased adrenergic activation, indicating a need for non-carbohydrate energy sources (Burke *et al.*, 1990; Robin *et al.*, 1981; Nordenström *et al.*, 1981; Vollenweider *et al.*, 1995). Thus, much effort has been made to further improve substrate utilization and reduce drawbacks associated with TPN, and much interest has been focused on the lipid component. The rationale for the use of lipid emulsions in parenteral feeding has so far been mainly twofold; a) to provide essential fatty acids and b) to provide a carbohydrate and insulin-independent energy-rich substrate. The lipid component consists in most emulsions for parenteral and enteral feeding, of long-chain triglycerides (LCT) which have proven to be a safe, effective and reliable as source of energy and essential fatty acids (Mascioli *et al.*, 1987). However, the use of LCT emulsions has been implicated as the cause of some metabolic and immunologic side-effects especially when used in stressed patients, which in turn has emphasized the need for alternative lipid sources (Michie and Guillou 1990; Sedman *et al.*, 1990; Monson *et al.*, 1988; Wan *et al.*, 1991; Blackburn 1992; Sedman *et al.*,

---

Correspondence: Anders Hyltander, M.D., Ph.D., Sahlgrenska University Hospital, Department of Surgery, S-413 45 Göteborg, Sweden. Tel: +46 31 601000; +46 31 604405 (direct); Fax: +46 31 41 7364.

1991). Lipid metabolism now represents an area of great scientific interest since information has emerged demonstrating fat as a metabolically active substrate which may offer metabolic advantages. Improved effects on nitrogen balance, positive effects on immunological functions including prostanoid metabolism, improved biochemical properties such as changed fatty acid patterns and blood viscosity are some important issues that have been addressed. A common denominator for achieving these goals has been related to the fatty acid composition of the lipid formulation. The development of esterification techniques leading to the introduction of structured triglycerides thus delineates a most important progress in lipid research enabling tailored fatty acid composition of lipid emulsions in order to achieve specific metabolic and possibly also pharmacologic effects in the future.

EFFECTS OF LIPID EMULSIONS ON IMMUNE FUNCTION

The immunologic cascade involves receptor-ligand interactions at the cell surface. Accordingly, the lipid composition of the cell membrane has been identified as a major determinant for an appropriate signal transduction evoked as a result of interactions between cytokines and growth factors with their respective receptors on the cell membrane (Mascioli et al., 1987). Thus, dietary fat can influence on the function of the immue system by altering the lipid composition of cellular membrane phospholipids. One possible mechanism behind a changed transmission across the cellmembrane, is a perturbation of the ratio of unsaturated/saturated fatty acids with changed physical and biochemical properties. Previous studies have demonstrated that administration of Ω-6 LCT containing lipid emulsions, which is part of most current complete TPN mixtures, can modify the biochemical composition of the cell membrane leading to interference with the receptor-ligand interaction. Interleukin-2 (IL-2) has been extensively studied *in vitro* experiments which have demonstrated a reduction of the cellular cytotoxic response to IL-2 in animals receiving LCT-containing lipid emulsions (Sedman et al., 1990; Monson et al., 1988). A reduction has also been found for IL-2 dependent processes such as the spontaneously occurring natural killer (NK) cell activity *in vivo*. It has been shown that the IL-2 molecule was prevented to bind to its ligand on the cell surface as thus prevented from internalization possibly due to a more rigid membrane structure. This may explain impaired IL-2 activated cellular cytotoxicity in patients receiving TPN with LCT containing lipid emulsions.

However, in other previous experimental studies, protective effects of LCT infusion in association with lipopolysaccharide, LPS, administration has been hypothesized (Read et al., 1995). LPS play a key role in the pathogenesis of gram-negative sepsis and reproduces in a dose-dependent manner the major features associated with septic shock (Glauser et al., 1991). Infusion of triglyceride-rich lipoproteins has been shown to attenuate inflammatory and pyrogenic responses to endotoxin and to improve survival (Ulevitch et al., 1979).

However, in studies on human volunteers, hypertriglyceridemia, achieved with infusion of a LCT-containing lipid emulsion, did not attenuate inflammatory responses to endotoxin administration measured as fever, leukocytosis or release of tumor necrosis factor. Some effects of LPS infusion were even potentiated such as release of interleukin-6 and 8 and neutrophil degranulation (van der Poll et al.,

1995). The disparate results may be explained by a several-fold higher plasma concentrations of triglycerides in the experimental studies (van der Poll *et al.*, 1995).

Altered eicosanoid metabolism is an important part of the response in immunomodulation events, since provision of LCT emulsions rich in Ω-6 fatty acids increase arachidonic acid production leading to increased production of 2-series of prostaglandins, A_2 thromboxanes and B_4 category of leucotrienes, all metabolites with pro-inflammatory effects (Wan *et al.*, 1991; Blackburn 1992). The inflammatory response diminishes proportionally to the reduction of LCT content when replaced with other lipid sources as for example medium chain triglycerides, MCT (Sedman *et al.*, 1991). However, the potentially positive effects on immune function associated with provision of MCT-based lipid emulsions compared with Ω-6 LCT emulsions, remain to be demonstrated in prospective clinical studies in critically ill patients.

MCT emulsions are associated with other advantages such as a more rapid clearance from the circulation than LCT emulsion due to the smaller molecular size and greater solubility (Babayan 1987; Lutz *et al.*, 1989). This may also contribute to a less tendency to deposition in liver or adipose tissue, but instead increased oxidation (Mascioli *et al.*, 1987; Geleibter *et al.*, 1983; Bach and Babayan 1982). MCT emulsions are independent of carnitine for transport into mitochondria for β-oxidation in contrast to LCT emulsions. However, carnitine deficiency has been demonstrated in less than 5% of a patient population suffering from critical illness and malnutrition (Wennberg *et al.*, 1992) and carnitine supplementation to patients with verified carnitine deficiency did not alter whole body oxidation of fatty acids (Lundholm *et al.*, 1988). Thus, carnitine dependency for complete oxidation does not seem to be a limiting factor for oxidation of LCT emulsions, as previously has been claimed. However, administration of acetyl-L-carnitine may be beneficial for support of cellular activities by means other than improving hemodynamic parameters (Gasparetto *et al.*, 1991). The positive effects of MCT emulsions on metabolism and immune function are, however, in part counteracted by significant side-effects since pure MCT solutions may be toxic and cause metabolic acidocis in larger doses, and do not contain essential fatty acids (Miles *et al.*, 1991; Cotter *et al.*, 1987; Christensen *et al.*, 1989).

STRUCTURED TRIGLYCERIDES

Hydrolysis of a mixture of LCT and MCT emulsions followed by random reesterification on the same glycerol backbone give a structured triglyceride as end product (Figure 1). This method has offered an unique tool to combine positive metabolic effects of both LCT and MCT emulsions and reduce adverse effects (Babayan, 1987; Moyer *et al.*, 1989). A more simple alternative is a physical mixture of both triglycerides. However, studies evaluating the metabolic effects of different lipid emulsions have demonstrated significant advantageous effects with structured triglycerides compared to physical mixtures of the same triglycerides (Mendez *et al.*, 1992; Mok *et al.*, 1984). As a consequence, a substantial body of evidence has emerged demonstrating beneficial effects of structured triglycerides instead of conventional LCT-based emulsions at least in various animal models (Mascioli *et al.*, 1989; Mascioli *et al.*, 1988; Kinsella and Lokesh, 1990; Lokesh *et al.*, 1992).

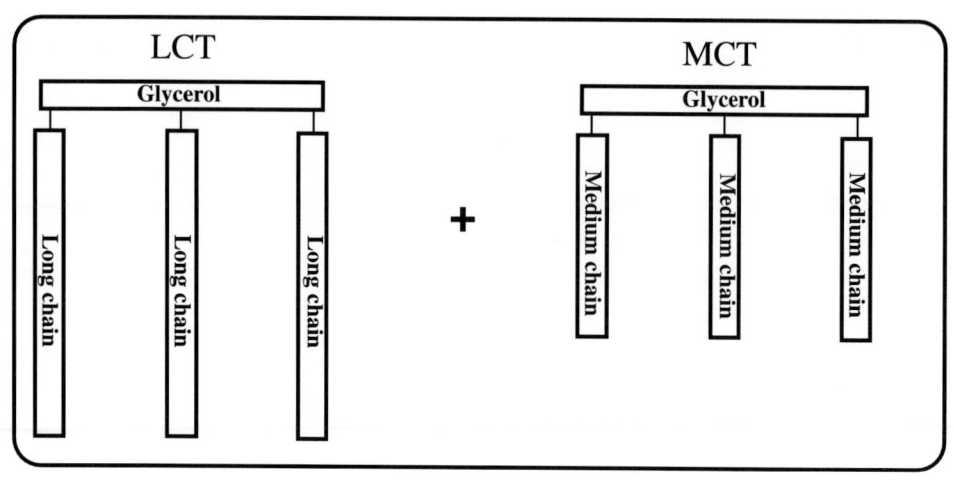

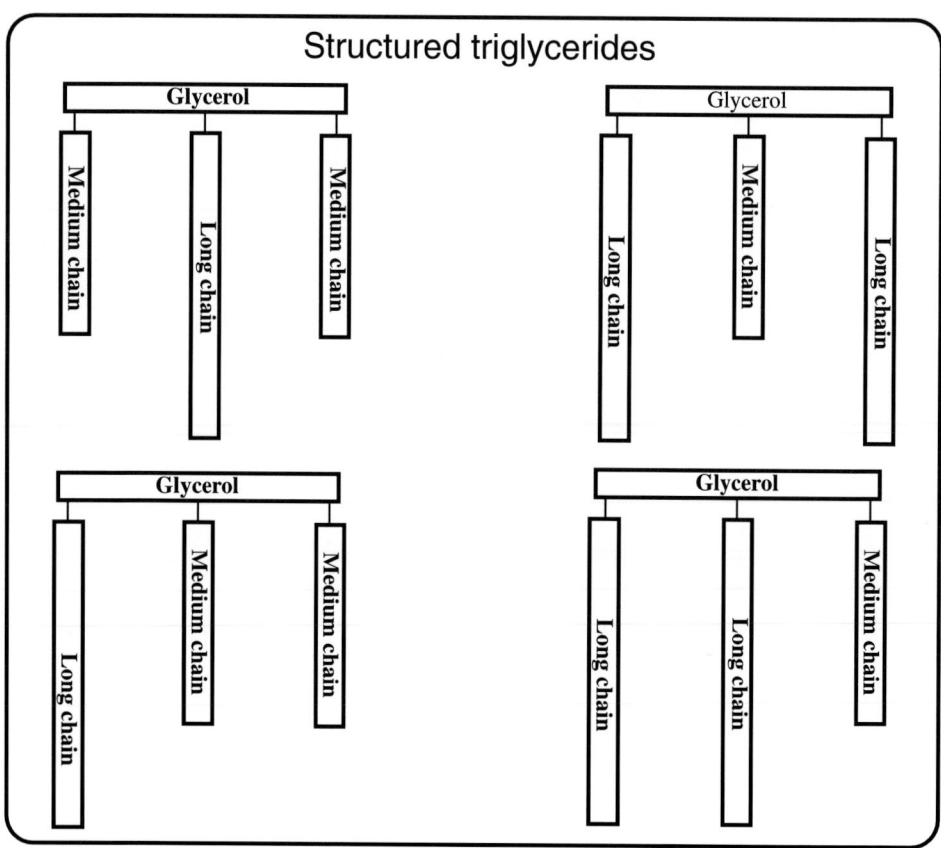

Figure 1 Schematic drawing of one kind of structured triglycerides. LCFA and MCFA on the back-bone of glycerol in six different molecules. The two molecules at the bottom exist in two stereoisomers each.

Biochemical Technology and Nutrition Pharmacology

The technique to synthesize structured triglycerides has indicated a new era with possibilities to use different sources of lipids for specific purposes and hereby create combinations of various fatty acids to reach specific metabolic and nutritional goals. One striking example is modification of the LCT component with the use of Ω-3 fatty acids instead of the most commonly used Ω-6 fatty acid, esterified with a MCT. The most frequently used Ω-3 fatty acids is fish oil. Ω-3 fatty acids have been used in numerous experimental studies demonstrating beneficial effects such as improvement in function of the reticulo endothelial system, RES, with additional benefits in protein metabolism (Mendez et al., 1992; Sobrado et al., 1985). Stressed animals receiving fish-oil showed improvements in protein metabolic parameters as well as cellular immunity compared to animals receiving LCT emulsions only (Alexander et al., 1986). Fish-oil feeding has also been reported to alter prostaglandin and leucotriene synthesis, producing less inflammatory 3-series of prostaglandins and 5-series of leucotrienes. This shift in eicosanoid metabolism would serve to reduce the proinflammatory reactions induced by sepsis or trauma (Kinsella and Lokesh, 1990; Lokesh et al., 1992; German et al., 1985; Nassar et al., 1987; Lee et al., 1985). The potential beneficial effects on the immune system are illustrated in studies demonstrating increased animal survival after toxin challenge. Guinea pigs in endotoxic chock receiving LCT's rich in n-6 poly unsaturated fatty acids, PUFA, demonstrated low survival rate. However, survival increased significantly when fish oil emulsions rich in n-3 PUFA were given (Mascioli et al., 1989; Mascioli et al., 1988). Ω-3 fatty acids offer advantages also in transplantation immunology. Fish-oil provision to recipient animals provided a significant protection against acute rejection with an increased allograft survival and reduced requirement for immunosuppressive drugs (Otto et al., 1990; Grimm et al., 1994). These effects seem also to be mediated by changes in eicosanoid metabolism in favor of less inflammatory metabolites (Leaf, 1988; Terano et al., 1985).

However, interference with inflammation is also generally associated with a decreased collagen deposition which may alter important reparative processes such as wound healing. This hypothesis has been addressed in experimental studies indicating that Ω-3 fatty acids may attenuate tensile strength, albeit without affecting collagen (Albina et al., 1993). There are no data available from clinical studies addressing this issue.

Lipid Emulsions and Tumorigenesis

Dietary fats are associated with tumor growth and a correlation has been demonstrated between amount of ingested fat and the incidence of solid tumors in colon and breast. It has also been shown that dietary fats may play an important role in promotion of malignant tranformation (Carroll and Braden, 1984; Reddy, 1981; Reddy, 1995). This information has lead to the hypothesis that interference with fat supply may modulate tumorigenesis and tumor growth. One of the cornerstones for this hypothesis is the previously described interference between dietary fat and phospholipid composition of cell membranes with subsequent effects on cytokine production and prostanoid synthesis and metabolism. Prostaglandins are potent immunomodulators and the synthesis of pro-inflammatory prostaglandins and leucotrienes is dependent on the composition of lipid emulsions used as previously has been demonstrated (Wan, Kanders et al., 1991; Blackburn, 1992). Dietary fat can either be stimulatory or inhibitory to tumor growth as has been demonstrated in experimental studies on nude mice. Animals fed a diet mainly consisting of linoleic acid which is a common component of commercially avaliable LCT-containing lipid emulsions stimulate tumor growth compared to administration of Ω-3 fatty acids (Welsch 1995). The anti-proliferative effects of administration of long-chain Ω-3 fatty acids have repeatedly been confirmed in several studies with experimental tumor models, including studies of metastasis (Carroll and Braden 1984; Welsch 1995). It must be emphasized that this information emerges exclusively from experimental studies on orally fed animals. These results have not been confirmed in clinical studies on humans, and there are no indications that intravenous administration of lipid emulsions to a considerable extent consisting of linoleic acid should promote malignant transformation in clinical practice. However, the results indicate a concept with great clinical potential, especially for treatment of diseases characterized by chronic and progressive inflammation and wasting, exemplified by cancer disease. The hypothesis that attenuation of the inflammatory response could be beneficial in such chronic diseases has gained support from a recently published placebo-controlled prospective, randomized clinical study on cancer patients with advanced disease (Lundholm et al., 1994). This study demonstrated for the first time that anti-inflammatory treatment given to cancer patients in advanced clinical state, significantly prolonged survival and maintained quality of life, indicating anti-inflammatory treatment as an important palliative treatment modality (Lundholm et al., 1994).

EFFECTS OF LIPID EMULSIONS ON RES FUNCTION

The reticuloenothelial system, RES, functions in the phagocytosis of foreign material and microorganisms in the bloodstream. It comprises, together with the neutrophils, the major antimicrobial system in the body. The majority, 80-90%, of the RES occurs in the liver and spleen with additional areas also in bone marrow and lungs (Saba, 1970). RES has been implicated with clerance of lipid particles when lipid emulsions have been infused indicating that provision of large amounts of fat could block the Kuppfer cells and impair RES clearance (Du Toid et al., 1978). Previous animal studies have also demonstrated that provision of LCT emulsions diminished bacterial uptake in the liver and spleen indicating impairment of the RES function (Sobrado et al., 1985; Hamawy et al., 1985). Human studies with infusion of labelled colloids as tracer have demonstrated reduced clearance of tracer in patients when receiving TPN containing fat emulsions consisting of LCT emulsions (Jensen et al., 1990). In the same study, infusion of a physical mixture of LCT/MCT, 25%/75% respectively, did not impair clearance rate when infused with identical rate as for the LCT-containing emulsion. This support MCT emulsions as advantageous since it may enable adequate metabolism of lipid emulsion without RES dysfunction (Jensen et al., 1990). This hypothesis has also gained support from experimental studies with sepsis and injury models (Mok et al., 1984; Maiz et al., 1984). Thus from a theorethical point of view, replacement of LCT with MCT could be beneficial in critically ill or septic patients and in patients receiving long-term TPN. However, the impairment of clearance rate associated with infusion of LCT emulsions in these studies was dose dependent and it must be emphasized that the infusion rate of lipid emulsion was several times higher than used in standard TPN with continuous and simultaneous infusion of all substrates. Continuous infusion regimens with "all-in-one" systems offer other metabolic advantages in patients in the postoperative course after major surgical procedures since it improves energy balance and nitrogen economy compared to sequential or intermittent infusions (Hyltander et al., 1993; Sandström et al., 1995b). Based on available data from randomized human studies, this infusion technique may theoretically be beneficial also when RES function is considered. However, no data are at present available from human studies of RES function and structured triglycerides.

STRUCTURED TRIGLYCERIDES IN CLINICAL PRACTICE

There are numerous experimental studies reporting on metabolic and immunologic effects of various types of structured triglycerides in trauma, cancer disease and sepsis, all with promising results indicating beneficial effects. However, so far data from human studies have been scarce. Structured triglycerides made from LCT, (Ω-6 fatty acids), and MCT, have been evaluated clinically in our institution (Sandström et al., 1993a). The random location and distribution of the various fatty acids used, is illustrated in Figure 1. The safety and tolerance of LCT/MCT structured triglycerides was evaluated in postoperative patients receiving TPN after major surgical procedures. Patients were randomly assigned to receive a conventional TPN admixture with 20% glucose and 0.2 g amino acid nitrogen and either lipid emulsion consisting of LCT (Intralipid) or structured triglyceride (fat emulsion 73403) both emulsions from Pharmacia Parenterals, Sweden. The weight ratio of MCT to LCT was 40:60 corresponding to a molar ratio of 50:50. Non-protein calories corresponding to 100% of resting energy expenditure, REE, was provided. The emulsion consisting of structured triglycerides was well tolerated and could safely be provided to patients following major surgical procedures (Sandström et al., 1993a). No signs of CNS toxicity were noted. Neither were there any tendencies of ketosis or significant increases in blood lipids (Sandström et al., 1993a). In a following study, also on postoperative patients after major surgery, we demonstrated for the first time in man that provision of structured triglycerides was associated with a higher whole body lipid oxidation rate than LCT in metabolically stressed postoperative patients (Sandström et al., 1995a). Lipid oxidation rate was statistically significantly higher with structured triglycerides, accounting for either the lipid amount in grams, or the caloric value (Figure 2). The increased oxidation rate was achieved without any significant change in resting energy expenditure. Previous animal studies have demonstrated improved nitrogen balance when structured triglycerides with a MCT/LCT ratio of 60:40 or higher were used (Gollaher et al., 1992). However, overall nitrogen economy was not affected by the type of lipid emulsions used in the present study, with a weight ratio MCT/LCT of 40:60. Whether the ratio MCT/LCT is critical for nitrogen balance must be addressed in future human studies with sufficiently long equilibrium periods to allow valid nitrogen or protein accretion measurements. It is likely that the positive effect of structured triglycerides in the study was due to a rapid plasma clearance including increased avaliability for

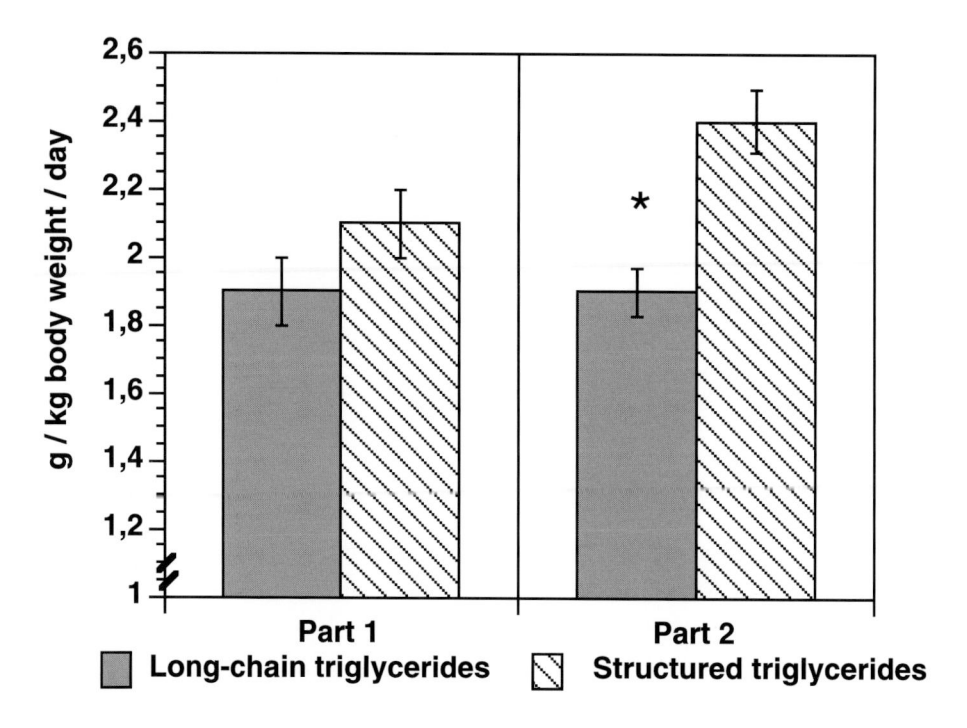

Figure 2 Whole body lipid oxidation rate per kg body weight in patients following major surgical operations. Mean values ± SE. * = p < 0,01. Fat oxidation was derived from measurements of gas exchange during lipid infusions. In the study marked Part 1 patients were provided with 1 g fat/kg b.w./day and calories corresponding to 80% of resting energy expenditure (REE) (55). Part 2 refers to a study where patients were provided 1,5 g fat/kg b.w./day and calories corresponding to 120% of REE. (56).

oxidative processes with minimal thermic effects, on whole body energy expenditure (Sandström et al., 1995a). These findings agree with the original metabolic and biochemical concept for structured triglycerides. Our results provide evidence to support that structured triglycerides may represent a next generation of intravenous fat emulsions that may be clinically advantageous to either conventional LCT or MCT/LCT emulsions.

In a previous, randomized, clinical study with 300 patients undergoing major surgical procedures, we addressed the hypothesis that TPN infusion postoperatively was superior to hypocaloric glucose infusion. All patients were randomized to receive on a daily basis either TPN with non-protein calories corresponding to 120% of REE (glucose.fat 70:30%), or only glucose infusions covering basal glucose needs (250–300 g) until oral intake was restored. The provision of calories in daily amounts not exceeding recommendations accepted of most clinicians, was accompanied by an excretion of significant amounts of glucose, 10–30 g/day, in the urine in both study groups. This was achieved in spite of normal plasma glucose concentrations in non-diabetic patients, indicating a changed renal threshold for glucose excretion (Sandström et al., 1993b). This finding was confirmed in a recent study on the impact of various TPN infusion kinetics on energy and nitrogen balances in postoperative patients after identical surgical procedures (Sandström et al., 1995b).

All patients were randomly assigned to receive non-protein calories corresponding to 100% of REE either as sequential infusion with glucose infusion during the night and fat/amino acids during the day, or simultaneous infusion of all substrates either intermittent or continuously. All study groups excreted glucose in the urine in spite of this moderately hypocaloric infusion regimen with plasma glucose concentrations within normal range (Sandström et al., 1995b). Thus, to avoid such complications, it is likely that the amount of glucose infused, should be further reduced and an alternative energy source as lipids may be used.

Derivation of Whole Body Lipid Oxidation

The traditional calculations of whole body carbohydrate and fat oxidation are based on equations described by Lusk (1917) and de Weir (1949) and are based on the assumption that starch and long-chain triglycerides are used for oxidation. The equations read:

Lipid oxidation rate = 2,432 V_{O2} − 2,432 V_{CO2} − 1,94 U_N (g lipids/day)
Energy expenditure = 5,50 V_{O2} + 1,76 V_{CO2} − 1,99 U_N (kcal/day)

However, the use of of structured triglycerides demand that special attention be paid to theoretical considerations when oxidation and energy expenditure are calculated since these lipids consist of fatty acids of various lengths on the same glycerol molecule. Calculations of whole body lipid oxidation rate, and energy expenditure must therefore be done with modified formulas when using structured triglycerides since the differences in chain length between LCT and MCT causes differences in the stoichiometric equations of fatty acid oxidation, and the fact that the caloric value of MCT is somewhat lower than that of LCT. For calculation of substrate oxidation and energy expenditure (EE) basic chemical variables as stoichiometric equations, caloric values and equivalent gas volumes for oxidation of glucose, fat, and amino acids must be known. The equation of Lusk, used without modification, when using structured triglycerides, will result in an underestimation of lipid oxidation rate in the magnitude of 10%. De Weir's equation is more robust to changes in fuel composition. Without modification de Weir's formula will overestimate energy expenditure by less than 1%.

The structured triglycerides used by us (fat emulsion 73403, Pharmacia Parenterals, Sweden) were composed of equal amounts of long-chain triglycerides and medium-chain triglycerides. The medium-chain triglycerides were made up of 8 carbon fatty acids and 10 carbon fatty acids. The ratio between 8 and 10 carbon fatty acids was 2,78/1. Oxidation of 8 carbon molecules yields the following reaction:

$C_8H_{16}O_2 + 11O_2 \rightarrow 8H_2O + 8CO_2$. The molar weight of this molecule is 144g.
11 moles of oxygen have the volume (liters) of 11 * 22,4 = 246,4
Oxidation of one gram of $C_8H_{16}O_2$ requires 246,4/144 = 1,711 liters of oxygen and produces 1,244 liters of CO_2.

Oxidation of 10 carbon molecules yields the following reaction:

$C_{10}H_{20}O_2 + 14O_2 \rightarrow 10H_2O + 10CO_2$. The molar weight of this molecule is 172g.
14 moles of oxygen have the volume (liters) of 14 * 22,4 = 313,6. Oxidation of one gram of $C_{10}H_{20}O_2$ requires 313,6/172 = 1,823 liters of oxygen and produces 1,302 liters of CO_2.

A weighed gas volume equivalent average of 2,78/1, which compensates for the different molar ratios of medium-chain fatty acids within medium-chain triglycerides, and then a straight 1/1 average with gas volume equivalents of long-chain triglycerides and medium-chain triglycerides compensates for the fact that the structured triglycerides used in our clinical studies was a mixture of equal molar amounts of LCT and MCT. This two-stage average gives the following equivalents:

Gas volume equivalents of 1 g of substrate:

Substrate	O_2	CO_2
Glucose (G)	0,746	0,746
Structured triglyc. (F_{ST})	1,880	1,343
Urea nitrogen (U_N)	6,04	4,89

Normally the gas volume equivalent of starch instead of glucose is used in metabolic calculations. This is correct for patients on oral diets, but not for patients on intravenous therapy, where glucose is the only carbohydrate used. With these equations V_{O2} and V_{CO2} can be written as:

$V_{O2} = 0,746\ G + 1,880\ F + 6,04\ U_N$
$V_{CO2} = 0,746\ G + 1,343\ F + 4,89\ U_N$

These two equations are solved for F or G and the result multiplied by 1,44 (unit conversion V_{O2} and V_{CO2}, liters/day → ml/min.)

The formula for lipid oxidation rate of structured triglycerides can be written as:
$F_{ST} = 2,68\ V_{O2} - 2,68\ V_{CO2} - 2,14\ U_N$ (modified equation of Lusk)

The formula for glucose oxidation rate can be written as:

$G = 6,79\ V_{CO2} - 4,85\ V_{O2} - 2,71\ U_N$;

where F_{ST} = lipid oxidation rate in g/day. G = glucose oxidation rate in g/day. V_{O2} = oxygen consumption in ml/min. V_{CO2} = carbon dioxide production in ml/min. U_N = urine nitrogen in g/day.

The caloric value for glucose (G) is 3,74 kcal/g. It is 8,75 kcal/g for structured triglycerides of corresponding composition (F_{ST}), and for urea nitrogen (U_N) it is 27 kcal/g. Energy expenditure (EE) is obtained by taking the sum of oxidation rates multiplied by the caloric value of each substrate:

$EE = 3,74\ G + 8,75\ F_{ST} + 27\ U_N$

By substituting G and F_{ST}

$EE = 5,32\ V_{O2} + 1,95\ V_{CO2} - 1,86\ U_N$ (modified equation of de Weir)

FUTURE USE OF STRUCTURED TRIGLYCERIDES

Results from our studies on stressed patients demonstrate that structured LCT/MCT triglycerides can safely be provided without risk for clinical or metabolic side effects (Sandström et al., 1993a). Moreover, lipid oxidation rate was significantly elevated compared to conventional LCT-based lipid emulsions, and it was associated with lower thermogenic effects (Sandström et al., 1995a). This indicates that structured triglycerides are energy-rich substrates that are rapidly available for oxidative processes with minor metabolic burden on the organism. The necessity for a substrate for intravenous use independent of glucose and insulin has recently been emphasized (Sandström et al., 1993b). These findings, together with previously described adrenergic stimulation of glucose infusion (Nordenström et al., 1981; Vollenweider et al., 1995; Mascioli et al., 1987), underline the need for alternative rapidly available energy sources than glucose. Based on information from our recent clinical studies on LCT/MCT emulsions, structured triglycerides represent an interesting alternative, especially in stressed patients (Sandström et al., 1993a; Sandström et al., 1995b).

REFERENCES

Albina, J.E., Gladden, P., Walsh, W.R. (1993) Detrimental effects of an omega-3 fatty acid-enriched diet on wound healing. *J. Parenter. Enteral. Nutr.*, **17**, 519–521.

Alexander, J.W., Saito, H., Trocki, O., et al. (1986) The importance of lipid type in the diet after burn injury. *Ann. Surg.*, **204**, 1–8.

Babayan, V.K. (1987) Medium chain triglycerides and structured lipids. *Nutr. Sup. Serv.*, **6**, 26–29.

Bach, A.C. and Babayan, V.K. (1982) Medium-chain triglycerides: an update. *Am. J. Clin. Nutr.*, **36**, 950–962.

Blackburn, G.L. (1992) Nutrition and inflammatory events: highly unsaturated fatty acids (Ω-3 vs Ω-6) in surgical injury. *Proc. Soc. Exp. Biol. Med.*, **200**, 183–188.

Burke, J.F., Wolfe, R.R., Mullany, C.J., et al. (1979) Glucose requirements following burn injury. *Ann. Surg.*, **190**, 274–285.

Carroll, K.K. and Braden, I.M. (1984) Dietary fat and mammary carcinogenesis. *Nutr. Cancer*, **6**, 254.

Christensen, E., Hagve, T.A., Grønn, M., et al. (1989) Beta oxidation of medium chain (C_8, C_{14}) fatty acids studied in isolated liver cells. *Biochim. Biophys. Acta*, **1004**, 187–195.

Cotter, R., Taylor, C.A., Johnson, R. (1987) A metabolic comparison of a pure long-chain triglyceride lipid emulsion (LCT) and various medium-chain triglyceride (MCT)-LCT combination emulsions in dogs. *Am. J. Clin. Nutr.*, **45**, 927–939.

de Weir, J. (1949) New methods for calculating metabolic rate with special reference to protein metabolism. *J. Physiol.*, **109**, 1–9.

Du Toid, D.F., Villet, W.T., Heydenrych, J. (1978) Fat emulsion deposition in mononuclear phagocytic system. *Lancet*, **2**, 898.

Gasparetto, A., Corbucci, G.G., DeBlasi, R.A. et al. (1991) Influence of acetyl-L-carnitine infusion on haemodynamic parameters and survival of ciculatory-shock patients. *Int. J. Clin. Pharm. Res.*, **11**, 83–92.

Geleibter, A., Torbay, N., Bracco, E.F., et al. (1983) Overfeeding either medium chain triglyceride diet results in diminished deposition of fat. *Am. J. Clin. Nutr.*, **37**, 1–4.

German, J.B., Lokesh, B., Bruckner, G.G., et al. (1985) Effect of increasing levels of dietary fish oil on tissue lipids and prostaglandin synthesis in the rat. *Nutr. Res.*, **5**, 1393–1407.

Glauser, M.P., Zanetti, G., Baumgartner, J.D., et al. (1991) Septic shock: pathogenesis. *Lancet*, **338**, 732–736.

Gollaher, C.J., Swenson, E.S., Mascioli, E.A., et al. (1992) Dietary fat level as determinant of protein-sparing actions of structured triglycerides. *Nutrition*, **8**, 348–353.

Grimm, H., Tibell, A., Norrlind, B., et al. (1994) Lipid mediated modification of rat heart allograft survival. *Transpl. Int.*, **7**, 247–52.

Hamawy, K.J., Moldawer, L.L., Georgieff, M., et al. (1985) The effect of lipid emulsions on reticuloendothelial system function in the injured animal. *JPEN J. Parenter. Enteral. Nutr.*, **9**, 559–565.

Hyltander, A., Arfvidsson, B., Körner, U., et al. (1993) Metabolic rate and nitrogen balance in patients receiving bolus intermittent total parenteral nutrition infusion. *JPEN J. Parenteral Enteral. Nutr.*, **17**, 158–168.

Jensen, G.L., Mascioli, E.A., Seidner, D.L., et al. (1990) Parenteral infusion of long and medium — chain triglycerides and reticuloendothelial system function in man. *JPEN J. Parenter. Enteral. Nutr.*, **14**, 467–471.
Kinsella, J.E., Lokesh, B. (1990) Dietary lipids, eicosanoids and the immune system. *Crit. Care Med.*, **18**, S94–S113.
Leaf, A. (1988) Effects of n-3 fatty acids on reocclusion after angioplasty. *Semin. Thromb. Hemost.*, **14**, 290–292.
Lee, T.H., Hoover, R.L., Williams, J.D., et al. (1985) Effects of dietary enrichment with eicosapentaenoic and docosahexaenoic acids on *in vitro* neutrophil and monocyte leucotriene generation and neutrophil function. *N. Engl. J. Med.*, **312**, 1217–1223.
Lokesh, B., LiCari, J., Kinsella, J. (1992) Effect of different dietary triglycerides on liver fatty acids and prostaglandin synthesis by mouse peritoneal cells. *JPEN J. Parenter. Enteral. Nutr.*, **16**, 316–321.
Lundholm, K., Gelin, J., Hyltander, A., et al. (1994) Anti-inflammatory treatment may prolong survival in undernourished patients with metastatic solid tumors. *Cancer Res.*, **54**, 5602–5606.
Lundholm, K., Persson, H., Wennberg, A. (1988) Whole body fat oxidation before and after carnitine supplementation in uremic patients on chronic hemodialysis. *Clin. Physiol.*, **8**, 417–426.
Lusk, G. (1917) *The elements of the science of nutrition*, 3rd ed. Philadelphia: W.B. Saunders.
Lutz, O., Lave, T., Frey, A, et al (1989) Activities of lipoprotein lipase and hepatic lipase on long- and medium-chain triglyceride emulsions used in parenteral nutrition. *Metabolism*, **38**, 507–513.
Maiz, A., Yamazaki, K., Sobrado, J., et al. (1984) Protein metabolism during total parenteral nutrition in injured rats using medium-chain triglycerides. *Metabolism*, **33**, 901–904.
Mascioli, E.A., Iwasa, Y., Trimbo, S., et al. (1989) Endotoxin challenge after menhaden oil diet: effects on survival of guinea pigs. *Am. J. Clin. Nutr.*, **49**, 277–282.
Mascioli, E.A., Leader, L., Flores, F., et al. (1988) Enhanced survival to endotoxin in guinea pigs fed IV fish oil emulsion. *Lipids*, **213**, 623–625.
Mascioli, E.A., Bistrian, B.R., Babayan, V.K., et al. (1987) Medium chain triglycerides and structured lipids as unique nonglucose energy sources in hyperalimentation. *Lipids*, **22**, 421–423.
Mendez, B., Ling, P.R., Nawfal, W.I., et al. (1992) Effects of different lipid sources in total parenteral nutrition on whole body protein kinetics and tumor growth. *JPEN J. Parenter. Enteral. Nutr.*, **16**, 545–551.
Michie, H. and Guillou, P.J. (1990) Biological response modifiers in cancer therapy. *Clin. Oncol.*, **2**, 347–353.
Miles, J.M., Cattalini, M., Sharbrough, F.W., et al. (1991) Metabolic and neurologic effects of an intravenous medium-chain triglyceride emulsion. *JPEN J. Parenter. Enteral. Nutr.*, **15**, 37–41.
Mok, K.T., Maiz, A., Yamazaki, K. (1984) Structured medium-chain and long-chain triglyceride emulsions are superior to physical mixtures in sparing body protein in the burned rat. *Metabolism*, **33**, 910–915.
Monson, J.R., Sedman, P.C., Ramsden, C.W., et al. (1988) Total parenteral nutrition adversely influences tumour-directed cellular cytotoxic responses in patients with gastrointestinal cancer. *Eur. J. Surg. Oncol.*, **14**, 935–943.
Moyer, E., Wennberg, A., Ekman, L., et al. (1989) A metabolic comparison between MCT, MCT/LCT and structured lipids. *Clin. Nutr.*, **8**, 83.
Nassar, B.A., Manku, M.S., Huang, Y.S., et al. (1987) The influence of dietary marine oil (Polepa) and evening primrose oil (Efamol) on prostaglandin production by the rat mesenteric vasculature. *Prostaglandins Leucotrienes Med.*, **26**, 253–263.
Nordenström, J., Jeevanandam, M., Elwyn, D.H., et al. (1981) Increasing glucose intake during total parenteral nutrition increases norepinephrine excretion in trauma and sepsis. *Clin. Physiol.*, **1**, 525–534.
Otto, D.A., Kahn, D.R., Hamm, M.W., et al. (1990) Improved survival of heterotopic cardiac allografts in rats with dietary n-3 polyunsaturated fatty acids. *Transplantation*, **50**, 193–198.
Read, T.E., Grunfeld, C., Kumwenda, Z., et al. (1995) Triglyceride-rich lipoproteins improve survival when given after endotoxin in rats. *Surgery*, **117**, 62–67.
Reddy, B.S. (1981) Dietary fat and its relationship to large bowel cancer. *Cancer Res.*, **41**, 3700–3705.
Reddy, B.S. (1995) Nutritional factors and colon cancer. *Crit. Rev. Food Sci. Nutr.*, **35**, 175–190.
Robin, A.P., Askanazi, J., Cooperman, A., et al. (1981) Influence of hypercaloric glucose infusion on fuel economy in surgical patients: a review. *Crit. Care Med.*, **9**, 680–686.
Saba, T.M. (1970) Physiology and pathophysiology of the reticuloendothelial system. *Arch. Intern. Med.*, **126**, 1031–1052.

Sandström, R., Hyltander, A., Körner, U., *et al.* (1993a) Structured triglycerides to postoperative patients: A safety and tolerance study. *JPEN J. Parenter. Enteral. Nutr.*, **17**, 153–157.

Sandström, R., Drott, C., Hyltander, A., *et al.* (1993b) The effect of postoperative intravenous feeding (TPN) on outcome following major surgery evaluated in a randomized study. *Ann. Surg.*, **217**, 185–195.

Sandström, R., Hyltander, A., Körner, U., *et al.* (1995a) Structured triglycerides were well tolerated and induced increased whole body fat oxidation compared with long-chain triglycerides in postoperative patients. *JPEN J. Parenter. Enteral. Nutr.*, **19**, 381–386.

Sandström, R., Hyltander, A., Körner, U., *et al.* (1995b) The effect on energy and nitrogen metabolism by either continuous, bolus or sequential infusion of a defined total parenteral nutrition formulation in patients after major surgical procedures. *JPEN J. Parenteral Enteral. Nutr.*, **19**, 333–340.

Sedman, P.C., Somers, S.S., Ramsden, C.W., *et al.* (1991) The differential effects of lipid emulsions on lymphocyte function during total parenteral nutrition. *Br. J. Surg.*, **78**, 1396–1399.

Sedman, P.C., Ramsden, C.W., Brennan, T.G., *et al.* (1990) Pharmacological concentrations of lipid emulsions inhibit interleukin-2 dependent lymphocyte responses *in vitro*. *JPEN J. Parenter Enteral. Nutr.*, **14**, 12–17.

Sobrado, J., Moldawer, L.L., Pomposelli, J.J., *et al.* (1985) Lipid emulsions and reticuloendothelial system function in healthy and burned guinea pigs. *Am. J. Clin. Nutr.*, **42**, 855–863.

Terano, T., Salmon, J.A., Moncada, S. (1985) Antiinflammatory effects of eicosapentaenoic acid: relevance to icosanoid formation. *Adv. Prostaglandin Thromboxane Leucotriene Res.*, **15**, 253–255.

Ulevitch, R.J., Johnston, A.R., Weinstein, D.B. (1979) New function for high density lipoproteins. Their participation in intravascular reactions of bacterial lipopolysaccharides. *J. Clin. Invest.*, **64**, 1516–1524.

van der Poll, T., Braxton, C.C., Coyle, S.M., *et al.* (1995) Effect of hypertriglyceridemia on endotoxin responsiveness in humans. *Infect. Immun.*, **63**, 3396–400.

Vollenweider, L., Tappy, L., Owlya, R., *et al.* (1995) Insulin-induced sympathetic activation and vasodilation in skeletal muscle. Effects of insulin resistance in lean subjects. *Diabetes*, **44**, 641–645.

Wan, M-F., Kanders, B.S., Kowalchuk, M., *et al.* (1991) Omega-3 fatty acids and cancer metastasis in humans. *World Rev. Nutr. Diet*, **66**, 477–487.

Welsch, C.W. (1995) Review of the effects of dietary fat on experimental mammary gland tumorigenesis: role of lipid peroxidation. *Free Radic. Biol. Med.*, **18**, 757–773.

Wennberg, A., Hyltander, A., Sjöberg, Å., *et al.* (1992) Prevalence of carnitine depletion in critically ill patients with undernutrition. *Metabolism*, **4**, 165–171.

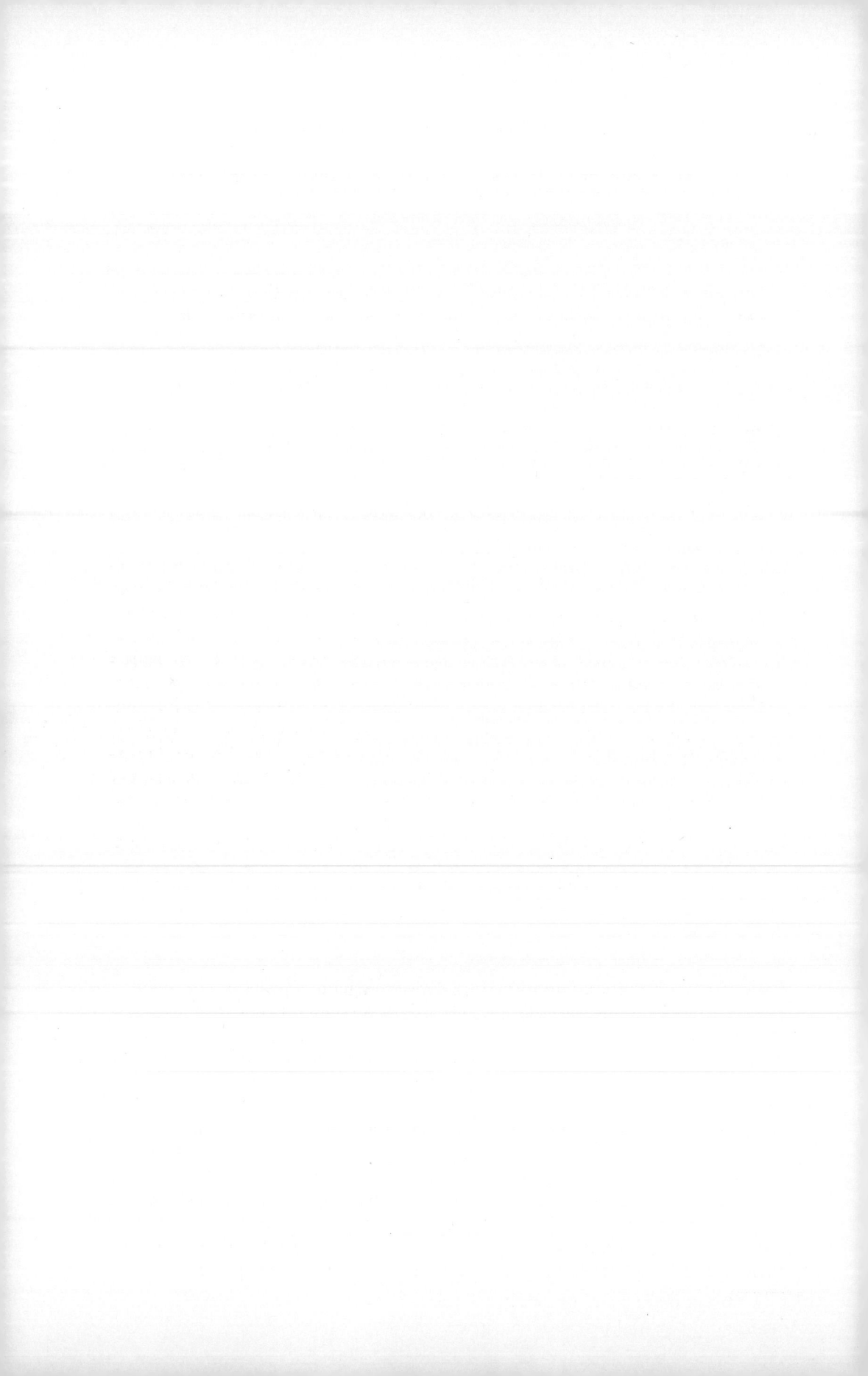

3. PARTICLE-SIZING TECHNOLOGIES FOR SUBMICRON EMULSIONS

R.J. HASKELL, J.R. SHIFFLETT and P.A. ELZINGA

Pharmaceutical Development, Pharmacia & Upjohn, Inc., 7000 Portage Road, Kalamazoo, Michigan 49001, USA

INTRODUCTION

Utility of Emulsions

Lipid emulsions have long been used in the parenteral delivery of energy and essential fatty acids for nutritional purposes (Hallberg *et al.*, 1966). Recent work has dwelled on the composition of the oil phase with the relative merits of medium-chain, long-chain, and structured triglycerides being the focal point of research in this area (Ulrich *et al.*, 1996; Nordenström *et al.*, 1995). Emulsions have also come under increasing scrutiny as a means of delivering pharmacologically active compounds that are intractable from a formulation perspective. When compared to conventional formulations, emulsion systems can display reduced irritancy, increased solubility of the drug, as well as the potential to increase shelf life and modify the bioavailability of the active compound (Mizushima 1996; Sakeda *et al.*, 1995; Collins-Gold *et al.*, 1990). However, the extent to which the aforementioned benefits can actually be realized are highly dependent upon the methods and materials used to manufacture the emulsion as well as the drug itself. Hence the design of parenteral emulsions is a complicated process requiring accurate feedback from the analytical function on how different design parameters affect the observable aspects of the final product.

Chapter Outline

This chapter will first provide a background on particle sizing and its relevance to the development of emulsion-based drug delivery systems in general. The question of what it means to measure the particle size of a complicated system such as a parenteral emulsion will then be addressed. Next, various methods that are applicable to characterizing these systems will be discussed on a method by method basis. Emphasis will be placed on identifying a phenomenological understanding of the various methods as a means of determining to what extent a given technique is appropriate to the problem at hand and what sort of reliable information can be extracted. Some analytical methods, e.g., CZE, LC, NMR, etc., which are either so common that they are covered elsewhere in the literature or have limited applicability to the problem at hand, will be discussed in a briefer format. Examples from the authors' laboratory or the current literature using emulsions, liposomes, or pharmaceutically relevant microparticulates will be introduced as appropriate. The chapter will conclude with the demonstration of a multi-method approach applied to formulation problems in the authors' laboratory.

Characterization

One of the prime physical characteristics of multiphase systems such as lipid emulsions is the size and shape of the particle distribution. A complete description of the particle size distribution (PSD) accounts for the entire colloidal mass present. However, no single experiment is capable of providing such information because the requisite dynamic range is not present in any one method. There are two areas of particular concern to those developing submicron emulsions. First is the nature of the size population in the submicron range itself. Well-formed emulsions should display a narrow PSD having a mean diameter ranging from 100–400 nm. The second area of interest is the greater than 1 μm range, since an increase in the number of particles of this size can be an indicator of physical instability as well as presenting a possible safety liability (Washington et al., 1993a).

Generating data on these two physical characteristics is important to achieving a complete understanding of the system at hand, which in turn can be used as feedback to rational formulation design. For example, the underlying physical processes that take place as an emulsion is processed are quite complicated (Dickinson, 1994) but, unfortunately, inaccessible to direct observation in general. The only information available to the user is that derived from characterizing the finished product. Thus, when process parameters such as time, temperature, pressure, equipment type, and sterilization conditions are modified in an attempt to optimize their values, particle sizing is one of the main characteristics employed as a response (Lashmar et al., 1996; Mbela et al., 1995). The results from a particle determination can be fed back into the design process in which formulation parameters, such as choice of co-surfactant, are adjusted to reduce the presence/formation of these larger particles. Processing can also be monitored in an real-time fashion via observation of emulsion characteristics. Particle size is one of the methods best suited to such in-line/near-line measurements (Wiese et al., 1993; Nicoli et al., 1991). Indispensable feedback on choices of emulsion components such as oils, surfactants, and co-surfactants is also provided by observing the PSD of the finished product.

Stability

Lipid emulsions are made up of oil droplets suspended in water, the former phase being surrounded by an emulsifying layer of surfactant. Their long-term physical stability is based upon the unfavorable kinetics towards coalescence produced when submicron particles are formed (Müller et al., 1993a). Hence a stable emulsion should retain the submicron PSD observed upon its production. Any changes in the PSD over time are indicative of poor physical stability. The number of particles present in the greater than 1 μm range can also be used as an indication of physical decomposition of the emulsion as the smaller droplets flocculate and/or coalesce to form larger entities. Small increases in particle number density in this size range can be of value in determining shelf life. The presence of such particles can also be an indication that the emulsion was improperly formed initially, e.g., insufficient energy in the emulsification process, low membrane stability, inadequate inter-particle electrostatic repulsion, etc.

Table 1 Population described by a set of cubes with n_i members of edge length l_i in each of the ith size classes (Finsey et al., 1991a).

Size Class (i)	Number (n_i)	Edge (l_i)	Volume ($v_i = n_i^3$)
1	5	2	8
2	6	3	27
3	3	4	64
4	2	7	343
5	1	10	1000

Safety

In addition to the aforementioned stability issues, particle size is also relevant to assessing the safety of a given emulsion formulation. Large particles present in emulsion formulations have been associated with pulmonary emboli, which in some cases have lead to fatal results (Hulman, 1995; Hill et al., 1996). It should be noted, however, that most of the *in-vivo* studies designed specifically to address the issue of size-related safety have been restricted to non-extrudable particles. In addition, reasonably large oil droplets have been observed in lipid emulsions intended for parenteral nutrition with no apparent ill effects in patients (Koster, et al., 1996; Washington et al., 1993b). However, drug-loaded emulsions may introduce an additional concern because of the possibility that precipitated drug may be present or that the drug molecules may interact with the lipid entities present in a manner that causes large agglomerations of colloidal material.

GOALS OF PARTICLE SIZING

Defining The Question

Measuring and describing the PSD of a complicated system such as a parenteral emulsion is not the simple process that it might seem at first. The following example, taken directly from the literature (Finsy et al., 1991a), clearly describes this problem. Imagine a vial containing a population of cubes as described in Table 1: 5 cubes with an edge dimension of 2, 6 with edge 3, etc. Note that the volumes of each of these cubes can be easily calculated by cubing the edge dimension. The goal of an analyst might be to determine an average dimension. If an analytical approach, such as microscopy, sensitive to the edge dimension is used, then the average linear dimension can be calculated according to

$$\bar{l}_1 = \frac{\sum_i n_i l_i}{\sum_i n_i}$$

where l_i is the edge dimension of each cube in the ith size class, and n_i is the number of cubes in that class. The result for l_1 using the data in Table 1 is 3.78. If an analytical approach sensitive to a volume measurement, such as weighing, were to be used, then the average linear dimension would be calculated according to

$$\bar{l}_2 = (\bar{v})^{1/3} = \left[\frac{\sum_i n_i v_i}{\sum_i n_i} \right]^{1/3}$$

where v_i is the volume dimension of each ith size class cube. The value of l_2 that results is 4.92 — clearly a different value than that obtained via microscopy, but equally valid in terms of the manner in which it was calculated. However, we find that the apparent paradox does not exist if instead the polydisperse system of one vial with 5 different types of cubes, the cubes are separated into each of 5 vials according to size. In this case, then as long as the contents of each via are measured independently, the values of l_1 and l_2 are the same for each vial. This agreement is a consequence of the monodispersity of the contents of each of these vials.

Several items are of note in this example (Finsy et al., 1991a). First, the population that exists in the vial containing all of the cubes can only be fully described by a complete assessment of everything in the vial, i.e., the data in Table 1 itself. Second, different experimental techniques provide results that are consistent with their principal of operation. The variation of results between techniques for a given sample do not necessarily imply that there is something "wrong" with the results. Third, a vastly improved understanding of the system at hand is obtained if more than one technique is used as a characterization tool. In the example above, using only one method would not have revealed the polydispersity associated with the vial containing all of the cubes. Fourth, certain analytical techniques may be preferable to others depending on what it is the investigator want to learn about the sample. For example, if the potential for adsorption is of interest, then use of a method that directly measures a surface area mean would be advisable.

Dependence of Result on the Method

The above example clearly demonstrates that the answer to the question of "What is the right particle size?" depends on the nature of the physical system under examination as well as the methods employed as a probe of size. In most cases, the term "right" is best defined in terms of how the measurement is being made. That is, the "right" answer is one that is consistent with the appropriate application of an analytical method to the system at hand. For example, using light scattering to size particles in a dispersion which is too concentrated to allow operation in the single scattering mode will produce an answer, but it will not be the "right" one because, unless special precautions are taken, optically dense samples produce scattering artifacts that generate corrupt results. The issue of whether the information provided by a given sizing experiment, light scattering in this example, is relevant even when properly implemented is a second issue that should also be considered.

Another, finer, example of this principle is one in which two independent observations of particle sizing are made via light scattering at two different scattering angles. As will be demonstrated in a following section, if the sample is polydisperse in size, then these two observations will produce different value for particle size. In this case, however, both answers are "right" in the sense that they each result from a faithful application of the underlying physical phenomenon. The apparent discrepancy results from the fact that proper compensation for the factors giving rise to angular dependence in light scattering is not taken into account when the results are interpreted.

This second scenario exemplifies the point that, in contrast to seeking the "right" answer, it is frequently a more effective approach to clearly define beforehand what is really being sought after, e.g., effect of processing passes on particle size, or freeze-thaw cycles on large particle formation. In this way one can ensure that the methods chosen are appropriate to the sample and the proper analytical techniques are applied. It may even be determined that an absolute value for size is not needed to address a certain question, but rather, a comparison between samples is sufficient to answer the question at hand. An example is shown by Bock et al. (1994) where particle size, as determined by Fraunhofer diffraction, is shown to drop for emulsions exposed to an increasing number of passes through a homogenizer at various pressures. Even though this method may not be the best suited for accurately measuring submicron particle size, the effects of processing parameters is clearly revealed in the results. Indeed, the results lose little of their value even if the analytical response is converted to a non-specific parameter such as "average size". Clearly, the success of such a proactive approach necessitates close coordination between the analytical and pharmaceutical aspects of a development project to assure that the required information is obtained.

DEFINITION OF TERMS

Matching Methods and Results

Of course a determination of particle size is not complete until the results are reported. There are many ways of describing the PSD, with mean size, median size, number average, and histograms being some examples. Terms such as number average, volume average, etc., will not be discussed in this chapter beyond what is necessary, as there are extensive definitions available elsewhere (Murphy, 1984). It is important to note here, though, that most methods have a result that is "native" to the technique, and from this result others can be calculated. For example, since microscopy directly measures the particles, the "native" results produced is a number-weighted distribution because the actual numbers of different particles are counted. A volume-weighted distribution can be calculated as well. However, these calculations can be carried out only after some assumptions, such as those concerning particle shape, are made. The simplest assumption is that of a sphere, in which case, calculating a volume-average becomes a matter of geometry. There is an important distinction between the two averages, however. If the assumptions regarding particle shape turn out to be invalid, then it is possible to have the situation where a number-average (the "native" result) is consistent with reality, but the volume-average (the calculated result) is not, even though both values arise from the same data set. Another example is light scattering: intensity measurements "natively" generate size measurements based upon the distribution of mass within the particle, radii of gyration, whereas size measurements from NMR lead to a z-average. The two should not compared directly, but can interconverted if assumptions about the particle morphology are made.

Distribution Definitions

Particle size distributions can be defined in terms of moments. The kth moment of a size distribution is defined as

$$M_k = \sum_i d_i^k n_i$$

where d_i is the diameter of particles in the ith "slice" of the distribution and n_i is the number of particles in that slice. The formalism of moments is very useful in allowing the calculation of more familiar terms. Hence, the number-average diameter of a distribution is defined as

$$D_N \equiv D_{1,0} = M_1/M_0$$

and the volume-average diameter is defined as

$$D_V \equiv D_{3,0} = M_3/M_0$$

The area average diameter, $D_{2,0}$, is defined in a similar manner as are other less common measurements such as $D_{3,2}$.

INTEGRATION OF ANALYTICAL APPROACH

When presented with a novel system to analyze, it is tempting to choose the methods with which the investigator either is most familiar or has come to rely upon due to past experience. However, it is important to keep in mind that each method will respond to the sample in a manner consistent with the underlying physical phenomena upon which the method depends. Thus the final result observed, mean particle size or an estimate of the PSD, will be influenced by the analytical method used and/or the particular manner by which it is implemented.

For example, dynamic light scattering is frequently employed as a means of determining whether or not an emulsion is well-made (Müller et al., 1993b). The implicit assumption is that if an emulsion is poorly-formed and/or unstable it will possess and/or generate particles substantially larger than those that make up the bulk of the submicron colloidal mass. This effect is expected to reveal itself via an increase in observed size in the submicron population. Unfortunately, this logic breaks down because, dynamic light scattering is not capable of detecting small numbers of larger particles in the presence of large number of smaller species. This

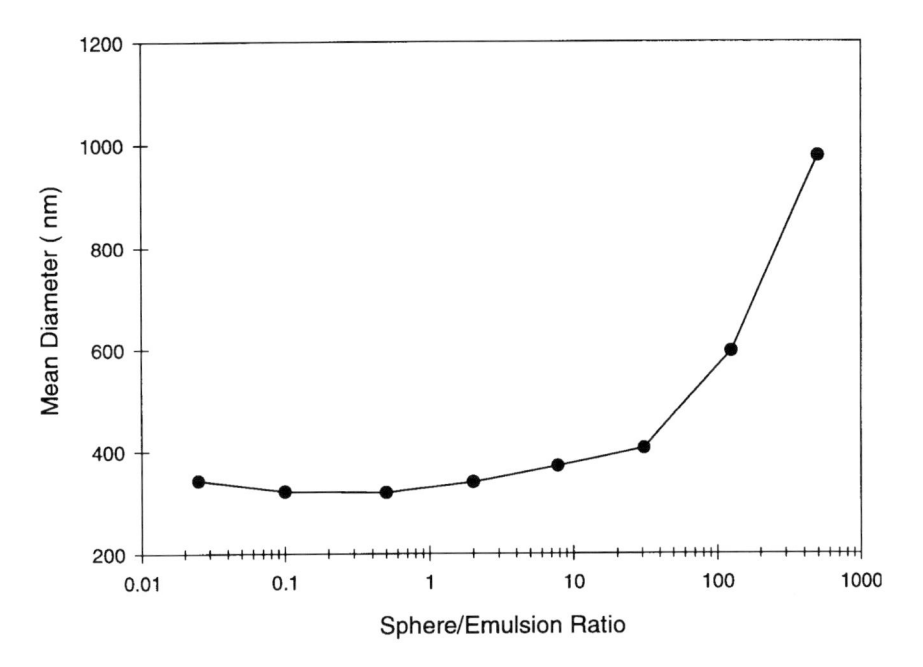

Figure 1 Effect of the addition of increasing amounts of 1 µm latex spheres to a solution of Liposyn II on diameter measured by dynamic light scattering. The experiment was conducted with a BI-200SM goniometer (Brookhaven Instruments; Holtsville, NY) using 514.5 nm laser light (95-4; Lexel Laser; Fremont, CA) and a 256-channel autocorrelator (BI-2030; Brookhaven Instruments). Data analysis was carried out via a 4th-order Cumulants fit (Koppel, 1972).

is demonstrated in Figure 1 where the mean size of an emulsion sample, as determined by dynamic light scattering, is measured as increasing amounts of 1 µm particulate standard are added. A significant increase in mean size is not observed until 2% solids have been added. Hence, all samples containing lesser amounts of large particles would have been determined to be equivalent — a situation that is clearly not the case. Any formulation optimization based solely on these light scattering results would be seriously compromised.

Another example is one in which two separate solutions containing monodisperse particle populations of different diameter, 50 and 300 nm, are analyzed via dynamic light scattering. Figure 2 shows that the relative scattering intensity of the population from the first sample, containing 50 nm particles decreases slowly as the scattering angle increases. However, the size value determined by the measurement will not be a function of angle. This is because the population is monodisperse so that no matter at which angle the light is collected, only light scattered from 50 nm particles strikes the detector. The same observation is true for the second solution, though the measured value will reflect the 300 nm diameter in this case. It is also noted in Figure 2 that the relative scattering intensity for this larger population is a function of scattering angle as well — a stronger dependence than for the 50 nm samples. However, if the two solution are mixed, thus making the sample polydisperse, the measured size becomes dependent upon angle. Comparison of the relative

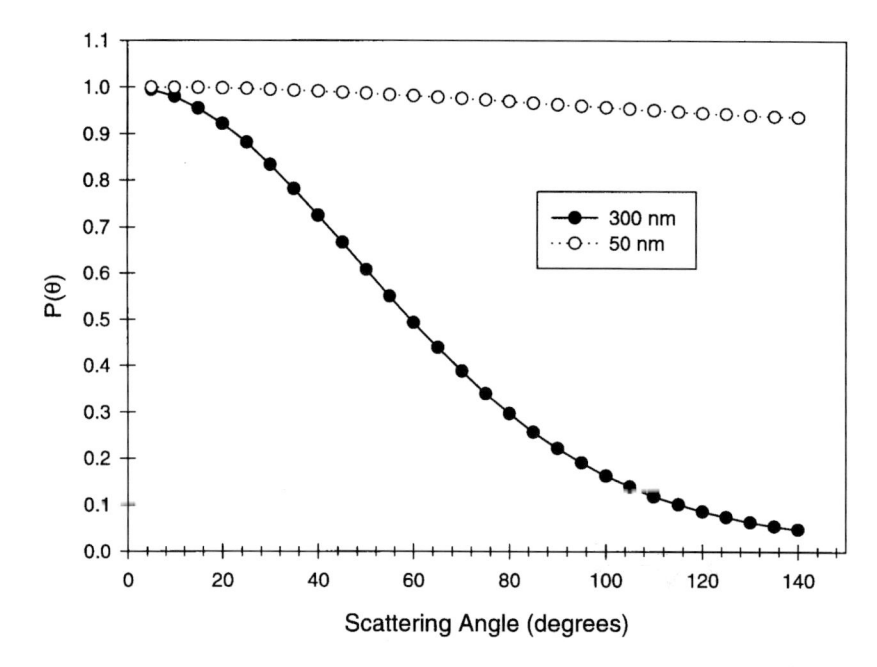

Figure 2 Plot of normalized Rayleigh-Gans-Debye particle scattering function, $P(\theta)$, versus scattering angle assuming a solid sphere (Table 4).

scattering intensities for the two particle populations as a function of angle reveals that low angle scattering from the larger particles contributes to the overall signal in greater proportion than is the case at higher scattering angles. The consequence of this differential contribution is that the value reported by the dynamic light scattering depends upon the scattering angle, but *only* in the case of a polydisperse sample. Hence the final result of an analysis may not only depend upon what measurement technique is employed, but exactly how the method was implemented.

Thus we note that a successful analytical approach is designed keeping in mind that no single method is capable of providing a wholly complete understanding of particle size distributions that straddle the 1 μm size range. For example, Table 2

Table 2 Effect of shaking on a colloidal dispersion of 10% MCT emulsified using 1.2% soy lecithin. DLS data collected using the fiber optic probe described in the text, 514.5 nm light, and a 256 channel autocorrelator. Data analysis carried out via the method of cumulants (Koppel, 1972). Obscuration-SPOS data collected using HIAC/Royco Model 3000 detector.

HIAC		Conditions	DLS (nm)	
No. Particles	% of Initial		Mean	Width
1500	100	Initial	170 ± 6	58 ± 13
3600	240	Heat Sterilized	169 ± 3	60 ± 7
80200	5300	Shaken for 1.5 hours	173 ± 6	48 ± 30
114600	7600	Shaken for 6.0 hours	176 ± 7	42 ± 39

shows that shaking of an emulsion does not appear to have an effect on the mean particle size as assessed by dynamic light scattering. However, a single particle counting method, such as light obscuration, reveals that the population of particles in the 2–6 μm range increases markedly with such treatment. The conclusion is that the submicron population remains largely unperturbed while a number of these small particles combine to form larger entities. Whether these entities are the result of flocculation, coalescence, or some other phenomenon cannot be determined without input from another method, such as microscopy, that is more responsive to morphology.

In order to pursue the development of submicron emulsions, a panel of techniques and approaches is required that, when used as a combined resource, can characterize the particles size distribution on a range from 5–10 nm to 5–10 μm. No single method is capable of providing a complete description of the physical structure of these systems, hence a variety of non-orthogonal technical approaches need to be pursued in order to achieve an adequate understanding. A similar philosophy has been employed for examining protein structure, another complex system, with good results (Havel *et al.*, 1990).

The following aspects of the individual methods should be considered when they are applied to multiphase systems:

Compatibility: Establish the suitability of individual methods for the analysis of specific samples. For example, the high surfactant loads used in non-diluted submicron suspensions may preclude the use of conventional light scattering, however, light obscuration techniques may remain unaffected.

Complementary: Establish the extent to which specific methods provide unique feedback on the particle characteristics. The cooperative use of the dynamic light scattering and light obscuration methods in characterizing stressed lipid emulsions (Table 2) is an example of such synergism. On the other hand, electrozone and light obscuration techniques may prove to be largely redundant.

Qualitative vs. Quantitative: Determine the extent to which specific methods can provide absolute information regarding the particle population and which are more suited to relative measurements. An example of the former might be electron microscopy whereas sedimentation field-flow fractionation may be an example of the latter.

CLASSIFICATION OF METHODS

Since the measurement of particle size and particle size distribution can be dependent upon the observation method employed, it is useful when discussing a variety of techniques to categorize them based upon their underlying similarities. Taking this approach, the list of techniques available to address the problem at hand can be subdivided into three categories as follows:

Ensemble

Methods in this category use an experimental protocol in which the sample is observed in its entirety, and then information about the particles giving rise to the instrumental response is extracted from the data set. This extraction is carried out by inverting the mathematical equations used to relate the particle population's physical characteristics to the observed signal. For example, the pattern of light impinging on the detector of a laser diffraction instrument is a consequence of the propagation of photons through the analyte and is thus interpreted based on the diffraction phenomena taking place therein. Under certain conditions the effect that the sample characteristics have on the observed pattern can be quantitatively modeled via Fraunhofer theory. Through inversion of the model's equations, specific information about the particle population, such as size, is derived. Other examples of this class of methods are dynamic light scattering, intensity light (Mie) scattering, turbidimetry, ultrasonic spectroscopy, dielectric spectroscopy, NMR, and small-angle X-ray scattering.

Because of the fact that these methods observe the entire sample at once, they multiplex the data collection process, and thus tend to be among the most rapid available, providing high sample throughput. Their speed makes them well suited to such high volume applications as quality control or statistically-based process optimization protocols. However, accuracy of the final result depends upon the appropriateness of the model employed and the effect that experimental noise has on the mathematics utilized in the inversion process. Should such a model fail to take into account all of the relevant physical phenomena present in the sample, the final result may be compromised — sometimes with little indication of the fact to an unwary operator. Another difficulty is the issue of dynamic range. Since the entire sample is viewed at once, the instrument settings and experimental protocol are adjusted to accommodate the sample as a single entity — conditions which may not be appropriate for the characterization of individual components within, e.g., a few large particles in the presence of many small ones.

Direct Counting

These methods include those that observe individual particles one at a time, identify specific characteristics of each one, and thus builds up a database of information about the sample. This database is then sorted according to a parameter of interest, such as size, to generate a complete understanding of the sample. For particle sizing purposes such a picture is usually reported as a histogram of population versus size. Because these methods observe each particle separately, some are capable of delivering information that goes beyond a size distribution, extending to such characteristics such as shape or morphology. Methods in this category include single particle optical sensing via either scattering or obscuration, microscopy, and electrolyte displacement.

If used responsibly, these methods are potentially among the most accurate available because each particle is individually inspected and results sorted accordingly. Thus, for example, the average value of size is calculated from a detailed knowledge of the sample, i.e., the histogram, rather than from a data inversion as is the case with ensemble methods. That is not to say that these methods are immune from artifacts, however. For them to attain their potential in characterizing unknown samples, it must be confirmed that the measurement process is valid, e.g., lack of coincidence or sample preparation effects.

The characteristic that makes these methods accurate is also the source of their main drawback. That is, because they examine each colloidal particulate, they can be very time consuming. In some cases, technology can be brought to bear on this problem. For example, computerized image analysis can greatly increase the throughput of a microscopy-based analysis as well as removing subjective observations of the analyst from the measurement process. However, a more insidious concern is one of sampling. It is impractical to consider examining *every* particle in a sample on an individual basis no matter how fast the process. A 2 mL sample of a 20% oil-in-water emulsion contains in excess of 10^{16} particles if one assumes a completely monodisperse size population having a mean diameter of 400 nm. Even counting at 8,000 particles per second it would take almost 5,000 years to carry out the task to completion! Thus the problem: How many particles need to be counted before one can be assured that a representative sample has been taken? This is of particular concern in the case of coalesced material where particles having a very low number population but very high contribution to volume are produced or in situations, such as electron microscopy, where the sample preparation is laborious. In a case where the particle size distribution is well-modeled by a mathematical function, e.g., log-normal, a rigorous statistical argument can be used to address this concern. That is, detailed knowledge of the well-characterized center of the distribution can be used to calculate values for less populated size ranges. However, when such a model cannot be shown to be applicable, the only answer is to count as many particles as is practical, assume reasonable counting statistics, e.g., Poisson, and report an estimate of error.

Separation

This final class of methods includes those that separate the sample into specific components. These components are then sequentially detected and their size inferred based on a mathematical understanding of the process that produced the separation. In the case where such an understanding is lacking or incomplete, a calibration procedure can be used instead or the separated components can themselves be analyzed as fractions using an ensemble or single counting method. This latter approach is particularly useful, because it essentially allows the sample to become its own calibrant. An example of this self-calibration will be described in the section on field-flow fractionation. This ability to calibrate, which minimizes the need for a complete modeling of the separation process as long as the calibrant is well-matched to the sample, is one of the main benefits of the separation methods. Another is the fact that once the separation analysis is complete, one possesses sample fractions than can be used for other purposes, such as zeta potential or drug content determination. Examples of separation methods include size exclusion and hydrodynamic chromatography, capillary zone electrophoresis, sedimentation, and various forms of field-flow fractionation.

The speed with which analyses can be executed varies depending upon the particular method employed as well as the nature of the sample. Capillary zone electrophoresis experiments can be relatively rapid whereas sedimentation-based experiments can take hours. However, even the fastest of these method is more time consuming than most ensemble approaches. Another drawback is that the behavior of the on-line schemes employed as detectors of the separated components must be well-characterized in order for the final size distribution results to be quantitative. For example, a conventional line-source detector placed at the end of a size exclusion column will convolute absorbance, scattering, and turbidimetric data thus rendering the response no longer solely proportional to concentration. This difficulty can be addressed by better modeling of the detector response or using a detection scheme more suited to the task, such as static light scattering.

It can be argued that the single counting category is just the separation category extended to the case wherein the resolution is taken to the most extreme, i.e., particle-by-particle, degree. While separation is indeed taking place in the single counting methods, the separation is not dependent upon the size characteristics of the particles involved. Rather, the particles are selected randomly and the process of sorting based on size takes place on the data set *after* the particles have been observed. Indeed, randomness is essential if the sampling issue discussed above is to be properly addressed.

It is also worth noting that the techniques actually employed are frequently combinations of the above classifications. The instance of a static light scattering detector attached to a chromatographic separation is an example of melding separation and ensemble approaches. Another example is microscopic analysis of fractions collected from a flow field-flow fractionation run.

DYNAMIC LIGHT SCATTERING

As an analytical technique for characterizing submicron particle populations, dynamic light scattering (DLS), also known as photon correlation spectroscopy (PCS), quasi-elastic light scattering (QELS), or intensity fluctuation spectroscopy (IFS) has achieved a wide reputation (Komatsu et al., 1995; Finsy, 1994; Phillies, 1990). However, it is also subject to misuse and is not the panacea it is sometimes thought to be. Therefore, a significant amount of discussion will be devoted to this method.

Instrumentation

In order to adequately discuss the experimental issues surrounding DLS, it is first necessary to describe the experimental configuration and physical background of the method. Figure 3 presents, in simplest terms, the basic elements of a DLS system. A sample cell is rigidly held in the path of a focused laser beam and light scattered from components within the solution is collected at an angle, θ, defined by the position of a detector with respect to the beam and cell. Light from a small region of the sample solution is imaged onto the surface of the photodetector via the use of slit and lens combinations. The photocurrent is then digitized and fed to a shift register (the autocorrelator) that generates the autocorrelation function (ACF). Details of the autocorrelator itself are beyond the scope of this chapter, but they are well-described elsewhere (Weiner, 1984a).

It is the ACF that constitutes the experimental response in DLS. In order for a DLS system to provide accurate data the laser should be of sufficient power to provide an adequate flux of scattered photons, have a stable mode structure, and

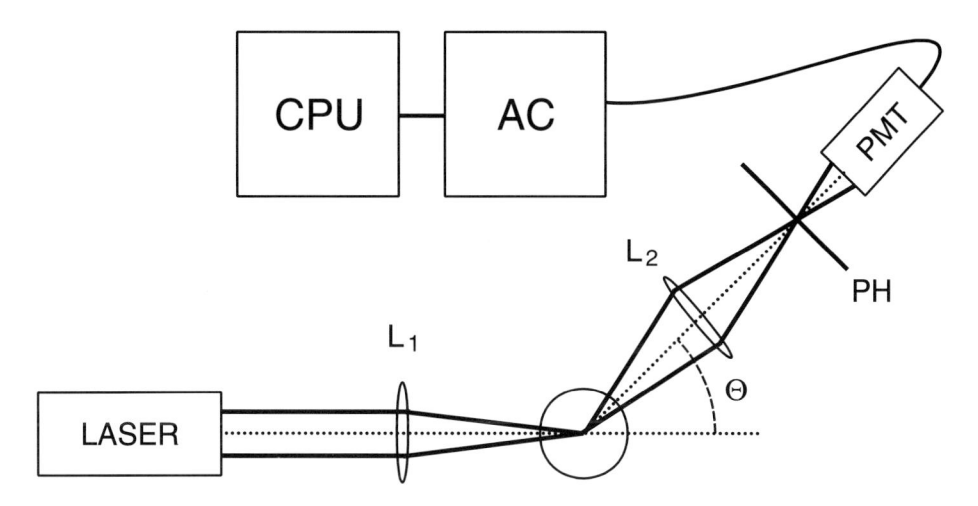

Figure 3 Diagram of a typical DLS instrument. Laser light is focused via lens, L_1, onto a sample. Light scattered at an angle, θ, is imaged onto a pinhole, PH, via lens L_2. Changing the diameter of the pinhole determines the volume of solution optically sampled. The photocurrent generated by light striking the photomultiplier (PMT) is amplified and passed to the autocorrelator (AC) which generates the autocorrelation function, $G^{(2)}$. Data acquisition and analysis are under the control of a computer (CPU).

be rigidly positioned. Instruments capable of making measurements at multiple angles should compensate for stray light (flare) at low angles, have a detection system that is easily aligned as well as robust procedures for confirming the accuracy of that alignment. Detection optronics should be sensitive in addition to possessing low background (dark counts) and dead times. Most commercial devices possess an optical configuration similar to that described in the figure, however, the extent to which the individual elements are apparent to, or in the control of, the user varies significantly among manufacturers.

Phenomenological Background

The intensity of light scattering from particles present in the small volume sampled by the instrument's optics is a function of wavelength, scattering angle, particle size, and the relative refractive index of the particle and surrounding medium. Shown in Figure 4 is an diagram describing the isotropic scattering of light from an isolated particle in solution. If a second particle is placed near the first, light scattered from the two produce an interference pattern that is a function of angle. Thus, if one was to move the detector around the particles in a circular fashion, the result would be alternating increases and decreases in photocurrent as the detector moved from regions of constructive interference into regions of destructive interference and back again. In reality what happens is the reverse of this scenario, but the result is the same: the particles move while detector remains fixed. As a given particle diffuses within the observed volume the light it scatters interferes with that scattered by its neighbors. The interference alternates between constructive and destructive

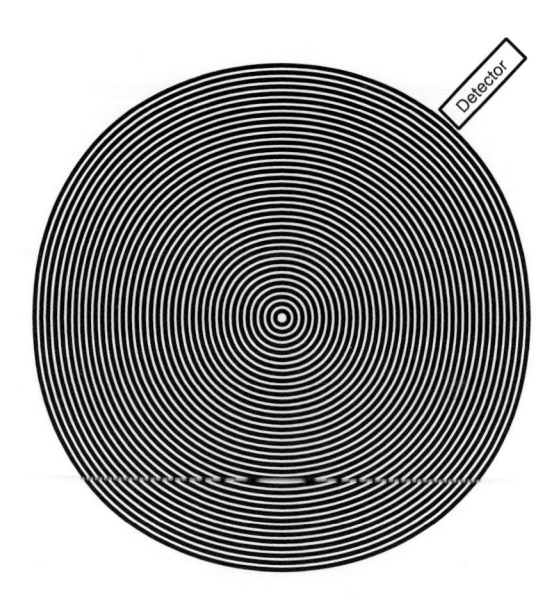

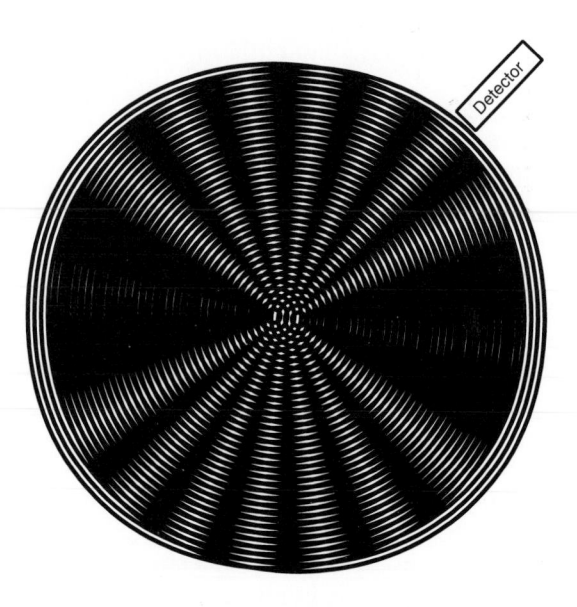

Figure 4 Upper: scattering of waves by a isotropic scatterer leads to symmetric distribution of energy about the sample and to a constant flux of light on the detector. Lower: interference pattern generated by scattering from two isotropically scattering particles. Relative motion of these two particles will lead to fluctuating intensity at the detector.

as the particles diffuse with respect to each other thus leading to a fluctuation in the overall scattered intensity. Rapidly moving particles, which are *assumed* to be doing so because they are small, lead to rapid changes in light scattering intensity. Likewise, larger particles, which are assumed to have smaller diffusion coefficients, result in intensity fluctuations of lower frequency.

Mathematical Background

This fluctuating intensity is observed by the detector as a spatial average because optical slits are located at a distance from the scattering volume. The fluctuation as measured by the autocorrelator is termed the second-order ACF, $G^{(2)}$, and is mathematically described via an exponential in time. The second-order ACF can be related to the normalized first-order ACF, $g^{(1)}$, via Equation 1

$$G^{(2)}(\tau) = a + b|g^{(1)}(\tau)|^2 + \varepsilon(\tau) \tag{1}$$

where τ is time, a is the baseline, b is an instrumental parameter that is an indication of the efficiency of the data collection process and possesses values ranging from 0 to 1.0, and ε is the experimental error. $g^{(1)}$ is also an exponential,

$$g^{(1)}(\tau) = \exp[-\Gamma\tau] \tag{2}$$

and has a decay constant, Γ, that is proportional to the translational diffusion coefficient, D,

$$\Gamma = DK^2 \tag{3}$$

via the scattering vector, K,

$$K = \frac{4\pi n}{\lambda}\sin\left(\frac{\theta}{2}\right) \tag{4}$$

where θ is the scattering angle of Figure 3, n is the index of refraction of the solution, and λ is the wavelength of light. If non-interacting, spherical particles of radii r are assumed, the Stokes-Einstein relationship can be used to extract the size via

$$D = \frac{k_b T}{6\pi\eta r} \tag{5}$$

where k_b is Boltzmann's constant, η is the dynamic viscosity of the suspending medium, and T is the temperature. Note that the particle size is not being measured directly, rather this parameter is calculated from the diffusion coefficient. Hence, any sample characteristic in addition to size that can affect the diffusion coefficient, such as electrostatic repulsion, if uncompensated for in the calculations, can lead to an incorrect measurement.

Experimental Details

As mentioned above, $g^{(1)}$ is an exponential decay in time. The "sample time", τ, defines the temporal spacing between individual data points and the "duration time" defines the length of time that the ACF is sampled. Both of these parameters are under the control of the user, although current instrumentation usually allows the former to be automatically selected if desired. The baseline is a particularly important parameter which can be either directly measured via autocorrelator channels positioned at long delay times or calculated from the average scattered intensity.

To assure precise measurements devoid of systematic, error certain conditions must be satisfied. First, samples should be free of extraneous matter, such as dust, which can originate from inadequately cleaned sample cells, diluent, or solution transfer lab ware. Large and erratic differences between the measured and calculated baseline can be a symptom of such contamination. Second, the samples should be sufficiently dilute so that multiple scattering effects are not occurring. In the case of very concentrated solutions, such as lipid emulsions, photons will be prevented from even reaching the sample volume imaged by the detector because of the high optical density. In this case the experiment is clearly compromised. However, in the situation where the solution is sufficiently concentrated that photons scatter off of more than one particle between their entering and leaving the cell, the photon count rate may be very high, but the decay of $g^{(1)}$ will reflect a convolution of particle and photon diffusion, and thus lead to an underestimation of particle size. Third, for experiments operating in homodyne mode, light not scattered off of diffusing particles, e.g., that reflected from a cell wall, must be prevented from reaching the detector. Uncompensated detection of such light (heterodyning) will lead to an overestimation of particle size. Fourth, there must be a sufficient number scattering particles to ensure that the photon count rate is not affected by shot noise and thus allow an accurate determination of $G^{(2)}$. There also must be enough particles to assure that the intensity fluctuations are due to interference between the particles and not due to an actual variation in the number density as particles diffuse in and out of the imaged volume.

Multiple Scattering and the Use of Fiber Optics

There are several approaches that have been taken to avoid the difficulties associated with highly scattering samples. The first and simplest approach is to dilute the sample to the point where such multiple scattering artifacts are not encountered. This approach has the disadvantage of possibly causing the sample to be contaminated with signal-producing substances, e.g., particulates. In addition for samples that are concentration sensitive, such dilution could produce an undesirable change in the nature of the system being studied. The former disadvantage can be dealt with by careful sample preparation technique, but in systems such as micelles or colloidal aggregates, the latter issue becomes a real limitation (Dorshow et al., 1983). Other approaches include the use of dual-angle or two-laser experimental configurations which are difficult to align (Phillies, 1981), and employing thin sample cells to reduce the likelihood of multiple scattering.

A variation on this last approach can be implemented through the use of fiber optics (Auweter et al., 1985). The basic idea is to use an optical fiber to deliver

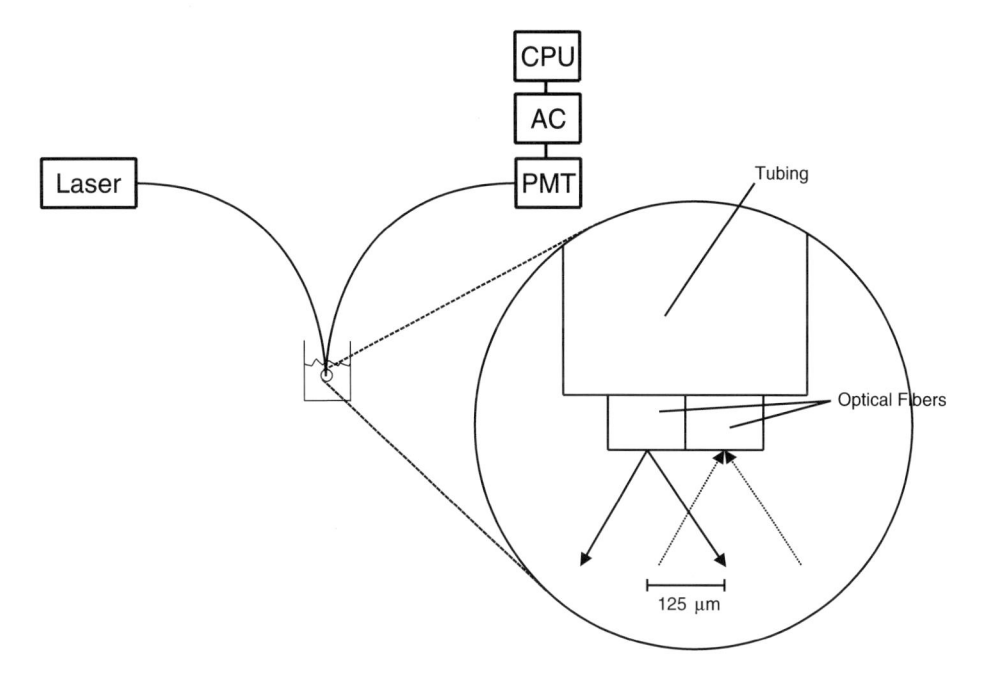

Figure 5 Schematic of the fiber-optic quasielastic light scattering (FO-QELS) probe built in the authors' laboratory. Light of 514.5 nm from an air-cooled laser is coupled into a single mode fiber with a 40× microscope objective. The opposite end of the fiber is stripped and embedded along with a second fiber into a piece of stainless steel tubing or an autosampler needle. Light exits the first fiber, is back-scattered off of material present in solution back into the second fiber. The scattered light passes through this collection fiber and into a PMT housing. Note that the volume region optically sampled by the probe is that defined by where the field of views of the two fibers overlap.

incident light directly into the sample. The same fiber or a second fiber located a few microns distant from the first, collects the scattered light and delivers it to a suitable detector. DLS optical arrangements based on fiber optics have been reported in the literature for some time (Macfayden et al., 1990), and they exist in two varieties. The first uses the same fiber to both deliver to and collect light from the sample and the second uses separate fibers, one for each purpose. The single fiber option has the advantage of being simpler to construct and providing the shortest possible path length, but has the disadvantage of allowing varying amounts of incident light to mix with scattered light (Van Der Meen et al., 1993). As noted above, this kind of optical contamination leads to experimental artifacts if it occurs in an irreproducible manner. Such a device was commercially available for a short time, but has since been removed from the market for this very reason. The dual fiber probe is more difficult to construct because the fiber tips at the sample end must be rigidly held at defined geometries with respect to each other, but is immune from the aforementioned intrinsic optical mixing problem (Dhadwal et al., 1991).

The overall layout of a fiber optic quasielastic light scattering (FO-QELS) spectrometer constructed in the author's laboratory is shown in Figure 5. The ends

(15 cm) of two single-mode fibers (model F-SA-10; Newport; Fountain Valley, CA) were stripped of their protective polymer jacket using methylene chloride and then blackened with ink from a permanent marker. The fibers were then cleaved at both ends with a knife (model F-CL1; Newport) using the scribe-and-break method. One end of each fiber was inserted into the barrel of a 0.42 mm i.d. autosampler needle (part no. 460952; Gilson; Middleton, WI) which had the point cut off prior to use. Two-component epoxy cement (Permatex Quick Set Epoxy; Loctite; Ontario, Canada) was applied to the fibers at the needle flange as they were inserted into the needle being careful to ensure that no glue obstructed the actual tips of the fibers. This insured that the fibers were securely attached to each other and the needle, over the entire length of the needle.

Special care was taken to position the ends of the fibers at, or just inside, the tip of the needle. The fibers at the flange end of the needle fit through a short piece of stainless steel tubing (model U-101; Upchurch Scientific) which was glued to the flange to provide mechanical rigidity at the point where the fibers entered the needle. The flange was then affixed inside the cap of an HPLC fitting (model F-301x; Upchurch Scientific), and a metal nut loosely screwed onto the fitting to add weight. The needle sleeve (part B49243; Gilson), but *not* the needle, was attached to the needle-tubing fitting (part 410160; Gilson) with another HPLC fitting (model F-301x; Upchurch Scientific), the threads of which had been cut to the 1 cm length of the needle-tubing fitting. The needle, with fibers, fit inside the needle sleeve and was free to slide up or down. The whole needle assembly was attached to the auto-sampler (model 231; Gilson) in the normal fashion.

Flexible PEEK HPLC tubing was then slipped over the length of each of the long portions of fiber optic extending from the end of the stainless steel tubing opposite from the fiber tips. One of the fibers was placed in a chuck attached to a single mode fiber coupler (model F-915; Newport). Light at 514.5 nm from an air-cooled argon ion laser (model 543-AP; Omnichrome; Chino, CA) was launched into the fiber using the coupler via a 40X microscope objective. The other fiber was inserted into another piece of stainless steel HPLC tubing which was inserted, via a fiber chuck, into the end of the photomultiplier-amplifier-discriminator housing provided with the autocorrelator (model BI-2030; Brookhaven Instruments; Holtsville, NY) spectrometer used for data collection.

Accuracy and precision of the probe are demonstrated by determining the apparent diameter of a solution of latex particle standards. Figure 6 shows the results of these experiments for 109 nm spheres and a water-in-oil emulsion containing 10% Miglyol 810 as the lipophilic phase. Samples were used neat and then diluted by successive factors of 2. Both plots, particularly Figure 6a show a sigmoidal shape in which the reported diameter of the particles in undiluted or slightly diluted samples are underestimated while those of highly diluted samples are overestimated. It has been demonstrated that multiple scattering events will cause an anomalously rapid decay in the autocorrelation function (Sorensen *et al.*, 1976). Through Equations 3 and 5 it can be seen that such a perturbation will lead to an overestimate of the diffusion coefficient and thus an underestimate in the particle size. Even though the 180° scattering geometry renders the probe insensitive to these effect unless three or more sequential scattering events occur (Sorensen *et al.*, 1976), the highly concentrated solutions possess a large enough particle density that even the micron-scale path length afforded by the dual-fiber probe is insufficient to prevent

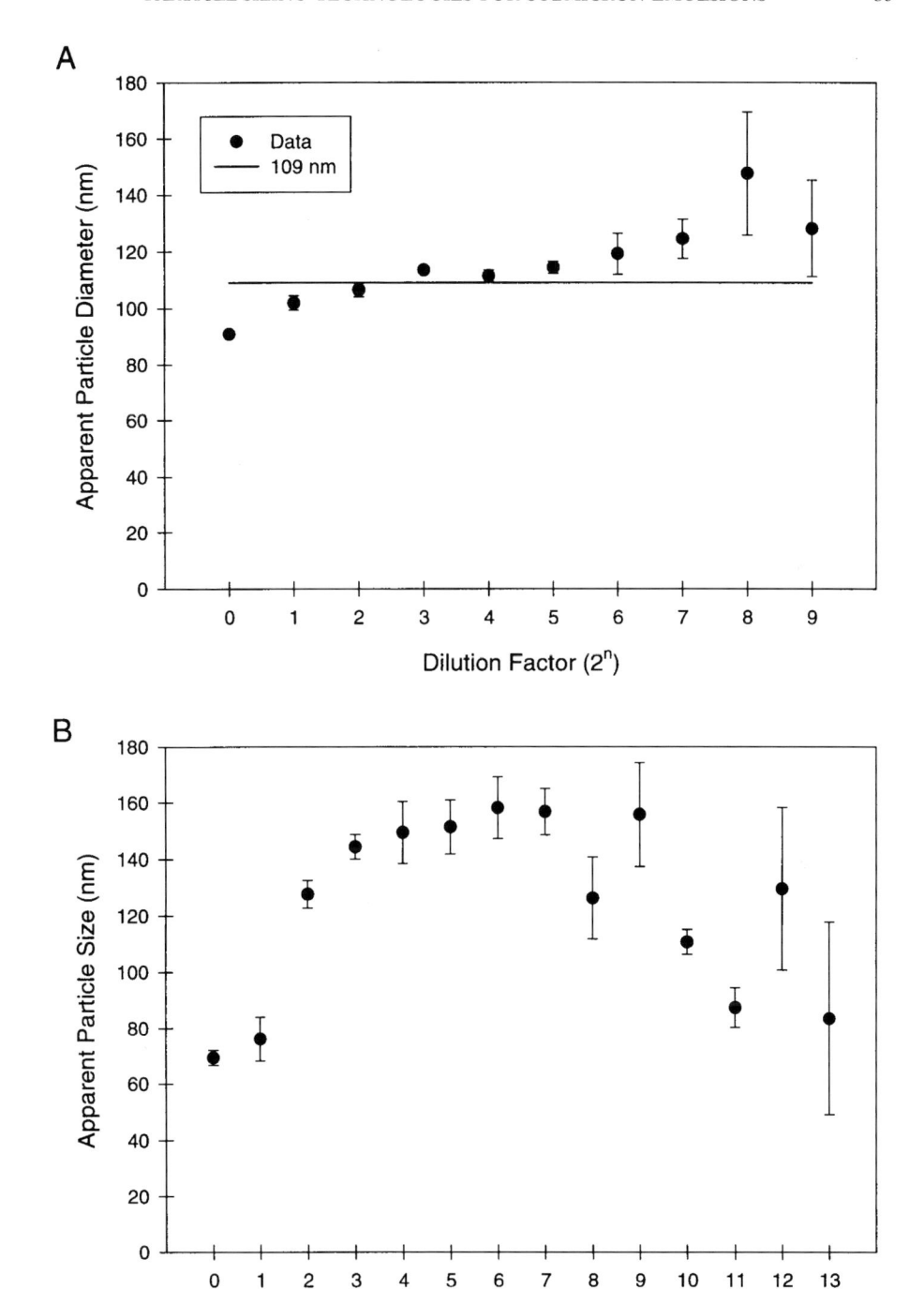

Figure 6 Concentration dependence of sample solutions as monitored by the FO-QELS probe upon successive water dilutions, a) 109 nm diameter latex spheres (Duke Scientific; Palo Alto, CA), b) 10% MCT o/w emulsion.

such occurrences. For highly dilute solutions, the particle size is overestimated because the diffusion coefficient extracted from the autocorrelation function is artifactually low. This error is the result of stray light reflecting from the bottom of the autosampler vial that only starts to occur as the sample becomes less optically dense as it is diluted.

Other laboratories employing a similar design for a DLS fiber optic probe report autocorrelation functions that are symptomatic of an ineffective control of coherence areas (Dhadwal et al., 1991). Values of β (see Equation 6) no higher than 0.1 were said to be obtainable in these studies. The source of this inefficiency was thought to be due to the very poor overlap between the fields of view of the two optical fibers which in turn was a consequence of inefficient geometry resulting from having the two fibers fixed collinearly at the probe tip. The authors reported much higher values of β for a design in which the metal tip served to hold the fibers at 157° with respect to each other, thus leading to greater overlaps in the fields of view. Using this configuration, β values of 0.9 were obtained. However, this increase in β was obtained at the expense of much greater complexity in construction. In addition, the fragile nature of the fibers requires that such a design have a probe diameter substantially larger than that of an autosampler needle.

While the collinear arrangement reported on here does not make maximal use of the number of scattered photons present, β values in excess of 0.7 are regularly obtained when using it to examine solutions such as those reported on elsewhere (Dhadwal et al., 1991). In addition, the higher scattering angle obtainable with the collinear probe theoretically makes it more resistant to multiple light scattering effects. The design described in the present report is also unique in that it can be constructed quickly from readily available off-the-shelf materials. The total cost of materials for the probe itself is around $100 US.

Data Analysis

After data collection, the most significant challenge is to convert $G^{(2)}$ into an estimate of the particle diffusion coefficient. A number of numerical routines can be employed to carry out this task. The basis for these routines will be described below starting with those that require no prior information about the sample.

The normalized first-order ACF can be derived from $G^{(2)}$ via

$$\left[\frac{G^{(2)}(\tau)-a}{a}\right]^{0.5} = b^{0.5}g^{(1)}(\tau) = b^{0.5}\exp[-\Gamma\tau] \qquad (6)$$

Taking the logarithm of both sides of this equation leads to a linear plot shown from which both G and b are extracted from the slope and intercept respectively. Signal-to-noise, a/b ratio, "beta", and efficiency are all terms directly related to b, which as described above, is an instrumental parameter and is directly related to the principle of coherence. A "strong" DLS signal will have a large value for b which is the same thing as saying that there is a large difference in photon counts between the first and last channels in the ACF.

Only in the case of a single exponential will the above extraction procedure lead to acceptable results. Such a circumstance arises when the particle size distribution is monodisperse as is the case for a sample of latex sphere standards. Graphical presentations of residuals and quantitative estimates of error, such as χ^2, are invaluable tools in determining whether such a model is appropriate to the sample at hand. *Assuming that neither the experimental artifacts discussed above nor normalization errors are in play*, then the failure of a single exponential model to fit the data is an indication that the sample is polydisperse in some fashion, i.e., a broad and/or multimodal distribution. This can be described in discrete or continuous mathematical forms by

$$g^{(1)}(\tau) = \sum_{i=1}^{n} c_i \exp(-\Gamma_i \tau) + \varepsilon(\tau) = \int_0^\infty C(\Gamma)\exp(-\Gamma\tau)d\Gamma + \varepsilon(\tau) \qquad (7)$$

A wide range of numerical routines are available to address such situations. The simplest approach is the method of cumulants first proposed by Koppel (1972). In this method, the logarithm of Equation 6 is expanded about Γ and then the above procedure is followed resulting in

$$\ln(g^{(1)}(\tau)) = 0.5\ln(b) - \overline{\Gamma}\tau + \frac{K_2 \tau^2}{2} - \frac{K_3 \tau^3}{6} + \ldots \qquad (8)$$

where $\overline{\Gamma}$ is the mean decay rate and K_n are the nth moments of the distribution for an nth "order" fit. Clearly this equation collapses to the monodisperse model if the higher order moments are set to zero. When examining data, the expansion serves to account for curvature in the $\ln(g^{(1)}(\tau))$ plot or, equivalently, non-exponential behavior in $G^{(2)}$. The polydispersity index, defined as K_2/Γ^2, is a convenient means of describing this deviation. The parameters of mean particle size and width can then be applied to a predefined distribution function, e.g., Gaussian, for presentation. However such an analysis should *not* be taken as evidence that the DLS data indicates such a function is appropriate. Given the error always present in the experimental data, see Equation 1, estimates of moments beyond K_2 are not easily obtained. Based on the evaluation of χ^2, higher order fits are sometimes able to give a better estimate of $\overline{\Gamma}$, however. Note that the use of the cumulant model implies nothing about the modality of the population distribution.

With the advent of widely available user-friendly nonlinear fit routines it is possible to dispense with the logarithmic transformations and fit directly to $g^{(1)}$. Indeed it should be possible to avoid the normalization procedure entirely and fit directly to the non-normalized ACF, $G^{(1)}$, allowing the baseline, a, to become an optimizable fit parameter. This has the benefit of avoiding the systematic errors that arise when taking the square root of Equation 6, but the drawback of consuming an additional degree of freedom.

A careful propagation of error through the calculations leads to estimates of uncertainties that can be applied to the derived values. In our experience we have found that the resulting error intervals are well below those found experimentally by collecting individual functions and taking a statistical average of the result — even when differences in duration times are taken into account. It is highly likely that the source of these anomalously low calculated error estimates is the presence of correlated noise between the data points of the ACF. Such a topic is well beyond the scope of this presentation, however, but has been dealt with in the literature (Haskell et al., 1985).

As alluded to above, the first-order cumulant fit is identical to a single exponential model. Another approach is to fit the data to a multiple exponential decay. This involves fitting the discrete form of Equation 7 to $g^{(1)}$ with the use of fitting software capable of nonlinear optimization. Note that when a small number of terms is used, i.e., $n \leq 3$, the adoption of this model carries with it an implicit assumption about the structure of the size distribution. For instance, the choice of $n = 2$ indicates that two discrete size populations are considered to be most appropriate *a priori*. Such fitting can be carried out with commercially available software. If a number of samples are to be examined then it is most appropriate to optimize for one set of Γ_i values across all of them and allow only the values c_i values to vary. SPLMOD is capable of carrying out fits in this manner (Provencher et al., 1983).

This above approach is the simplest example of forcing a physical model, e.g., bimodal, trimodal, etc., on the system being studied in order to achieve improved statistical results. A good fit of the data with such a model does *not* constitute proof of its accuracy, only that the data is consistent with the model. Additional confidence can be placed in the selection if there is prior knowledge about the sample that can provide some direction as to the appropriate choice.

A variation on the multiple exponential model is the singular value reconstruction method. The use of singular values has been available for quite a while in the form of partial least squares analyses for quantitative infrared spectroscopy, however, the approach has been applied to DLS only recently (Finsy et al., 1989). In this method a matrix of exponential factors is constructed and then decomposed into component eigenvectors. These eigenvectors are then assessed and retained based upon the additional information content that each cumulatively accounts for in the original ACF. The number of retained functions is thus clearly defined in a statistical sense, and the arbitrary decision regarding the number of populations does not have to be made. A major limitation of this method, however, is that the sample times must be constant across the entire ACF.

The remaining methods all require implicit assumptions about the nature of the solution before the numerical analysis can be applied. Thus, their use injects a certain degree of uncertainty into the analysis. All of these methods assume a preselected range for the discrete Γ_i values employed in the continuous form of Equation 7 that remain fixed during the analysis. Each of the Γ_i values represents a "grid point" and the set of c_i, one associated with each of these points, are the fitted parameters and thus as a group constitute the solution to the problem. The spacing interval between the grid points can be linear, geometric (exponential sampling) (Ostrowsky et al., 1981), or logarithmic (CONTIN). In principle, one could use a nonlinear algorithm that attains an optimum based upon a least squares analysis to find the solution set of c_i. This approach reduces essentially to a multiple exponential fit in which n is allowed to become very large, e.g., 80. Unfortunately, given the error term in Equation 1, such fits are quite unstable and result in distributions that depend upon the number and range of grid points chosen, vary widely from data set to data set, and can yield negative (non-physical) solutions.

The latter case of negative solutions can be avoided by forcing the condition of $c_i \geq 0$ on all of the grid points. This restriction tends to dampen some of the grid point dependency and is the defining characteristic of the non-negative least squares

(NNLS) approach available with many commercial instruments (Lawson *et al.*, 1974). Another tactic, implemented in CONTIN, is to impose an additional requirement of smoothness or "parsimony" on the solution by requiring that the second-derivative of the solution changes slowly throughout the solution set (Provencher, 1982).

It should be re-emphasized that, while under reasonable conditions they do provide stable mathematical solutions, these approaches either require the user to define the range of possible answers, e.g., number/range of grid points, ahead of time or impose arbitrary restrictions during the analysis, e.g., parsimony. Our lab generally uses the unbiased results of a cumulants analysis to define the grid points thus making the up-front decisions less dependent on the subjective whims of the operator.

Comparisons of Data Reduction Methods

Some studies have been carried out with the goal of comparing the plethora of data analysis routines currently available (Finsy *et al.*, 1992). The conclusion has been similar to that advocated for submicron particle sizing in this chapter: A number of approaches should be applied, the results from which are contrasted and compared with each other in order to arrive at a reasonable understanding. In general, however, the mean of a monodisperse population can be determined with reasonable accuracy while widths can be estimated much less so (Weiner *et al.*, 1987). Confidence drops precipitously with highly polydisperse or multimodal systems. The literature is replete with examples in which DLS has been used to characterize submicron emulsions (Ricard, *et al.*, 1996; Mehta *et al.*, 1992; Müller *et al.*, 1992). Mean diameter is the most frequently reported parameter, however little information is supplied about the derived width of the population. Statistical parameters providing some information on the quality of the data fits are rarely reported.

STATIC LIGHT SCATTERING

Static light scattering (SLS), also referred to as classical or intensity light scattering, rather than monitoring the time evolution of light, involves measuring the absolute intensity of light scattered from an irradiated sample. This relatively simple measurement belies the more detailed underlying phenomena that render the technique useful. In particular, the angular dependence of the scattered light is monitored over a broad range of scattering geometries. The resulting data is then fit to a model in which particle size and sometimes particle size distribution are the variable parameters.

Data Models

Selection of the appropriate model for the system at hand is a key factor in determining not only the accuracy of the final result, but also the mathematical complexity of the data analysis. There are several models available, with the choice between them depending upon the extent to which the colloidal particle perturbs the electric field of the impinging photons. This perturbation is a function of the

Table 3 Influence of particle radius (r), wavelength of light (λ), and refractive index of the particle (n_2) and suspending medium (n_1) on the choice of appropriate scattering model (Chýlek et al., 1995).

Model	Requirements
Rayleigh	$\dfrac{2\pi r}{\lambda} \ll 1, \quad \dfrac{2\pi r}{\lambda}\left|\dfrac{n_2}{n_1}-1\right| \ll 1$
Rayleigh-Gans-Debye	$\left|\dfrac{n_2}{n_1}-1\right| \ll 1, \quad \dfrac{2\pi r}{\lambda}\left|\dfrac{n_2}{n_1}-1\right| \ll 1$
Mie	$\dfrac{2\pi r}{\lambda} \gg 1, \quad \left|\dfrac{n_2}{n_1}-1\right| \ll 1$
Geometrical	$\dfrac{2\pi r}{\lambda} \gg 1, \quad \dfrac{2\pi r}{\lambda}\left|\dfrac{n_2}{n_1}-1\right| \gg 1$

particle size, wavelength of light, and relative refractive index of the particle and suspending medium. Table 3 shows how these parameters interact to determine the applicable model (Chýlek et al., 1995). Certainly, one could use the most complete, i.e., Mie, model to describe even the least perturbing system, but only at the expense of decreased convenience which would in turn limit the analytical utility of the technique.

In its most general form, the intensity of scattered light, I, is a function of the intensity of incident light, I_0, the number of scattered particles, N, the mass of those particles, M, and scattering factors $P(q, m, r)$ and $S(q)$ via

$$I(q) \propto I_o NM^2 S(q) P(q, m, r) \qquad (9)$$

where q is the scattering vector described in the section on DLS, m is the refractive index of the particle compared to that of the medium, and r is the particle radius. The information imbedded in P is of particular interest as this describes the angular dependence that is the experimental observable, and the particle size, which is the desired result. $S(q)$ describes the pattern of light generated by the interference of light scattered off of neighboring particles and as such represents a dynamic light scattering event "frozen" in time.

Rayleigh Scattering

Rayleigh scattering represents the case in which the particles are sufficiently small that $P \approx 1$ (Kratochvíl, 1987). In this case, light scattering becomes invariant as a function of angle (isotropic) and depends only on particle concentration, molecular weight, and change in refractive index with concentration. For visible wavelengths of light, this regime represents particle radii on the order of 10 nm, hence this case is useful for characterizing molecular polymers, but not colloidal systems.

Table 4 RGD scattering form functions for a variety of different particle morphologies where r is the particle radius, R is the outer radius of the shell, d is the thickness of the shell, and q is the scattering vector.

Shape	$P(q, m, r)$
Solid Sphere	$\left[\left(\dfrac{3}{X^3}\right)(\sin X - X\cos X)\right]^2$, $X = qr$
Thin Shell	$\left[\dfrac{\sin(qr)}{qr}\right]^2$
Spherical Shell	$\left[\left(\dfrac{3}{X_o^3 - X_i^3}\right)(\sin X_o - X_o\cos X_o - \sin X_i + X_i\cos X_i)\right]^2$, $X_o = qR$, $X_i = q(R-d)$

Rayleigh-Gans-Debye Scattering

Rayleigh-Gans-Debye (RGD) theory represents the next level of complexity brought about by the fact that the particles are of sufficiently large size and/or differ in refractive index from that of the suspending medium, so that the approximation of $P \approx 1$ becomes invalid. Specific forms of this scattering function for common particle types are presented in Table 4. An example is presented in Figure 2 in which the form factor for solid particles of diameter 300 nm and 50 nm are shown as a function of scattering angle. This angular dependence clearly discriminates between the two sizes and thus forms the basis for a sizing technique.

There are several items to be noted when examining Table 4 and the functions the entries represent. First, complete application of the intensity light scattering method requires that the analyst know something about the colloidal system ahead of time. That is, if experimental data is to be used to determine size via RGD theory, then a specific entry from the table must be selected, which in turn implies an assumption of particle morphology. The effect of the scattering form function on scattered light can be substantial as shown by van Zanten et al. (1994) in which the function for two systems made up of particles having the same radius but different internal structures, i.e., solid versus coated sphere, are presented. Second, it is noted that refractive index is not a parameter that influences the form factors. Thus, even though shape has to be pre-defined, refractive index does not, which simplifies the problem to a certain extent and rendering the analysis somewhat less arbitrary. Third, the equations are simple enough to be handled by straightforward fitting algorithms such as those present in commonly available non-linear curve-fitting software packages. This simplicity is of considerable benefit compared with Mie scattering, as will be seen below. Fourth, it must be emphasized that these form factors assume monodisperse size distributions — a condition that is almost certainly not the case for real emulsion samples. To account properly for polydispersity, the size distribution, $G(r)$, needs to be substituted for the size parameter, r, and an integral taken over dr. This adds significantly to the complexity of the mathematics and renders the inversion from scattered intensity to size unstable to the presence of noise in the experimental data.

Mie Scattering

A mathematically exact description of vertically polarized incident light scattered from spherical particles is available in the Mie scattering model via

$$S = \sum_{n=1}^{\infty} \frac{2n+1}{n(n+1)} \{a_n \pi_n(\cos\theta) + b_n \tau_n(\cos\theta)\}(-1)^{n+1} \quad (10)$$

where the angular data is included in the functions

$$\pi_n(\cos\theta) = \frac{P_n^{(1)}(\cos\theta)}{\sin\theta}$$

$$\tau_n(\cos\theta) = \frac{d}{d\theta} P_n^{(1)}(\cos\theta)$$

with $P_n^{(1)}$ defined as the Legendre polynomial. Further angular dependence as well as dependence on size, shape, and relative refractive index are present in the scattering coefficients, a_n and b_n. Any further detailed discussion of the mathematical relationships endemic to Mie scattering are well beyond the scope of this discussion, but are available for review in numerous references (van de Hulst, 1981; Kerker, 1969).

Appropriate selection of equations based on Mie theory will require the analyst to make all of the same assumptions about the colloidal particles as were necessary when applying the RGD model — although values for real and imaginary refractive indexes of the particle and real refractive index of the suspending medium are needed as well. The infinite sum of Equation 10, makes Mie calculations troublesome, however, several routines written in FORTRAN (Bohren et al., 1983) and Pascal (Zijp et al., 1993) are publicly available to carry out these calculation. Even so, it should be noted that use of these programs assume that the scattering particles are solid spheres — the simplest model possible.

Because it makes use of absolute intensity measurements, the technique is experimentally challenging in terms of instrumental design and sample preparation. The optical alignment of the instrumentation must be stable, robust, and easily aligned. Angular variation in the data, that can easily mask or distort the experimental signal, can be generated by even small misalignments in the optical train. Goniometer and multiangle (phtotodiode-based) instruments are both used in the field (Egelhaaf et al., 1996; Weiner, 1984a; Haller et al., 1983), and while the former is easier to construct, it is less stable, and because only one angle is observed at a time, data collection is much slower. In addition, the multiangle instruments tend to be more capable of probing lower scattering angles. Even with a state-of-the-art diode instrument, absolute intensity measurements are rarely made. Instead, the intensity of light scattered from a known calibrant, such as toluene is used as a reference to which all sample data is compared. Great care needs to be taken during preparation of the sample to avoid contamination with even trace quantities of particulates. Such contamination can lead to noisy data as well as excessive scattering at low angles.

The need for correct selection of particle scattering functions and optical parameters is an appropriate concern if it is necessary to determine absolute parameters

Table 5 Theoretical correlation between data calculated via Mie theory (Zijp et al 1993) and then fit using RGD employing the solid sphere form factor as defined in Table 4. The wavelength of light, particulate real refractive index, particulate imaginary refractive index, and media real refractive index were specified to be 514.5 nm, 1.4, 0.0, and 1.33 respectively. Scattering was calculated from 35 to 140 degrees in 5 degree increments. Data in the table fits to a linear model with a correlation coefficient of 0.99998 and an F-ratio in excess of 1.4×10^5.

Mie Diameter (nm)	Fit to RGD (nm)
54.0	72.2
102.0	136.1
204.0	274.3
364.0	493.8
500.0	681.3

for the size distribution mean and width. However, it is useful at times to consider if it is really necessary to determine absolute values if the analysis calls for only a comparison of samples. For example, Table 5 shows that when a monodisperse size distribution of solid spheres is assumed, there is a strong correlation between full application of Mie theory to that of the simpler RGD approach.

The utility of this correlation to the experimentalist is demonstrated in Figure 7. This figure shows the SLS data for four 25% lipid emulsions containing increasing

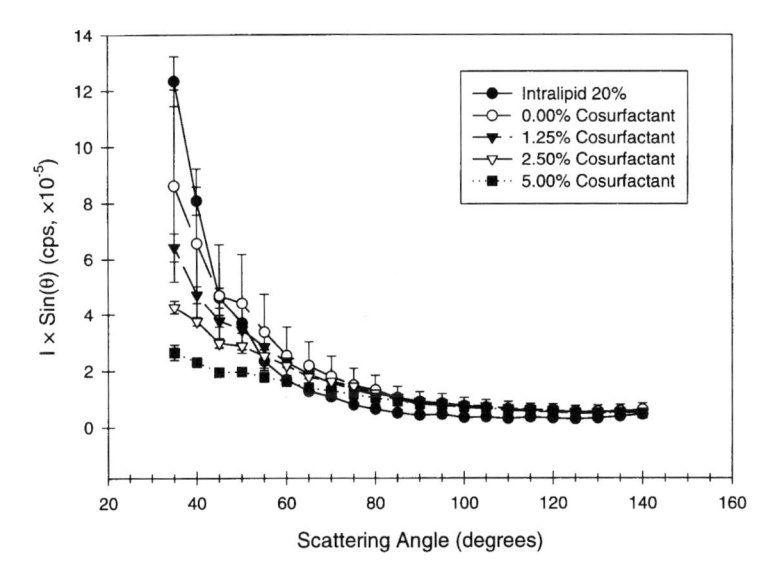

Figure 7 Static light scattering data collected of 25% MCT o/w emulsions using the apparatus described in the caption of Figure 3. Samples were diluted $1:5 \times 10^5$ in water with the emulsions being prepared with a) 0.0%, b) 1.25%, c) 2.5%, d) 5.0% cosurfactant.

Table 6 Results of intensity light scattering on o/w emulsions. Angular-dependent intensities from solutions diluted $1:5 \times 10^5$ in water was collected with a BI-200SM goniometer (Brookhaven Instruments; Holtsville, NY) operating at scattering angles from 35 to 140 degrees in 5 degree increments using 514.5 nm light. Data was fit to an RGD model using the solid sphere form factor from Table 4. A Mie equivalent was then determined using the correlation in Table 5. Error intervals determined from the standard deviation of 5 independent runs of each sample.

Sample	RGD (nm)	Mie (nm)
0.00% cosurfactant	409 ± 15	301 ± 11
1.25% cosurfactant	367 ± 13	271 ± 10
2.50% cosurfactant	307 ± 8	227 ± 6
5.00% cosurfactant	265 ± 5	196 ± 4
Intralipid 20%	585 ± 16	430 ± 12

amounts of a cosurfactant. Comparisons of the data with the plots of Figure 2 clearly indicates that additional cosurfactant changes the angular scattering of light in a manner consistent with a reduction in particle size. This trend can be quantified by fitting the data to Equation 9 in which $P(q)$ selected from Table 4 is that for a solid sphere. The correlation of Table 5 can be used to estimate the real diameter from the apparent diameter extracted from the fits to the RGD theory's equations. The results are shown in Table 6.

This approach is worth considering if the original question is: Does the addition of cosurfactant change the mean diameter of emulsions particles in a consistent manner? This approach is not valid if the question is: What is the size of the particles present in these samples? It is worth noting that frequently, the latter question is the one that gets asked whereas it is the answer to the former question that supplies the desired information in the context of formulation development.

There are a number of caveats that must be taken into account when using this approach to data analysis. The first caveat stems from the assumption of solid spheres. This assumption allows both the Mie and RGD calculations to be simplified, but only at the expense of distancing the final result, from the "true" value of the mean because "real" emulsion particles are better modeled as coated spheres. Second, the morphology of the particle population is assumed to be homogeneous. That is, all of the colloidal particles present in the sample are assumed to possess the same structure, be it solid sphere, thin shell, etc. Just because a distribution is monodisperse in size does not say anything about whether it is homogeneous or not. Furthermore, not only is it necessary that the morphology of the particle population be homogeneous, but that this homogeneity not be influenced by other parameters of the experiment — the addition of cosurfactant in this case. If, in the case of this example, addition of cosurfactant simultaneously leads to the generation of a higher proportion of liposomes, then the analysis may be faulty. Indeed, even a direct application of full Mie theory may be inadequate in such a situation. A third concern is that the functions for $P(q, m, r)$ described above and used in the Mie calculations assume monodispersity. One possibility is to make the substitution of $G(r)dr$ for r as has been done for RGD modeling (Strawbridge et al., 1994), and is the source of much active research in the field (Shortt, 1994; Finsy, 1991b). Both vesicles (Wang et al., 1995; van Zanten, 1994) and emulsions have been examined (Schnablegger et al., 1993).

Clearly, while SLS can generate useful information, quantitative assessment of the results can depend on exactly how the experiment was conducted — the data analysis steps in particular. Therefore, whatever method is chosen to extract sizing information from the light scattering data, a report on the experiments conducted is not complete until the full details of the calculations are described.

FRAUNHOFER DIFFRACTION

Fraunhofer, also known as far-field, diffraction takes advantage of the redirection of light waves that occurs when a sample containing small particles is irradiated from an infinite distance. This same phenomenon is responsible for the diffraction pattern generated by light passing through a single slit or fringes observed around rain droplets on one's eyeglasses. Via this process light scattered from particles placed in the path of monochromatic plane waves will combine to form a bright image at a distant detector at certain scattering angles, whereas at other angles the light destructively interferes to produce a region devoid of light.

The phenomenon is put to practical use via a simple optical scheme. A lens serves to deliver plane waves from a light source, placed at a distance less than infinity, to a fluid-borne sample. A second lens, placed on the opposite side of the sample, serves to focus the forward-scattered waves onto a detector surface, σ. The light source is usually a helium-neon laser, chosen because of the monochromatic and coherent nature of irradiation it produces. The ubiquitous use of a laser in this role has lead to the technique also being referred to as laser diffraction. The pattern of light on the detection plane is digitized via the use of photosensor elements placed at various positions with the intent of unambiguously capturing the scattering pattern. The placement of these detectors is frequently used as a means by which competing instrument manufacturers discriminate amongst themselves. Note that the source and detector are placed at conjugate focal planes, thus satisfying the requirement that incident and scattered light behave as plane waves.

Size information is derived via the inversion of

$$I(\theta) = I(0) \frac{\alpha^4 \lambda^2}{16\pi^2} \left[\frac{2 J_1(\alpha \sin \theta)}{\alpha \sin \theta} \right]^2 \qquad (11)$$

where $I(0)$ is the intensity of the incident light, $I(\theta)$ is the intensity of light scattered at an angle θ, J_1 is the first order Bessel function, $\alpha = \pi d/\lambda$, d is the particle diameter, and λ is the wavelength of light. As for the other ensemble methods, if the sample is polydisperse in size, then a functional dependence must be substituted for the α term in Equation 11. Inversion of this equation to solve for the size parameters

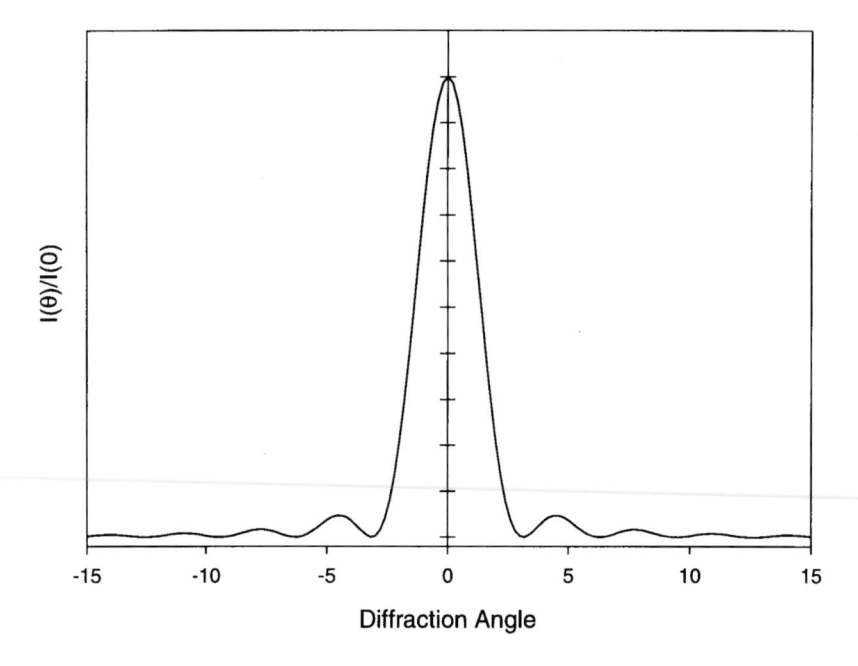

Figure 8 Airy disk function representing a cross-section of the diffraction pattern generated by the presence of micron-sized particles in the sample chamber of a Fraunhofer diffraction instrument. The oscillations "move" towards the central maximum as the particle size increases, whereas they expand outwards in the opposite case. Eventually the loss of features occurring in the latter incidence necessitates monitoring intensity at higher angles.

is the source of active research in the field (Agrawal et al., 1993; Huzarewicz et al., 1991).

The image at the focal plane, σ, has the general appearance of the function shown in Figure 8, and is circularly symmetric about the optical axis defined by the incoming light beam. The pattern corresponds to the Fourier transform of the spatial distribution of matter in the sample itself, hence L_2 is sometimes referred to as the Fourier lens. Because of this Fourier relationship, as the particle size drops the pattern becomes more diffuse with the distances between successive intensity maxima increasing. Conversely, as the particle size increases, the inter-maxima spacing goes down. In order to assure that a given diffraction pattern is spread over a significant fraction of the detector surface, the focal length of L_2, and hence the distance between it and σ, must be appropriately matched to the sizes of particles present in the sample.

Comparison with Intensity Light Scattering

It is worth considering Fraunhofer diffraction in comparison to intensity light scattering. Fraunhofer theory is strictly applicable only to those particles possessing a diameter substantially greater than the wavelength of incident light (De Boer et al., 1987; Weiner, 1984b). For the purposes of the commonly used laser sources, this condition is satisfied if the particle diameter exceeds 1 μm. Use of the theory also assumes that there is no direct interaction of the light with the scattering centers, e.g., absorption, hence there is no need for prior knowledge of the index of refraction — real or imaginary. If the index of refraction of the particles is extremely high, though, then the lower size range for which Fraunhofer theory is appropriate is increased. In the case of lipid emulsions, where the real index of refraction approximates 1.4 and the imaginary refractive index is very small, this limitation is of no concern.

Note, however, that the above size requirement places the vast bulk of the emulsion particle population below the accessibility of the Fraunhofer theory and thus any diffraction instrument based solely upon it cannot be said to produce accurate sizing results for such samples. Light diffraction instrumentation can be used to examine such samples, but only if Mie theory as described in the above section is applied to the data collected from the image plane. Indeed, most commercial instruments now possess the capability of using Mie theory, however, the rigor with which the calculations are carried out varies. In so doing, these instruments cease to do Fraunhofer diffraction and have become intensity light scattering spectrometers instead. In addition, it must be recalled that if Mie calculations are to be employed, values for the real and imaginary index of refraction are required, and the final results obtained will be no better than the quality of these inputs.

Instrumental limitations come into play as well. As Figure 2 shows, unless very high scattering angles are measured, the ability to examine the size of very small particles, i.e., less than 200 nm in diameter, is reduced regardless of the completeness of the theory used. In principal, accuracy in characterizing particles in this size region should be improved by taking advantage of the scattering dependence on wavelength and polarization state of the incident light (Harfield, 1991). Doing so has been demonstrated to increase substantially resolution when characterizing submicron systems (Schuhmann *et al.*, 1995).

As with intensity light scattering, the presence of too many scattering centers in the sample leads to artifactual results in laser diffraction (Hirleman, 1988). This multiple scattering tends to spread light over a broader region of the image plane, and because of the Fourier relationship discussed above, this leads to an underestimate of the particle size. In contrast to intensity light scattering, however, optimal signal to noise is achieved in laser diffraction when 30–50% of the light is blocked by the sample. Should that level of obscuration be taking place in an intensity or dynamic light scattering experiment, the results would certainly be skewed.

Diffraction instrumentation is commonly available in the laboratory because of its prevalence in determining the particle size of pharmaceutical solids and aerosols. Hence, in spite of the limitations of the method, Fraunhofer diffraction has enjoyed great popularity as a primary tool for characterizing submicron emulsions during formulation development. Indeed, with the inclusion of Mie capability, and as long as one is at least as interested in comparing similar samples with like refractive index, as one is in determining the absolute size parameters of a distribution, Fraunhofer is a valuable tool because of its rapid sample throughput and reproducibility. The stability of emulsions to various cations, amino acids and other additives have been probed using this method (Washington *et al.*, 1992a). Another application has been as a means of determining the effects of processing on the particle size distribution (Bock et al., 1994). Both of these studies represent appropriate applications of the method as a relative measurement since it is not expected that the optical properties of the particles will change substantially. Experiments conducted where the results of various of sizing methods are compared have shown that laser diffraction is not capable of detecting the early onset of coalescence or flocculation (Washington et al., 1992a) nor does is provide complete agreement with microscopy (Jokela et al., 1990) or electrolyte displacement (Brewer et al., 1995; Michoel, 1991).

TURBIDIMETRY

Turbidimetry is the measurement of light loss due to its blockage by the presence of a population of particles. This effect is due to the physical blocking of light by the individual particles and is not to be confused with absorption. In the latter case, light loss occurs because energy is transferred from the impinging photons into the constituents of the particle. Simple geometry suggests that the amount of light blocked by a given particle should be dependent on its cross section according to straightforward equations, thus leading to the possibility of a simple sizing method. While this statement is true for large particles, the relationship between size and blockage becomes more complex when the sizes of the particles approach that of the wavelength of the light. Indeed, at that point, turbidity, which by definition is measured at a 0° angle, is the complement to light scattering and is fully described by

$$\tau(\lambda_0) = \frac{\pi}{4} \int_0^\infty Q_{ext}(\lambda_0, D) D^2 f(D) dD \tag{12}$$

where Q_{ext} is the extinction (blocking) efficiency, D is the particle diameter, λ_0 is the wavelength of light, and $f(D)\,dD$ is the function describing the particle size distribution. Note that Q_{ext}, derived from Mie theory (Kerker, 1969) via

$$Q_{ext} = \frac{\lambda^2}{2\pi^2 r^2} \sum_{l=1}^{\infty} (2l+1)(|a_l|^2 + |b_l|^2) \tag{13}$$

is dependent upon optical constants such as the wavelength of incident light and the real and imaginary relative refractive index of the blocking particles in a manner similar to that employed in intensity light scattering. Note also that the same sort of mathematical complexities found in intensity light scattering, i.e., infinite sums, etc., are present in the equations that fully describe turbidimetry. This complexity describes the strong, oscillatory dependence of Q_{ext} on particle size and wavelength, which suggests that a particular particle size can be unambiguously identified via an interpretation of the data in terms of $Q_{ext}(\lambda, r)$. This possibility is realized, however, only as long as the particles are large enough to be outside the Rayleigh regime.

Data Analysis

Particles small compared to the wavelength of light can be sized using a simpler relationship, specifically

$$\left(\frac{\tau}{\phi}\right) = 24\pi^3 \left(\frac{(n^2-1)}{(n^2+2)}\right) \frac{V_V}{\lambda^4} \tag{14}$$

where ϕ is volume fraction of colloidal solute present, n is the index of refraction, and V_V is the volume-average volume for the particle size distribution (Kerker, 1969). Application of Equation 14 is the most common form of turbidimetry in which a measurement is made at one wavelength and the size is extracted. Note, however, that this equation requires that ϕ be known which is effectively the same as requiring that the concentration of the sample be evaluated ahead of time. This requirement emphasizes the fact that the turbidimetric signal is a function of both particle size *and* particle concentration. Hence, it is impossible to unambiguously determine one unless the other has been defined using another method. One must be cautious in using this method with colloids that have the potential to flocculate or coalesce, since such processes can lead to changes in both parameters simultaneously.

Another approach is to take advantage of the strong wavelength dependence inherent in Q_{ext}. A clear example of this dependency is described in the literature (Kourti, 1991). Size dependent information is available if the experiment is conducted in a manner complementary to light scattering. In the light scattering experiment it is the angular dependence of scattered light at a given wavelength that is monitored, where as in turbidimetry, the angle is kept constant (at 0°) and the wavelength is allowed to vary. This latter experiment, then, is the equivalent of collecting a "spectrum" of the colloidal solution where light loss is occurring due to turbimetric effects rather than absorption. However, were absorption to be occurring, then the final result would be in error since the conversion of the turbidity spectrum to a size population does not take absorption effects into account. Thus, in order to make use of this approach to characterize droplet size in an emulsion care must be taken to assure that light-absorbing species are not present in the formulation. This is of particular concern in the case of colored degradation products which could form over time.

This wavelength-dependent approach has been demonstrated as a means of determining particle size in colloidal suspensions made up of latex particles. This has been accomplished in several ways. One method (Eliçabe et al., 1989) involves reducing Equation 12 to the form of a Fredholm integral and then treating the data in a discreet form. This leads to

$$\tau(\lambda_i) = \sum_{j=1}^{n} a(\lambda_i, D_j) f(D_j) \tag{15}$$

in which the i and j indices span the wavelength of the spectrum and the n slices of the size distribution, respectively. The elements of the matrix relating $f(D_j)$ to $\tau(\lambda_i)$ are the a_{ij}. Note that the choice of n is left to the discretion of the analyst. This is written in vector form with the explicit inclusion of error

$$\underline{\tau} = \underline{\underline{A}}\underline{f} + \underline{\varepsilon} \tag{16}$$

where $\underline{\varepsilon}$ is the error in the turbidity data, $\underline{\tau}$.

Unfortunately, the problem of extracting size information from the turbidity spectrum through the inversion of Equation 16 is identical to that discussed in the context of both dynamic and intensity light scattering. Thus, results of the method are sensitive to the presence of experimental noise, $\underline{\varepsilon}$. In addition, the inversion problem becomes more complex when the sample is polydisperse and/or multimodal thus leading to potentially unstable results. Regularization techniques have been employed with reasonable success (Eliçabe, 1990) as they have with the other ensemble approaches. Better results are forecast when an equation analogous to Equation 12 is used to describe light scattering data, $i(\lambda_i)$, that is also collected, and both equations are solved simultaneously for f (Eliçabe, 1996).

Another approach, involving substituting diffraction theory for Mie theory in the determination of Q_{ext}, leads to the generation of an equation in which the size distribution is defined in terms of the derivative of the turbidity with respect to wavelength (Wang, 1996). The derivatives of the turbidity spectra are calculated via the widely-available Savitzky-Golay filter and the result inverted via Fourier transform to extract the size distribution, $f(r)$. This method has been tested via numerical simulation and appears to be capable of reconstructing bimodal size distributions in the presence of 10% noise, however performance for size distributions with means below 1000 nm was not investigated.

Instrumentation

One of the most appealing facets of the turbidimetric approach is the simplicity of the experimental technology. In most cases, a conventional absorption spectrophotometer can be employed to collect the data. A diode array-based instrument is particularly useful in that it allows an entire turbidity spectrum to be collected at once — a considerable advantage when the very short term stability of an emulsion is being investigated. A drawback of this sort of instrument, compared to more sophisticated single wavelength instruments which employ multiple slits, is the reduced ability to prevent low-angle light scattering from reaching the detector. Such a capability is essential since the turbidimetric equations discussed above are developed assuming that such signal has been eliminated, i.e., pure turbidimetry. The simplicity of the measurement makes the technique appealing for simple experiments in which the production of large particles in a stressed emulsion is used as a testing screen (Schuhmann et al., 1993; Rubino, 1990).

Turbidimetry can be applied as an on-line method in which values for the specific turbidity, τ/c, where c is the concentration of particles, for particles of various sizes are precalculated using Equation 14 and stored a look-up table (Kourti et al., 1990). Flowing sample then passes through the detector and the collected values for the specific turbidity are converted to particle size using the tabulated data. While being very easy to implement, there is the danger that if the relative refractive index or particle refractive index, composition, on concentration changes unexpectedly, then the reported values for size will be in error.

ULTRASOUND SPECTROSCOPY

One method that has received recent attention in the sizing of emulsion droplets is ultrasound, or acoustic spectroscopy. In this approach the experimental behavior of sound waves through colloidal media is fit to a mathematical model in which particle size is one of the variable parameters.

Background and Theory

The passage of sound through a fluid media occurs via the propagation of compression waves. Such waves involve the generation of alternating regions of high and low density within the sample, with the distance between maxima (or minima) being defined as the wavelength. As with all wave phenomena, their translational behavior is described via a simple equation involving frequency, propagation velocity, and attenuation (McClemments et al., 1996a). In the case of ultrasonics this description is formalized via

$$\left(\frac{k}{2\pi f}\right)^2 = \rho \kappa \tag{15}$$

where f is the sound wave frequency, ρ is the density, κ is the adiabatic compressibility, and k is the "wave number" of the propagating fluid. This last parameter contains the observable properties unique to the sample, the propagation velocity, c, and the attenuation coefficient, α, according to

$$k = \frac{2\pi f}{c} + i\alpha \tag{16}$$

Attenuation can occur via the conversion of sound energy into the fluid media as heat, due to either absorptive phenomena or processes that perturb susceptible chemical equilibria, or via the scattering of sound waves off of colloidal material. For the purposes of particle sizing in such media it is the scattering losses that are of most interest. As long as the particles much smaller than the wavelength of the 0.1–200 MHz sound waves typically employed, the propagation constant can be described as

$$\left(\frac{K}{k_1}\right)^2 = \left(1 - \frac{3\varphi i A_0}{k_1^3 r^3}\right)\left(1 - \frac{9\varphi i A_1}{k_1^3 r^3}\right) \tag{17}$$

where k_1 is the corresponding constant for the continuous phase, ϕ is the volume fraction of the discontinuous phase, and r is the particle radius. Comparing this equation to Equation 15 it is demonstrated that the first term on the right hand side corresponds to an effective density, ρ_{eff}, and the second term to an effective adiabatic compressibility, κ_{eff}. The above size requirement is easily met in submicron emulsions used in parenteral formulations. A_0 and A_1 are coefficients termed the "scattering coefficients", and describe the attenuation of ultrasonic energy due to scattering effects. These secondary ultrasonic waves are generated by the particles as they pulsate and physically move back and forth in response to the incident energy. The scattering coefficients are functions of temperature and frequency which are experimental parameters, and density, specific heat capacity, thermal conductivity, and coefficients of volume expansion which are thermophysical parameters. These dependencies are fully described elsewhere (McClements *et al.*, 1996a).

Instrumental

Instrumental requirements for the experiment are rather straightforward (McClemments, 1996b). The sample cell contains transducers that generate the sound waves and collect the transmitted energy. In some configurations, the same transducer is employed for both purposes, in which case the opposite side of the cell is pressed into service as a reflective surface redirecting the sound wave back towards its original source. Frequently more than one source/detector pair are required order to cover the necessary range of acoustic frequencies. Measurement of the ultrasonic velocity is a simple manner of noting the time an emitted wave takes to travel the known distance from its source until it is detected. Attenuation is determined relative to a calibrant for which the attenuation coefficient is known. Suitable electronics for production of the ultrasonic pulses and digitization of the collected energy are also required.

The data itself can be collected in several ways. The first involves sending a pulse of energy between the source and detector and measuring c and α. This process is repeated for as many frequencies as one has the need or patience to collect. In a modification of this approach, Fourier analysis is employed to extract the frequency-dependent information collected from the results of sending a very short high-energy burst through the sample. This method has the chief benefit of reducing the number of frequencies through which the ultrasonic emission must be scanned. A final technique is to set up a standing wave within the sample cell, the characteristics of which are determined by physically moving the opposite side of the cell wall with respect to the source/detector. Noting the wall placement as minima and maxima in signal intensity occur during this scanning provides the experimental response.

Applications

One of the simplest applications of ultrasonic spectroscopy to emulsions is its use to monitor creaming phenomena. In this case the source and detector are placed on opposite sides of the sample vessel and a reading is taken. Additional measurements are then taken as the source/detector pair is then moved vertically along the vessel. In this way a spatial profile of the sample is presented. This profile may be reported as a plot in which the *x*-axis corresponds to vertical displacement along the sample and the *y*-axis reports on particle concentration. Definition of the ordinate axis is accomplished via a calibration step using appropriate standards rather than using equations of the type listed above. As long as the difference in density between the droplet and the continuous phases are not too large, this relationship between attenuation and concentration is expected to be linear through 30% (v/v) (Herrmann *et al.*, 1996). While this application does not involve the determination of particle size directly, it can be used to monitor flocculation — a purpose for which particle size methods are frequently employed. In addition, this method has the advantage of being capable of monitoring formulations within their final package. It should be noted, however, that using rate of creaming as an estimate of flocculation or stability can be misleading since the flocculation process can occur within seconds, whereas the creaming that results may take hours or longer to form. Hence it is possible to derive an overly-optimistic estimate of stability from these sorts of measurement.

Direct determination of particle size using ultrasound is carried out by determining normalized values for effective velocity, effective adiabatic compressibility, or effective density, calculated from the terms in Equation 17 as a function of $rf^{0.5}$ and comparing them with the experimentally derived values (McClemments, 1996b). Next, rather than trying to invert the pertinent equations, the difference between observed and calculated plots are minimized by allowing the estimate of particle size, r, to vary using non-linear fitting algorithms. The value of r for which an optimum is obtained constitutes the determination of particle size by this method. The problem becomes decidedly more complex for colloids that are polydisperse in size.

The ultrasonic method has the advantage of being very simple to implement instrumentally. This simplicity makes it well-suited to a production environment where material in a process stream can be directly observed by placing that stream between source and sensor. In addition, direct calibration of the response as described in the application to flocculation above, allows for its quantitative use in an on-line mode in which an emulsion is characterized. In contrast to turbidimetry, ultrasonic spectroscopy is compatible with concentrated colloids hence obviating the need for dilution of the emulsion before analysis. Disadvantages of the ultrasonic method include the need for pre-determined thermophysical quantities, if particle size is to be directly determined, and a sensitivity to the presence of bubbles in the sample. Indeed, from the standpoint of scattering phenomena within the sample, bubbles display the same behavior as emulsion droplets, and thus can lead to artifacts in the data. Equipment to carry out these sorts of determinations via ultrasonic spectroscopy is only just becoming commercially available.

SINGLE PARTICLE OPTICAL SENSING

Overview

One of the most useful techniques available for the characterization of submicron emulsions is single-particle optical sensing (SPOS). The physical basis for the measurement, as diagrammed in Figure 9, is to categorize the size of individual particles as they pass through a sensor based on the changes in signal their presence induces in an optical detector. A light beam is passed through a flowing liquid sample stream. Particles passing through the beam interact with the light thus leading to a transient change in the detector signal. After assumptions about the particle refractive index and shape are made, the magnitude of the signal change can be directly related to the size of the particle present. The capability of the detection electronics (analog-to-digital conversion and comparator circuitry) to discriminate between signal decreases of different magnitudes, coupled with the internal

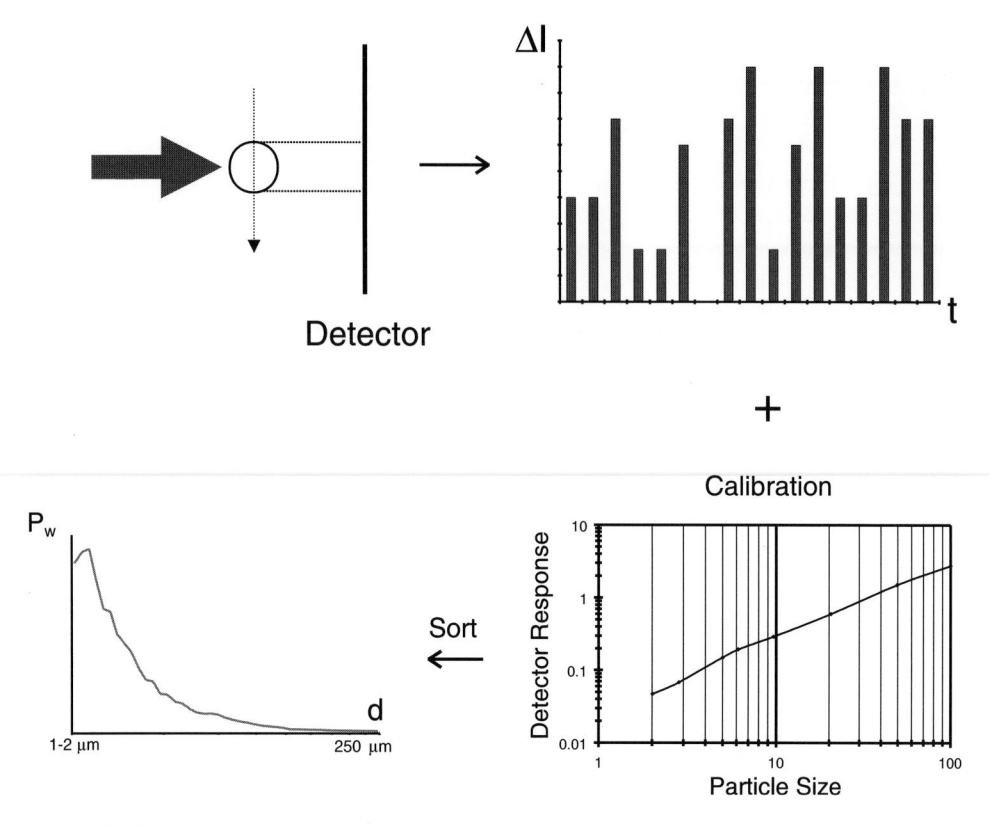

Figure 9 Schematic diagram of a SPOS experiment. See text for details. Note the logarithmic nature of the axes in the calibration step.

dimensions of the sensor itself, determines the ability of the instrument to characterize and resolve the distribution of particle sizes. The result is a sorting of photocurrent changes into different "bins" which in turn leads to the generation of a histogram that represents the distribution of particle sizes present in the total sample that has passed through the sensor.

It is this last attribute that places this analytical approach in the direct counting category. That is, when the technique is properly applied, each particle is detected individually. If enough particles are sampled, one has a complete understanding of the particle size distribution without the need to apply mathematical models to extract the results from the experimental data. Thus, uncertainties associated with the ensemble methods are dispensed with when SPOS techniques are applied. Since most implementations of SPOS apply to particles of diameter greater than 1 μm, the approach is useful because it can provide an indication of physical decomposition of the emulsion as the smaller droplets flocculate and/or coalesce to form larger entities.

This is not to say that the approach is devoid of difficulties. The first problem is a direct consequence of the above process, that is, since each particle is being inspected one at a time, the entire process can be extremely time consuming.

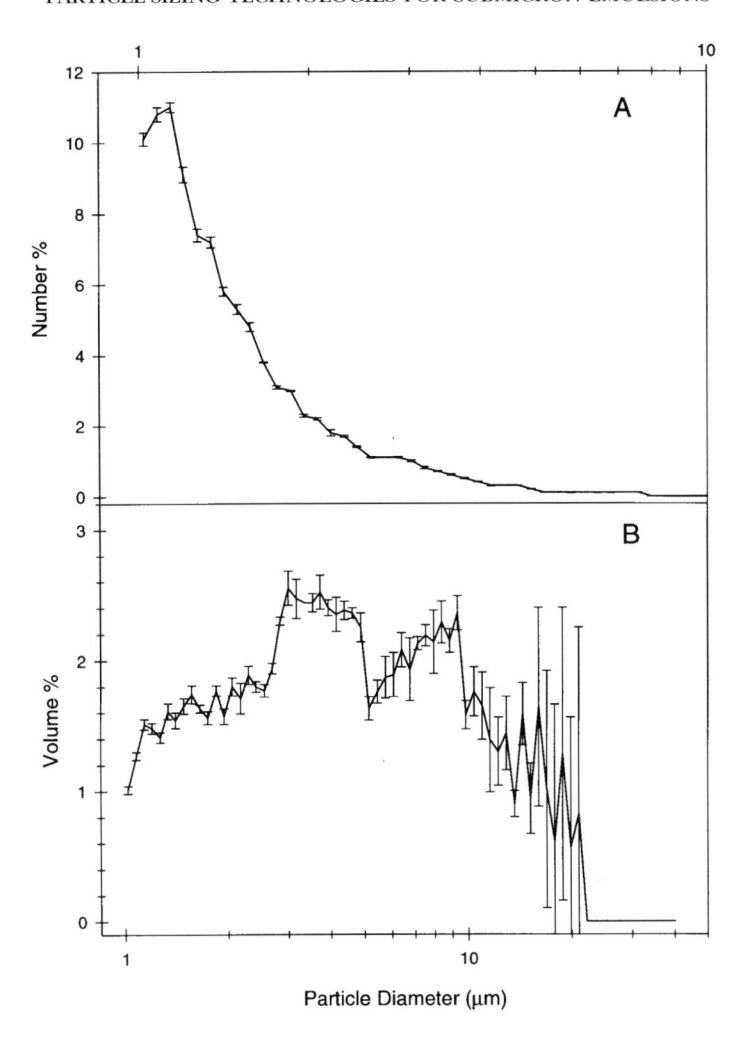

Figure 10 Comparison of the a) number, and b) volume percent of a sample of microparticulate drug as determined by an obscuration-SPOS instrument (Accusizer 770/770A; Particle Sizing Systems; Santa Barbara, CA). A particle count rate of 8,000 cps or less was maintained. Note that the error bars, as determined by triplicate measurements, demonstrate the uncertainty associated infrequently-sampled particle sizes. In the SPOS approach the number population is directly measured and the volume percent is calculated assuming a spherical particle shape.

Furthermore, particles on the extremes of the size distribution have by their very nature, a low probability of being detected since there are not many of them present in the original sample. This is of particular concern for particles that populate the large-size end of the size distribution. Such particles represent a small number fraction of colloidal phase, but may represent a very large volume fraction because of the cubed relationship between size and volume. Unfortunately, the presence of just such difficult-to-detect particles may be important indicators of emulsion quality (Müller et al., 1993a). An example is shown in Figure 10 in which the upper-size fraction of a particle population represents a small number fraction, but a large volume. Also shown are the experimentally-derived uncertainties associated with the different particles size bins. It is noted that the uncertainties increase dramatically as the number fraction drops. Thus the problem comes down to one of sampling: enough particles must pass through the detector to ensure that the resulting measured size distribution is a representative description of those that did *not* pass through. Good experimental procedure includes a protocol for estimating an uncertainty level associated with the final result. In the absence of a protocol allowing this parameter to be determined experimentally, perhaps due to a limitation in sample availability, some consideration should be given to applying a model of appropriate counting statistics as an approximation.

The second problem is related to the nature of the measurement itself. The above description of the process assumes that the solution is sufficiently dilute so that only one particle is present in the light beam at one time. If the number density of the particles in the solution delivered to the sensor becomes too high, then there may be more than one particle interacting simultaneously with the light. This "coincidence event" leads to the misinterpretation of these few small particles as arising from one particle equivalent in size to their sum. The result is that the measured population is skewed to large sizes compared to that of the actual population. Dilution experiments can be carried out to validate the absence of this situation because such artifacts lead to a nonlinear dependence on concentration when particle counts are plotted against the volume of the sample aliquot. This topic and others will be discussed in more detail below after some attention is given to describing characteristics of the instrumentation.

A final problem is the possibility that the passage of particles through a narrow flow stream could perturb the results. This is of particular concern for emulsion droplets which could deform during the observations step and hence lead to erroneous results. If the technique is used for assessing the presence of flocs, the stability of the species to the passage through the sensor should be evaluated (Gibbs, 1982).

Light Blockage

SPOS can be implemented in one of two ways, with the differences between them defined by the means with which the light-particle interaction is detected: blockage or scattering. The first approach involves placing a photodetector on the opposite size of the fluid flow from the light source, and measuring the shadow cast by the particle as it passes through the light beam. As for all so-called "obscuration" devices, the quantity measured directly by the sensor is a decrease in photocurrent generated by the particle's passage. The magnitude of the decrease is presumed to be proportional in some fashion to the cross section (diameter) of the particle. However, particularly for particles in the 1–10 μm range, the physical mechanism leading to this decrease is a combination of geometric obscuration, and diffraction/scattering, with the relative contributions of each being dependent on particle size and composition itself. Hence the relationship is between the observable (voltage decrease) and output (size) is not determined absolutely by the device, but is derived from a calibration step. Monodisperse polystyrene latex spheres having diameters from

2 to 100 μm are useful size calibrants. Standards having a known particle number density are available as well.

The obscuration technique is limited to particles greater than 1 μm in size because the passage of single particles with a diameter smaller than this value do not result in a sufficiently large decrease in photocurrent to be reproducibly evaluated. This final item represents a significant area for current instrumentation development and will be discussed further below. Instrument controlling software then presents the data in a variety of forms using user-defined weighting parameters if so desired.

Light Scattering

Another approach to SPOS is to take advantage of the light scattering taking place when the particle passes through the light beam in the sensor (Sommer, 1991). In this case, light scattered at a given angle is collected and then digitized, sorted, and reported on in the same manner as is done with the obscuration instruments. The primary advantage of this approach is the improved sensitivity to small particles inherent in the physical process of light scattering as compared to obscuration. These advantages derive from 1) the fact that individual submicron particles do not posses enough cross section to generate a reproducible obscuration signal whereas the same particle will generate copious scattering, and 2) the scattering signal is being detected against a background devoid of signal, whereas in obscuration the goal is to measure a small change in a large signal (similar to the difference between fluorescence and absorbance). The consequence of these advantages is that particles as small as 50 nm in diameter can be individually detected.

While the detection capabilities are impressive, there are disadvantages of the light scattering SPOS approach as well. First, the design of the light scattering sensors is decidedly more complex than that of their obscuration counterparts (Kollenberg *et al.*, 1992). This complexity serves to eliminate stray light, account for particles passing through different parts of an inhomogeneous light beam, and eliminate cavitation which produces a signal indistinguishable from that of a passing particle. In addition to the additional expense these design considerations imply, the light scattering sensors are significantly less robust and are more difficult to maintain than their obscuration counterparts. Second, as discussed in a previous section, the intensity of scattered light is intimately dependent upon characteristics of the sample particle such as microstructure, shape, imaginary and real refractive indexes. As a result, calibration of the size scale becomes even more of a necessity, but at the same time the ability to match samples with appropriate standards becomes more challenging (Martin *et al.*, 1992).

Third, when using these instruments, the analyst quickly discovers that the world is full of particles on the 100 nm size scale, and that generating a water supply in the laboratory with sufficiently low particle counts to be useful for sample delivery is a demanding task. Continuously-generated 0.1 μm filtered water and a HEPA filter-equipped laminar flow hood were found to be required in the author's laboratory. The fourth difficulty derives from the fact that these instruments were originally designed for the purpose of particle contaminant detection in the already clean fluid systems used in the semiconductor industry (Hango *et al.*, 1991). Hence, factors of dilution in the 10^6–10^8 range are required if the individual droplets in the submicron population of a parenteral emulsion are to be directly monitored. The effect of such extreme dilution on the sample size population needs to be considered when the results are interpreted. Also deriving from the instruments' semiconductor heritage is a fifth drawback which is that the sampling equipment is cumbersome, i.e., more suited to in-line than batch measurements in a laboratory setting, and the number of size-specific channels is limited to 16.

Comparisons

Light obscuration first became commonly used in the form of the "HIAC", an instrument designed to measure particulate contamination in parenteral solutions (Backhouse *et al.*, 1987). However, the problem at hand is to detect and characterize particles that are inherent to the sample and thus may be present in large numbers. Since that time a number of different instruments utilizing this mode of measurement have become available, but one of them is unique in several ways in its ability to characterize emulsions (Nicoli *et al.*, 1992). First, it has the capability to monitor large total volumes of solution because of the pump delivery system employed. This allows the accurate monitoring of particle number densities that populate the edge of the size distribution. Syringe-based models have a limited total volume capacity which is disadvantageous since the statistical uncertainties associated with individually counting small numbers of large particle becomes unacceptably high. However, the aforementioned configuration allows a sample to be continuously diluted with clean solvent until the total count rate drops to a preset value below which there is assurance that coincidence events can be avoided. For the intended purpose of examining particle systems containing 10–30% solids with uncharacterized size populations, this "autodilution" feature results in substantial time savings as well as a higher level of confidence in the results obtained. The ability to sample large volumes allows particle counting to continue until sufficient particle counts are obtained. Second, the comparator circuitry allow the discrimination of particle sizes from 16 to as high as 512 channels. Instruments such as the HIAC are limited to the 8–16 range. However, it is important to differentiate between the number of channels possessed by a given instrument and the actual size resolution obtained (Holve, 1995).

Coincidence Problems

As described above, SPOS sensors are subject to negative quantitation errors when the particle number concentration climbs to the point where the statistical probability of more than one particle being present in the detector volume becomes significant (Knapp *et al.*, 1994). Unlike the "traditional" application of these instruments to determining trace levels of particulates in solution, e.g., USP procedure 788, examination of systems such as emulsions involves samples with much larger number concentrations of particles, and hence the potential for generating artifactual data is much higher. A particular concern exists for systems in which most of the PSD is present at submicron diameters — sizes below the nominal detection limit of obscuration sensors. While *individual* particles cannot be detected by these sensors, should many such particles be present in the sensor simultaneously, they could reduce the detector photocurrent to the point where a false signal is generated. For

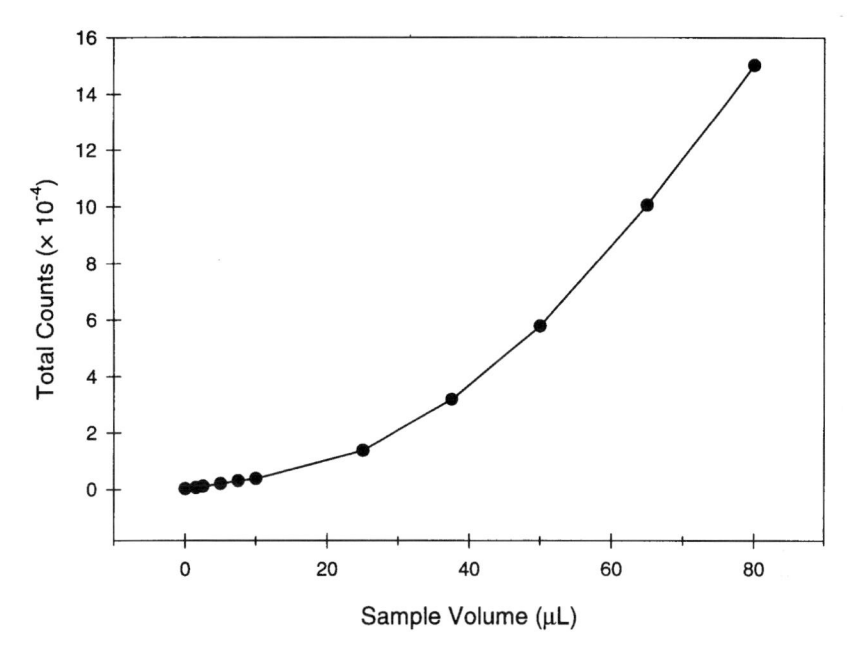

Figure 11 Demonstration of the effect of coincidence counting events on size intervals greater than those corresponding to the size of the particles themselves. Addition increasing volumes of 595 nm diameter particles to the sample vessel leads to the appearance of signal in an instrument (Accusizer 770/770A; Particle Sizing Systems) with a detection limit of approximately 1.5 μm.

emulsion samples, the population of submicron particles is sufficiently high that conditions in which 2, 3, 4 or more submicron particles could be present in the sensor are easily obtained. Indeed, the "better" the emulsion, i.e., the lower the ratio of micron to submicron droplets, the more likely artifacts from the submicron PSD become because more sample is required to get statistically valid counts of the micron-sized species.

Figure 11 clearly shows an example of the phenomenon. Polystyrene latex spheres of 0.5 μm diameter (Polysciences) were added to an obscuration-SPOS mixing flask at increasing levels to generate a plot of total counts as a function of sample volume. In principle, there should be no particles in these samples large enough to be individually detected by the sensor, thus any signal that is generated would have to be due to coincidence counting events involving the submicron particles. The figure indicates that such events are taking place and that they lead to a non-linear functional dependence.

Clearly it is necessary to understand the effects occurring in the sensor, and more importantly, identify data characteristics that indicate a given data set may be distorted by coincidence effects. A sample of 1.9 μm diameter polystyrene latex spheres was used to model an emulsion. Figure 12 shows that it has the qualitative distribution associated with submicron systems: a strong central peak with a "tail" to larger sizes although the size-axis is shifted to the micron size range, thus assuring that the entire PSD of the sample can be detected directly by the sensor.

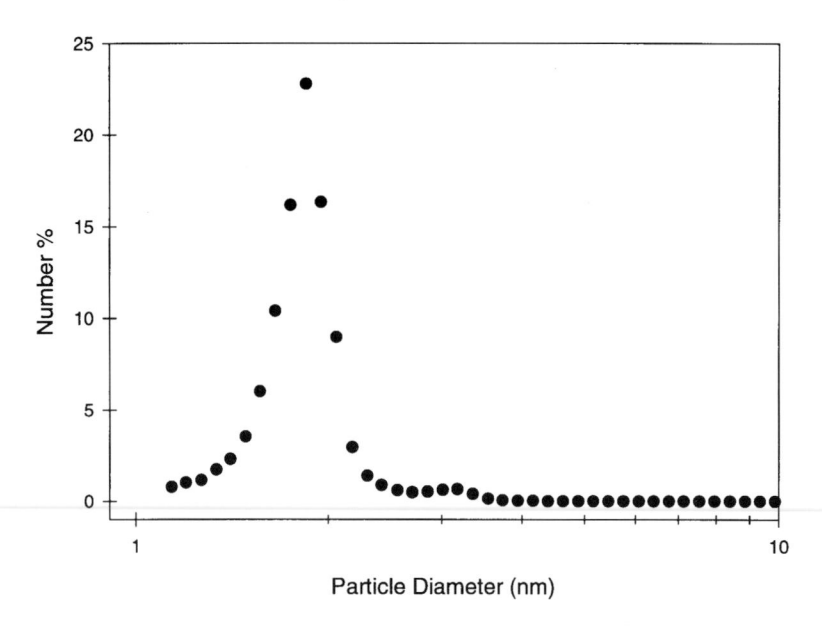

Figure 12 Population of latex spheres having a nominal diameter of 1.9 µm (Polysciences; Warrington, PA) as determined by obscuration-SPOS (Accusizer 770/770A; Particle Sizing Systems). Count rate was kept at less than 6,000 cps to ensure the absence of coincidence effects which would distort the measured shape of the PSD.

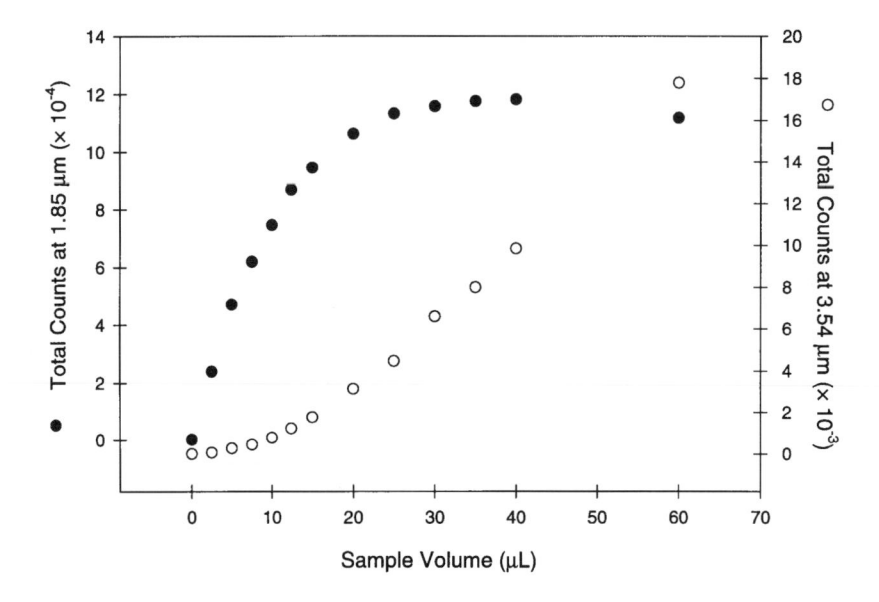

Figure 13 Effect of coincidence counting at two sizing intervals on increasing volume samples of the latex described in Figure 12. The autodilution feature of the instrument was disabled thus allowing count rates in excess of 25,000 cps. The negative deviation from linearity, indicative of coincidence counting is demonstrated at the 1.85 µm sizing interval whereas the complementary effect occurs at 3.54 µm.

Increasing amounts of these spheres were analyzed via obscuration-SPOS with the autodilution feature disabled to generate the plot shows in Figure 13. It is noted that the PSD mode is at 1.85 μm (Figure 12) and that, for samples in excess of a few microliters, the corresponding size bin displays the negative departure from linearity that is a defining characteristic of coincidence effects (Figure 13). As the sample aliquot increases, the incidence of multiple counting rises to the point where particles that should contribute to the histogram at the 1.85 mm space do not do so. Clearly, these particles sensor generate a signal, but where is the evidence of their passage? Examination of the 3.54 μm size bin (Figure 13) displays a complementary curvature in which the plot deviates in a positive direction from linearity in a manner similar to that seen previously (Figure 11). It is no coincidence that 3.54 is roughly twice 1.85. Indeed, the stronger the negative deviation observed at 1.85 μm becomes as more sample is added, the stronger is the positive deviation observed at 3.54 μm. Therefore, the question of the "missing" particles is answered: They "appear" in a size corresponding to their simultaneous presence in the sensor. Thus, the signal arising in the 3.54 μm bin arises in large part from the "spilling over" of signal from the bin counting particles of half the size (or other combinations of particle sizes that sum to an effective diameter of 3.54 μm, though given the narrow PSD of the sample such other combinations are less likely). This same phenomenon is responsible for the production of signal from a sample consisting of 0.595 μm particles (Figure 11). Note that Figure 11 displays the same positive curvature as is seen in Figure 13 suggesting that the observed signal in the former is due to coincidence effects and not due to the actual presence of larger particles.

In the case of an emulsion system, the model described above constitutes a clear warning that the submicron PSD can affect substantially the results derived from examining larger particles even when the former are not individually detectable. It is also demonstrated that for a given particle size, negative deviation from linearity is indicative of a loss of signal due to coincidence counting effects at that size whereas positive deviations result from coincidence events occurring at bins corresponding to smaller size particles. Hence, a complete study of colloidal particles using the SPOS approach should include a thorough investigation of linearity with respect to sample aliquot size as a means of demonstrating the absence of coincidence events. This recommendation is equally valid for both light scattering and obscuration-based sensors.

MICROSCOPY

Frequently cited as the reference method for particle sizing, microscopy is often the first method that comes to mind when considering options for techniques that rely on the principle of single particle counting (Cooke, 1996). There are good reasons for this popularity, but its use must be placed in the context of both the problem at hand and the other methods available. There are many discussions of the fundamentals of microscopy available elsewhere, so the following will be limited to a brief overview, discussion of options, and some examples from the literature.

Optical Microscopy

The general equation that describes the possibility of observing small particles via microscopy is

$$d = \frac{0.612\lambda}{NA} \qquad (18)$$

where d is the minimum distance between two resolvable points, λ is the wavelength of impinging radiation, and NA is the numerical aperture of the observing optics. In the case of emulsions, d would also correspond to the diameter of the smallest droplet possible that could be accurately sized. Numerical apertures of 1.1 are obtainable for non-immersion objectives, thus corresponding to a minimum size of 280 nm for 500 nm light, however, this value represents a theoretical optimum — 800 nm is the practical limit, particularly if the images are to be of quality sufficient for use in particle sizing. This limitation is due to the optical physics upon which the technique is predicated. Instrumental modifications like those associated with dark-field (or "ultra") microscopy serve to increase the method's ability to *detect* smaller particles, but do not enhance the ability to size them.

There are several points to make about Equation 18. First, is that choice of wavelength can help determine the resolution capability. Thus, using ultraviolet light can lead to the sizing of smaller particles. However, employing such wavelengths of light necessitate the use of quartz optics in the microscope which increases significantly the cost of instrumentation. However, this line of argument serves as the basis for electron microscopy where the wave-like attribute of electrons is employed to improve dramatically the resolution capability. Increasing the numerical aperture of the objective is another possibility for enhancing performance. However, maximal NA values of 1.3–1.5 are only obtainable with oil-immersion objectives which would not be an option for the o/w emulsions under consideration here.

Several other concerns, not specifically addressed in the above equation, need to be discussed. First is that the smaller particles observable by optical microscopy are also subject to Brownian motion. Diffusion coefficients for a 800 nm particle are on the order of 2.5×10^{-5} cm^2/sec. For practical purposes this diffusion serves to make these smaller particles appear as a shimmering haze, which renders the method unusable for sizing particles less than 2 μm in diameter. The influence of Brownian motion on particle sizing can be substantially reduced by use of a high-flux light source (Müller, 1991). This enables pictures to be taken with small exposure times which serves to stroboscopically "freeze out" diffusion. Another concern is that the depth of field, the region of sample normal to the focal plane that is in focus at one time, is reduced as the magnification is increased. This reduction decreases the number of particles that can be observed at one time, and is related to the issue of sampling which will be discussed in more detail below.

Thus the use of optical microscopy is limited to the size range associated with the upper region of the particles present in a parenteral emulsion formulation. This does not mean the technique is not useful, however. As will be shown below for microscopy and other some single-particle counting methods, significant and unique information about the behavior of the submicron population of an emulsion can be derived from observing the larger particles that result from processes such as flocculation and coalescence.

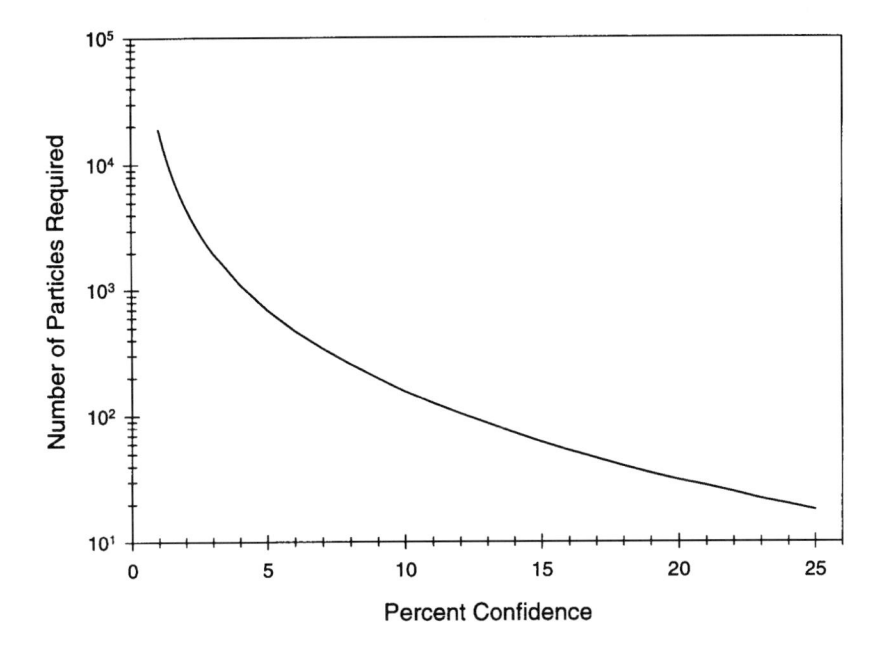

Figure 14 Plot of uncertainty in sizing accuracy as a function of particles counted via microscopy according to Hastedt et al. (1995).

Electron Microscopy

As mentioned above, reduction of the wavelength of incident radiation leads directly to a decrease in the minimum size observable. An electron accelerated to 10 kV has an associated deBroglie wavelength of less than a nanometer. Thus, the first benefit of electron microscopy is clear: The capability to directly observe all sizes of particles present in a submicron emulsion. Transmission electron microscopy (TEM), in which the electron beam is detected after it has passed through the sample, allows particles as small as 1 nm to be observed, though procedures for rendering the droplets opaque to the electrons must be employed. Scanning electron microscopy (SEM), in which electrons reflected from a beam rastered across the sample are monitored, can only resolve features to the 10 nm scale. However, this minimum size range is more than adequate for the emulsion samples under consideration, and SEM also possesses a greater depth of field than TEM.

Statistical Concerns

Microscopy is the penultimate method for single particle counting of emulsions since each droplet is individually observed and inspected. However, what makes the method so precise also serves to emphasize its greatest limitation, namely that of obtaining a statistically relevant sample of emulsion droplets. Figure 14 shows the number of particles that have to be counted in order to define a normal population mean to a given degree of confidence. Clearly, the requirements go up steeply as the need for confidence increases. For example, to obtain a 98% confidence for the mean size of a population while counting at one particle per second would take

1.5 hours. Note that this calculation does not take into account the time required to prepare multiple samples needed to carry out this analysis. Even if a 90% confidence were deemed sufficient, in which case only 150 particles need to be counted, multiple samples should be prepared to avoid the possibility of anomalies in any one sample preparation skewing the results. Finally, it should be emphasized that the figure is referring to determination of a population mean. Accurately determining a width for the population would require more effort, and defining subtle features, i.e., the growth of shoulders on the mean distribution, would be more demanding still. Any report of size derived from microscopy should include an estimate of error, and a detailed account of the number of droplets and samples observed. On the other hand, microscopy is the only method of determining the morphology of the sample droplets discussed in this samples. This is a valuable characteristic and is emphasized in some examples presented below.

In principal, these statistical requirements are not a concern, but the analysis must be carried out in a reasonable time. Hence, the analyst must balance the need for accuracy with the time available per sample against each other to arrive at a protocol that is efficient while still providing relevant feedback to formulation development.

Sample Preparation

Sample preparation for optical microscopy is relatively straightforward. Undiluted sample is placed on a slide, covered with a slip and then directly observed. A graticule can be used to calibrate either the optics of the microscope or to serve as a visual reference against which size can be estimated. The processes then reduces to one in which size measurements for multiple observations are recorded and tabulated to generate a final result. In order to satisfy the statistical requirements outlined above, this can be a tedious process. Either semi-automated (where the droplet is identified and defined by the operator and tabulated by the instrumentation) or fully automated (where the entire process is carried out by software algorithms) image analysis approaches can serve to alleviate the tedium, increase sample throughput, and increase the number of droplets observed per sample. If particular pattern recognition algorithms are used, then the source and basis for their use should be specified.

Sample preparation for electron microscopy is more problematic than is the case for optical methods. First, in order to allow the passage of electrons through the instrument, the sample must be maintained under vacuum. This requirement clearly precludes the observation of *in situ* samples, and necessitates a pretreatment step to stabilize the droplets against the harsh environment. Second, the sample must be electrically conductive so that charge imparted by the impinging electrons does not build up and lead to a perturbation in the electron beam and ultimately distort the image. This conductivity can be intrinsic to the sample or afforded by the preparation. Frequently, the concerns of both issues can be resolved simultaneously with an appropriate sample preparation technique. Unfortunately, such treatment of the sample may lead to processes that distort the sample and thus lead to inaccuracies in sizing. For example, one sample preparation method (du Plessis *et al.*, 1986) calls for embedding the lipid particles in bubble-free agar followed by fixation with OsO$_4$. The matrix containing the particles is then sliced and the exposed surface is examined. While the physical stabilization problem is addressed, there is the concern than the slicing plane may not, indeed probably will not, bisect each droplet. This would lead to an underestimation of size. Another option is to fix the droplets directly with a material, such as OsO$_4$ or malachite green and gluteraldehyde, that are opaque to the electron beam (Harris *et al.*, 1991; Hamilton-Attwell, *et al.*, 1987). This avoids the potential hazards of using a cross section, but the droplets may become distorted as they sit on the sample mount. Use of SEM provides a three-dimensional image of the specimen whereas the TEM micrographs reveal less morphological information, but are equally useful for sizing (du Plessis *et al.*, 1988).

As mentioned above, one of the distinct advantages of microscopy it its ability to determine the morphology of the droplets themselves. In the case of optical microscopy, because of resolution limitations, the analyst is generally restricted to examining the remains of a coalescence event. However, electron microscopy possesses sufficient resolution to allow the particles that make up the bulk of the size distribution themselves to be observed directly. For example, the presence of liposomal material in soybean emulsions has been unambiguously confirmed via TEM of negatively-stained samples (Rotenberg, *et al.*, 1991; Groves *et al.*, 1985). In another study, the presence of multi-layered objects suggesting the formation of w/o/w emulsions in commercial nutritional emulsions was demonstrated (Li *et al.*, 1994).

In order to take maximal advantage of this capability the sample needs to be prepared via freeze-fracture. In this method the sample is rapidly frozen with the goal of rendering the droplets structurally intact and robust for the next step. The frozen sample is then fractured to expose the surfaces of interest, and then coated with a metal such as Pt-C. The original material is then washed away and the metal material, serving as a negative image, is mounted and observed in the microscope. While being capable of providing very high quality images, the technique requires specialized equipment for the freezing and metal evaporation steps, is time-consuming, and quite expensive (Chapman *et al.*, 1986; Menold *et al.*, 1972). When applied to lipid emulsions, however, the technique is capable of providing impressive images (Levy *et al.*, 1994; Li *et al.*, 1994).

FIELD-FLOW FRACTIONATION

Field-flow fractionation (FFF), in particular sedimentation FFF (SdFFF), has demonstrated the ability to separate particles based on their size and has been applied to the investigation of submicron lipid emulsions with great success (Caldwell *et al.*, 1989; Li *et al.*, 1994; Levin *et al.*, 1994). Successful characterization of the particles was achieved when DLS was used to determine the size of the eluted fractions (Li *et al.*, 1993a) so that appropriate corrections for the density of the submicron particles could be applied (Li *et al.*, 1994; Levin *et al.*, 1995). Separations have been carried out using both constant (Caldwell *et al.*, 1989; Li *et al.*, 1993; 1994) and gradient gravitational fields (Levin *et al.*, 1994; 1995a).

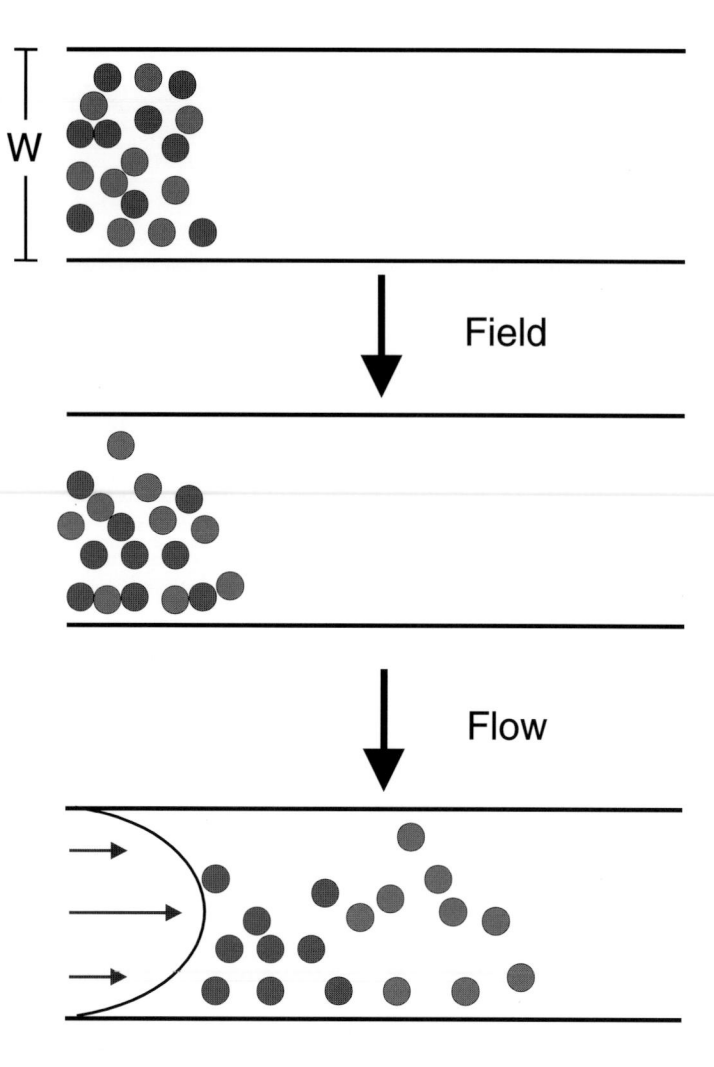

Figure 15 Diagram of the FFF process. Analytes placed in a channel of width, w, are exposed to a force that differentially interacts with the populations present. Application of a laminar flow, which possesses a parabolic profile, serves to cause those populations less affected by the force to elute earlier. The amount of time between application of the force and the eluting flow defines the relaxation time.

Background

FFF refers to a class of separation technologies in which analytes are separated based upon their relative positions in a laminar flow (Giddings, 1981). The analytes' response to a perpendicularly applied force field determines the position that they take up in these laminar flow lines and thus determines the rate at while they are eluted. The process is described pictorially in Figure 15. Samples are placed in a thin channel having a height on the order of hundreds of microns, a width on the order of centimeters, and a length on the order of tens of centimeters. Figure 15 shows an edge-on perspective of the situation immediately after sample introduction into the channel. A force field is applied in a direction perpendicular to the ultimate elution flow and serves to separate the various sample components based on some property that is sensitive to this field, e.g., charge, hydrodynamic size, or buoyancy in the case of an electrical, flow, or gravitational field, respectively. The time from the initial application of the field to that at which equilibrium has been reached depends upon the nature of the field and its interaction with the analytes, and is termed the "relaxation time". After this time has elapsed, a flow of solvent along the length of the channel is introduced while the original force-field continues to be applied. The choice of flow rate, solvent viscosity, and channel design together serve to cause this eluting flow to take on laminar characteristics with the distributions of flow velocities possessing a parabolic front. Those sample components forced into the bottom (or top) of the channel by the perpendicular field elute at a slow rate consistent with flow velocities present in that part of the channel. On the other hand, those components less affected by the applied field sample (on average) the faster flow velocities present in the center of the channel and hence elute at the beginning of the "fractogram".

In the case of SdFFF, the cross-field is gravitational and artificially generated by rapidly spinning the flow channel which itself is positioned along the inner wall of a centrifuge drum. Separation takes place based on the buoyancy of the sample present in the channel which is in turn dependent upon both size and density of the sample components, the latter relative to that of the elution fluid. As will be demonstrated below, FFF can be used to discriminate based on one characteristic, e.g., size, even though the actual basis for the interaction of the sample with the cross field is based on another characteristic, i.e., buoyancy, providing the two properties are quantitatively related to each other. However, one must be alert to situations in which the elution time may not be reflecting this assumed relationship, and thus careful scrutiny of the instrument response is always prudent to avoid misinterpreting the data.

Sedimentation FFF (SdFFF)

SdFFF is one of the more developed FFF techniques in which the retention mechanisms are well understood (Caldwell, 1984). This understanding allows the elution times to be rigorously related to physical properties through a parameter, λ, which describes the sensitivity of the analyte to the cross field. The experimental observable for the FFF experiment is the elution volume, V_e, for the various components as determined via peak position on the fractogram. Generally this is reported in relation to the void volume of the channel, V_o, via

$$R = \frac{V_o}{V_e} \tag{19}$$

so that late eluting peaks are associated with lower values of R. R in turn is related to λ by

$$R = 6\lambda \left[\coth\left(\frac{1}{2\lambda}\right) - 2\lambda \right] \tag{20}$$

The equations developed up to this point are independent of the type of cross field employed and, in the absence of steric and lift forces, apply to all forms of FFF. In the particular case of SdFFF, the relationship between gravitational force and sedimentation leads to Equation 21.

$$\lambda = \frac{6kT}{d^3 \Delta \rho G \pi w} \quad (21)$$

where $\Delta \rho$ is the difference in density between the particle and the suspending medium, G is the acceleration of the artificially generated gravitational field, and d is the diameter of the particle. Rearranging Equation 21 to

$$d^3 \Delta \rho = \frac{6kT}{\lambda G \pi w} \quad (22)$$

shows how results are derived from the experimental observations. R is determined via Equation 19 using V_e, which is extracted from the fractogram's x-axis since the flow rate is known, and V_o, which is an instrumental constant determined by injecting a non-retained substance. Solution of Equation 20 for λ leads to a value that can be used in conjunction with the instrumental (G, w) and physical constants (k, T) of Equation 22 to determine $d^3 \Delta \rho$.

There are several important points to make about the relationship described in Equation 22. First, since the gravitational field affects the particles only through their buoyancy, which is a function of both volume (size) *and* density, the dimensions of the particles cannot be unambiguously determined unless their density is independently measured. Conversely, the particle density cannot be determined via SdFFF unless the size of the eluting particles is already known. However, if it can be confirmed that the density of the particles is constant across a series of samples, then comparison of the resulting fractograms is a useful means of comparing particle size distributions without making absolute determinations. Finally, in situations where it may not be possible to measure absolute quantities directly, the technique can still be employed as a means of separating the sample into portions whose particle size can be determined by another method such as DLS. Such a fractionation process is of great utility because DLS is not adept at characterizing the particle population of unfractionated samples with a complex size distribution (Finsy et al., 1992). Indeed, the combination of fractionation and DLS allows the independent determination of particle size required for the density measurements and can be used to "calibrate" the elution profile as described above. Such an approach has met with great success (Li et al., 1993a; Levin et al., 1995).

A convoluting process can occur if the particles being analyzed are large, i.e., >1 μm. In this case the particles, regardless of dimension, are pressed against the wall of the channel and depending upon their diameter protrude into the elution flow profile to differing but nonetheless substantial degrees. Larger particles protrude further into the profile and thus sample a greater average flow velocity as they roll/bounce along the channel wall. The final result is that the elution ordering of samples is reversed from the expected case such that larger particles elute *earlier* than those that are smaller. This mode of separation constitutes a variation on SdFFF that is termed steric FFF (SFFF). While SFFF is a valid means of separating particles

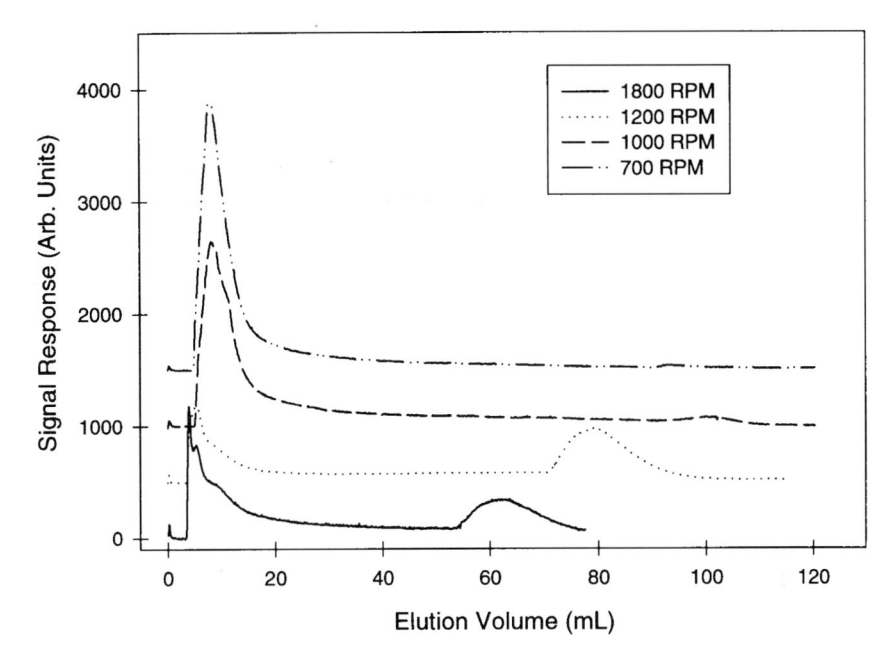

Figure 16 SdFFF fractograms collected for 3 μL injections of a 25% Miglyol 810 emulsion for rotational frequencies of 700, 1000, 1200, and 1800 rpm. Water, supplied via a peristaltic pump at 1 mL/min after a 30 minute relaxation interval, was used as the elution fluid. Detection was carried out via a UV HPLC detector operating at 254 nm.

(Caldwell, 1984) it is important to note that the experimental conditions used are identical to those employed for SdFFF. Therefore, care must be taken when examining uncharacterized systems to assure that the actual mode of fractionation taking place is adequately understood.

As an example, Figure 16 shows the fractograms collected for 3 μL injections of a 25% Miglyol 810 emulsion for rotational frequencies of 700, 1000, 1200, and 1800 rpm. All of the fractograms are characterized by an early spike that corresponds to elution of non-retained material, an asymmetric peak that corresponds to material that fractionated according to SdFFF processes, and a late eluting fraction that is only released from the channel when the gravitational acceleration is set to zero. The appearance of these fractograms are consistent with those collected from lipid emulsions by others using a constant gravity field (Caldwell *et al.*, 1989; Li *et al.*, 1993a; 1994).

It is worth noting the dependence of the fractogram shape on G. Increasing the spin frequency increases the area of the late eluting peak while simultaneously decreasing the area of the void and retained peaks. Apparently, as G increases, the particles are forced closer to the wall on average, where the elution flow is low. Particles with a large enough value of $d^3\Delta\rho$ are pushed so close to the wall that their elution is effectively arrested and thus they only elute when the drum is stopped and are thus allowed to diffuse into faster flow streams. Lower values of G do not force these large $d^3\Delta\rho$ particles as close to the wall thus they elute earlier in the fractogram rather than eluting in the "field-off" peak. Note that there appears to be no spin frequency that leads to appreciable amounts of material being eluted in the 20–50 minute region. This suggests a low dynamic range for the resolution such that a given setting of G is only optimum for a limited portion of the total analyte population. In this scenario adjusting G serves mostly to cause material to shift back and forth between eluting early to eluting in the field-off peak. This is analogous to balancing a length of wood on a razor blade. Most of the wood is either on one side or the other, i.e., elutes early or late, while very little of the wood is actually on the blade itself, i.e., elutes in the 20–50 minute range.

The above discussion assumes application of a constant value of G throughout the experiment to the separation channel, thus being somewhat analogous to isocratic chromatography. The analog to gradient chromatography also exists in which the applied gravitational field is allowed to vary in time as the analysis proceeds. In most cases the gravitational field is decreased over time which allows species that interact strongly with the field to elute much earlier, and thus with a narrower peak width, than they would otherwise. This approach is particularly useful in the analysis of highly polydisperse systems such as submicron emulsions. The example suggests that better results would be obtained using such a gradient in which the spin rate is slowly decreased during the course of the run. Indeed such an approach, called "power programming", has been successfully applied in the analysis of lipid emulsions, and yielded high resolution fractograms (Levin et al., 1994). A drawback of power programming, however, is that the relationship between elution, R, and physical characteristics of the particles becomes much more complex than the constant power approach so that the simple equations described above no longer apply (Williams et al., 1994).

Other Forms of FFF

In addition to SdFFF, which employs gravity as the cross-field, other forms of FFF exist (Giddings, 1995) some of which may be applicable to the characterization of emulsions. Electrical FFF (EFFF) involves the use of an electrical field to discriminate between particles within the sample based upon surface charge via the following dependence

$$\lambda = \frac{kT}{\mu f E} \qquad (23)$$

where μ is the electrophoretic mobility, f is the friction coefficient, and E is the electrical field strength (Schimpf et al., 1995). In EFFF the fractionation channel is constructed from graphite blocks which are coated to reduce porosity and then polarized to produce the electric field.

Separation based upon hydrodynamic size is possible via Flow FFF (F^4) in which

$$\lambda = \frac{kT}{3\pi \eta d_h U} \qquad (24)$$

where η is the viscosity of the suspending medium, d_h is the hydrodynamic diameter, and U is the linear cross-flow velocity. In F^4 the channel is made up of a permeable material through which additional suspension media passed, thus generating a cross flow (Theilking *et al.*, 1995). This method has the great advantage of having the elution be related predominantly to size.

Detection

As mentioned above, the separation taking place may not be based on the assumed principle of the method. On-line or near-line detection can resolve such ambiguity if an appropriate detection scheme is used. For example, DLS can determine the size of particles that elute thus enabling a reliable calibration of the time/volume-axis even when power programming is employed, as well as allowing the density of eluting particles to be determined. Furthermore, while DLS is not the method of choice for extracting accurate size parameters from populations that are multimodal or highly polydisperse, fractionation of the sample by the FFF ensures that the sample delivered to the detector is reasonably monodisperse, thus increasing the reliability of light scattering result. In this way both the separation and detection techniques are used in a synergistic manner to the benefit of results derived from both.

Care must be exercised to ensure that the detection scheme does not produce convoluted results itself. Chromatographic absorbance detectors are frequently pressed into service in FFF. However, in addition to correcting the output for Mie scattering, it must be remembered that this signal is a convolution of droplet size with droplet concentration. Therefore, concentration information, either through an off-line analysis or another serially-placed concentration-specific detector, must be obtained as well if a size determination is to be made. More promising than the use of an absorbance detector is the application of multi-angle intensity light scattering detectors (Theilking *et al.*, 1995). Such devices collect light at many angles simultaneously, thus allowing concentration-independent calculations like those described in the corresponding section above to be made on the particles as they elute. Again, the fractionation afforded by the immediately preceding separation step is of great benefit. In addition, the sensitivity inherent in intensity measurements allows the method to be employed on-line as compared to DLS, which is carried out on collected fractions.

Examples

The following example demonstrates the utility of such a combination. The first step is to plot the size, obtained via DLS, versus the elution volume for each fraction. Figure 17 shows such a plot obtained for samples of soy lecithin-emulsified 10% Miglyol 810 using the fractions collected from the corresponding fractograms. It is clear that the data points generate two essentially linear plots. For those samples that are analyzed using the same FFF conditions if overlapping plots are observed, the size versus elution time calibration should be transferable from fractogram to fractogram. It is interesting to note that the sample with the deviant plot is one that had been kept at −20°C whereas the others were stored at 4°C. The plots in Figure 17 suggest that freezing the sample profoundly changes the nature of the emulsion droplets. Another example is presented in Figure 18. The corresponding plots for samples in which the drug is present and absent do not overlap thus the calibrations do not transfer and the fractograms cannot be directly compared. Apparently the

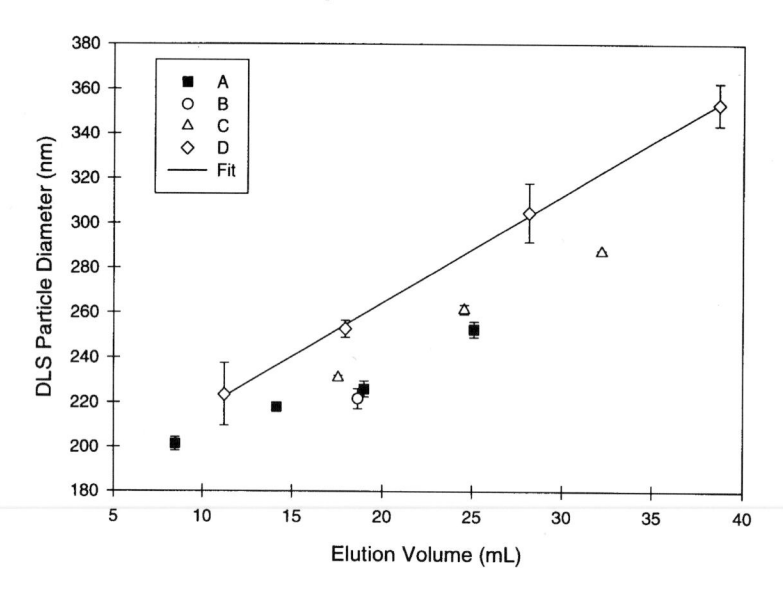

Figure 17 Particle diameter of 2 mL fractions collected from SdFFF fractionation of 10% Miglyol emulsions emulsified with soy lecithin. Control (A), control spiked with centrifuge-derived infranatant (B), and control spiked with centrifuge-derived cream (C) all stored at 4°C, and control stored at −20°C (D). Particle size was determined via DLS using a helium-neon laser operating at 632.8 nm, with a 90° scattering geometry defined by a BI-20SM goniometer. The autocorrelation function was collected with a 72-channel BI-2030AT (Brookhaven) autocorrelator. Data analysis carried out using a second-order cumulants fit.

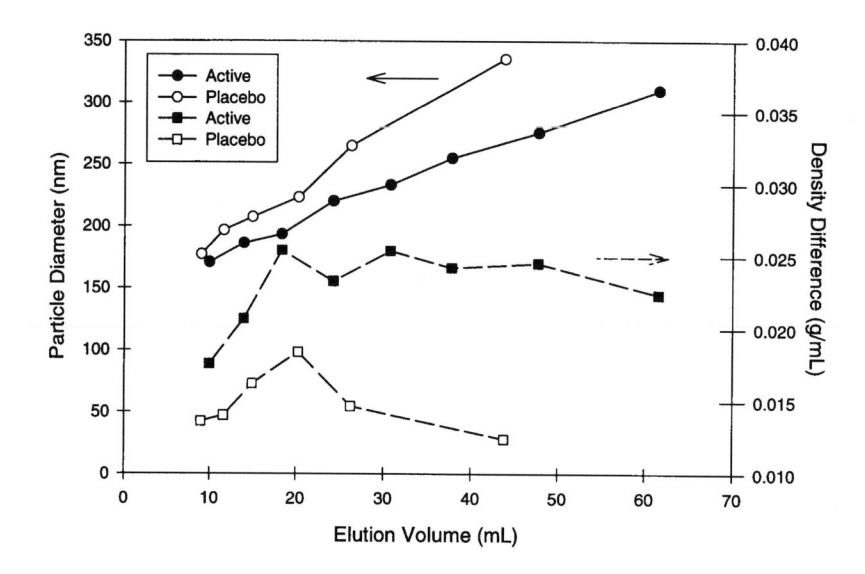

Figure 18 Particle diameter of 2 mL fractions collected from SdFFF fractionation of active and placebo 20% Miglyol emulsions emulsified with egg lecithin. The density difference, $\Delta\rho$, was calculated as described in the text.

presence of drug in the emulsion changes the nature of the droplets in some substantive fashion. Note that an uncritical comparison of the raw fractograms of these two samples would lead to an erroneous interpretation of the data.

Using the DLS-derived value for particle size, d, and λ from the retention data, in Equation 22 allows the determination of $\Delta\rho$ for the collected fractions. Figure 18 shows a plot of $\Delta\rho$ versus elution volume for two emulsions samples: an active and a placebo. There are two items of note in this figure. The first item is that there is a large difference between the drug-containing and vehicle emulsion with the former being larger. Since the emulsion droplets are less dense than water, i.e., they float upon centrifugation, the value of $\Delta\rho$ is negative with respect to the suspending medium, and the particles of the drug-containing emulsion must be less dense than those of the vehicle emulsion. Note that this implies the particles move towards the inner wall of the fractionating channel during the relaxation step. The second item is that the value of $\Delta\rho$ is relatively constant for V_e from 10–50 mL suggesting that the density differences may be independent of size.

OTHER METHODS

There are a number of other methods that are either just emerging as viable analytical techniques or have only recently been applied to colloidal/emulsion systems. In other cases, these methods have been superseded by alternative techniques. A brief description of each is presented along with some literature references that may serve as a guide for possible future studies.

Ensemble Methods

Dielectric Spectroscopy

In much the same way that the propagation of sound waves through a colloidal medium can be used to determine size via ultrasonic spectroscopy, the dielectric properties of such as system can be evaluated via monitoring the passage of electromagnetic radiation (Sjoblom et al., 1994). The magnitude and frequency dependence of the radiation's attenuation and phase behavior of can be modeled using equations in which size is one of the parameters. The technique is only just emerging as a method of characterizing pharmaceutical colloids (Smith et al., 1995).

Nuclear Magnetic Resonance

Most frequently employed for structural characterization of materials and molecules, NMR has also been applied to particle sizing. The variation in chemical shift induced is monitored when a magnetic field gradient is placed across the sample, and the time dependence of this variation is measured through the pulsed-field gradient spin echo (PFGSE) data collection sequence. The decay of the spin echo as a function of field strength is directly related to the diffusion coefficient of the species associated with the given spectral peak. The particle size is then extracted from the diffusion coefficient (Soederman et al., 1996; Li et al., 1992). Therefore, as for DLS, a rapid decay is associated with a faster diffusion coefficient which is in turn assumed to be indicative of a smaller particle size. Thus, all of the concerns about non-size related phenomena affecting the diffusion coefficient apply with this method as is the case with DLS. The NMR approach has the disadvantage of requiring significant amounts of time on expensive equipment. However, it possess the advantage of the molecular specificity associated with high resolution NMR. In order to assume that the result is indicative of the size of the colloid, however, it must be confirmed that the spin echo decay is due to overall motion of the particle and not local motion of the individual molecules within. This specificity has also been employed in morphological studies of lipid-based particulates through diffusion-ordered 2D spectroscopy (DOSY) methods (Hinton et al., 1993).

Separation Methods

Size Exclusion Chromatography (SEC)

Size exclusion is the process by which sample is passed through a column packed with porous beads. Small particles can "partition" into the pores more effectively that the larger particles which are excluded from such small regions. Hence the elution time is inversely proportional to the particle size. This method has been applied to colloidal systems such as liposomes (Lesieur et al., 1993) and latex particles (Kourti et al., 1987), but the dependence of the retention time on the rigidity of the membrane calls into question if the separation process is taking place via exclusion solely or whether there are some extrusion processes occurring as well (Ollivon et al., 1986). This latter process would lead to underestimates of particle size. Calibration of the elution time to size using standards is necessary. Differences in non-specific interactions of the emulsion components with the stationary phase compared with those for the standard can lead to anomalous results. Analyzing collected fractions with orthogonal methods such as DLS, as is done with FFF, has been successful (Huve et al., 1994).

Hydrodynamic Chromatography (HDC)

Separation via this method takes place via the relative displacement different sample populations experience in a laminar flow induced by a narrow channel. Small particles are more effective at sampling the slower flow lines, hence they are eluted later. The narrow channel can be either the interstitial paths present in a packed bed of *nonporous* material or that present in a narrow capillary. When the latter approach is used the technique is frequently referred to as capillary hydrodynamic fractionation (CHDF). In principle use of a capillary instead of a packed bed should avoid the possibility of the deformable emulsion droplets extruding through small spaces and thus producing anomalous results. A crude implementation of HDC has been demonstrated as a means of separating liposomes (Cebamanos et al., 1990), but more recent work using CHDF has proved capable of characterizing various submicron systems (DosRamos et al., 1991).

Disk Centrifuge

Characterization of colloidal systems has also been accomplished via use of the disk centrifuge (Bowen et al., 1993; Gill et al., 1992). In this method a spinning disk of suspending media is prepared and a sample introduced. Sedimentation of the analyte is then monitored via scattering/attenuation and standard relationships are used to calculate size, hence calibration is not required if the necessary input parameters are available. A variation on this method is one in which the sample is premixed with the suspending media and loss of the particles from the solution is monitored as the particles "spin out" as specified by their size and relative density. This approach is mandatory when examining lipid emulsions because their constituent droplets are less dense than any suspending medium that would be chemically compatible. A benefit of this "homogeneous start" is that the presence of any material remaining in the spin fluid at the conclusion is readily detected. Thus, unlike some methods, such as Fraunhofer diffraction or the various chromatographic techniques, one has an immediate indication of what is *not* getting analyzed.

Capillary Zone Electrophoresis (CZE)

In this approach an electroosmotic flow is established in a narrow capillary via the application of high voltage to an electrolyte-containing solution. Charged analyte present in the capillary flow are attracted towards either the anode or cathode depending upon the sign of that charge. However, their passage is counterbalanced to various extents by the electroosmotic flow depending upon their charge/size ratio. The induced flow profile in CZE is not parabolic in nature, rather it is that of a plug. Thus, even though the process is occurring in a capillary, size separation is taking place via electrophoretically-determined mobility (of which size is one aspect) rather than intrinsic diffusion as is takes place in CHDF. Since charge as well as size is relevant in determining elution time, a calibration step is required. Latex spheres and liposomes have been separated successfully via this method (Roberts *et al.*, 1996; Peterson *et al.*, 1992).

Single Counting Methods

Electrolyte Displacement

In the technique of electrolyte displacement, also known as electrozone or "Coulter" counting, particles are hydrodynamically pulled through a micron-sized orifice across which a current has been induced by the application of an electric field. Changes in the electric current induced by the passage of individual particles are monitored, the changes sorted according to size, and the resulting histogram related to particle size. This final step is possible due to a preceding calibration step using reference standards. Thus the method is highly analogous to light obscuration with the electric current taking the role of the light source — both fluxes being disturbed in a size-dependent fashion by the passage of colloidal material (Washington, 1992b). The orifice size used must be appropriate to the expected size of the particles in order to assure that a significant, easily measured current change occurs upon their passage. For parenteral emulsions, this requires the use of very small orifices which are easily plugged. Even with this configuration, particle diameters below 2 μm cannot be measured. The biggest drawback of the method is the required use of an electrolyte solution to maintain the flow of current. Usually in the with ionic strengths in the 0.15 range, such solutions are generally not compatible with colloidal systems, such as o/w emulsions, that rely on electrostatic interactions to maintain their physical stability. Although electrolyte displacement was one of the first techniques applied to particle sizing of emulsions (Matthews, 1971), it has largely been replaced by either Fraunhofer diffraction — a questionable substitution given the dissimilarity of the two methods — or obscuration-based SPOS (Li *et al.*, 1993b; Cham *et al.*, 1989).

EXAMPLES OF COMBINED METHODS

Principals of the Approach

As mentioned earlier in this chapter, the use of multiple techniques in the size characterization of submicron emulsions is a synergistic approach. There are several situations where this approach is appropriate. In the first situation, having results from different methods provides a greater degree of assurance that the results extracted from any single technique are accurate. This approach may involve more effort and expense than is necessary for answering some formulation development questions. In such cases, it may be more appropriate to use two methods on the first sample to establish that the overall sample characteristics and only one method on those that remain. However, in other cases, where the size must be determined on an absolute basis, as in characterizing a reference standard, this multifaceted approach is indispensable. In a second situation, information that is not obtainable by one technique, and would be missed if only that one technique were chosen, can be extracted if complementary methods are used. In both scenarios, the synergism is realized fully only if the various techniques employed are based on fundamentally different principles and/or are selected from the different classifications, i.e., ensemble, etc., listed above. For example, choosing intensity light scattering as a second method would not be a significant improvement if the first method was Fraunhofer diffraction. However, if the first method was SPOS based on light scattering, then the potential for additional information and/or confirmation is greatly enhanced. An example of each of these situations from experiences in the author's laboratory will be presented.

Example: Effect of Cosurfactant on Emulsion Particle Size

In the first example, the goal was to determining the effect that a lipid cosurfactant had on the size distribution of a 25% MCT lipid emulsion in which the primary surfactant was egg phospholipid. To accomplish this task a series of emulsions was produced with increasing amounts of the cosurfactant and samples subjected to particle size characterization. It was hoped that the addition of the cosurfactant would lead to an increase in the ability of the emulsion to accommodate drug. While it was assumed there would be a concomitant decrease in the mean size of the droplet size distribution, this could not be guaranteed *a priori*, nor was it known what the effect might be on high-size tail of the population.

The analytical techniques of FO-QELS, Fraunhofer diffraction, and scattering SPOS were employed as a means of extracting the desired information. For comparison purposes, a sample of Intralipid 20% was also examined as a control. Table 7 shows the results of the DLS experiment from which several items are worth noting.

Table 7 Sizing information for samples of Intralipid 20%, and four MCT o/w emulsions. DLS data collected from solutions diluted 1:50 with water using the fiber optic probe described in the text and a 256-channel autocorrelator (BI-2030, Brookhaven Instruments; Holtsville, NY). Data analysis was carried out via a 4th-order Cumulants fit (Koppel, 1972). Laser diffraction was carried out using a Mastersizer-S (Malvern Instruments; Southborough, MA).

Sample	FO-QELS Diameter (nm) Mean	S.E.	FO-QELS Width (nm) Mean	S.E.	Laser Diffraction (nm) Mean
Intralipid 20%	264	19	148	48	420
0.00% Cosurfactant	161	5	56	13	320
1.25% Cosurfactant	154	4	58	3	300
2.50% Cosurfactant	145	5	42	13	260
5.00% Cosurfactant	135	5	42	10	240

First, is that the mean of the submicron distribution appears to be dropping in a statistically significant manner as a function of added cosurfactant, but that the differences between the MCT emulsions as a group and Intralipid are much greater. Second, is that little can be said based upon this data as to whether there is a reduction in the width of the size distribution. The values for the width are slightly lower for those emulsions that contain additional cosurfactant, but the standard errors associated with these values suggest that these differences are not well defined.

The Fraunhofer diffraction results for the population mean, also tabulated in Table 7, are clearly in agreement with those of DLS with respect to the trend, i.e., increasing surfactant concentration leading to decreasing size with the size of particles in the Intralipid being substantially larger. However, the absolute values do not agree at all. Calculation of the mean can depend upon the shape of the distribution from which it arises. The cumulants method used in the DLS calculations does not explicitly define a functional dependence for the result, however, the inversion implemented in the laser diffraction system produces a distribution, as shown in Figure 19. This figure implies that not only is the mean decreasing as surfactant is added, but the distribution increasingly tails to the lower size range as well. This observation of tailing by the Fraunhofer method may account for some of the difference in measured size means when compared to DLS. Exacerbating this issue is the fact that the Fraunhofer experiment is carried out exclusively at small scattering angles, whereas the geometry of the FO-QELS experiment restricts observation to very high angles. As noted in Figure 2, larger particles scatter preferentially in the forward direction, hence one would expect that the diffraction method be more sensitive to the presence of these larger entities. The fact that both methods show the same trend implies that it is the entire distribution that is being reduced in size as cosurfactant is added, not just some portion thereof.

The report of mean and width obtained from DLS is relatively low in information content compared that contained in the plots in Figure 19. Since this means that there are substantially fewer degrees of freedom left in the residuals of the Fraunhofer calculations, a critical issue becomes the extent to which the shapes of the reported

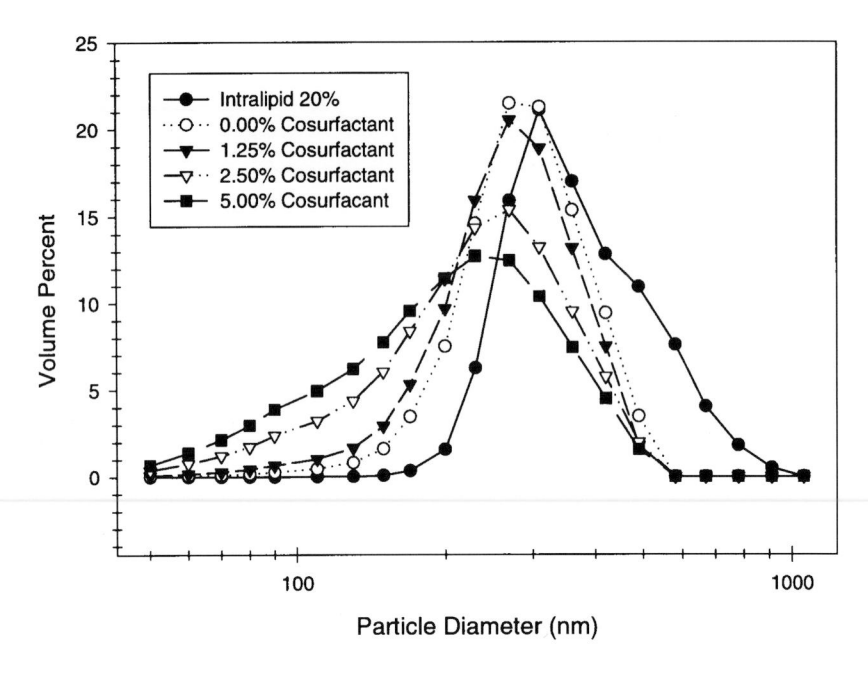

Figure 19 Size populations of droplets present in 25% MCT emulsions emulsified with 1.2% egg lecithin and increasing amounts of cosurfactant as reported by Fraunhofer diffraction (Mastersizer S; Malvern Instruments; Southborough, MA). The analysis of Intralipid 20% is presented as a comparison.

size distribution can be taken as truth. To address this concern samples of the cosurfactant-free MCT emulsions were spiked with increasing amounts of latex spheres standards possessing a nominal diameter of 595 nm. As shown in Figure 20, the presence of this material becomes apparent in the form of a shoulder between 500 and 600 nm in the distribution. These results suggest at least some confidence can be placed in the reported shapes of Figure 19. However, execution of the experiment brought up a difficult problem. Since Mie calculations were used to carry out the inversions, values for real and imaginary index of refraction were required. It is not clear in this situations where dissimilar samples are mixed together, whether the refractive index of the oil or latex is most appropriate. Thus, even the results reported in Figure 20 need to be viewed with some caution.

The final method employed was scattering SPOS. The detector employed in this case was one with a 200 nm diameter lower cut-off. Figure 21 shows the number distributions obtained for the same samples; volume distributions were calculated assuming that the droplets were spherical — a reasonable assumption for lipid emulsions. Once again, a trends towards decreasing size with increasing cosurfactant content is observed, and Intralipid is notably different from the other emulsions. Recall that since this method is classified as a direct counting technique, there is no concern that the reported shape of the size distribution is due to mathematical instabilities or underlying assumptions. Thus, the results of these figures are remarkable because they are reporting directly on the shape of the submicron distribution. Indeed, for the Intralipid 20% emulsion the distribution can be observed

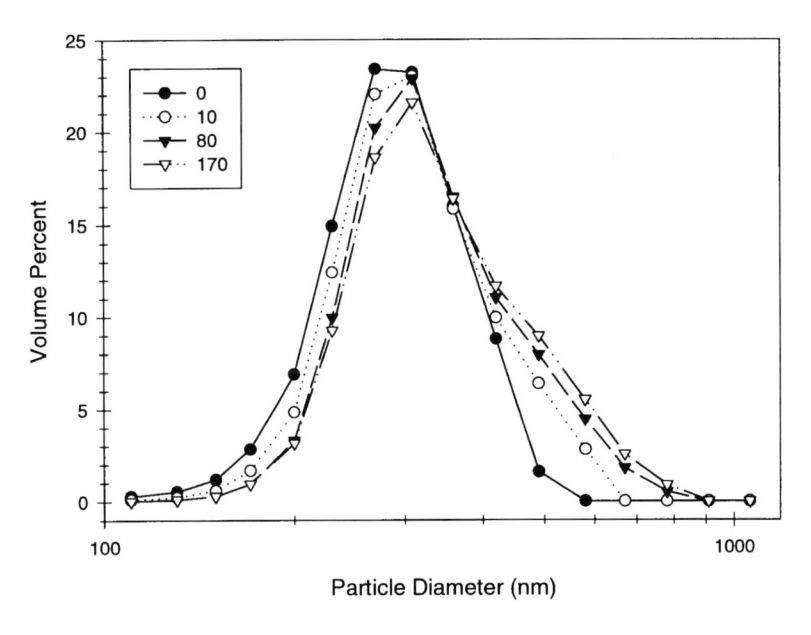

Figure 20 Fraunhofer diffraction-derived size populations of droplets present in 25% MCT lecithin-emulsified emulsion of Figure 19 spiked with increasing volumes of (μL) latex solution containing 595 nm diameter particles.

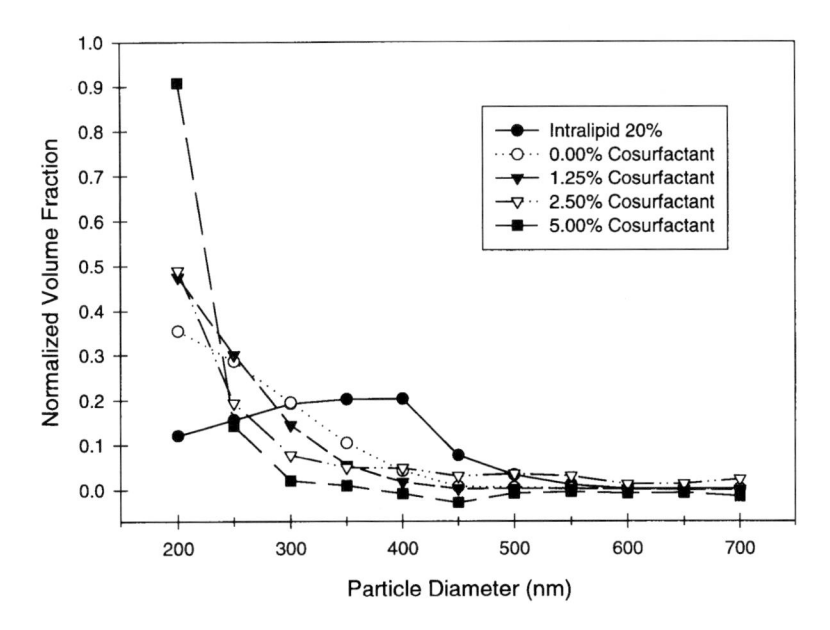

Figure 21 Size populations of droplets present in 25% MCT emulsions emulsified with 1.2% egg lecithin and increasing amounts of cosurfactant as reported by the light scattering SPOS method employing a 0.2 μm detector (Liquilaz; Particle Measuring Systems; Boulder, CO). The analysis of Intralipid 20% is presented as a comparison. Samples were diluted by a factor of 4.5×10^8 before passage through the detector.

on both sides of the volume-averaged mean. Tabulated results of mean are not reported for this method because it was impossible to do so since, even in the case of Intralipid 20%, the figures clearly show that significant portions of the particle size distribution reside below the sizing limit of the instrument.

Based on the above results several items are clear. First, as confirmed by all three methods, the MCT emulsions possess particles that are substantially smaller in size from those in Intralipid. Second, the addition of a cosurfactant serves to reduce appreciably the mean of the distribution, with additional cosurfactant leading to additional size decrease. Even so, however, the choice of oil phase, i.e., MCT versus LCT, has a greater influence on size than the cosurfactant. Third, because of the offset between the means determined by the forward scattering Fraunhofer and backscattering DLS measurements, it is concluded that there is a substantial size polydispersity present in all of the samples. The actual means are most likely similar to those determined via DLS. The scattering SPOS results strongly contradict the values for the means produced by laser diffraction. If the size distributions determined via Fraunhofer (Figure 19) were correct in an absolute sense, then there should be a much greater SPOS particle count in the 250-350 nm region than are actually observed. It is speculated that the overestimation in size by laser diffraction is due to the limitation of the Mie calculations and the lack of high-angle data.

Example: Interaction of Emulsions with Plasma

A second example is one in which the influence of plasma interactions with drug-delivering lipid emulsions became of interest. *In vivo* rat studies of a series of cosurfactant-containing o/w emulsions indicated that there was a substantial build-up of lipid, detected via histological methods, in the capillaries of the lungs. Chemical analysis of the lungs themselves demonstrated a preponderance of the triglyceride used in the oil phase, but none of the cosurfactant. It was also noted that unless at least 6.25% cosurfactant was present, no pulmonary build-up was observed. Since the cosurfactant itself was never directly observed in the chemical analysis, it was conjectured that it was indirectly responsible for the observations through encouraging deposition of the oil phase in the lung. Interaction of the lipid emulsions with the plasma was one possible mechanism by which this might occur. Therefore, *in vitro* experiments examining changes in the particle size distributions that occur upon the introduction of EDTA-stabilized rat plasma to a series of cosurfactant-containing lipid emulsions were undertaken.

Four methods were chosen to carry out the characterizations: turbidimetry, FO-QELS, FO-ILS, obscuration-SPOS, and optical microscopy. Turbidimetry was used as a rapid initial screen, DLS and ILS were chosen as means of exploring the submicron population, SPOS was used to look for evidence of flocculation and/or coalescence, while microscopy was employed as a way of determining the morphology of these larger entities. Four 25% o/w MCT-based emulsions containing increasing amounts of cosurfactant were used as the test samples while samples of 20% Intralipid was used as a control. The exact preparation protocols varied slightly in order to accommodate the requirements of various methods employed.

Samples for turbidimetry were prepared by mixing rat plasma and the emulsion sample containing the most cosurfactant in ratios of 1:1, 2:1, 4:1, 8:1, 16:1, and 32:1 using water as a balance to maintain a constant volume among the preparations.

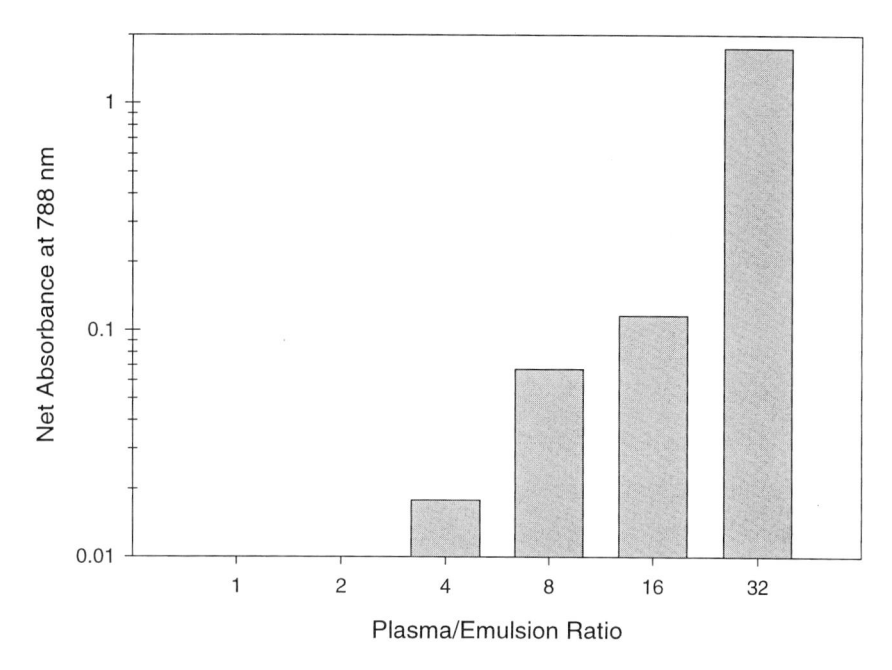

Figure 22 Turbidimetric assessment of 25% MCT emulsion mixed and incubated with increasing ratios of EDTA-stabilized rat plasma (see text). Measurements carried out using a 1 cm spectrophotometer cell and a diode array spectrophotometer (HP8450A; Hewlett-Packard; Palo Alto, CA). Results indicate a substantial change in the colloidal system as the level of plasma is raised.

The mixtures were incubated for one-half hour at 37°C, and then diluted to 1 mL with water and transferred to a spectrophotometer cell with which the "absorbance" was determined at 788 nm. The far-red wavelength was chosen to assure that the extinction signal would not have an absorption component. Figure 22 shows that there is clear positive correlation between plasma concentration and turbidity. The results of this experiment were not intended to provide a quantitative estimate of particle size, but were clear indicators that more detailed experiments were in order.

Samples for DLS and ILS were prepared as above except that all of the emulsion samples were examined, only 0:1 (control), 8:1, 16:1, and 32:1 ratios were employed, and after incubation the samples were only diluted to 500 μL. Both light scattering experiments were carried out by dipping the fiber optic probe into the diluted, but still opaque, samples. Figure 23 shows the results of the DLS experiments as a plot of particle diameter as a function of plasma:emulsion ratio for the different emulsion samples. For the control emulsion there is a clear decrease in droplet size with increasing cosurfactant much as there was in the above example. This trend has disappeared for the samples containing the maximum amount of plasma so that the sample containing the most cosurfactant shows a marked increase in mean particle size. Note that the samples containing lesser amounts of cosurfactant display only a limited size increase in response to the higher level of plasma. It is also observed that Intralipid shows a substantial plasma-dependent effect as well.

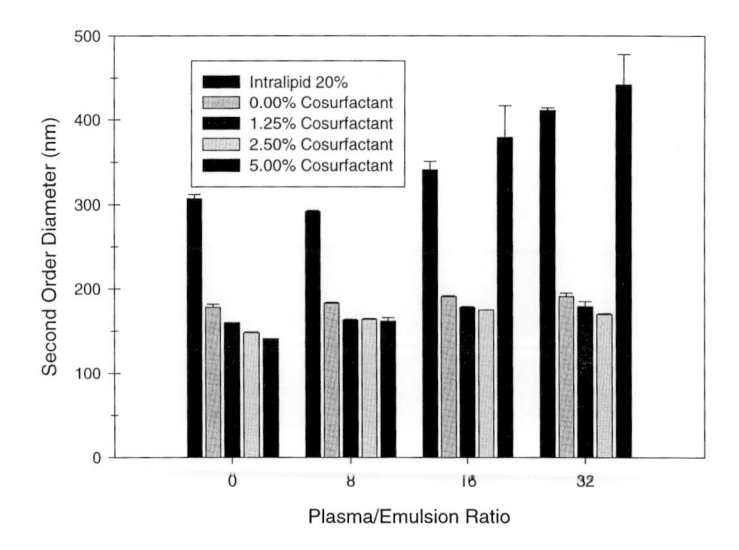

Figure 23 Size populations of droplets present in 25% MCT emulsions emulsified with 1.2% egg lecithin and increasing amounts of cosurfactant, and then mixed and incubated with rat plasma (see text). DLS measurements were carried out with the fiber optic probe described in the text using 514.5 nm laser light (95-4; Lexel Laser; Fremont, CA) and a 256-channel autocorrelator (BI-2030; Brookhaven Instruments). Data analysis employed a 2nd-order Cumulants fit (Koppel, 1972).

ILS data were collected simultaneously with the DLS data over a 60-second integration time. The results are shown in Figure 24 as a plot of backscattered intensity as a function of sample type and plasma content. The plot is at first difficult to interpret until the rational behind Figure 2 is recalled. Larger particles scatter

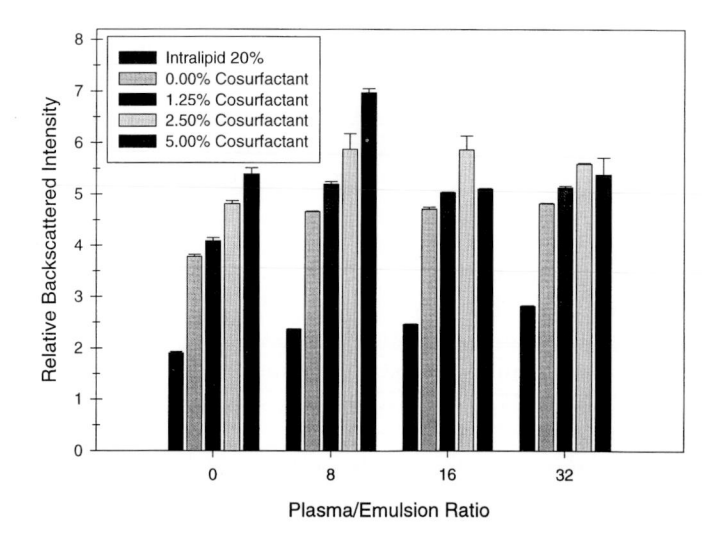

Figure 24 Backscattered intensity simultaneously collected with the DLS data of Figure 23 (see text for discussion).

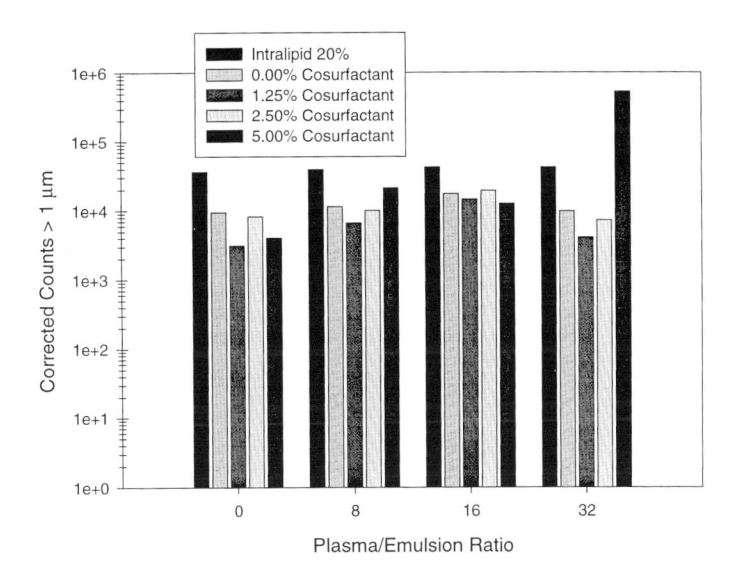

Figure 25 Light obscuration-SPOS (Accusizer 770/770A; Particle Sizing Systems) data collected of the samples described in Figure 23 and in the text.

aniosotropically so that for a given incident intensity less light is observed at high angles as a opposed to the forward direction. Therefore, since the fiber optic collects data near 180 degrees, the low signal associated with the non-plasma-containing Intralipid sample compared to that of the MCT emulsions is a consequence of the presence of smaller emulsion droplets in the latter. This is consistent with the DLS data.

The identical argument is applicable in describing the increase in scattered intensity with increased plasma content. However, as additional plasma is used in the sample preparation, the trend reverses so that the relationship appears to roll over on itself. This is clear evidence for the increase in particle size in those samples with greater amounts of cosurfactant and plasma.

Obscuration-SPOS data was collected by taking 100 μL samples of the diluted mixtures prepared as above and adding them to the 50 mL of water present in the sampling flask of the instrument. Data was collected for 1 minute. Figure 25 shows the results in a format similar to that used for the ILS and DLS data. The response is recorded as number of particles (counts) sized as greater than 1.0 μm per measurement. In the absence of plasma, Intralipid contains the greatest number of these larger particles — an observation consistent with the fact that LCT is the oil phase and no cosurfactants are employed. The high-cosurfactant sample containing the 32:1 plasma:emulsion ratio displays a substantial increase in large particles. However, it is also noted that these higher levels of plasma have little effect on the other emulsions examined.

The above DLS and ILS results lead to the conclusion that the submicron population of MCT-containing emulsions increases when plasma is present. However, this increase is highly dependent on the amount of cosurfactant present in the emulsion and plasma present in the preparation. Of particular note is that there

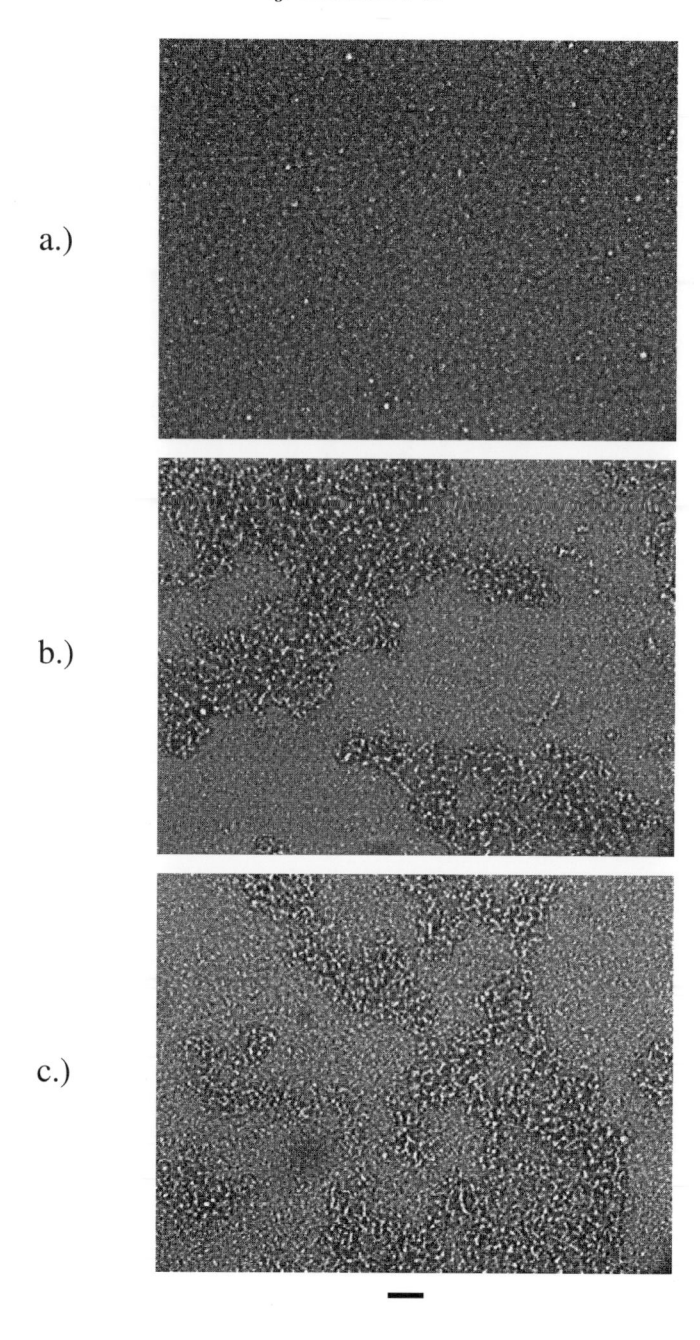

10 μm

Figure 26 Transversely illuminated sample of emulsion magnified 500X (BH-2; Olympus; Tokyo, Japan). Image was collected with a television camera (JE3012/A; Javelin Electronics; Torrance, CA) and thence digitized (Snappy; Play International; Rancho Cordova, CA). a.) Intralipid 20% alone, b.) 4 minutes after mixing with rat plasma, c.) 13 minutes after mixing with plasma.

are clear no-effect levels of plasma and cosurfactant for this large particle generation: near 8:1 for the former and 2.5% for the latter. The LCT-containing, cosurfactant-absent emulsion does not display the sudden change in population effect as a function of plasma or cosurfactant content — it is more gradual and much weaker instead. Obscuration-SPOS implies that an increase in 1 μm and larger particles is observed as well, but only for the sample containing the most cosurfactant and plasma.

Optical microscopy experiments were carried out as a means of gaining a better understanding for the mechanisms that might be taking place in the samples. 2 μL drops of emulsion and plasma were placed next to each other on a microscope slide. A cover slip was then placed on both droplets. This event constituted the beginning of the experiment as the placement of the slip served to bring the two liquids in contact with each other in a well-defined space. This region of the slide was then observed over time with the results stored as a digitized video image.

Figure 26 shows the appearance of Intralipid 20% as a function of time. The emulsion clearly has the contains some larger particles and the addition of plasma initiates a flocculation process that in turn leads to the formation of large clumps of material. Figure 27 shows a similar sequence for the MCT emulsion containing no surfactant. Even after only 10 seconds small chain-like entities have formed, but the process is still limited to flocculation. As shown in Figure 28, the presence of 2.5% cosurfactant produces the same small chains at short time, but at longer time points coalescence has occurred. A video recording of the process clearly shows that the coalesced material arises directly from the flocs. For samples containing 5% cosurfactant (Figure 29), coalescence is prevalent at early times as well. Indeed, this process is so rapid that the chains are never observed, presumably because they are too unstable toward coalescence.

The microscopy results serve to enhance those obtained by the other methods. The DLS/ILS results are taken of samples that have been diluted by a factor of 250 in comparison to neat emulsion, and the SPOS samples are diluted another 500-fold. It is noted that of all the methods, SPOS shows an effect on the high-plasma, high-cosurfactant sample only. Microscopy indicates that coalescence is the main large particle-generating mechanism for the 5% cosurfactant emulsion — a process that cannot be reversed by dilution and is this thus still visible via SPOS. The process by which large entities are produced in the 1.25% cosurfactant emulsion is flocculation. These flocs appear to be reversible since only slight effects are observed via DLS and ILS, and none are observed via SPOS.

The results from the *in vitro* experiments are consistent with the observations made during the *in vivo* tests. It is clear that the presence of cosurfactant results in a flocculation/coalescence process which could in turn lead to a lipid deposition in the small capillaries present in the lung. It must be noted that the *in vitro* experiments are not conclusive proof that this process is occurring in the rats. However, both models are suggestive of mechanisms that do not demonstrate perturbation of the lipid emulsions unless a critical level of cosurfactant is present. In addition, the *in vitro* studies lead to the development of a laboratory-based screen that has potential for use in further formulation development.

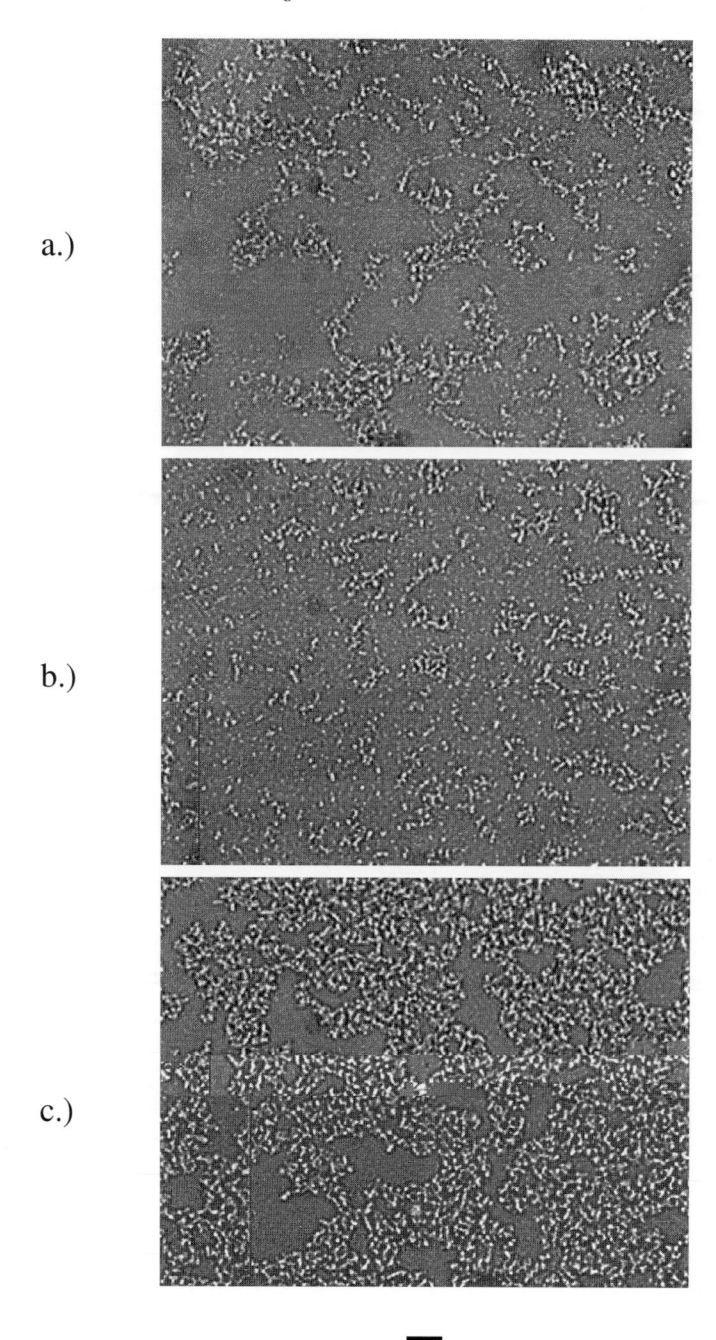

10 µm

Figure 27 As for Figure 26, but with 25% MCT emulsion stabilized with 1.2% egg lecithin and no cosurfactant: a.) 10 seconds, b.) 4 minutes, and c.) 10 minutes after mixing with rat plasma.

PARTICLE-SIZING TECHNOLOGIES FOR SUBMICRON EMULSIONS 91

a.)

b.)

10 µm

Figure 28 As for Figure 26, but with 25% MCT emulsion stabilized with 1.2% egg lecithin and 2.5% cosurfactant: a.) 30 seconds, and b.) 19 minutes after mixing with rat plasma.

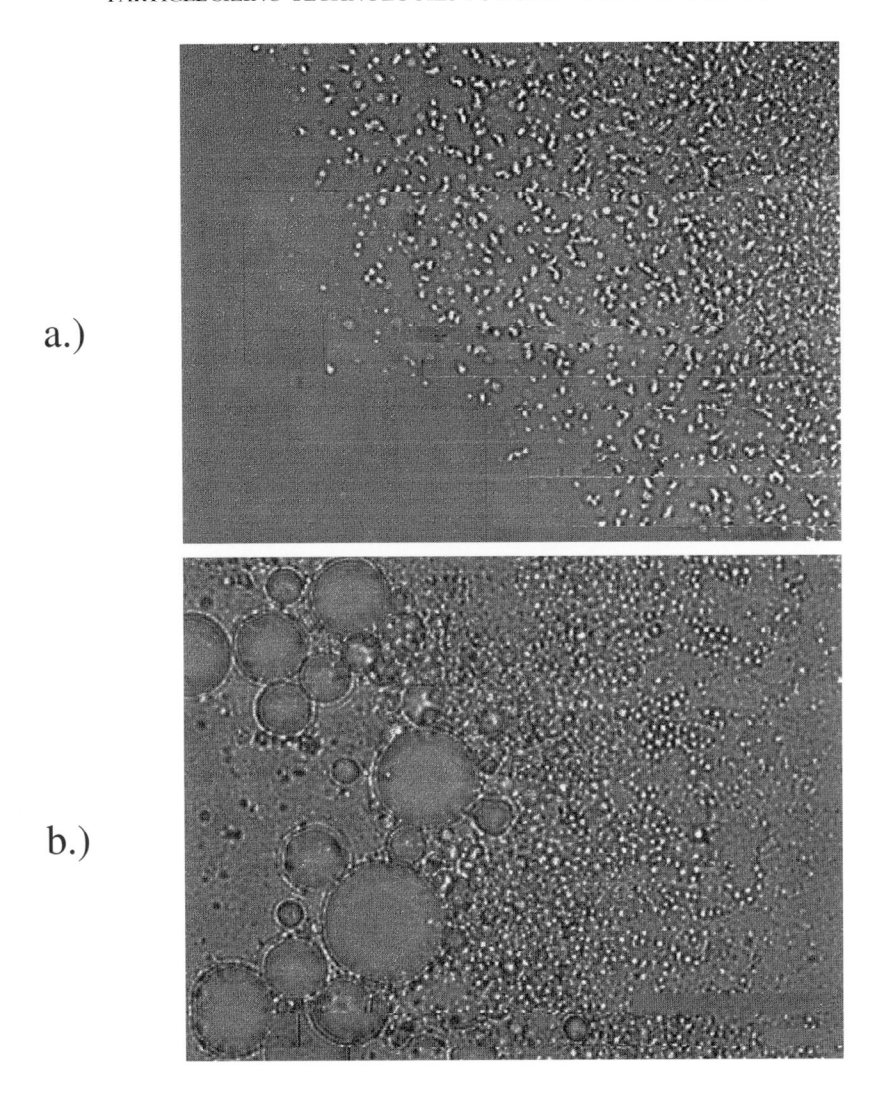

Figure 29 As for Figure 26, but with 25% MCT emulsion stabilized with 1.2% egg lecithin and 5.0% cosurfactant: a.) 3 minutes, and b.) 15 minutes after mixing with rat plasma.

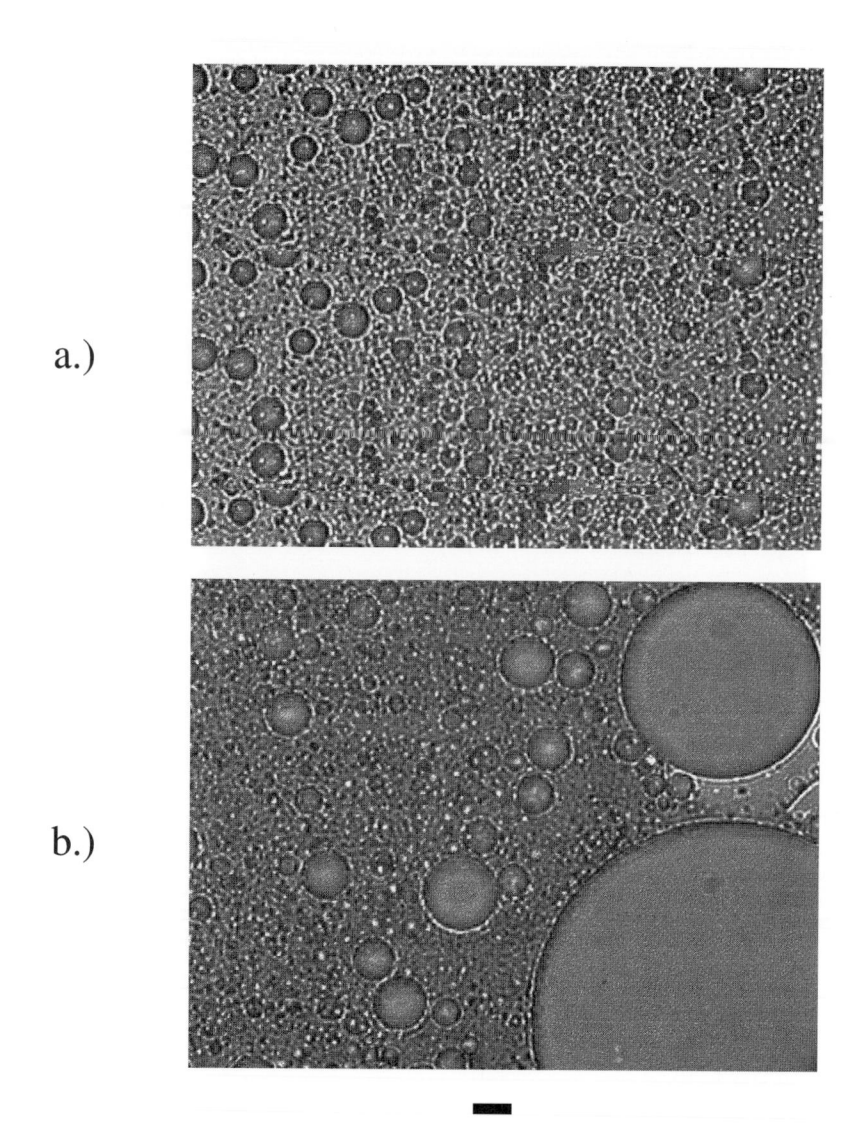

ACKNOWLEDGEMENTS

The authors would like to express heir appreciation for Professor Karin Caldwell, Department of Bioengineering of the University of Utah, and Professor Bradley Anderson and Dr. Jaimin Li, Department of Pharmaceutics of the University of Utah for their assistance and the use of their facilities in which the FFF experiments discussed in this report were conducted.

REFERENCES

Agrawal, Y.C., Pottsmith, H.C. (1993) Optimizing the Kernel for Laser Diffraction Particle Sizing. *Appl. Opt.*, **32**, 4285–4287.
Auweter, H., Horn, D. (1985) Fiber-Optic Quasielastic Light Scattering of Concentrated Dispersions. *Journal of Colloid and Inter Sci.*, **105**, 399–409.
Backhouse, C.M., Ball, P.R., Booth, S., Kelshaw, M.A., Potter, S.R., McCollum, C.N. (1987) Particulate Contaminants of Intravenous Medications and Infusions. *J. Pharm. Pharmacol.*, **39**, 241–5.
Bock, T.K., Lucks, J., Kleinebudde, P., Müller, R.H., Müller, B.W. (1994) High Pressure Homogenisation of Parenteral Fat Emulsions — Influence of Process Parameters on Emulsion Quality. *European J. Pharm. Biopharm.*, **40**, 157–160.
Bohren, C.F., Huffman, D.R. *Absorption and Scattering of Light by Small Particles*. New York: Wiley-Interscience.
Bowen, P., Dirksen, J.A., Humphrey-Baker, R., Jelinek, L. (1993) An Approach to Improve the Accuracy of Sub-Micron Particle Distribution Measurement Using the Horiba CAPA-700. *Powder Technol.*, **74**, 67–71.
Brewer, E., Ramsland, A. (1995) Particle Size Determination by Automated Microscopical Imaging Analysis with Comparison to Laser Diffraction. *J. Pharm. Sci.*, **84**, 499–501.
Caldwell, K.D. (1984) Field-Flow Fractionation of Particles. In *Modern Methods of Particle Size Analysis*, edited by H.G. Barth, pp. 211–250. New York: Wiley.
Caldwell, K.D., Li, J. (1989) Emulsion Characterization by the Combined Sedimentation Field-Flow Fractionation-Photon Correlation Spectroscopy Methods. *J. Colloid Interf. Sci.*, **132**, 256–268.
Cebamanos, F., Vila, A.O., Dieguez, Figueruelo, J., Molina, F.J. (1990) Modified Hydrodynamic Chromatography and its Application to Liposomes. *J. High Res. Chromatogr.*, **13**, 583–584.
Cham, T.M., Yu, H.M., Tung, L.C. (1989) Counting of Microspheres in Electrolytes and Parenteral Solutions. *Drug Dev. Ind. Pharm.*, **15**, 2441–54.
Chapman, R.L. Staehelin, L.A. (1986) Freeze-Fracture (-Etch) Electron Microscopy. In *Ultrastructure Techniques for Microorganisms*, edited by H.C. Aldrich, W.J. Todd, pp. 213–239. New York: Plenum.
Chýlek, P., Li, J. (1995) Light Scattering by Small Particles in an Intermediate Region. *Opt. Commun.*, **117**, 389–394.
Collins-Gold, L.C., Lyons, R.T., Bartholow, L.C. (1990) Parenteral Emulsions for Drug Delivery. *Adv. Drug Del. Rev.*, **5**, 189–208.
Cooke, P.M. (1996) Chemical Microscopy. *Anal. Chem.*, **68**, 333–378.
De Boer G.B.J., De Weed, C., Thoenes, D., Goossens, H.W.J. (1987) Laser Diffraction Spectrometry: Fraunhofer Diffraction Versus Mie Scattering. *Part. Charact.*, **4**, 14–19.
Dhadwal, H.S., Ansari, R.R., Meyer, W.V. (1991) A Fiber-Optic Probe for Particle Sizing in Concentrated Suspensions. *Rev. Sci. Instrum.*, **62**, 2963–2968
Dickinson, E. (1994) Emulsions and Droplet Size Control. In *Controlled Particle, Droplet and Bubble Formation*, edited by D.J. Wedlock, pp. 189–216. Oxford: Butterworth-Heinemann.
Dorshow, R.B., Bunton, C.A., Nicoli, D.F. (1983) Comparative Study of Intermicellar Interactions Using Dynamic Light Scattering. *J. Phys. Chem.*, **87**, 1409–1416.
DosRamos, J.G., Silebi, C.A., (1991) Size Analysis of Simple and Complex Mixtures of Colloids in the Submicrometer Range Using Capillary Hydrodynamic Fractionation. *ACS Symp. Ser.*, **472**, (Part. Size Distrib. 2), 292–307.
du Plessis, J., Tiedt, L.R., van Wyk, C.J., Ackerman, C. (1986) A New Transmission Electron Microscope Method for the Determination of Particle Size in Parenteral Fat Emulsions. *Int. J. Pharm.*, **34**, 173–174.

du Plessis, J., Tiedt, L.R., Kotze, A.F., van Wyk, C.J., Ackerman, C. (1988) A Transmission Electron Microscope Method for Determination of Droplet Size in Parenteral Fat Emulsions Using Negative Staining. *Int. J. Pharm.*, **46**, 177–178.

Eliçabe, G.E., García-Rubio, L.H. (1989) Latex Particle Size Distribution from Turbidimetry Using Inversion Techniques. *J. Colloid Interf. Sci.*, **129**, 192–200.

Eliçabe, G.E., García-Rubio, L.H. (1990) Latex Particle Size Distribution from Turbidimetric Measurements. Combining Regularization and Generalized Cross-Validation Techniques. *Adv. Chem. Ser.*, **227** (Polym. Charact.), 83–104.

Eliçabe, G., Frontini, G. (1996) Determination of the Particle Size Distribution of Latex Using a Combination of Elastic Light Scattering and Turbidimetry — A Simulation Study. *J. Colloid. Interf. Sci.*, **181**, 669–672.

Egelhaaf, S.U., Schurtenberger, P. (1996) A Fiber-Optics-Based Light Scattering Instrument for Time-Resolved Simultaneous Static and Dynamic Measurements. *Rev. Sci. Instrum.*, **67**, 540–545.

Finsy, R., de Groen, P., Deriemaeker, L., van Laethem, M. (1989) Singular Value Analysis and Reconstruction of Photon Correlation Data Equidistant in Time. *J. Chem. Phys.*, **91**, 7374–7383.

Finsy, R., De Jaeger, N. (1991a) Particle Sizing by Photon Correlation Spectroscopy Part II: Average Values. *Part. Part. Syst. Charact.*, **8**, 187–193.

Finsy, R., Geladé, E., Joosten, J. (1991b) Maximum Entropy Inversion of Static Light Scattering Data for the Particle Size Distribution by Number and Volume. In *Advances in Measurements and Control of Colloidal Processes*, edited by N. De Jaeger, R. Williams, pp. 401–420. Oxford: Heinemann.

Finsy, R., De Jaeger, N., Sneyers, R., Geladé, E. (1992) Particle Sizing by Photon Correlation Spectroscopy Part III: Mono and Bimodal Distributions and Data Analysis. *Part. Part. Syst. Charact.*, **9**, 125–137.

Finsy, R. (1994) Particle Sizing by Quasi-Elastic Light Scattering. *Adv. Colloid Interf. Sci.*, **52**, 79–143.

Gibbs, R.J. (1982) Floc Breakage During HIAC Light-Blocking Analysis. *Environ. Sci. Technol.*, **16**, 298–9.

Giddings, J.C. (1981) Field Flow Fractionation. *Anal. Chem.*, **53**, 1170A-1178A.

Giddings, J.C. (1995) Measuring Colloidal and Macromolecular Properties by FFF. *Anal. Chem.*, **67**, 592A-598A.

Gill, M., Armes, S.P., Fairhurst, D., Emmett, S.N., Idzorek, G., Pigott, T. (1992) Particle Size Distributions of Polyaniline-Silica Colloidal Composites. *Langmiur*, **8**, 2178–2182.

Groves, M.J., Wineberg, M., Brian, A.P.R. (1985) The Presence of Liposomal Material in Phosphatide Stabilized Emulsions. *J. Disp. Sci. Technol.*, **6**, 237–243.

Hallberg, D., Schuberth, O., Wretlind, A. (1966) Experimental and Clinical Studies with Fat Emulsion for Intravenous Nutrition. *Nutr. Dieta*, **8**, 245–281.

Haller, H.R., Destor, C., Cannell, D.S. (1983) Photometer for Quasielastic and Classical Light Scattering. *Rev. Sci. Instrum.*, **54**, 973–983.

Hamilton-Attwell, V.L., du Plessis, J., van Wyk, C.J. (1987) A New Scanning Electron Microscope (SEM) Method for the Determination of Particle Size in Parenteral Fat Emulsions. *J. Microsc.* **145**, 347–349.

Hango, R.A., Clancy, T.P., Eldred, B.J. (1991) Particle Counting. Examination of Particles Less Than 0.1 μm in Semiconductor Pure Water by SEM and On-Line Particle Counting Methods. *Ultrapure Water*, **8**, 44–48.

Harfield J.G. (1991) Methodology for the Particle Size Analysis of Pigments Using a PIDS [Polarization Intensity Differential Scattering] Enhanced Laser Diffraction Analyzer. *Surf. Coat. Int.*, **74**, 446–452.

Harris, R., Horne, R. (1991) Negative Staining. In *Electron Microscopy in Biology: A Practical Approach*, edited by J.R. Harris, pp. 203–227. Oxford: IRL.

Haskell, R.C., Pisciotta, G.L. (1985) Problems of Channel Correlation and Statistical Bias in Photon-Correlation Spectroscopy," *J. Opt. Soc. Am. B*, **2**, 714–720.

Hastedt, J.E., Franklin, M.L. (1995) Physical Characterization of Multi-Phase Systems by Microscopic Techniques. *37th Annual International Industrial Pharmaceutical Research and Development Conference*, Merrimac, June 1994.

Havel, H.A., Chao, R.S., Haskell, R.J., Thamann, T.J. (1990) Investigations of Protein Structure with Optical Spectroscopy: Bovine Growth Hormone. *Anal. Chem.*, **61**, 642–650.

Herrmann, N., Boltenhagen, P., Lemarechal, P. (1996) Experimental Study of Sound Attenuation in Quasi-Monodisperse Emulsions. *J. Phys. II*, **6**, 1389–1403.

Hill, S.E., Heldman, L.S., Goo, E.D.H., Whippo, P.E., Perkinson, J.C. (1996) Fatal Microvascular Pulmonary Emboli From Precipitation of a Total Nutrient Admixture Solution. *J. Paren. Ent. Nutr.*, **20**, 81–87.

Hinton, D.P., Johnson, C.S. (1993) Diffusion Ordered 2D NMR Spectroscopy of Phospholipid Vesicles: Determination of Vesicle Size Distributions. *J. Phys. Chem.*, **97**, 9064–9072.

Hirelman, E.D. (1988) Modeling of Multiple Scattering Effects in Fraunhofer Diffraction Particle Size Analysis. *Part. Part. Syst. Charact.*, **5**, 57–65.

Holve, D.J. (1995) How Many Channels Are Enough for Particle Size Analysis? *Am. Lab.*, **27**, 25–27.

Hulman, G. (1995) The Pathogenesis of Fat Embolism. *J. Pathology*, **176**, 3–9.

Huve, P., Verrecchia, T., Bazile, D., Vauthier, C., Couvreur, P., (1994) Simultaneous Use of Size Exclusion Chromatography and Photon Correlation Spectroscopy for the Characterization of Poly(lactic acid) Nanoparticles. *J. Chromatogr. A*, **675**, 129–139.

Huzarewicz, S., Stewart, G.W., Presser, C. (1991) Application of the Singular Value Decomposition to the Inverse Fraunhofer Diffraction Problem. *NIST Spec. Publ.*, **813** (Proc. Int. Conf. Liq. Atomization Spray Syst., 5th, 1991), 341–348.

Jokela, P., Fletcher, P.D.I., Aveyard, R., Lu, J.R. (1990) The Use of Computerized Microscopic Image Analysis to Determine Emulsion Droplet Size Distributions. *J. Colloid. Interf. Sci.*, **143**, 417–426.

Kerker, M. (1969) *The Scattering of Light and Other Electromagnetic Radiation*. New York: Academic Press.

Knapp, J.Z., Abramson, L.R. (1994) A New Coincidence Model for Single Particle Counters, Part I: Theory and Experimental Verification. *J. Pharm. Sci. and Technol.*, **48**, 110–134.

Kollenberg, R.G., Veal, D.L. (1992) Optical Particle Monitors, Counters, and Spectrometers: Performance Characterization, Comparison, and Use. *J. IES*, **35**, 64–81.

Komatsu, H., Kitajima, A., Okada, S. (1995) Pharmaceutical Characterization of Commercially Available Intravenous Fat Emulsions: Estimation of Average Particle Size, Size Distribution and Surface Potential Using Photon Correlation Spectroscopy. *Chem. Pharm. Bull.*, **43**, 1412–1415.

Koppel, D.E. (1972) Analysis of Macromolecular Dispersity in Intensity Correlation Spectroscopy: The Method of Cumulants. *J. Chem. Phys.*, **57**, 4814–4820.

Koster V.S., Kuks, P.F.M., Lange, R., Talsma, H. (1996) Particle Size in Parenteral Fat Emulsions, What Are the True Limitations? *Int. J. Pharm.*, **134**, 235–238.

Kourti, T., Penlidis, A., MacGregor, J.F., Hamlielec, A.E. (1987) Measuring Particle Size Distribution of Latex Particles in the Submicrometer Range Using Size-Exclusion Chromatography and Turbidity Spectra. In *Particle Size Distribution Assessment and Characterization*, edited by T. Provder, pp. 242–255. Washington: ACS.

Kourti, T., MacGregor, J.F., Hamielec, A.E. (1990) Particle Size Determination Using Turbidimetry: Capabilities, Limitations and Evaluation for On-line Applications. *Polym. Mater. Sci. Eng.*, **62**, 301–5.

Kourti, T., MacGregor, J.F., Hamielec, A.E. (1991) Turbidimetric Techniques. Capability to Provide the Full Particle Size Distribution. *ACS Symp. Ser.*, **472** (Part. Size Distrib. 2), 2–19.

Kratochvíl, P. (1987) *Classical Light Scattering From Polymer Solutions*. Amsterdam: Elsevier.

Lashmar, U.T., Richardson, J.P., Erbod, A. (1996) Correlation of Physical Parameters of an Oil in Water Emulsion with Manufacturing Procedures and Stability. *Int. J. Pharm.*, **125**, 315–325.

Lawson, C.L., Hanson, R.J. (1974) *Solving Least Squares Problems*. Englewood Cliffs: Prentice-Hall.

Lesieur, S., Grabielle-Madelmont, C., Paternostre, M., Ollivon, M. (1993) Study of Size Distribution and Stability of Liposomes by High-Performance Gel Exclusion Chromatography. *Chem. Phys. Lipids*, **64**, 57–82.

Levin, S., Stern, L., Ze'evi, A., Levy, M.Y. (1994) Characterization of Submicrometer Emulsions Using Sedimentation Field-Flow Fractionation with Power Programming. *Anal. Chem.*, **66**, 368–377.

Levin, S., Klauser, E. (1995) Measurement of Size Distribution and Density of a Pharmaceutical Fat Emulsion, Using Field-Programmed Sedimentation Field-Flow Fractionation (SdFFF). *Pharm. Res.*, **12**, 1218–1224.

Levy, M.Y., Schutze, W., Fuhrer, C., Benita, S. (1994) Characterization of Diazepam Submicron Emulsion Interface: Role of Oleic Acid. *J. Microencapsulation*, **11**, 79–92.

Li, J., Caldwell, K.D., Anderson, B.D. (1993a) A Method for the Early Evaluation of the Effects of Storage and Additives on the Stability of Parenteral Fat Emulsions. *Pharm. Res.*, **10**, 535–541.

Li, J., Caldwell, K.D. (1994) Structural Studies of Commercial Fat Emulsions Used in Parenteral Nutrition. *J. Pharm. Sci.*, **83**, 1586–1592.

Li, X., Cox, J.C., Flumerfelt, R.W. (1992) Determination of Emulsion Size Distribution by NMR Restricted Diffusion Measurement. *AIChE J.*, **38**, 1671–1674.

Li, L.C., Sampogna, T.P. (1993b) A Factorial Design Study on the Physical Stability of 3-in-1 Admixtures. *J. Pharm. Pharmacol.*, **45**, 985–7.

Macfayden, A.J., Jennings, B.R. (1990) Fibre-Optic Systems for Dynamic Light Scattering — A Review. *Opt. Laser Technol.*, **22**, 175–187.

Martin, M., Heintzenberg, J. (1992) Calibration of an Optical Counter for Liquid-Borne Particles. *J. Aerosol Sci.*, **23**, 373–378.

Matthews, B.A. (1971) The Use of the Coulter Counter in Emulsion and Suspension Studies. *J. Pharm. Sci.*, **6**, 29–34.

Mbela, T.K.M.N., Ludwig, A. (1996) Physical Properties and Stability Evaluation of Submicron Mefloquine Emulsions. *S.T.P. Pharma Sciences*, **5**, 225–231.

McClemments, D.J., Coupland, J.N. (1996a) Theory of Droplet Size Distribution Measurements in Emulsions Using Ultrasonic Spectroscopy. *Coll. Surf. A*, **117**, 161–170.

McClemments, D.J., (1996b) Principles of Ultrasonic Droplet Size Determination in Emulsions. *Langmiur*, **12**, 3454–3461.

Mehta, R.C., Head, L.F., Hazrati, A.M., Parr, M., Rapp, R.P., DeLuca, P.P. Fat Emulsion Particle Size Distribution in Total Nutrient Admixtures. *Am. J. Hosp. Pharm.*, **49**, 2749–2755.

Michoel, A. (1991) Comparative Particle Size Measurements Using the Electrical Sensing Zone and Laser Diffraction Methods. A Collaborative Study. In *Advances in Measurements and Control of Colloidal Processes*, edited by N. De Jaeger, R. Williams, pp. 369–387. Oxford: Heinemann.

Mizushima, Y. (1996) Lipid Microspheres (Emulsions) as a Drug Carrier — An Overview *Adv. Drug Del. Rev.*, **20**, 113–115.

Menold, R., Luttage, B., Kaiser, W., Schmidt, A. (1972) Cold Fracture Technique for Study of Suspensions and Emulsions. *Chem. Ing. Tech.*, **44**, 1226–1231.

Müller, R.H., Heinemann S. (1992) Fat Emulsions for Parenteral Nutrition I: Evaluation of Microscopic and Laser Light Scattering Methods For The Determination of Physical Stability. *Clin. Nutr.*, **11**, 223–236.

Müller, R.H., Heinemann S. (1993a) Emulsions for Intravenous Application II. Destabilization and Stabilization in Fat Emulsions. *Pharm. Ind.*, **55**, 948–953.

Müller, R.H., Heinemann S. (1993b) Fat Emulsions for Parenteral Nutrition II: Characterisation and Physical Long-Term Stability of Lipofundin MCT/LCT. *Clin. Nutr.*, **12**, 298–309.

Murphy, C.H. (1984) *Handbook of Particle Sampling and Analysis Methods*, Verlag, Weinheim.

Nicoli, D.F., Kourti, T., Gossen, P., Wu, J.S., Chang, Y.J., MacGregor, J.F. (1991) Online Latex Particle Size Determination by Dynamic Light Scattering. Design for an Industrial Environment. *ACS Symp. Ser.*, **472** (Part. Size Distrib. 2), 86–97.

Nicoli, D.F., Wu, J. S., Chang, Y. J., McKenzie, D. C., Hasapidis, K. (1992) Automatic, High-Resolution Particle Size Analysis by Single-Particle Optical Sensing. *Amer. Lab.*, **24**, 39–44.

Nordenström, J., Thörne, A., Olivecrona, T. (1995) Metabolic Effects of Infusion of Structured-Triglyceride Emulsion in Healthy Subjects. *Nutrition*, **11**, 269–274.

Ollivon, M., Walter, A., Blumenthal, R. (1986) Sizing and Separation of Liposomes, Biological Vesicles, and Viruses by High-Performance Liquid Chromatography. *Anal. Biochem.*, **152**, 262–274.

Ostrowsky, N., Sornette, D., Parker, P., Pike, E.R. (1981) Exponential Sampling for Light Scattering Polydispersity Analysis. *Optica Acta*, **28**, 1059–1070.

Peterson, S.L., Ballou, N.E. (1992) Effects of Capillary Temperature Control and Electrophoretic Heterogeneity on Parameters Characterizing Separations of Particles by Capillary Zone Electrophoresis. *Anal. Chem.*, **64**, 1676–1681.

Phillies, G.D.J. (1981) Experimental Demonstration of Multiple Scattering Suppression in Quasielastic Light Scattering Spectroscopy by Homodyne Coincidence Techniques. *Phys. Rev. A*, **24**, 1939–1943.

Phillies, G.D.J. (1990) Quasielastic Light Scattering. *Anal. Chem.*, **62**, 1049A-1057A

Provencher, S.W. (1982) A Constrained Regularization Method for Inverting Data Represented by Linear Algebraic or Integral Equations. *Comp. Phys. Commun.*, **27**, 213–227.

Provencher, S.W., Vogel, R.H. (1983) Regularization Techniques for Inverse Problems in Molecular Biology. In *Numerical Treatment of Inverse Problems in Differential and Integral Equations*, edited by P. Deuflhard, E. Hairer, pp. 304–319. Boston: Birkhäuser.

Ricard, C., Fortune, R., Florent, M., Bardet, L. (1996) Mean Particle Size and Particle Size Distribution of Fat Emulsions, Stability Parameters for the Preparation of Total Nutrient Mixtures. *J. Clin. Pharm.*, **15**, 72–80.

Roberts, M.A., Locascio-Brown, L., MacCrehan, W.A., Durst, R.A. (1996) Liposome Behavior in Capillary Electrophoresis. *Anal. Chem.*, **68**, 3434–3440.

Rotenberg, M., Rubin, M., Bor, A., Meyuhas, D., Talmon, Y. (1991) Physicochemical Characterization of Intralipid Emulsions. *Biochim. Biophys. Acta*, **1086**, 265–272.

Rubino, J.T. (1990) The Influence of Charged Lipids on the Flocculation and Coalescence of Oil-in-Water Emulsion. I: Kinetic Assessment of Emulsion Stability. *J. Parent. Sci. Tech.*, **44**, 210–215.

Sakeda, T., Hirano, K. (1995) O/W Lipid Emulsions for Parenteral Drug Delivery 2: Effect of Composition on Pharmacokinetics of Incorporated Drug. *J. Drug Targeting*, **3**, 221–230.

Schimpf, M.E., Caldwell, K.D. (1995) Electrical Field-Flow Fractionation for Colloidal and Particle Analysis. *Amer. Lab*, **27**, 64–68.

Schnablegger, H., Glatter, O. (1993) Simultaneous Determination of Size Distribution and Refractive Index of Colloidal Particles from Static Light Scattering Experiments. *J. Colloid Interf. Sci.*, **158**, 228–242.

Schuhmann, V.R., Mehnert, W., Müller, R.H. (1993) Coulter Counter-Based Coalescence Assay for the Determination of Emulsion Stability After Electrolyte Addition. *Pharm. Ind.*, **55**, 701–704.

Schuhmann, V.R., Müller, R.H. (1995) Analysis of Disperse Systems by Light Scattering Methods. Comparison of Mie Evaluation With and Without Polarization Intensity Differential Scattering Technology. *Pharm. Ind.*, **57**, 579–584.

Shortt, D.W. (1994) Measurement of Narrow-Distribution Polydispersity Using Multi-Angle Light Scattering. *J. Chromatogr. A*, **686**, 11–20.

Sjoblom, J., Skodvin, T., Jakobsen, T., Dukhin, S.S. (1994) Dielectric Spectroscopy and Emulsions — A Theoretical and Experimental Approach. *J. Disp. Sci. Technol.*, **15**, 401–421.

Smith, G., Duffy, A.P., Shen, J., Olliff, C.J. (1995) Dielectric Relaxation Spectroscopy and Some Applications in the Pharmaceutical Sciences. *J. Pharm. Sci.*, **84**, 1029–1044.

Soederman, O., Balinov, B. (1996) NMR Self-Diffusion Studies of Emulsions. *Surfactant Sci. Ser.*, **61** (Emulsions and Emulsion Stability), 369–392.

Sommer, H.T. (1991) Performance of Optical Particle Counters: Comparison of Theory and Experiment. *Proc. — Inst. Environ. and Sci.*, **37**, 425–432.

Sorensen, C.M., Mackler, R.C., O'Sullivan, W.J. (1976) Depolarized Correlation Function of Light Double Scattered from a System of Brownian Particles. *Phys. Rev. A*, **14**, 1520–1532.

Strawbridge, K.B., Hallett, F.R. (1994) Size Distributions Obtained from the Inversion of I(Q) Using Integrated Light Scattering Spectroscopy. *Macromolecules*, **27**, 2283–2290.

Theilking H., Roessner, D., Kulicke, W.M. (1995) On-Line Coupling of Flow Field-Flow Fractionation and Multiangle Light Scattering for the Characterization of Polystyrene Particles. *Anal. Chem.*, **67**, 3229–3233.

Ulrich, H., Pastores, S.M., Katz, D.P., Kvetan, V. (1996) Parenteral Use of Medium Chain Triglycerides: A Reappraisal. *Nutrition*, **12**, 231–238.

van de Hulst (1981) *Light Scattering By Small Particles*. New York: Dover.

Van Der Meen, P., Bogaert, S.M., Vanderdeelen, J., Baert, L. (1990) Accurate Determination of the Short Time Self Diffusion Coefficient by Fiber Optic Quasielastic Light Scattering: New Methods for Correcting the Homodyne Effect. *J. Colloid Interf. Sci.*, **160**, 117–126.

van Zanten, J.H., Monbouquette, H.G. (1994) Phosphatidylcholine Vesicle Diameter, Molecular Weight and Wall Thickness Determined by Static Light Scattering. *J. Colloid Interf. Sci.*, **165**, 512–518.

Wang, J., Hallet, F.R. (1995) Vesicle Sizing by Static Light Scattering: A Fourier Cosine Transform Approach. *Appl. Opt.*, **34**, 5010–5015.

Wang, J., Hallet, F.R. (1996) Spherical Particle Size Determination by Analytical Inversion of the UV-Visible-NIR Extinction Spectrum. *Appl. Opt.*, **35**, 193–197.

Washington, C., Sizer, T. (1992a) Stability of TPN Mixtures Compounded from Lipofundin S and Aminoplex Amino-Acid Solutions: Comparison of Laser Diffraction and Coulter Counter Droplet Size Analysis. *Int. J. Pharm.*, **83**, 227–231.

Washington, C. (1992b) *Particle Size Analysis in Pharmaceutics and Other Industries, Theory and Practice*. New York: Horwood.

Washington, C., Ferguson, J.A., Irwin, S.E. (1993a) Computational Prediction of the Stability of Lipid Emulsions in Total Nutrient Admixtures. *J. Pharm. Sci.*, **82**, 808–812.

Washington, C., Koosha, F., Davis, S.S. (1993b) Physicochemical Properties of Parenteral Fat Emulsions Containing 20% Triglyceride: Intralipid and Ivelip. *J. Clin. Pharm. Ther.*, **18**, 123–131.

Weiner, B.B. (1984a) Particle Sizing Using Photon Correlation Spectroscopy. In *Modern Methods of Particle Size Analysis*, edited by H.G. Barth, pp. 93–116. New York: Wiley.

Weiner, B.B. (1984b) Particle and Droplet Sizing Fraunhofer Diffraction. In *Modern Methods of Particle Size Analysis*, edited by H.G. Barth, pp. 135–172. New York: Wiley.

Weiner, B.B., Tscharnuter, W.W. (1987) Uses and Abuses of Photon Correlation Spectroscopy. In *Particle Size Distribution Assessment and Characterization*, edited by T. Provder, pp. 48–61. Washington: ACS.

Wiese, H., Horn, D. (1993) Fiber-Optic Quasielastic Light Scattering in Concentrated Dispersions: The On-Line Process Control of Carotenoid Micronization. *Ber. Bunsenges. Phys. Chem.*, **97**, 1589–1597.

Williams, P.S., Giddings, J.C. (1994) Theory of Field-Programmed Field-Flow Fractionation with Corrections for Steric Effects. *Anal. Chem.*, **66**, 4215–4228.

Zijp, J.R., ten Bosch, J.J. (1993) Pascal Program to Perform Mie Calculations. *Opt. Eng.*, **32**, 1691–1695.

4. BIOFATE OF FAT EMULSIONS

MAKIYA NISHIKAWA, YOSHINOBU TAKAKURA and MITSURU HASHIDA

Department of Drug Delivery Research, Graduate School of Pharmaceutical Sciences, Kyoto University, Sakyo-ku, Kyoto 606-8501, Japan

INTRODUCTION

For over 40 years, fat emulsions have been used in parenteral nutrition for patients who are unable to obtain adequate calories from food. Several commercial products, for example Intralipid®, are marketed in many countries. Such emulsions are injectable formulations of triglyceride oils emulsified with phospholipids in an aqueous solution, with a mean diameter of 200–300 nm. More recently, fat emulsions have also been used as drug carriers for lipophilic drugs whose intravenous administration in an aqueous solution is hampered due to their insufficient solubility (Collins-Gold et al., 1990; Davis et al., 1987; Singh and Ravin, 1986). Emulsions can solubilize considerable amounts of lipophilic drugs in the hydrophobic domain of the oil core. Compared to liposomes, which are widely and extensively investigated as carriers for hydrophobic drugs as well as hydrophilic ones, emulsions can be produced in a large industrial scale, and are relatively stable and biocompatible (Hansrani et al., 1983). Emulsion formulations of lipophilic drugs such as prostaglandin E_1, diazepam and non-steroidal anti-inflammatory drugs have been developed and marketed (Collins-Gold et al., 1990; Mizushima, 1996).

After entering the body, fat emulsions encounter various events. Figure 1 briefly summarizes the biofate of fat emulsions after intravenous administration. They will be taken up by both target and non-target tissues depending on their particulate

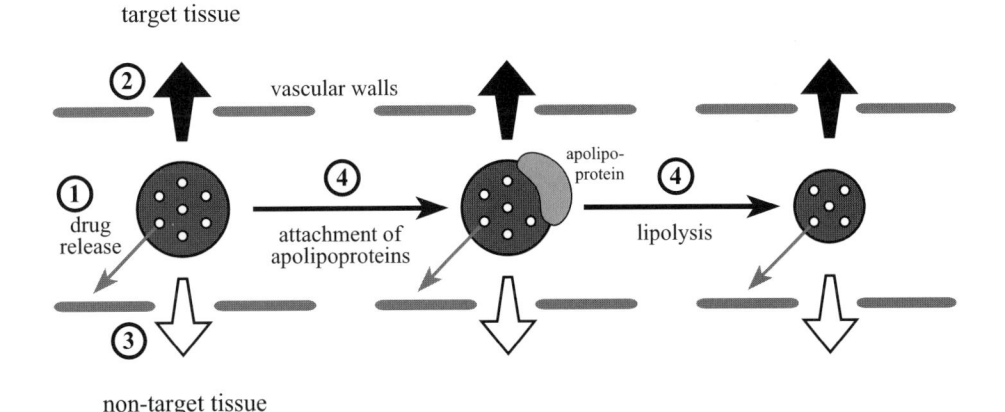

Figure 1 Biofate of fat emulsions after intravascular administration. The *in vivo* disposition of fat emulsions and incorporated drugs are determined by (1) release of drugs, (2) uptake by target tissues, (3) uptake by non-target tissues and (4) catabolism pathways of fat emulsions.

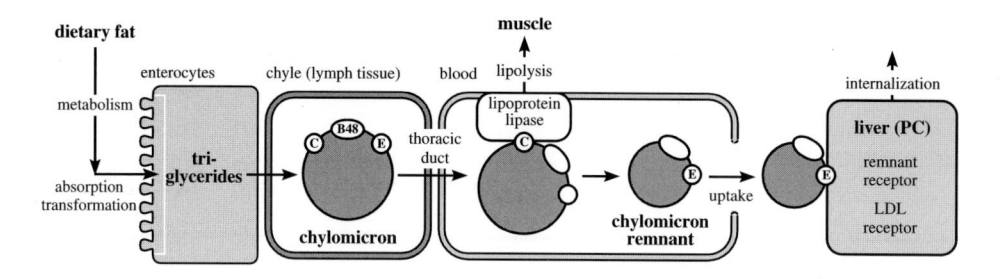

Figure 2 Absorption and metabolism of dietary fat. Triglycerides are delivered to the chyle where they are incorporated into chylomicrons. Chylomicrons enter the blood compartment via the thoracic duct. During circulation, the triglycerides of chylomicrons are rapidly hydrolyzed by lipoprotein lipase existing on endothelial surfaces, which produces chylomicron remnants. These remnants are cleared by the liver by the remnant or the LDL receptor.

properties as well as the anatomical and physiological characteristics such as the type of the endothelial wall in each tissue. Phagocytic uptake by the mononuclear phagocyte system would often be an obstacle for the use of fat emulsions as drug carriers. In addition, fat emulsions would acquire apolipoproteins from lipoproteins followed by the lipolysis as fat-sorting particles. Such catabolism would endow them with different particulate characteristics, and consequently alter their *in vivo* disposition profiles. The release property of incorporated drugs is also an important factor determining the disposition of drugs. In this chapter, the biofate and eliminating mechanisms of fat emulsions in the body are reviewed in relation to factors affecting their recognition in the body such as the particle size and the composition. Finally, the drug delivery with emulsion formulations is discussed based on the lipophilicity of drugs.

MECHANISMS FOR ELIMINATION OF FAT EMULSIONS

Metabolism and Transport as Natural Fat Particles

Intravenously administered fat emulsions would be handled by the body as naturally-occurring fat-sorting particles. Dietary fat is taken up by the enterocytes in the intestine and packaged into chylomicrons (Tso, 1985; Tso and Balin, 1986) (Figure 2). These triglyceride-rich particles are secreted into the lymph and subsequently enter the blood circulation via the thoracic duct. After entering the blood circulation, the triglycerides of chylomicrons is known to be rapidly hydrolyzed by lipoprotein lipase on the surface of endothelial cells (Bengtson and Olivecrona, 1980). Lipoprotein lipase is highly expressed in adipose tissue, heart, and skeletal muscles. The released fatty acids are transported predominantly into adipose tissue and muscle cells (Peterson *et al.*, 1985). A major difference between fat emulsions and chylomicrons is the absence of apolipoproteins on the surface of the emulsions. However, when injected intravenously, some emulsions are considered to immediately acquire several apolipoproteins in plasma. Erkelens *et al.* (1979) reported that an emulsion formulation (Intralipid®) captures apolipoprotein Cs within minutes after an infusion in man. Apolipoprotein CII is known to facilitate the lipolysis of emulsions by lipoprotein lipase (Goldberg et al., 1990). In addition, the attachment of apolipoprotein E would greatly alter the *in vivo* distribution of fat emulsions since the protein is a ligand for the apolipoprotein E-specific receptors on the liver parenchymal cells (Mahley and Hussain, 1991).

Once emulsions acquire apolipoproteins, they would undergo the metabolic and transport pathways of lipoproteins. Redgrave et al. (1992) investigated the lipolysis of emulsions having different compositions of phospholipids. When incubated with rat plasma, a formulation emulsified with 1-palmitoyl-2-oleoylphosphatidylcholine (POPC) acquired three-fold more apolipoprotein Cs than ones emulsified with dipalmitoylphosphatidylcholine (DPPC) or egg yolk sphingomyelin (EYSM), which resulted in more rapid lipolysis of triolein in the POPC-stabilized emulsion both *in vitro* and *in vivo*. Bennett Clark and Derksen (1987) also studied the effects of phospholipid composition of emulsions on their lipolysis. An emulsion formulation with egg yolk phosphatidylcholine (EYPC), a chylomicron model, was rapidly lipolyzed by lipoprotein lipase of rat heart homogenate, while a formulation with distearoylphosphatidylcholine (DSPC) was hardly hydrolyzed. The surface fluidity of emulsion particles could be important on the lipolysis of emulsions by lipoprotein lipase; the surface of DSPC emulsion is expected to be solid at 37°C. Experiments using dimyristoylphosphatidylcholine (DMPC) stabilized emulsions confirmed the importance of the surface fluidity on the lipolysis rate by lipoprotein lipase; when emulsions have fluid surfaces, apolipoprotein CII and/or lipoprotein lipase can easily bind to the surface and the hydrolysis of triglycerides is accelerated. The core composition of emulsions also affects their lipolysis rate *in vivo*. Handa et al. (1994) reported that the addition of cholesteryl oleate (CO) retards the lipolysis of triglycerides in emulsions. Lipolysis results in the reduction of the particle size of fat emulsions (Umezawa et al., 1991) and consequently affects the *in vivo* distribution characteristics of fat emulsions after intravenous administration.

The hydrolysis of chylomicron by lipoprotein lipase produces a much smaller particle called chylomicron remnant, which is relatively enriched in cholesterol and apolipoprotein E (Lakshmann et al., 1981; Redgrave, 1970). These remnants are rapidly cleared from the circulation by the liver either via the remnant receptor on the liver parenchymal cells (Arbeeny and Rifici, 1984; De Groot et al., 1981) which is suggested to be mediated by apolipoprotein E (Beisiegel et al., 1989; Floren and Nilsson, 1987), or via the low density lipoprotein (LDL) receptor (Ishibashi et al., 1996; Redgrave and Maranhao, 1985) which is mediated by both apolipoprotein B_{100} and apolipoprotein E (Brown and Goldstein, 1986). Borensztajn et al. (1988) reported that more than 80% of the radiolabeled chylomicron remnant was recovered in the liver at 4 min after intravenous injection in rats. After lipolyzed *in vivo*, emulsions are also likely to be taken up by the liver; this uptake should be mediated by apolipoprotein E (Bijsterbosch and Van Berkel, 1990; Mahley, 1988; Zhang et al., 1992). Oswald and Quarfordt (1987) reported that apolipoprotein E significantly increases the uptake of emulsions by rat hepatocytes *in vitro*. When emulsions emulsified with EYPC, dioleoylphosphatidylcholine (DOPC), DMPC or POPC and having rapid lipolysis rates were injected intravenously, ^{14}C-CO label, which remains within particles even after the lipolysis of emulsions, was mainly accumulated in the liver (Bennett Clark and Derksen, 1987; Lenzo et al., 1988; Redgrave et al., 1992). About 90% of ^{3}H-cholesteryl hexadecylether, a non-metabolizable marker of emulsion particles, was accumulated in the liver at 4 h after the injection of the emulsion formulation composed of soy bean triglycerides and EYPC (Handa et al., 1994).

To escape the elimination pathways of naturally-occurring lipoproteins, therefore, fat emulsions should be free from apolipoproteins. Selection of the composition of emulsions would accomplish this end. On the other hand, when the liver parenchymal cells are the target, the hepatic uptake pathway of chylomicron remnant mediated by the apolipoprotein E would be utilized as a mechanism for targeted drug delivery with fat emulsions.

Recognition by the Mononuclear Phagocyte System

When recognized as foreign by the body, fat emulsions can be scavenged by the mononuclear phagocyte system. Studies dealing with the disposition of Intralipid® demonstrated the presence of fat droplets in mononuclear phagocytes in the liver, spleen, and lungs (Friedman et al., 1978; Van Haelst and Sengers, 1976). Takino et al. (1993) investigated the biodistribution of an emulsion formulation (Intralipid®) radiolabeled with ^{14}C-CO in mice. After intravenous injection, the emulsion was rapidly disappeared from the plasma and the most of the administered dose was recovered in the liver. The apolipoprotein-associated uptake by the liver parenchymal cells could be involved in this hepatic uptake, but a significant fraction should be

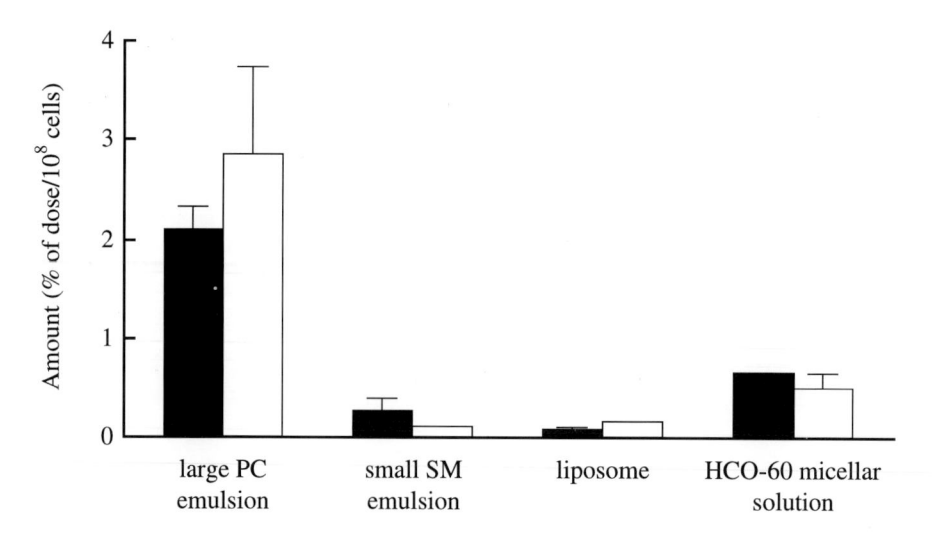

Figure 3 Intercellular distribution of various formulations labeled with ^{14}C-cholesteryl oleate injected in single-pass rat liver perfusion systems. Each formulation was administered into the portal vein of the perfused liver. After 1 min, the liver was perfused with a buffer containing collagenase and the liver cells obtained were separated into parenchymal cells (*closed bar*) and nonparenchymal cells (*open bar*). Results are expressed as the mean ± S.D. *large PC emulsion*, an emulsion formulation with a diameter of about 280 nm and a composition of egg yolk phosphatidylcholine (EYPC): soybean oil = 0. 12: 1; *small SM emulsion*, an emulsion formulation with a diameter of about 100 nm and a composition of EYPC: egg yolk sphingomyelin (EYSM): soybean oil = 0.7: 0.3: 1; *liposome*, a formulation with a diameter of about 100 nm and a composition of EYPC: EYSM = 0.7: 0.3; *HCO-60 micellar solution*, a micellar solution solubilized with polyoxyethylene hydrogenated castor oil.

phagocytosed by Kupffer cells in the sinusoid of the liver. This was confirmed by the single-pass rat liver perfusion experiments in which serum- and albumin-free buffer was used as a perfusate (Takino et al., 1995). Although there was no lipoproteins in the perfusate, more than 70% of ^{14}C-CO injected with an emulsion formulation with a mean diameter of 250 nm was extracted by the liver, indicating an extensive uptake of the emulsion within a single passage. Fractionation of the liver cells into parenchymal cells (PC) and nonparenchymal cells (NPC) including Kupffer cells showed a higher accumulation of ^{14}C-CO in the NPC fraction (Figure 3). On the other hand, a liposome and an emulsion formulations having smaller particle size (about 100 nm in diameter) and EYSM in their compositions, were hardly taken up by the liver, supporting the extensive phagocytic uptake of large emulsions by Kupffer cells. In addition, about 70% of both ^{14}C-CO and ^{3}H-TO of DSPC-stabilized emulsion was recovered in the liver within 1 min after injection although the emulsion was not hydrolyzed by lipoprotein lipase as described above (Bennett Clark and Derksen, 1987). The mononuclear phagocyte system would be involved in the removal of the DSPC-stabilized emulsion particles from the circulation.

Several factors are known to affect the recognition of particles like liposomes by the mononuclear phagocytes (Scherphof, 1991). In the following section, the importance of the particle size and composition of fat emulsions is discussed in relation to their *in vivo* distribution patterns after intravenous injection.

BIODISTRIBUTION OF FAT EMULSIONS AND FACTORS AFFECTING IT

After intravenous injection, fat emulsions show diverse distribution patterns depending on their particle size and compositions. Figure 4 shows the distribution profiles of two emulsion formulations after intravenous injection in mice (Takino et al., 1994). Although the profiles of emulsion particles, which were traced with ^{14}C-CO, are different among the two formulations, the liver and the spleen are the organs mainly contributing the elimination of the emulsions from the blood circulation. The recognition mechanisms in these organs described in the above section should be involved in the uptake of the emulsions. However, the rate and extent of the uptake by these organs are affected by several factors of fat emulsions. Here, the biodistribution, mainly profiles in the plasma elimination and the liver accumulation, are reviewed in relations to the properties of fat emulsions.

Fat Emulsions as Nutrients

Today, there are several commercially available fat emulsions used as intravenous high-calorie nutrient fluids. These products are a series of formulations of purified soybean oil, purified safflower oil, or medium-chain triglycerides, emulsified with purified egg or soya phospholipids. Their particle sizes are around 160–400 nm in diameter and their surfaces are negatively-charged (Komatsu et al., 1995; Lutz et al., 1989a) although larger droplets can be detected in commercially available emulsions (Koster et al., 1996). Lutz et al. (1989a) reported that the mean diameter of particles in the 20% emulsions is larger than that in the 10% emulsions and the diameter in long-chain triglyceride (soybean oil) emulsions is greater than that in medium-chain triglyceride emulsions. However, these particle properties of fat emulsions will

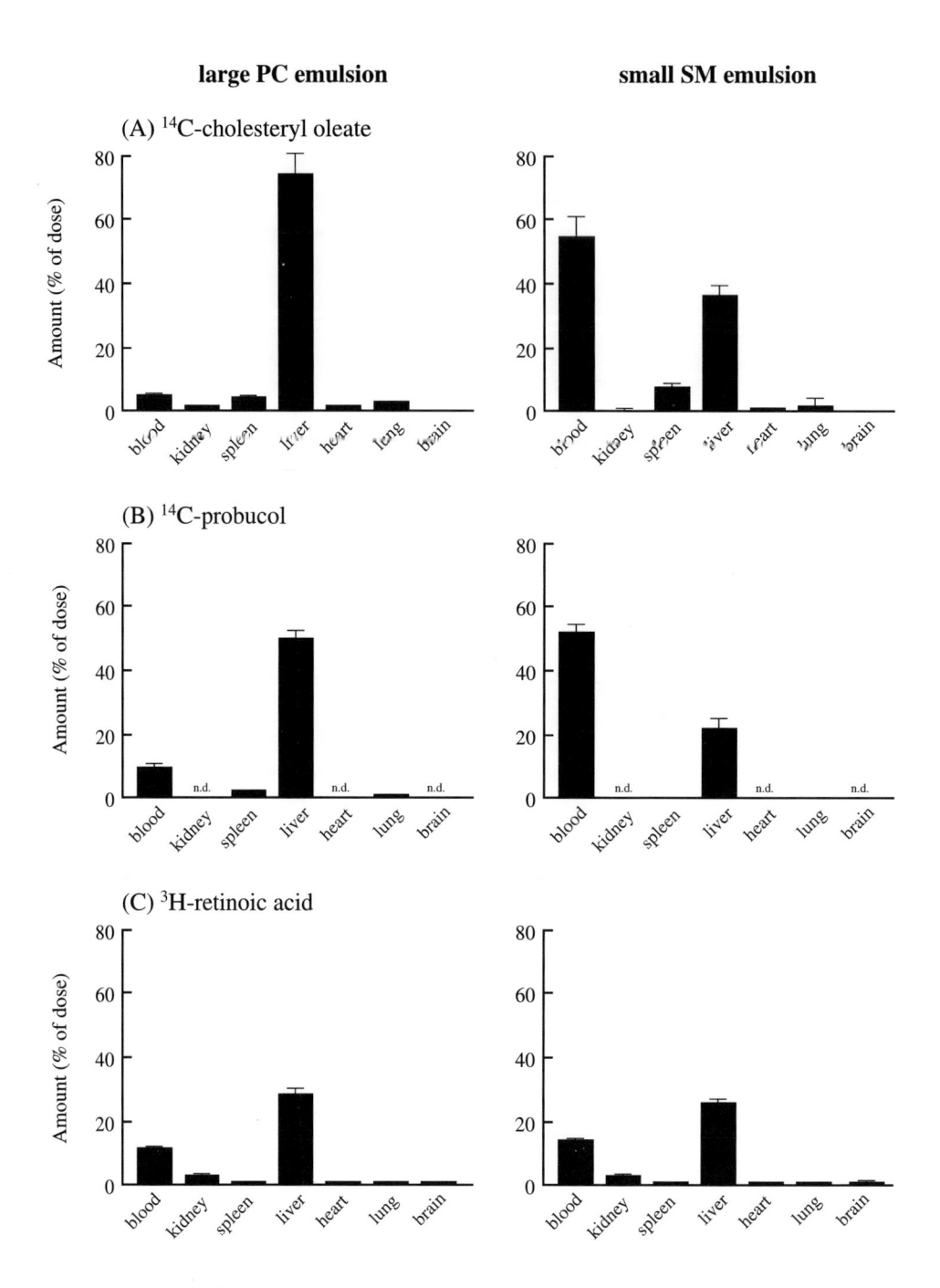

Figure 4 Biodistribution of fat emulsions and incorporated drugs after intravenous injection in mice. Mice were injected with emulsions containing ^{14}C-cholesteryl oleate (logPC$_{oct}$ = 18.3), ^{14}C-probucol (10.7) or ^{3}H-retinoic acid (6.61) and the tissues were sampled at 30 min after the injection. Results are expressed as the mean ± S.D. The characteristics and compositions of the emulsions are listed in Table 2. *n.d., not determined.

Table 1 Factors affecting the metabolism as lipoproteins, the recognition by the Mononuclear Phagocyte System (MPS) and the elimination from the blood circulation of fat emulsions after parenteral administration

	Metabolism as lipoproteins		Recognition by MPS		Elimination from the blood circulation	
	poor	extensive	poor	extensive	slow	rapid
Particle size	large	small	small	large	small	large
Emulsifier	DPPC* DSPC SM	EYPC	DPPC SM	DSPC	DPPC SM	EYPC DSPC
Oil phase	LLL	MMM			LLL	MMM

* DPPC, dipalmitoylphosphatidylcholine; DSPC, distearoylphosphatidylcholine; SM, sphingomyelin; EYPC, egg yolk phosphatidylcholine; LLL, long-chain triglycerides (e.g. soybean oil); MMM, medium-chain triglycerides.

change with time. Washington and Davis (1987) studied the effect of aging on the zeta-potential of a fat emulsion. The zeta-potential of the emulsion was −47 mV at the beginning then became more negative with time probably due to the production of fatty acids. Such change in the characteristics of emulsions would influence their *in vivo* distribution after intravenous injection.

The *in vivo* disposition of fat emulsions administered as nutrients, as well as administered as drug carriers, would depend on the particle properties such as the size, zeta-potential, and compositions of phospholipids and oil phase which may vary among different products and the batches of each product. A remarkable difference is observed in the administration dose of fat emulsions between the cases used as nutrients and as drug carriers; a dose for nutrients should be much higher than that for drug carriers. Boberg *et al.* (1969) found that the removal of triglycerides follows first-order kinetics within the physiologic plasma levels of triglycerides, while at higher concentrations the clearing mechanisms become saturated and are independent of plasma concentrations.

Factors Affecting the Biodistribution of Fat Emulsions

Fat emulsions would be handled by the body as fat-sorting lipoproteins or foreign particles. The properties of emulsions determine the rate and extent of their recognition (Table 1). Such characteristics of fat emulsions also determine other processes in the body such as the transport through the blood vessels, and consequently determine the *in vivo* fate of fat emulsions.

Particle size

The size of particulate carriers is known to influence both the phagocytic uptake by the mononuclear phagocyte system (Allen and Everest, 1983; Liu *et al.*, 1991; Senior *et al.*, 1985) and the binding of apolipoproteins to emulsions (Connelly and Kuksis, 1981). Furthermore, the particle size is a major determinant of the transfer to extravascular spaces from the blood compartment. The capillaries of the vascular

Table 2 Particle properties and *in vivo* pharmacokinetic parameters of emulsion formulations

Formulation	Composition[a]	Diameter[b] (nm)	AUC[c] (% dose·h/ml)	Organ distribution clearance (µl/h)[c]		
				liver	spleen	lung
large PC emulsion	EYPC/SO (0.12: 1)	278 ± 67	2.76	26800	1340	845
small PC emulsion	EYPC/SO (1: 1)	102 ± 28	10.5	2340	163	7.1
small SM emulsion	EYPC/EYSM/SO (0.7: 0.3: 1)	103 ± 20	16.9	658	49.1	29.2

[a] EYPC, egg yolk phosphatidylcholine; EYSM, egg yolk sphingomyelin; SO, soybean oil.
[b] The mean diameter (± S.D.) was measured by a dynamic laser scattering method.
[c] AUC (area under the blood concentration-time curve) and organ distribution clearances were calculated for the initial phase of experiment until 30 min after injection.

system can be classified into three categories: the continuous, the fenestrated and the discontinuous (sinusoidal) ones (Bundgaard, 1980). Particulate carriers including fat emulsions are considered to pass through capillaries and reach extravascular cells only in organs having discontinuous capillaries such as the liver, spleen and bone marrow. In such tissues, the extravasation of particles should be regulated by their size since the largest pores in the capillary endothelium is reported to be about 100 nm (Wisse, 1970). In addition, tumor capillaries have unique characteristics in their structures and functions in comparison with normal tissues such as muscle (Jain, 1987; Takakura and Hashida, 1995), which results in the enhanced distribution of particulate carriers to tumor tissues (Gabison *et al.*, 1990; Wu *et al.*, 1993; Yuan *et al.*, 1995). The distribution of emulsions within a tumor tissue was also regulated by the size of particulate carriers (Nomura *et al.*, 1995).

Takino *et al.* (1994) investigated the *in vivo* distribution of fat emulsions having different particle sizes: A large emulsion formulation was prepared by diluting Intralipid® 10% with the same volume of water and it has the diameter of about 280 nm and the lipid composition of EYPC: soybean oil = 0.12: 1 (Table 2). A small emulsion was prepared by mixing the same amount of EYPC and soybean oil followed by sonication to have a diameter of around 100 nm. ^{14}C-CO was selected as a tracer of the particles and incorporated into the emulsions since it is not released from carriers due to its sufficiently high lipophilicity (Takino *et al.*, 1993). After intravenous injection in mice, the large emulsion was rapidly disappeared from the blood and about 60% of the dose was recovered in the liver within 10 min (Figure 5). The decrease in the size of emulsions reduced the hepatic uptake and prolonged the blood circulation time. The pharmacokinetic analysis revealed that the small emulsion has 8–100 times smaller organ distribution clearances in the liver, spleen and lungs and about 4 times larger the area under the plasma concentration-time curve (AUC) value than the large emulsion (Table 2). The disappearance rate from plasma is also different among fat emulsions having diameters larger than 300 nm. An emulsion formulation with a diameter of about 500 nm eliminated more rapidly than one with a particle size of about 300 nm (Lutz *et al.*, 1989a). Even if emulsions are prepared with components which prolong the

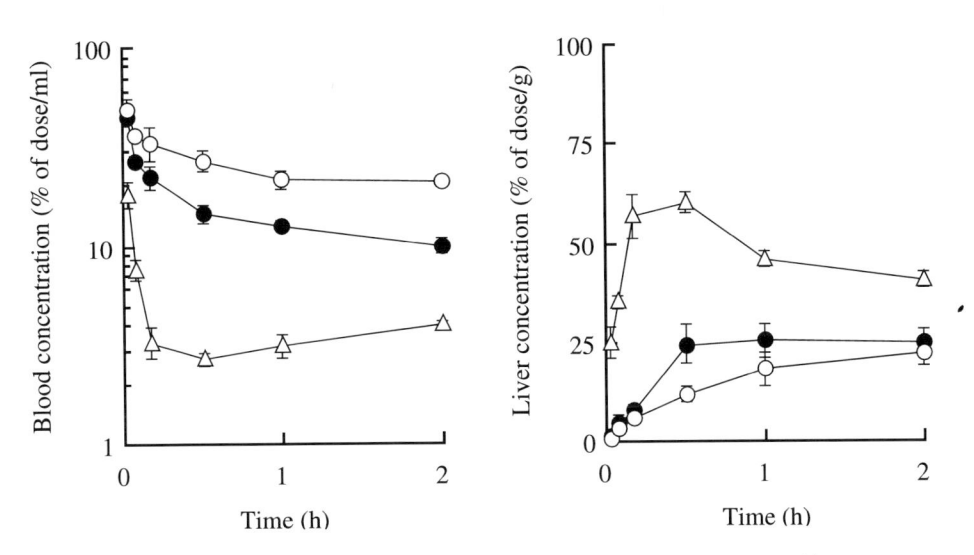

Figure 5 Blood and liver concentrations of emulsion particles labeled with ^{14}C-cholesteryl oleate after intravenous injection in mice. Each point represents the mean ± S.D. △, large PC emulsion (egg yolk phosphatidylcholine (EYPC): soybean oil = 0. 12: 1, 280 nm); ●, small PC emulsion (EYPC: soybean oil = 1: 1, 100 nm); ○, small SM emulsion (EYPC: egg yolk sphingomyelin: soybean oil = 0.7: 0.3: 1, 100 nm).

plasma circulation, the particle size will still affect the *in vivo* disposition of emulsions. Lundberg *et al.* (1996) reported the effect of the particle size of emulsions composed of TO, DPPC, polysorbate 80, and polyethylene glycol-modified phosphatidylethanolamine on the elimination from plasma. After intravenous injection in mice, the smallest emulsion formulation (50 nm in diameter) was superior to other formulations (100 and 175 nm) on the survival in plasma.

The rate of lipolysis would be also affected by the particle size of emulsions. A rapid lipolysis was observed *in vivo* for an emulsion composed of polyoxyethylene-(60)-hydrogenated castor oil (HCO-60) and dioctanoyldecanoylglycerol with a diameter of about 130 nm compared with other emulsions having larger particle size and the same components (Kurihara *et al.*, 1996a).

Emulsifier and other additives localizing on the surface of fat emulsions

The emulsifier determines the surface properties of fat emulsions and influences the *in vivo* disposition of emulsions. Some emulsions are formulated with only one emulsifier but others are prepared by mixing two or more emulsifiers. Lenzo *et al.* (1988) investigated the disposition of emulsions stabilized with either EYPC, DOPC, DMPC, DPPC or POPC. Although all emulsion formulations were prepared to be about 150 nm in diameter, the elimination rate from plasma in rats depended on the kind of phospholipid of each formulation. An emulsion formulation emulsified with DPPC showed the lowest elimination rate from plasma determined with ^{14}C-CO. On the contrary, EYPC- and POPC-stabilized emulsions were most rapidly cleared. DPPC-stabilized emulsion would remain in the circulation due to its poor ability to be metabolized by lipoprotein lipase. However, DSPC-stabilized emulsion was much more rapidly eliminated from plasma than DPPC-stabilized emulsion (Redgrave et al., 1992), although DSPC-stabilized emulsions were hardly lipolyzed by lipoprotein lipase (Bennett Clark and Derksen, 1987). At 30 min after the injection of DSPC-stabilized emulsion in rats, about 60 and 15% of the dose of ^{14}C-CO were recovered in the liver and spleen, respectively, indicating an extensive uptake by the mononuclear phagocytes in these organs. The difference between the disposition profiles of DPPC- and DSPC-stabilized emulsions, both of which are hardly catalyzed by lipoprotein lipase before their tissue uptake, could be explained by the surface fluidity of these emulsions (Lenzo et al., 1988). In the case of liposomes, however, a formulation of DSPC and cholesterol was known to act as a long-circulating liposome which is hardly recognized by the mononuclear phagocytes (Senior, 1987).

Sphingomyelin (SM) is considered to stabilize the membrane structure of liposomes (Schmidt et al., 1977) and the addition of SM to liposomes has been reported to be effective in reducing their clearance by the mononuclear phagocyte system (Allen and Chonn, 1987; Senior and Gregoriadis, 1982; Tokunaga et al., 1988). SM also prolongs the circulation time of fat emulsions in vivo. Takino et al. (1994) investigated the effect of egg yolk SM (EYSM) addition on the disposition of emulsions composed of soybean oil and EYPC. By replacing the 30% of EYPC by EYSM, a prolonged retention of the emulsion in plasma and reduced distribution clearances in the liver and spleen were observed (Table 2, Figure 5). The effect of SM on increasing the AUC of the emulsions depended on the proportion of SM in the mixture of phospholipids. The higher the proportion of EYSM added to the EYPC-stabilized emulsions is, the longer the retention time in plasma after intravenous injection is due to reduced hepatic and splenic uptake (Redgrave et al., 1992). Cholesterol is another well-known compound which potentially influences the elimination rate of liposomes (Senior, 1987). Handa et al. (1994) observed a difference between the plasma clearances of emulsions composed of only EYPC and triglyceride (20: 20 in molar ratios) and of EYPC, triglyceride and cholesterol (20: 20: 8.7). The plasma retention after intravenous injection in rats was longer for the cholesterol-containing emulsion formulation than for the formulation without cholesterol.

Addition of surfactants with large hydrophilic moiety can often reduce the uptake of fat emulsions by the mononuclear phagocyte system. Block copolymers of polyoxyethylene and polyoxypropylene are known to prolong the circulation of fat emulsions in plasma and poloxamines (polyoxyethylene-polyoxypropylene-ethylene diamine block copolymer) or poloxamers (polyoxyethylene-polyoxypropylene block copolymer) are used to prolong the circulation time of particulate carriers (Illum and Davis, 1987; Illum et al., 1987; Jeppsson and Rossner, 1975). The blood clearance of a poloxamine 908-emulsified formulation of soybean oil was much slower than that of a EYPC-emulsified formulation (Illum et al., 1989). A phosphatidylethanolamine derivative with polyethylene glycol (PEG-PE) is widely used to increase the plasma retention of particulate carriers such as liposomes (Allen et al., 1991; Klibanov et al., 1990; Woodle and Lasic, 1992), polystylene microspheres (Dunn et al., 1994) and nanospheres (Gref et al., 1994). Recently, the addition of PEG-PE to emulsion formulations is investigated as a coemulsifier to prolong their circulation time (Lundberg et al., 1996; Wheeler et al., 1994). Liu and Liu (1995) studied the effect of the chain length of PEG on PEG-PE and found that PEG-PE having a PEG chain with 2,000 in molecular weight is most effective on prolonging the circulation time of emulsions. Addition of HCO-60, a derivative of hydrogenated castor oil containing PEG, was also reported to prolong plasma circulation of emulsions (Kimura et al., 1986). The increase in the circulation time of particles by the addition of these PEG-containing compounds would be explained by the increased hydrophilicity of the emulsion surface and/or the formation of a steric barrier. These compounds also decrease the lipolysis of fat emulsions (Kurihara et al., 1996b) and prevent the uptake by the mononuclear phagocytes (Papahadjopoulos et al., 1991).

The composition of materials localizing on the emulsion surface also determines the surface charge at once. Most emulsion formulations such as Intralipid® are negatively charged (Komatsu et al., 1995) because of the presence of acidic phospholipids (Washington, 1990) and/or the production of free acid from lecithin and triglycerides (Washington and Davis, 1987). The addition of cationic lipids to emulsion formulations will drastically alter their surface charge and zeta potential. Elbaz et al. (1993) reported that the addition of stearylamine at a ratio of 0.3% (w/w) to an emulsion increased its zeta potential from −15 mV to about 20 mV. Although the surface charge or the zeta-potential of liposomes remarkably affects their biodistribution after intravenous administration (Aoki et al., 1995; Gregoriadis and Neerunjun, 1974), there is little work on the *in vivo* disposition of emulsions having cationic charge. Davis and Hansrani (1985) observed differences in the phagocytic uptake of fat emulsions having different zeta potentials by mouse peritoneal macrophages.

Oil phase

Oils and highly lipophilic compounds such as cholesteryl oleate (CO) form a core structure of a fat emulsion. Hydrolysis by the lipolytic enzymes and binding of apolipoproteins would depend on the composition of the oil phase of emulsions. Handa et al. (1994) studied the *in vivo* disposition of emulsions composed of soybean triglycerides (TG), TG and CO, or CO alone emulsified with EYPC after intravenous injection in rats. Although the TG emulsion labeled with ^{3}H-cholesteryl hexadecylether was rapidly eliminated from plasma, the addition of CO to the emulsion retarded the plasma clearance. Furthermore, complete replacement of the core TG by CO resulted in an enhanced prolongation of the plasma retention of the emulsion, probably due to the suppression of the lipolysis. The source of vegetable oils can also influence the disposition of fat emulsions. Brouwer et al. (1993) observed a slow elimination rate from plasma for an olive oil (monounsaturated fatty acids)-containing emulsion compared to that for a soybean oil (polyunsaturated fatty acids) emulsion.

The effects of chain length of triglycerides are also extensively investigated. Some fat emulsions in the market are composed of medium-chain triglycerides (MCT) instead of long-chain triglycerides (LCT) such as soybean oil. The constituent fatty acids of LCT are longer than 12 in the carbon length, while those of MCT are between 6 and 12. After intravenous administration, MCT-based emulsions were cleared faster than LCT-based emulsions from plasma (Lutz et al., 1989a, 1989b). More rapid lipolysis of MCT within the blood circulation than LCT is reported (Hultin et al., 1994; Johnson et al., 1990), and which would explain the difference in the disposition of emulsions. Recently, structured lipids possessing fatty acids with a different length at 1 and 3 positions of triglycerides (1,3-specific triglycerides) are investigated as core materials of fat emulsions. Hedeman et al. (1996) prepared three types of emulsion formulations with different oil phases: soybean oil (C_{16}-C_{18}, long-chain triglyceride: LLL), a structure lipid with medium-chain fatty acids (C_8-C_{10}) in the 1,3 positions (MLM), and a structure lipid with short-chain fatty acids (C_4) in the 1,3 positions (SLS). After intravenous injection in rats, the SLS-based emulsion labeled with ^{14}C-CO had a smaller elimination rate from the plasma than those of the MLM and LLL emulsions.

Attachment of homing devices

When particulate carriers have structures or ligands which are selectively recognized by a specific cell type, they can be used as carriers for targeted delivery of drugs. Antibody-mediated delivery of anticancer agents incorporated in 'immunoliposomes' has been extensively studied although there are still many obstacles to be overcome in its successful application (Allen and Moase, 1996). Carbohydrate receptor-mediated endocytosis is another mechanism widely utilized for cell-specific delivery of liposomes (Moonis et al., 1993; Muller and Schuber, 1989; Tsuchiya et al., 1986), lipoproteins (Bijsterbosch and Van Berkel, 1990, 1992) and gene-cationic macromolecule complexes (Chowdhury et al., 1993; Perales et al., 1994; Wu and Wu, 1988). However, few targeting systems based on emulsion formulations have been attempted.

Iwamoto et al. (1991) studied the distribution of fat emulsions coated with cholesterol derivatives modified with either mannan, amylopectin or pullulan, and observed a higher accumulation of mannan-coated emulsions in the lung in guinea pigs. Rensen et al. (1995) reported the liver targeting of an antiviral drug incorporated in a fat emulsion complexed with recombinant apolipoprotein E. After intravenous injection of formulations labeled with ^{14}C-CO, the apolipoprotein E-containing emulsion accumulated in the liver particularly in the parenchymal cells. The accumulation reached to about 70% of the dose which was remarkably higher than that of the emulsion without the protein (30% of the dose), suggesting that such emulsions can be used as targetable carriers for lipophilic drugs to the liver parenchymal cells.

DRUG DELIVERY USING FAT EMULSIONS

Drug Retention in Fat Emulsions

In a fat emulsion-based drug delivery system, another issue should be important besides the disposition of fat emulsions: the drug retention in emulsion formulations. Even if an emulsion formulation shows a desirable *in vivo* disposition properties, rapid release of drugs will fail to increase the therapeutic potency of drugs. Although some lipophilic drugs such as prostaglandin E_1 (PGE_1) are reported to be delivered to tumor and inflamed tissues with emulsions (Mizushima, 1991; Mizushima et al., 1990), they are also rapidly released from fat emulsions upon incubation with human blood or serum and only 0.5–2% of PGE_1 was retained in the emulsion formulations after 5 min (Igarashi et al., 1992; Mizushima and Hoshi, 1993).

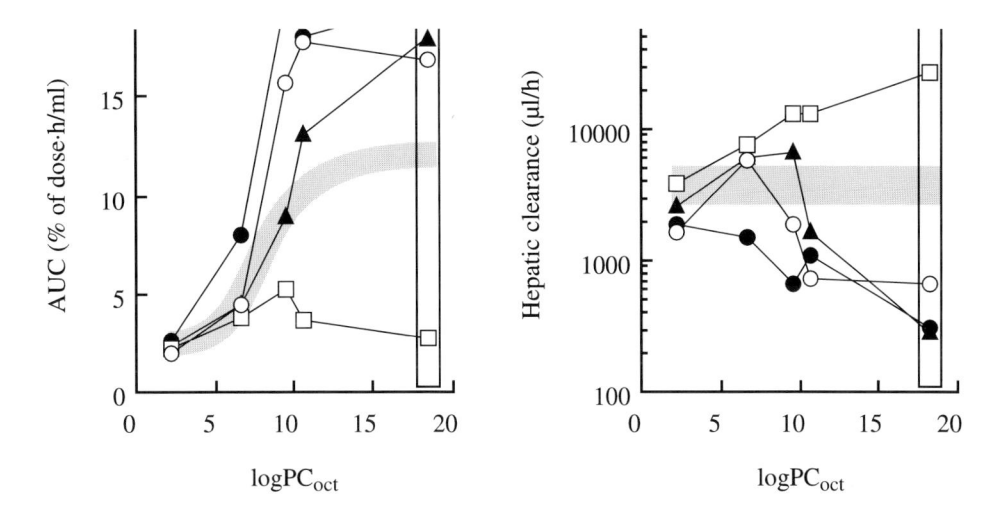

Figure 6 Effect of the lipophilicity of drugs on the area under the concentration-time curve (AUC) and the hepatic clearance after administration with various carrier systems. The *shadow zones* represent the intrinsic values of lipophilic drugs determined by the experiments using solution with mouse serum. The *long rectangles* indicate the intrinsic values of carrier systems labeled with ^{14}C-cholesteryl oleate. (□), large PC emulsion (egg yolk phosphatidylcholine (EYPC): soybean oil = 0. 12: 1, 280 nm); (○), small SM emulsion (EYPC: egg yolk sphingomyelin (EYSM): soybean oil = 0.7: 0.3: 1, 100 mu); (●) liposome (EYPC: EYSM 0.7: 0.3, 120 nm); (▲), HCO-60 micellar solution (20 nm). Results for ^{3}H-prostaglandin E$_1$ (logPC$_{oct}$ = 2.15), ^{3}H-retinoic acid (6.61), ^{14}C-cholesterol (9.46), ^{14}C-probucol (10.7) and ^{14}C-cholesteryl oleate (18.3) are plotted.

Takino *et al.* (1994) systematically investigated the *in vivo* disposition of drugs incorporated into three types of emulsion formulations in relation to their lipophilicity. Compounds having different logarithm of the *n*-octanol/water partition coefficient (logPC$_{oct}$) values, i.e. ^{3}H-PGE$_1$ (logPC$_{oct}$ = 2.15), ^{3}H-retinoic acid (6.61), ^{14}C-cholesterol (9.46), ^{14}C-probucol (10.7) and ^{14}C-CO (18.3) were used as model drugs. They were incorporated into small sized emulsions of about 100 nm in diameters with compositions of EYPC: soybean oil = 1: 1 (small PC emulsion) and EYPC: EYSM: soybean oil = 0.7: 0.3: 1 (small SM emulsion) and a large sized emulsion (about 280 nm) with a composition of EYPC: soybean oil = 0.12: 1 (large PC emulsion). The movement of ^{14}C-CO was considered to reflect that of emulsion particles due to its high lipophilicity. Although the emulsion formulations indicated diverse *in vivo* distribution properties depending on their composition and particle size, ^{3}H-PGE$_1$ and ^{3}H-retinoic acid showed common disposition profiles regardless of emulsion types (Figures 4 and 6). On the other hand, ^{14}C-cholesterol and ^{14}C-probucol showed disposition patterns similar to those of emulsion particles (^{14}C-CO) in all formulations. Therefore, drugs with logPC$_{oct}$ larger than 9 would be stably retained in emulsion formulations even after the administration into the body and the *in vivo* disposition of such drugs can be controlled by arranging the composition and particulate characteristics of emulsions. On the contrary, there would be few chances to control the *in vivo* behavior of drugs having lower lipophilicity. As shown in Figure 6, a liposome formulation composed of EYPC: EYSM = 0.7: 0.3 requires 6 or higher values in logPC$_{oct}$ of drugs to control their *in vivo* disposition properties, while a HCO-60 micellar solution can regulate the *in vivo* fate of drugs only with a logPC$_{oct}$ value of higher than 11. Therefore, with regard to the retention and disposition control of drugs, it can be concluded that emulsion formulations have an advantage over micellar solutions which are sometimes used as a solubilizer of highly lipophilic drugs. Sakaeda and co-workers (1994, 1995) also reported a rapid release of a drug (sudan II) with logPC$_{oct}$ value of 5.4 from emulsion formulations. Comparing with the administration in a form of plasma solution, the fat emulsion composed of soybean oil and EYPC increased the blood concentration of sudan II after intravenous injection. However, the plasma retention of sudan II was much lower than that of fat emulsions themselves determined by the plasma concentration of phospholipids and triglycerides. The soybean oil-emulsions emulsified with EYPC, HCO-60, or Pluronic F127 (polyoxyethylene-polyoxypropylene block copolymer) were eliminated from plasma with a half-life of 2–3 h, while sudan II incorporated in the emulsions was very rapidly released from the emulsions with a half-life of less than 1 min in all emulsions studied. Therefore, it can be concluded that higher lipophilicity of drugs should be required for stable retention in emulsion formulations.

Prodrug Approaches

As described above, emulsions require large logPC$_{oct}$ values or high lipophilicity for drugs to keep them in the particulate structures. One of the potential approaches to prolong the retention time in emulsions seems to increase the lipophilicity of drugs by chemical modifications. Based on this concept, Hashida and Sezaki (1983) presented a prodrug approach to control the disposition properties of drugs by incorporating into liposomes and emulsions (Figure 7). Although mitomycin C, an antitumor agent, could not be incorporated into an emulsion formulation, its lipophilic derivatives were efficiently formulated in the emulsion and an enhanced delivery to the regional lymph nodes was achieved after intramuscular injection (Sasaki *et al.*, 1984, 1985).

Recently, similar approaches which use a combination of physical device (fat emulsion) and chemical modification (increasing the lipophilicity) are investigated for improving targeted delivery of drugs. Lipophilic prodrugs could be retained in emulsion formulations than parent drugs. Mizushima *et al.* (1987) developed a methyl ester of isocarbacyclin, which showed a slower release from an emulsion formulation than the parent drug. A similar result was observed for PGE$_1$ and its prodrug, Δ^8-9-*O*-butyryl prostaglandin F$_1$ butyl ester (Igarashi *et al.*, 1992); 7–12% of the prodrug remained in the formulation after 5 min incubation at 37°C, while only 0.5–2% was retained for PGE$_1$. These derivatization approaches would be promising, but the *in vivo* release kinetics of such derivatives should be elucidated since more rapid release will occur in the presence of serum components than in buffers (Mizushima and Hoshi, 1993; Yamaguchi *et al.*, 1995). Van Berkel and co-workers derivatized an antiviral drug, iododeoxyuridine, into a lipophilic form, dioleoyliododeoxyuridine, and incorporated it into lipophilic particles (Bijsterbosch *et al.*, 1994; Rensen *et al.*, 1995). When incorporated into an emulsion formulation

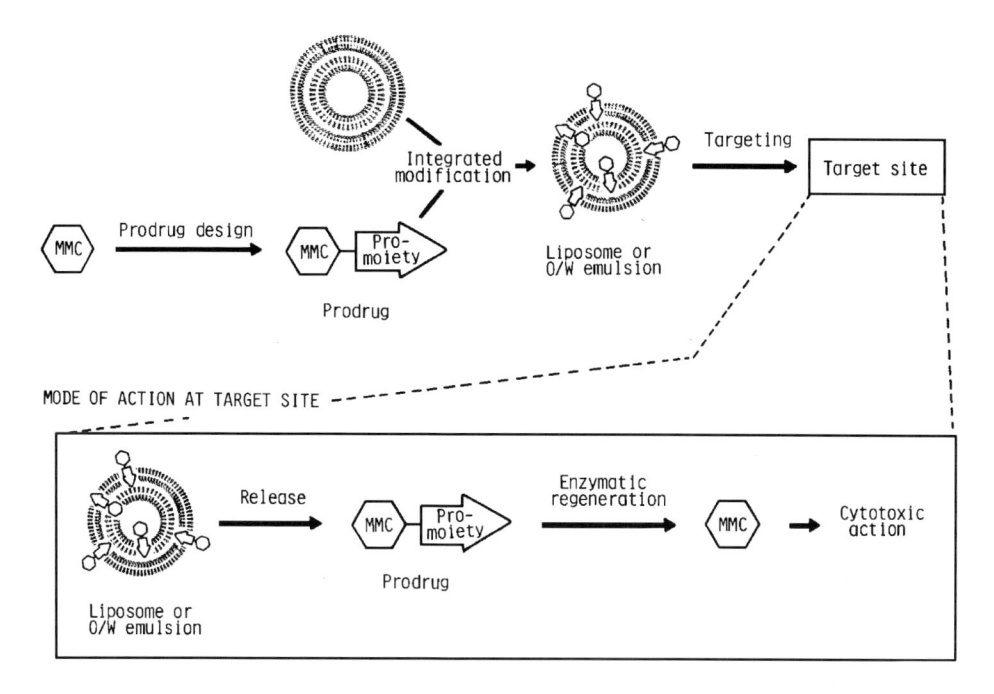

Figure 7 Schematic model showing the basic concept and mechanism of drug delivery systems consisting of a combination of physical devices (e.g. fat emulsion and liposome) and chemical modifications.

and administered in rats, ^{3}H-dioleoyliodododeoxyuridine showed a similar distribution profile to that of ^{14}C-CO, indicating that the derivative can be stably retained in the emulsion formulation.

CONCLUSIONS

Fat emulsions will be a promising drug delivery system which can solubilize considerable amounts of lipophilic drugs, control the *in vivo* disposition of incorporated drugs, and deliver drugs selectively to a target site. The optimization of drug delivery, however, can only be achieved when the characteristics of both emulsions and drugs are strictly regulated. If the purpose is not the targeted delivery to the liver parenchymal cells or to the mononuclear phagocytes, emulsions should be formulated not to be recognized by mechanisms for eliminating lipoproteins or foreign materials from circulation. The use of emulsifiers having large hydrophilic moiety will prevent such recognition to some extent. On the other hand, fat emulsions can mimic chylomicrons and can be utilized as a targetable carrier to the liver when complexed with ligands like apolipoprotein E. To regulate the *in vivo* disposition of drugs, they should be retained in emulsion formulations even after the administration in the body. Drugs with moderate lipophilicity (less than 6 in $\log PC_{oct}$) are rapidly released from emulsions, therefore the increase in the lipophilicity of drugs by chemical modification (prodrug) would be promising to achieve precise control of their *in vivo* disposition with emulsion formulations.

REFERENCES

Allen, T.M., Chonn, A. (1987) Large unilamellar liposomes with low uptake into the reticuloendothelial system. *FEBS Lett.*, **223**, 42–46.
Allen, T.M., Everest, J.M. (1983) Effect of liposome size and drug release properties on pharmacokinetics of encapsulated drugs in rats. *J. Pharmacol. Exp. Ther.*, **226**, 539–544.
Allen, T.M., Moase, E.H. (1996) Therapeutic opportunities for targeted liposomal drug delivery. *Adv. Drug Delivery Rev.*, **21**, 117–133.
Allen, T.M., Hansen, C., Martin, F., Redemann, C., Yau-Young, A. (1991) Liposomes containing synthetic lipid derivatives of polyethyleneglycol show prolonged circulation half-lives *in vivo*. *Biochim. Biophys. Acta*, **1066**, 29–36.
Aoki, H., Sun, C., Fuji, K., Miyajima, K. (1995) Disposition kinetics of liposomes modified with synthetic aminoglycolipids in rats. *Int. J. Pharm.*, **115**, 183–191.
Arbeeny, C.M., Rifici, V.A. (1984) The uptake of chylomicron remnants and very-low-density lipoprotein remnants by the perfused rat liver. *J. Biol. Chem.*, **259**, 9662–9666.
Beisiegel, U., Weber, W., Ihrke, G., Herz, J., Stanley, K.K. (1989) The LDL receptor-related protein is an apo E binding protein. *Nature*, **341**, 162–164.
Bengtson, G., Olivecrona, T. (1980) Lipoprotein lipase, some effects of activation of proteins. *Eur. J. Biochem.*, **106**, 549–555.
Bennett Clark, S., Derksen, A. (1987) Phosphatidylcholine composition of emulsions influences triacylglycerol lipolysis and clearance from plasma. *Biochim. Biophys. Acta*, **920**, 37–46.
Bijsterbosch, M.K., Van Berkel, T.J.C. (1990) Native and modified lipoproteins as drug delivery systems. *Adv. Drug Delivery Rev.*, **5**, 231–251.
Bijsterbosch, M.K., Van Berkel, T.J.C. (1992) Lactosylated high density lipoprotein: a potential carrier for the site-specific delivery of drugs to parenchymal liver cells. *Mol. Pharmacol.*, **41**, 404–411.
Bijsterbosch, M.K., Schouten, D., Van Berkel, T.J.C. (1994) Synthesis of the dioleoyl derivative of iododeoxyuridine and its incorporation into reconstituted high density lipoprotein particles. *Biochemistry*, **33**, 14073–14080.
Boberg, J., Carlson, L.A., Hallberg, D. (1969) Application of a new intravenous fat tolerance test in the study of hypertriglyceridaemia in man. *J. Atheroscler. Res.*, **9**, 159–169.
Borensztajn, J., Getz, G.S., Kotlar, T.J. (1988) Uptake of chylomicron remnants by the liver: further evidence for the modulating role of phospholipids. *J. Lipid Res.*, **29**, 1087–1096.
Brouwer, C.B., de Bruin, T.W.A., Jansen, H., Erkelens, D.W. (1993) Different clearance of intravenously administered olive oil and soybean-oil emulsions: role of hepatic lipase. *Am. J. Clin. Nutr.*, **57**, 533–539.
Brown, M.S., Goldstein, J.L. (1986) A receptor-mediated pathway for cholesterol homeostasis. *Science*, **232**, 34–47.
Bundgaard, M. (1980) Transport pathways in capillaries — in search of pores. *Ann. Rev. Physiol.*, **42**, 325–336.
Chowdhury, N.R., Wu, C.H., Wu, G.Y., Yerneni, P.C., Bommineni, V.R., Chowdhury, J.R. (1993) Fate of DNA targeted to the liver by asialoglycoprotein receptor-mediated endocytosis *in vivo*: prolonged persistence in cytoplasmic vesicles after partial hepatectomy. *J. Biol. Chem.*, **268**, 11265–11271.
Collins-Gold, L.C., Lyons, R.T., Bartholow, L.C. (1990) Parenteral emulsions for drug delivery. *Adv. Drug Delivery Rev.*, **5**, 189–208.
Connelly, P.W., Kuksis, A. (1981) Effect of core composition and particle size of lipid emulsions on apolipoprotein transfer of plasma lipoproteins *in vivo*. *Biochim. Biophys. Acta*, **666**, 80–89.
Davis, S.S., Hansrani, P. (1985) The influence of emulsifying agents on the phagocytosis of lipid emulsions by macrophages. *Int. J. Pharm.*, **23**, 69–77.
Davis, S.S., Washington, C., West, P., Illum, L., Liversidge, G., Sternson, L., Kirsh, R. (1987) Lipid emulsions as drug delivery systems. *Ann. N.Y. Acad. Sci.*, **507**, 75–88.
De Groot, P.H.E., Van Berkel, T.J.C., Van Tol, A. (1981) Relative contribution of parenchymal and non-parenchymal (sinusoidal) liver cells in the uptake of chylomicron remnants. *Metabolism*, **30**, 792–797.
Dunn, S.E., Brindley, A., Davis, S.S., Davies, M.C., Illum, L. (1994) Polystyrene-poly(ethylene glycol) (PS-PEG2000) particles as model systems for site specific drug delivery. 2. The effect of PEG surface density on the *in vitro* cell interaction and *in vivo* biodistribution. *Pharm. Res.*, **11**, 1016–1022.

Elbaz, E., Zeevi, A., Klang, S., Benita, S. (1993) Positively charged submicron emulsions — a new type of colloidal drug carrier. *Int. J. Pharm.*, **96**, R1–R6.

Erkelens, D.W., Brunzell, J.D., Bierman, E.L. (1979) Availability of apolipoprotein CII in relation to the maximal removal capacity for an infused triglyceride emulsion in man. *Metabolism*, **28**, 495–501.

Floren, C.H., Nilsson, A. (1987) Hepatic chylomicron remnant (apolipoprotein E) receptors. *Scand. J. Gastroenterol.*, **22**, 513–520.

Friedman, Z., Marks, K.H., Maisels, J., Thorson, R., Naeye, R. (1978) Effect of parenteral fat emulsion on the pulmonary and reticuloendothelial systems in the newborn infant. *Pediatrics*, **61**, 694–698.

Gabison, A., Price, D.C., Huberty, J., Bresalier, R.S., Papahadjopoulos, D. (1990) Effect of liposome composition and other factors on the targeting of liposomes to experimental tumors: biodistribution and imaging studies. *Cancer Res.*, **50**, 6371–6378.

Goldberg, I.J., Scheraldi, C.A., Yacoub, L.K., Saxena, U., Bisbaier, C.L. (1990) Lipoprotein apoC-II activation of lipoprotein lipase. *J. Biol. Chem.*, **265**, 4266–4272.

Gref, R., Minamitake, Y., Peracchia, M.T., Trubetskoy, V., Torchilin, V., Langer, R. (1994) Biodegradable long-circulating polymeric nanoparticles. *Science*, **263**, 1600–1603.

Gregoriadis, G., Neerunjun, D.E. (1974) Control of the fate of hepatic uptake and catabolism of liposome-entrapped proteins injected into rats. Possible therapeutic applications. *Eur. J. Biochem.*, **47**, 179–185.

Handa, T., Eguchi, Y., Miyajima, K. (1994) Effects of cholesterol and cholesteryl oleate on lipolysis and liver uptake of triglyceride/phosphatidylcholine emulsions in rats. *Pharm. Res.*, **11**, 1283–1287.

Hansrani, P.K., Davis, S.S., Groves, M.J. (1983) The preparation and properties of sterile intravenous emulsions. *J. Parent. Sci. Technol.*, **37**, 145–150.

Hashida, M., Sezaki, H. (1983) Specific delivery of mitomycin C: combined use of prodrug and spherical delivery systems. In S.S. Davis, L. Illum, J.G. McVie and E. Tomlinson, (eds.), *Microspheres and Drug Therapy. Pharmaceutical, Immunological and Medical Aspects*, Elsevier Science Publishers B.V., Amsterdam, The Netherlands, pp. 281–293.

Hedeman, H., Brøndsted, H., Müllertz, A., Frokjaer, S. (1996) Fat emulsions based on structured lipids (1,3–specific triglycerides): an investigation of the *in vivo* fate. *Pharm. Res.*, **13**, 725–728.

Hultin, M., Müllertz, A., Zundel, M.A., Olivecrona, G., Hansen, T.T., Deckelbaum, R.J., Carpentier, Y.A., Olivecrona, T. (1994) Metabolism of emulsions containing medium- and long-chain triglycerides or interesterified triglycerides. *J. Lipid Res.*, **35**, 1850–1860.

Igarashi, R., Mizushima, Y., Takenaga, M., Matsumoto, K., Morizawa, Y., Yasuda, A. (1992) A stable PGE$_1$ prodrug for targeting therapy. *J. Controlled Release*, **20**, 37–46.

Illum, L., Davis, S.S. (1987) Targeting of colloidal particles to the bone marrow. *Life Sci.*, **40**, 1553–1560.

Illum, L., Davis, S.S., Muller, R.H., Mak, E., West, P. (1987) The organ distribution and circulation time of intravenously injected colloidal carriers sterically stabilised with a block copolymer-poloxamine 908. *Life Sci.*, **40**, 367–374.

Illum, L., West, P., Washington, C., Davis, S.S. (1989) The effect of stabilising agents on the organ distribution of lipid emulsions. *Int. J. Pharm.*, **54**, 41–49.

Ishibashi, S., Perrey, S., Chen, Z., Osuga, J., Shimada, M., Ohashi, K., Harada, K., Yazaki, Y., Yamada, N. (1996) Role of the low density lipoprotein (LDL) receptor pathway in the metabolism of chylomicron remnants. A quantitative study in knockout mice lacking the LDL receptor, apolipoprotein E, or both. *J. Biol. Chem.*, **271**, 22422–22427.

Iwamoto, K., Kato, T., Kawahara, M., Koyama, N., Watanabe, S., Miyake, Y., Sunamoto, J. (1991) Polysaccharide-coated oil droplets in oil-in-water emulsions as targetable carriers for lipophilic drugs. *J. Pharm. Sci.*, **80**, 219–224.

Jain, R.K. (1987) Transport of molecules across tumor vasculature. *Cancer Metas. Rev.*, **6**, 559–593.

Jeppsson, R., Rossner, S. (1975) The influence of emulsifying agents and of lipid soluble drugs on the fractional removal rate of lipid emulsions from the bloodstream of the rabbit. *Acta Pharmacol. Toxicol.*, **37**, 134–144.

Johnson, R.C., Young, S.K., Cotter, R., Lin, L., Rowe, B. (1990) Medium-chain-triglyceride lipid emulsion: metabolism and tissue distribution. *Am. J. Clin. Nutr.*, **52**, 502–508.

Kimura, A., Yamaguchi, H., Watanabe, K., Hayashi, M., Awazu, S. (1986) Factors influencing the tissue distribution of coenzyme Q$_{10}$ intravenously administered in an emulsion to rats: emulsifying agents and lipoprotein lipase activity. *J. Pharm. Pharmacol.*, **38**, 659–662.

Klibanov, A.L., Maruyama, K., Torchilin, V.P., Huang, L. (1990) Amphipathic polyethylene glycols effectively prolong the circulation time of liposomes. *FEBS Lett.*, **268**, 235–237.

Komatsu, H., Kitajima, A., Okada, S. (1995) Pharmaceutical characterization of commercially available intravenous fat emulsions: estimation of average particle size, size distribution and surface potential using photon correlation spectroscopy. *Chem. Pharm. Bull.*, **43**, 1412–1415.

Koster, V.S., Kuks, P.F.M., Lange, R., Talsma, H. (1996) Particle size in parenteral fat emulsions, what are the true limitations? *Int. J. Pharm.*, **134**, 235–238.

Kurihara, A., Shibayama, Y., Yasuno, A., Ikeda, M., Hisaoka, M. (1996a) Lipid emulsions of palmitoylrhizoxin: effects of particle size on blood dispositions of emulsion lipid and incorporated compound in rats. *Biopharm. Drug Dispos.*, **17**, 343–353.

Kurihara, A., Shibayama, Y., Mizota, A., Yasuno, A., Ikeda, M., Sasagawa, K., Kobayashi, T., Hisaoka, M. (1996b) Lipid emulsions of palmitoylrhizoxin: effects of compositions on lipolysis and biodistribution. *Biopharm. Drug Dispos.*, **17**, 331–342.

Lakshmann, M.R., Muesing, R.A., LaRose, J.C. (1981) Regulation of cholesterol biosynthesis and 3–hydroxy-3-methylglutaryl coenzyme A reductase activity by chylomicron remnants on isolated hepatocytes and perfused liver. *J. Biol. Chem.*, **256**, 3037–3043.

Lenzo, N.P., Martins, I., Mortimer, B.-C., Redgrave, T.G. (1988) Effects of phospholipid composition on the metabolism of triacylglycerol, cholesteryl ester and phosphatidylcholine from lipid emulsions injected intravenously in rats. *Biochim. Biophys. Acta*, **960**, 111–118.

Liu, F., Liu, D. (1995) Long-circulating emulsions (oil-in-water) as carriers for lipophilic drugs. *Pharm. Res.*, **12**, 1060–1064.

Liu, D., Mori, A., Huang, L. (1991) Large liposomes containing ganglioside GM_1 accumulate effectively in spleen. *Biochim. Biophys. Acta*, **1066**, 159–165.

Lundberg, B.B., Mortimer, B.-C., Redgrave, T.G. (1996) Submicron lipid emulsions containing amphipathic polyethylene glycol for use as drug-carriers with prolonged circulation time. *Int. J. Pharm.*, **134**, 119–127.

Lutz, O., Meraihi, Z., Mura, J.-L., Frey, A., Riess, G.H., Bach, A.C. (1989a) Fat emulsion particle size: influence on the clearance rate and the tissue lipolytic activity. *Am. J. Clin. Nutr.*, **50**, 1370–1381.

Lutz, O., Lave, T., Frey, A., Meraihi, Z., Bach, A.C. (1989b) Activities of lipoprotein lipase and hepatic lipase on long- and medium-chain triglyceride emulsions used in parenteral nutrition. *Metabolism*, **38**, 507–513.

Mahley, R.W., Hussain, M.M. (1991) Chylomicron and chylomicron remnant catabolism. *Curr. Opin. Lipidol.*, **2**, 170–176.

Mahley, R.W. (1988) Apolipoprotein E: cholesterol transport protein with expanding role in cell biology. *Science*, **240**, 622–630.

Mizushima, Y. (1991) Lipo-prostaglandin preparations. *Prostagl. Leukotr. Essent. Fatty Acids*, **42**, 1–6.

Mizushima, Y. (1996) Lipid microspheres (lipid emulsions) as a drug carrier — An overview. *Adv. Drug Delivery Rev.*, **20**, 113–115.

Mizushima, Y., Hoshi, K. (1993) Recent advances in lipid microsphere technology for targeting prostaglandin delivery. *J. Drug Targeting*, **1**, 93–100.

Mizushima, Y., Igarashi, R., Hoshi, K., Sim, A.K., Cleland, M.E., Hayashi, H., Goto, J. (1987) Marked enhancement in antithrombotic activity of isocarbacyclin following its incorporation into lipid microspheres. *Prostaglandins*, **33**, 161–168.

Mizushima, Y., Hamano, T., Haramoto, S., Kiyokawa, S., Yanagawa, A., Nakura, K., Shintome, M., Watanabe, M. (1990) Distribution of lipid microspheres incorporating prostaglandin E_1 to vascular lesions. *Prostagl. Leukotr. Essent. Fatty Acids*, **41**, 269–272.

Moonis, M., Ahmad, I., Bachhawat, B.K. (1993) Mannosylated liposomes as carriers for hamycin in the treatment of experimental aspergillosis in balb/c mice. *J. Drug Targeting*, **1**, 147–155.

Muller, C.D., Schuber, F. (1989) Neo-mannosylated liposomes: synthesis and interaction with mouse Kupffer cells and resident peritoneal macrophages. *Biochim. Biophys. Acta*, **986**, 97–105.

Nomura, T., Yamashita, F., Takakura, Y., Hashida, M. (1995) Pharmacokinetic analysis of various lipid carrier systems after intratumoral injection in tissue-isolated tumors. *Proc. Int. Symp. Controlled Release Bioact. Mater.*, **22**, 420–421.

Oswald, B., Quarfordt, S. (1987) Effect of apoE on triglyceride emulsion interaction with hepatocyte and hepatoma G2 cells. *J. Lipid Res.*, **28**, 798–809.

Papahadjopoulos, D., Allen, T.M., Gabizon, A., Mayhew, E., Matthay, K., Huang, S.K., Lee, K.-D., Woodle, M.C., Lasic, D.D., Redemann, C., Martin, F.J. (1991) Sterically stabilized liposomes: improvements in pharmacokinetics and antitumor therapeutic efficacy. *Proc. Natl. Acad. Sci. USA*, **88**, 11460–11464.

Perales, J.C., Ferkol, T., Beegen, H., Ratnoff, O.D., Hanson, R.W. (1994) Gene transfer *in vivo*: Sustained expression and regulation of genes introduced into the liver by receptor-targeted uptake. *Proc. Natl. Acad. Sci. USA*, **91**, 4086–4090.

Peterson, J., Olivecrona, T., Bengtsson-Olivecrona, G. (1985) Distribution of lipoprotein lipase and hepatic lipase between plasma and tissues: effect of hypertriglyceridemia. *Biochim. Biophys. Acta*, **837**, 262–270.

Redgrave, T.G. (1970) Formation of cholesteryl ester-rich particulate lipid during metabolism of chylomicrons. *J. Clin. Invest.*, **49**, 465–471.

Redgrave, T.G., Maranhao, R.C. (1985) Metabolism of protein-free lipid emulsion models of chylomicrons in rats. *Biochim. Biophys. Acta*, **835**, 102–112.

Redgrave, T.G., Rakic, V., Mortimer, B.-C., Mamo, J.C.L. (1992) Effects of sphingomyelin and phosphatidylcholine acyl chains on the clearance of triacylglycerol-rich lipoproteins from plasma. Studies with lipid emulsions in rats. *Biochim. Biophys. Acta*, **1126**, 65–72.

Rensen, P.C.N., Van Dijk, M.C.M., Havenaar, E.C., Bijsterbosch, M.K., Kruijt, J.K., Van Berkel, T.J.C. (1995) Selective liver targeting of antivirals by recombinant chylomicrons — a new therapeutic approach to hepatitis B. *Nat. Med.*, **1**, 221–225.

Sakaeda (nee Kakutani), T., Hirano, K. (1995) O/W lipid emulsions for parenteral drug delivery. II. Effect of composition on pharmacokinetics of incorporated drug. *J. Drug Targeting*, **3**, 221–230.

Sakaeda (nee Kakutani), T., Takahashi, K., Nishihara, Y., Hirano, K. (1994) O/W lipid emulsions for parenteral drug delivery. I. Pharmacokinetics of the oil particles and incorporated sudan II. *Biol. Pharm. Bull.*, **17**, 1490–1495.

Sasaki, H., Takakura, Y., Hashida, M., Kimura, T., Sezaki, H. (1984) Antitumor activity of lipophilic prodrugs of mitomycin C entrapped in liposome or O/W emulsion. *J. Pharmacobio-Dyn.*, **7**, 120–130.

Sasaki, H., Kakutani, T., Hashida, M., Sezaki, H. (1985) Absorption characteristics of the lipophilic prodrug of mitomycin C from injected liposomes or an emulsion. *J. Pharm. Pharmacol.*, **37**, 461–465.

Scherphof, G.L. (1991) *In vivo* behavior of liposomes: interactions with the mononuclear phagocyte system and implications for drug targeting. In *Targeted Drug Delivery*, edited by R.L. Juliano, pp. 285–327. Berlin, Germany: Springer-Verlag.

Schmidt, C.F., Barenholz, Y., Thompson, T.E. (1977) A nuclear magnetic resonance study of sphingomyelin in bilayer systems. *Biochemistry*, **16**, 2649–2656.

Senior, J., Gregoriadis, G. (1982) Is half-life of circulating liposomes determined by changes in their permeability? *FEBS Lett.*, **145**, 109–114.

Senior, J., Crawley, J.C.W., Gregoriadis, G. (1985) Tissue distribution of liposomes exhibiting long half-lives in the circulation after intravenous injection. *Biochim. Biophys. Acta*, **839**, 1–8.

Senior, J. (1987) Fate and behavior of liposomes *in vivo*: a review of controlling factors. *Crit. Rev. Ther. Drug Carrier Syst.*, **3**, 123–193.

Singh, M., Ravin, L.J. (1986) Parenteral emulsions as drug carrier systems. *J. Parent. Sci. Technol.*, **40**, 34–41.

Takakura, Y., Hashida, M. (1995) Macromolecular drug carrier systems in cancer chemotherapy: macromolecular prodrugs. *Crit. Rev. Oncol. Hematol.*, **18**, 207–231.

Takino, T., Nakajima, C., Takakura, Y., Sezaki, H., Hashida, M. (1993) Controlled biodistribution of highly lipophilic drugs with various parenteral formulations. *J. Drug Targeting*, **1**, 117–124.

Takino, T., Konishi, K., Takakura, Y., Hashida, M. (1994) Long circulating emulsion carrier systems for highly lipophilic drugs. *Biol. Pharm. Bull.*, **17**, 121–125.

Takino, T., Nagahama, E., Sakaeda (*nee* Kakutani), T., Yamashita, F., Takakura, Y., Hashida, M. (1995) Pharmacokinetic disposition analysis of lipophilic drugs injected with various lipid carriers in the single-pass rat liver perfusion system. *Int. J. Pharm.*, **114**, 43–54.

Tokunaga, Y., Iwasa, T., Fujisaki, J., Sawai, S., Kagayama, A. (1988) Liposomal sustained-release delivery systems for intravenous injection. II. Design of liposome carriers and blood disposition of lipophilic mitomycin C prodrug-bearing liposomes. *Chem. Pharm. Bull.*, **36**, 3557–3564.

Tso, P. (1985) Gastrointestinal digestion and absorption of lipid. *Adv. Lipid Res.*, **21**, 143–179.

Tso, P., Balin, J.A. (1986) Formation and transport of chylomicrons by enterocytes to the lymphatics. Editorial review. *Am. J. Physiol.*, **250**, G715–G726.

Tsuchiya, S., Aramaki, Y., Hara, T., Hosoi, K., Okada, A. (1986) Preparation and disposition of asialofetuin-labelled liposome. *Biopharm. Drug Dispos.*, **7**, 549–558.

Umezawa, K., Karino, A., Hayashi, M., Tahara, K., Kimura, A., Awazu, S. (1991) Hepatic uptake of lipid-soluble drugs from fat emulsion. *J. Pharmacobio-Dyn.*, **14**, 591–598.

Van Haelst, U.J.G.M., Sengers, R.C.A. (1976) Effects of parenteral nutrition with lipids on the human liver. *Virchows Arch. B.*, **22**, 323–332.

Washington, C. (1990) The stability of intravenous fat emulsions in total parenteral nutrition mixtures. *Int. J. Pharm.*, **66**, 1–21.

Washington, C., Davis, S.S. (1987) Ageing effects in parenteral fat emulsions: the role of fatty acids. *Int. J. Pharm.*, **39**, 33–37.

Wheeler, J.J., Wong, K.F., Ansell, S.M., Masin, D., Bally, M.B. (1994) Polyethylene glycol modified phospholipids stabilize emulsions prepared from triacylglycerol. *J. Pharm. Sci.*, **83**, 1558–1564.

Wisse, E. (1970) An electron microscopic study of the fenestrated endothelial lining of rat liver sinusoids. *J. Ultrastruct. Res.*, **31**, 125–150.

Woodle, M.C., Lasic, D.D. (1992) Sterically stabilized liposomes. *Biochim. Biophys. Acta*, **1113**, 171–199.

Wu, G.Y., Wu, C.H. (1988) Receptor-mediated gene delivery and expression *in vivo*. *J. Biol. Chem.*, **263**, 14621–14624.

Wu, N.Z., Da, D., Rudoll, T.L., Needham, D., Whorton, A.R., Dewhirst, M.W. (1993) Increased microvascular permeability contributes to preferential accumulation of Stealth liposomes in tumor tissue. *Cancer Res.*, **53**, 3765–3770.

Yamaguchi, T., Fukushima, Y., Itai, S., Hayashi, H. (1995) Rate of release and retentivity of prostaglandin E_1 in lipid emulsion. *Biochim. Biophys. Acta*, **1256**, 381–386.

Yuan, F., Dellian, M., Fukumura, D., Leunig, M., Berk, D.A., Torchilin, V.P., Jain, R.K. (1995) Vascular permeability in a human tumor xenograft: molecular size dependence and cutoff size. *Cancer Res.*, **55**, 3752–3756.

Zhang, S.H., Reddick, R.L., Piedrahita, J.A., Maeda, N. (1992) Spontaneous hypercholesterolemia and arterial lesions in mice lacking apolipoprotein E. *Science*, **258**, 468–471.

5. DESIGN AND EVALUATION OF SUBMICRON EMULSIONS AS COLLOIDAL DRUG CARRIERS FOR INTRAVENOUS ADMINISTRATION

SHMUEL KLANG and SIMON BENITA

Department of Pharmaceutics, School of Pharmacy, The Hebrew University of Jerusalem, P.O. Box 12065, Jerusalem 91120, Israel

INTRODUCTION

Emulsions are heterogeneous systems in which one immiscible liquid is dispersed as droplets in another liquid. Such a system is thermodynamically unstable and is kinetically stabilized by the addition of one further component or mixture of components that exhibit emulsifying properties. The present International Union of Pure and Applied Chemistry definition of an emulsion is broader because it includes the possibility of several phases in an emulsion, including liquid crystalline phases: "In an emulsion, liquid droplets and/or liquid crystals are dispersed in a liquid". Depending on the nature of the diverse components and of the emulsifying agents, various types of emulsions can result from the mixture of immiscible liquids. Invariably, one of the two immiscible liquids is water, and the second is an oily substance, often a long chain triglycerides. Whether the aqueous or oil phase becomes the dispersed phase depends primarily on the emulsifying agents used and the relative amounts of the two liquid phases. Hence, an emulsion in which the oil is dispersed as droplets throughout the aqueous phase is termed an oil-in-water (O/W) emulsion. When water is the dispersed phase and oil is the dispersion medium, the emulsion is termed a water-in oil (W/O) type. All pharmaceutical emulsions designed for parenteral administration are of the O/W type.

Lipid emulsions were developed after World War II (Muller and Canham, 1965) to serve as an intravenous source of both calories and essential fatty acids. The wide and clinically well-accepted usage of emulsions for parenteral nutrition (as also emphasized in the first chapter of this book) has raised the possibility of using the oil phase of oil-in-water emulsion as a carrier of poorly water-soluble drugs for parenteral administration. However, there are other reasons listed in Table 1 why intensive research efforts have been concentrated for designing parenteral emulsions as a drug administration vehicle (Prankerd and Stella, 1990).

EMULSION DESIGN AND CHARACTERIZATION

Intravenous emulsions, like all parenteral products, are required to meet pharmacopoeial requirements (Benita and Levy, 1993). The emulsions must be sterile, isotonic, non-pyrogenic, non-toxic, biodegradable and stable, both physically and chemically. Furthermore, the particle size of the droplets needs to be below one micron, and generally ranges between 100–500 nm. With larger droplet size, potential oil embolism may occur (Wretlind, 1964; Levene *et al.*, 1980).

Table 1 Reasons for using medicated emulsions

Reason	Drug Sample
A. Solubilization of low water-solubility drugs	diazepam, vitamin A, vitamin E, propofol, dexamethasone palmitate.
B. Stabilization of hydrolytically susceptible compounds	lomustine, physostigmine salicylate
C. Prevention of drug uptake by infusion sets	diazepam, Perilla Ketone
D. Reduction of irritation, pain, or toxicity of intravenously administered drugs	amphotericin, diazepam, propofol
E. Potential for sustained release dosage forms	barbiturates, dexamethasone palmitate, physostigmine salicylate
F. Possible directed drug delivery to various organs	cytotoxic agents

Excipient Selection

To comply with the requirements for parenteral emulsion, careful selection of the excipients needs to be performed. Special attention should be given to two major excipients in the emulsion formulation — the oil and the emulsifier(s). A detailed description of the excipient specifications for parenteral emulsion was presented by Hansrani *et al.* (1983). Only the main aspects of the physicochemical properties of the excipients that should be considered will be outlined below.

Oil

In previous studies (Table 2) the oil phases of the emulsion were based mainly on long chain triglycerides (LCT) from vegetable sources (soybean, safflower and

Table 2 Some commercially available lipid emulsions

Trade Name	Oil Phase (%)	Emulsifier (%)	Other Components (%)
Intralipid (Kabi-Pharmacia)	Soybean 10 and 20	Egg lecithin 1.2	Glycerol 2.5
Lipofundin S (Braun)	Soybean 10 and 20	Soybean lecithin 0.75 or 1.2	Xylitol 5.0
Lipofundin (Braun)	Cottonseed 10	Soybean lecithin 0.75	Sorbitol 5.0
Lipofundin N (Braun)	Soybean and MCT (1:1) 10 and 20	Egg lecithin 0.75 and 1.2	Glycerol 2.5
Liposyn (Abbott)	Safflower 10 and 20	Egg lecithin 1.2	Glycerol 2.5
Abbolipid (Abbott)	Safflower and Soybean (1:1) 10 and 20	Egg lecithin 1.2	Glycerol 2.5
Lipovenos (Fresenius)	Soybean 10 and 20	Egg lecithin 1.2	Glycerol 2.5
Travemulsion (Travenol)	Soybean 10 and 20	Egg lecithin 1.2	Glycerol 2.5

cottonseed oils) (Davis et al., 1985; Boyett and Davis, 1989). The oils need to be purified and winterized to allow removal of precipitated wax materials after prolonged storage at 4°C. Known contaminants (hydrogenated oils and saturated fatty materials) should be minimized.

The use of medium chain triglycerides (MCT) in fat emulsion formulations grew extensively during the 70's (Bach et al., 1972; Guisard and Debry, 1972). These MCTs are obtained from hydrolysis of coconut oil and fractionation into free fatty acids that contain between 6 and 12 carbon atoms. The MCTs are esterified with glycerol and are 100 times more soluble in water than are LCTs. MCT has mostly been used in fat emulsions (Table 2) in combination with LCT (Turlan et al., 1983; Kolb and Sailer, 1984). MCT was also used in medicated emulsions owing to its increased ability to dissolve large concentrations of liposoluble drugs (Levy et al., 1990).

Emulsifier

Since emulsions are thermodynamically unstable systems, a mixture of surfactants should be added for better stability (Benita and Levy, 1993). Most of the known synthetic and efficient emulsifiers are toxic upon parenteral administration due to hemolysis. The most frequent emulsifiers used in parenteral emulsion formulation are: phospholipids (generally from egg yolk sources), block copolymers of polyoxyethylene polyoxypropylene (poloxamer) and, to a lesser extent, acetylated monoglycerides (Jeppsson, 1972a,b).

The main functions of the surfactants are to form a thin film in the interface, lower the surface tension, thus, preventing flocculation and coalescence of the dispersed phase. The most frequently emulsifiers used in parenteral administration are phospholipids from egg source (Hansrani et al., 1983; Prankerd and Stella, 1990; Benita and Levy, 1993). These phospholipids are mixture of two major components: phosphatidylcholine and phosphatidylethanolamine. Other phospholipids include phosphatidic acid and phosphatidylinositol. In some cases a second emulsifier and even a third emulsifier are needed to enhance the physical stability of the emulsion. Such a combination of emulsifiers in parenteral submicron emulsions is frequently defined as an emulsifying complex or complex emulgator. Other emulsifiers, such as the polyoxyethylene castor oil derivatives (Cremophors®) and polyoxyethylene sorbitans (Tweens®), are already approved by the various pharmacopoeias for parenteral administration and can therefore be considered for emulsion formulation design. However, it should be kept in mind that heat exposure following steam sterilization can alter the emulsifying ability by reducing aqueous solubility resulting in final phase separation.

The properties of the emulgator interfacial film are altered by the incorporation of liposoluble drugs. Thereafter, a stabilizer agent capable of localizing in the interfacial film should be added. Such molecules are generally amphipathic and are poor surface-active agents but can stabilize the film by enhancing molecular interactions and increasing electrostatic surface charge droplets. A well-known stabilizer is oleic acid or its sodium salt (Levy and Benita, 1991; Muchtar et al., 1992; Levy et al., 1994). Cholic acid, deoxycholic acid and their respective salts (Levy et al., 1993, 1995), cationic lipids such as stearylamine, oleylamine, (Korner et al., 1994; Zeevi et al., 1994; Klang et al., 1996), 3β-[N-(N', N'-dimethylaminoethane) carbamoyl] cholesterol (DC-Chol) (Liu et al., 1996; Hara et al., 1997) were also shown to markedly improve drug-incorporated emulsion stability.

Additives

Additives are needed to adjust to physiological pH and tonicity. Glycerol is most recommended as an isotonic agent, and can be found in almost every parenteral emulsion (Dawes et al., 1978; Washington et al., 1989; Washington, 1990). However xylitol and sorbitol are also being used as osmotic agents by some of the manufacturers of fat emulsions (Table 2). The pH is adjusted to the desired value with an aqueous solution of NaOH or HCl, depending on the value that should be reached. The pH of the emulsion is generally adjusted between 7 and 8 to allow physiological compatibility and maintain emulsion physical integrity by minimizing fatty acid ester hydrolysis of the MCT-LCT and phospholipids (Klang et al., 1996). Furthermore, emulsion stabilizers are often needed to preserve emulsions from oxidation or phase separation. While the first approach is easy to accomplish by adding antioxidants or reducing agents like tocopherol, desferoxamine mesylate and ascorbic acid, the second one is much more difficult to accomplish since it is related to interfacial degradation.

Drug

Submicron emulsions intended for parenteral administration are designed for the incorporation of lipophilic and hydrophobic drugs, which exhibits poor aqueous solubility. Inclusion of hydrophobic drugs in the innermost oil phase presents special problems related to the solubilization of the drugs. However these problems generally can be overcome by techniques such as the elevation of the temperatures and the use of additives to increase the oil solubility of hydrophobic drugs. The addition of other drugs to emulsions for iv application also resulted in reduced stability or cracking. The therapeutic applications of emulsions will be thoroughly described later on in this chapter.

Emulsion Preparation

The mean droplet size of i.v. emulsions must be smaller than the finest capillaries likely to be encountered in the vascular system, otherwise, a potential pulmonary embolism may occur. This risk is significantly greater in cases of neonates treated with parenteral fat emulsion nutrition. Thorough descriptions of the different technical approaches used to manufacturing submicron emulsions have been reported in the literature (Hansrani et al., 1983; Prankerd et al., 1990; Benita and Levy, 1993). From a review of the literature, it can be deduced that the conventional equipment e.g. electric mixers and mechanical stirrers, etc., show not only large droplet size but also a wide droplet size distribution. Therefore, irrespective of the preparation process, homogeneous submicronized emulsion formulation can be manufactured only if high pressure homogenizers are used (Benita and Levy, 1993).

Two approaches may be used for the preparation of medicated emulsions (Prankerd et al., 1990):

1. *De novo emulsification* of a drug-containing oil phase with an aqueous phase, employing a suitable emulsifying agent: It is desirable to incorporate the drug into the innermost phase of the emulsion in order to successfully exploit the advantages of an emulsion dosage form. Therefore, the type of emulsion to be used depends, to a large extent, upon the physicochemical properties of the drug. Inclusion of hydrophobic drugs in the oil phase presents special problems related to the solubilization of the drug, however these can generally be overcome by techniques such as elevation of temperature and the use of surfactants as previously mentioned. Usually, the whole preparation process is conducted in a laminar flow hood under a nitrogen atmosphere in case excipients and drugs sensitive to oxidation are used. Sterilization is normally achieved either by the use of a standard steam procedure (autoclaving) or by the maintenance of aseptic conditions during the entire preparation process, depending on the sensitivity of the active ingredients to elevated temperatures. Benita and Levy (1993) have reviewed the development of submicron emulsions as colloidal drug carrier systems and emphasized the need for physicochemical studies in the design and characterization of such systems. A schematic general description of the entire parenteral emulsion manufacturing process is depicted in Figure 1.

2. *Extemporaneous addition* of a concentrated sterile solution of the drug in a solvent such as dimethylacetamide or ethanol to a commercial i.v. fat emulsion such as Intralipid® or Liposyn®: These products contain either 10% w/w or 20% w/w of emulsified soybean oil (Intralipid®) or safflower oil (Liposyn®) with mean particle sizes of 0.3 µm. Some commercially available lipid emulsion formulations are depicted in Table 2. They are stabilized either with purified egg yolk or soybean lecithin and contain different osmotic agents to maintain isotonicity. The addition procedure must be performed with great care for the following two reasons:

a. To prevent precipitation of the drug in the aqueous phase of the emulsion
b. To prevent cracking of the emulsion.

This approach has been used successfully in preliminary animal and clinical studies with investigational cytotoxic agents but is not regarded a suitable procedure for routine use because of emulsion stability problems.

Emulsion Characterization

Droplet Size

Particle size distribution is one of the most important characteristics of an emulsion. For example, sedimentation and creaming tendencies during long-term and accelerated stability tests of an emulsion can be conventionally monitored by measuring the changes in the droplet size distribution. A wide range of particle sizes is found in emulsion systems, as evidenced by intravenous fat emulsions that should contain particles in the range of 50 nm–1 µm, and emulsions used as contrast media in computerized tomography that are 1–3 µm in size. Particles above 5 µm are clinically unacceptable because they cause the formation of pulmonary emboli (Burnham et al., 1983). These are sometimes present because of inefficient homogenization,

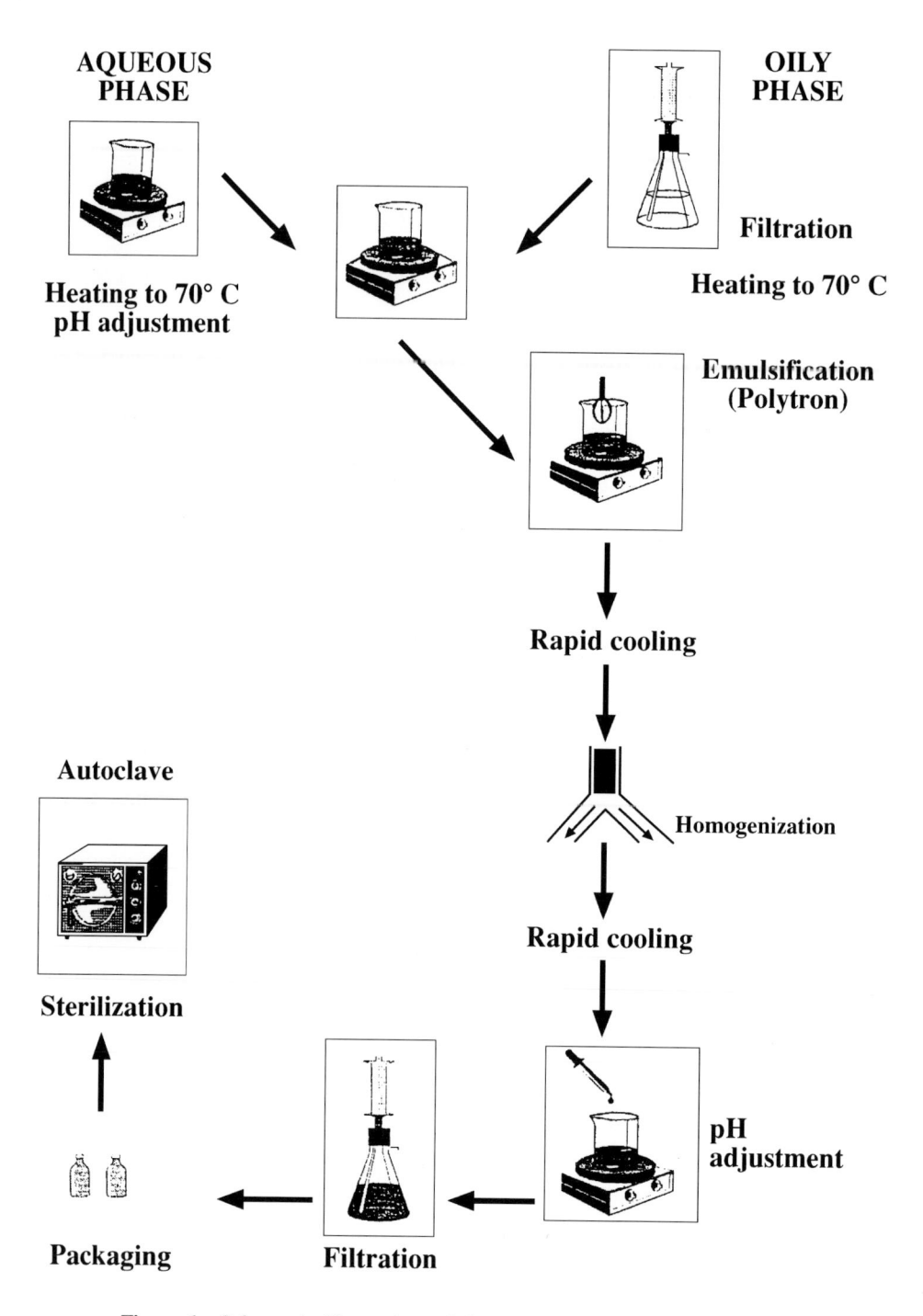

Figure 1 Schematic illustration of the emulsion preparation process.

or as a result of instability of the emulsion. Hence, it is necessary to size them even if they are present in small numbers. An exhaustive evaluation of the various methods used for characterizing particle size of submicron emulsions and its relevance to the emulsion-based drug delivery systems in general is provided in another chapter of the present book.

Droplet Surface Charge

The electrical charge on the emulsion droplets is measured using either a Zetasizer (Malvern, England) or the moving boundary electrophoresis technique, which has been shown to yield accurate electrophoretic mobility data (Hunter, 1981). The shape of an electrophoresis cell and the method to convert the electrophoretic mobility to zeta potential have been clearly reviewed (Benita et al., 1986).

Emulsifiers can stabilize the emulsion droplet ,not just by formation of a mechanical barrier, but also by producing an electrical (electrostatic) barrier or surface charge. The electrical surface charge of the droplets is produced by the ionization of interfacial film-forming components. The surface potential (zeta potential) of an emulsion droplet will be dependent upon the extent of ionization of the emulsifying agent. The ionization extent of some phospholipids comprised in lecithin is markedly pH-dependent (Bangham, 1968; Davis and Galloway, 1981; Davis, 1982).

Commercial lecithins are in fact a mixture of phospholipids which vary in composition. They may comprise phosphatidylcholine (PC) as the major component, zwitterionic in form, neutral over a wide pH range, together with negatively charged phospholipids such as phosphatidylethanolamine (PE) etc. In addition, other components such as cholesterol are present and may affect the interfacial film-charge extent.

Rydhag (1981) suggested that emulsion stabilization may be optimized by selection of commercial lecithin that contain appropriate amounts of negatively-charged and uncharged phosphatides, resulting in the formation of an interfacial lamellar liquid crystalline phase. Attempts were made to enrich a mixture of purified phospholipids with negatively-charged phosphatides following extraction and removal of neutral components, such as cholesterol, from a crude commercial lecithin product (Muchtar et al., 1991) by adding to the mixture of phospholipids a small quantity of negatively-charged phospholipids Washington et al., 1989; Washington, 1990). It is believed that emulsions prepared from such highly negatively-charged phospholipid compositions will exhibit high zeta potential values and will be less sensitive to the addition of small amounts of monovalent and divalent electrolytes (Rubino, 1990; Manning and Washington, 1992). Other authors have recently prepared emulsions stabilized by mixed emulsifying films containing phospholipids, nonionic surfactants and cationic lipids such as stearylamine, oleylamine or DC-Chol in order to confer an overall positive charge to the emulsified oil droplets (Klang et al., 1994; Liu et al., 1996). It is believed that these positively-charged submicron emulsions may alter the pharmacokinetic profile of selected incorporated drugs, and enhance localization of higher drug, DNA or antisenseoligonucleotide concentration in targeted organs or cells (Gershanik and Benita, 1996, Liu et al., 1996, Hara et al., 1997).

High zeta potential values (above 30 mV) should be achieved in most of the emulsions prepared in order to ensure a high-energy barrier which causes repulsion of adjacent droplets resulting in the formation of stabilized emulsions.

pH

It has already been shown that the main degradation pathway of fat emulsions led to the formation of the fatty acids which gradually reduce the pH of the emulsion (Hansrani et al., 1983; Herman and Groves, 1993). The initial pH of the emulsion might decrease progressively with time. However, this pH decrease can be controlled by adjusting the initial pH of the emulsion (Levy and Benita, 1991; Klang et al., 1996). Providing the initial adjusted pH is satisfactory, the hydrolysis rate of the phospholipids and triglycerides might be minimized. Therefore, the pH of the emulsion should be monitored continuously over the entire shelf life of the emulsion to detect detrimental free fatty acid formation.

Drug Content

As required for any dosage form, quantitative and sensitive methods of analysis should be applied to evaluate the chemical fate of the active ingredient in the emulsion formulation. It should be recalled that in medicated submicron emulsion the decomposition of the drug can be accelerated by micellar catalysis (Benita and Levy, 1993). Hence, further attention should be given in monitoring the chemical integrity of drugs in emulsions containing emulsifying agents. Consequently, a thorough study of the knowledge of the partitioning of the drug between the various emulsion phases is needed. Generally, ultrafiltration techniques are performed to achieve such objectives.

Stability Assessment

Accelerated tests

It should be emphasized that the stability results of accelerated tests based on temperature elevations generally do not reflect the actual stability of the emulsion when stored at normal temperatures. The large discrepancy observed between the predicted value and that obtained experimentally by various authors (Yalabik-Kas, 1985; Rieger, 1986) could be explained by the instability of the emulsion and the phospholipid decomposition at elevated temperatures. Emulsions subjected to temperature variations undergo dramatic physicochemical changes. Thus, long-term stability of emulsions and the subsequently induced protective effect versus sensitivity to drugs cannot be predicted from experiments carried out at high temperatures.

Therefore, among the various accelerated tests reported in the literature (Burnham et al., 1983; Hansrani et al., 1983; Yalabik-Kas, 1985), steam sterilization, excessive shaking and freeze-thaw cycles are generally used to "predict" the emulsion shelf life. These tests are considered most relevant to the stress conditions that emulsions may encounter during sterilization, transportation and aging.

The emulsions are packed in final packaging and subjected to the various accelerated tests described above. The pH, zeta potential, droplet size distribution and the drug content are evaluated before and after testing.

Long-term Tests

It is routine to determine the shelf life of a new product by storing it for various periods of time at elevated temperatures. The Arrhenius equation is commonly used to predict the shelf life.

Long-term stability studies of emulsions are conducted at various temperatures ranging from 4° to 50°C. The chemical (drug content) and physical (emulsion droplet size, creaming and pH, etc.) changes that might occur in the emulsion during storage are followed up over long periods of time. However, it must be noted that in the case of emulsions this can be erratic since the changes in temperature not only change the rate of the reaction, but could also destroy the physical stability of the emulsion.

As suggested by Rieger (1986) a realistic stability program to assess the normal shelf life of emulsions needs to be constructed according to predictions of normal conditions undergone by the specific emulsion formulation.

During the long testing period, the samples stored at various conditions should be observed critically for separation and monitored at reasonable time intervals for changes in the following characteristic properties: electrical conductivity, viscosity, particle size distribution, zeta potential, pH and chemical composition.

In addition to these physical measurements, a shelf life program for emulsions should include testing of the emulsion for the establishment of sterility and lack of pyrogens by validated, recognized microbiological methods. Furthermore, for further insight information regarding possible minor changes affecting emulsion integrity, new approaches for emulsion investigation and characterization using monolayer studies, transmission, scanning, freeze-fracturing microscope techniques, X-ray diffraction and fluorescence methods have been used and described elsewhere (Benita and Levy, 1993). It should be added that there was been an increase in the use of ^{31}P-NMR in the last few years due to its success as a novel non-invasive technique for emulsion phase characterization (Westesen and Wehler, 1992, 1993).

IN VITRO RELEASE KINETIC EXAMINATION

An accurate analysis of *in vitro* drug release from emulsion first requires a knowledge of the distribution of the drug in the various phases of the emulsion. The ultrafiltration technique at low pressure is generally used to determine the concentration of the unbound drug in the aqueous external phase of the emulsion by measuring drug concentrations in the aqueous ultrafiltrate at various filtrate volumes (Shimamoto *et al.*, 1973; Teagarden *et al.*, 1988), while maintaining the physical integrity of the dispersed system. The technique has been thoroughly described and reviewed by Benita and Levy (1993).

It is difficult to characterize drug release profile from a colloidal carrier owing to the physical obstacles attributed to the very tiny size of the dispersed particles. Various techniques were used to evaluate drug release from colloidal carriers, particularly from o/w submicron emulsions (Washington and Koosha, 1990). Attempts were made to elucidate the release mechanism by using the dialysis sac diffusion technique (Sasaki *et al.*, 1984; Ammoury *et al.*, 1989; Ammouri *et al.*, 1990) or by diffusion cells (Hashida *et al.*, 1980; Benita *et al.*, 1986; Miyazaki *et al.*, 1986). Washington (1990) claimed that in these techniques the carrier is never diluted with the release solution, and so the experiment is not performed under sink conditions. As a consequence, it does not measure the true release rate. Levy and Benita (1990) proposed the bulk-equilibrium reverse dialysis sac technique in order to avoid the enclosure of the submicron emulsion dispersion in a dialysis sac. However, the kinetic system proposed is only able to differentiate between colloidal drug delivery carriers releasing their contents over a period greater than one hour. A more rapid stringent test based on a centrifugal ultrafiltration technique in the absence of any physical membrane was also used (Ammoury *et al.*, 1990). All these tests were recently used to evaluate clofibride release from a submicron emulsion in order to avoid any controversial *in vitro* release kinetic deductions (Santos-Magalhaes *et al.*, 1991a,b, 1995). Finally the ultrafiltration technique at low pressure was also proposed for the evaluation of drug release profile from colloidal carriers such as submicron emulsions and nanoparticles (Magenheim *et al.*, 1993). Normally, the drug incorporated in the emulsion is liposoluble and exhibits limited aqueous solubility which may prevent sink conditions from prevailing. The low solubility of such drugs makes it difficult to create conditions of infinite dilution in an aqueous release medium. Addition of organic solvents or surface-active agents definitely improves the drug's solubility in release solutions, but it would be erroneous to predict the drug's behavior *in vivo* on the basis of its release profile in such solutions. However, lipophilic drugs bind with high affinity to blood proteins, mainly albumin (Goodman and Gilman, 1990). Olson *et al.* (1988) reported the use of human serum albumin to improve the solubility of lipophilic drugs such as diazepam, in aqueous injectable solutions. The increase in the aqueous solubility of diazepam and miconazole with albumin was also reported by Benita and Levy (1993). Furthermore, albumin solution as a release medium has a distinct advantage over other co-solvents, since it is a natural component, comprising part of the prevailing *in vivo* conditions. Thus, in an *in vitro* investigation of release rates of drugs from a carrier, the goal is to imitate expected *in vivo* conditions as much as possible. Release profile of a drug from a dosage form intended for i.v. administration is usually tested in aqueous buffered solutions with a pH value close to that of blood. Sometimes, albumin at concentrations ranging from 1 to 3% are added to the buffered solutions to ensure perfect sink conditions.

From a thorough review of the literature, it can be deduced that four main *in vitro* kinetic techniques have been used to evaluate the release of a drug from submicron emulsions following separation of part of the aqueous phase from the oil droplets and quantitative determination of the released drug in the aqueous phase.

Dialysis Sac Diffusion Technique

A detailed description of the technique was given elsewhere (Levy and Benita, 1990; Santos-Magalhaes *et al.*, 1991). A brief description will be reported here.

A given volume of the medicated emulsion should be placed in the dialysis sac, hermetically sealed and dropped into an appropriate sink solution. The entire system should be kept at 37°C with continuous magnetic stirring. Samples should be withdrawn from the sink solution at predetermined time intervals and assayed for drug content.

In preliminary studies, various authors (Benita *et al.*, 1986; Miyazaki *et al.*, 1986; Ammoury *et al.*, 1989; Ammoury *et al.*, 1990) tried first to evaluate the diffusion of the drug dissolved in appropriate solution through the membrane dialysis at adequate concentration. They usually reported that the drug diffused rapidly into the sink solution, indicating that the membrane is not a rate-limiting step under the experimental conditions used. However, the release of drugs from the emulsions is generally slower compared to the respective drug solutions.

Numerous investigators have pointed out various reasons explaining the drastic decrease in the release rate of a drug from the emulsions using the dialysis technique (Levy and Benita, 1990; Ammoury, 1990; Santos-Magalhaes *et al.*, 1991a,b). It was assumed that slow drug release through the dialysis membrane under very low drug gradient was the main factor which should have drastically reduced the drug release from the colloidal carriers, as compared to the large drug gradient when a given drug solution concentration is used (Levy and Benita, 1990).

Bulk-equilibrium Reverse Dialysis Sac Technique

To avoid the enclosure of the medicated emulsion in a dialysis bag, the emulsion is directly placed into an appropriate volume of stirred sink solutions, where numerous dialysis sacs containing one ml of the same sink solutions were previously immersed. The dialysis sacs should be equilibrated with the sink solution for a few hours prior to experiments, as recommended by the authors (Levy and Benita, 1990; Santos-Magalhaes *et al.*, 1991a,b, 1995). Again, at predetermined time intervals, a dialysis sac and 1 ml of the sink solution should be withdrawn, and the drug content of the dialysis sac and sink solution should be assayed. The kinetic experiments should be performed at 37°C under constant magnetic stirring. Upon drug emulsion immersion in the sink solution, an infinite dilution is achieved and a new equilibrium is re-established where drug is partitioned between the oily nanodroplets and the sink solution, which become the external phase of the emulsion without being separated from the oily droplets by any artificial membrane. The diffusion of the drug from the oily droplets to the sink solution will be governed by a true and real gradient existing between the oily and the new external aqueous phase. Drugs dissolved in the aqueous phase will then permeate into the dialysis sacs.

As previously reported, the percent drug released will be calculated from the ratio of drug concentration measured at predetermined time intervals in the dialysis bags versus the total concentration of the drug in the sink solution where oily nanodroplets are also present (Levy and Benita, 1990).

The release of drug from the emulsions and respective product into the sink solution was found to be rapid (Levy and Benita, 1990; Santos-Magalhaes *et al.*, 1991a,b, 1995). Practically all the drug is released in the sink solution within less than one hour. No difference in the release profiles of drug from the various dosage forms was observed at a given pH value. These observations were expected since a large dilution (x500) with an aqueous phase was performed. This leads to drug partition largely in favor of the aqueous phase, as was confirmed by the apparent partition coefficient data presented by the authors, who suggested that the overall kinetic process is governed rather by the oil-water partition rate of the emulsion, than by the diffusion rate of the drug through interfacial mixed emulgator film.

It is not yet possible to distinguish whether the drug release from the oily droplets is faster than the permeation rate of the dissolved drug through the dialysis membrane in the enclosed sink solution. This deduction was based on the similarity in the kinetic behavior yielded by the various pharmaceutical dosage forms.

Attempts were made to identify the actual release profile of a drug from a submicron emulsion by designing an *in vitro* kinetic experiment, devoid of any dialysis membrane, based on a centrifugal ultrafiltration technique.

Centrifugal Ultrafiltration Technique

This method was developed by Millipore Corp. (Bedford, MA, USA). The device, mainly based on an Eppendorf centrifuge tube separated from an enclosed tube by an ultrafiltration membrane, allows for separation of nanoparticles from microliter volumes of aqueous dispersion medium in a centrifuge (Ultra-free MC unit). This technique has been successfully applied by Ammoury et al. (1990) to evaluate the *in vitro* release profile of indomethacin from polylactic nanocapsules. Santos-Magalhaes et al. (1991a,b, 1995) adopted the method to evaluate clofibride release from either a submicron emulsion or nanocapsules. 1.0 ml of the clofibride emulsion was directly placed in 250 ml of a stirred buffer sink solution at 37°C. At given time intervals, 400 μl of the release solution, where the emulsion was dispersed, are deposited in the Ultra-free MC unit (10,000 NMWL, low protein binding membrane, PLGC type) which is subjected to centrifugation at $5000 \times g$ for 5 minutes. 50 μl of the ultrafiltrate are then withdrawn and assayed for clofibride content by the HPLC technique. The percent release of clofibride is calculated from the ratio of drug concentration in the ultrafiltrate versus the total concentration of clofibride in the release solution. This technique yielded rapid *in vitro* release profiles of clofibride from the emulsion. 75–90% of the clofibride content is released from the emulsion within 15 minutes, confirming that the kinetic process is probably controlled by the oil-water partition rate of the emulsion under perfect sink conditions. The kinetic results reported by Santos-Magalhaes et al. (1995) clearly exclude the use of submicron emulsions as colloidal controlled release delivery systems for any administration route where perfect sink conditions should prevail. However, this technique might suffer from the drawback that the marked centrifugal force needed to separate the ultrafiltrate from the nanodroplets might alter the emulsion integrity, resulting in a different drug phase distribution profile. Therefore, our laboratory attempted to adapt an ultrafiltration technique at low pressure for the purpose of evaluating drug release profiles for submicron emulsions (Magenheim et al., 1993).

Ultrafiltration Technique at Low Pressure

A certain volume of the medicated emulsion is placed in a stirred cell model 8200 (Amicon, Danvers, MA, USA) containing an adequate volume of sink solution (30–200 ml). At given time intervals aliquots of release medium are filtered through an ultrafiltration membrane (Amicon YM 10 or 100) using nitrogen gas at less than 0.5 bar. The lack of adsorption of the drug on the membrane has first to be established in prior experiments. The clear filtrate, collected at given time intervals, is then analyzed for drug content, using appropriate analytical methods.

It should be emphasized that other types of stirred ultrafiltration cells, such as the UP-110 model of Schleicher and Schuell (Dassel, Germany) could also be used, depending on the final volume of release sink solution needed. The UP model is suitable for release solutions ranging in volume from 200 to 1000 ml.

This approach was used by Benita and Levy (1993) to evaluate the release of diazepam from either a marketed emulsion product, Diazemuls® (Kabivitrum, Sweden) or from a submicron emulsion, the physicochemical properties of which were already reported (Levy and Benita, 1989). The release of diazepam from both emulsions was very rapid It was observed that within a few minutes most of the drug is released from both emulsions, as expected under perfect sink conditions. Moreover, no change in release between both emulsions and a hydroalcoholic solution of diazepam was noted, clearly indicating that the rate-determining step in the overall kinetic process is the partition of the drug in the dispersion system. These results are in agreement with the clinical studies which revealed that no difference in the pharmacokinetic profile of diazepam was noted when the hydroalcoholic marketed solution Valium® was compared to the marketed emulsion Diazemuls® following i.v. administration (Von Dardel et al., 1981). The release of miconazole from either a submicron emulsion or a marketed micellar aqueous solution was also very rapid under perfect sink conditions (Magenheim et al., 1993) confirming the kinetic behavior of diazepam release from the emulsion.

The *in vitro* release kinetic deductions which suggested that the drug release from an emulsion was rapid and mainly governed by a diffusion partition process should be restricted to lipophilic drugs with low log PC, if an attempt to correlate with *in vivo* results is made. Regarding the *in vivo* release kinetics of highly lipophilic drugs from emulsions, it should be pointed out that the drug may remain localized in the oil core despite infinite dilution in the bloodstream and the *in vivo* lipolytic metabolism of the emulsified triglyceride tiny droplets by lipases are likely to contribute to drug release and modification of the pharmacokinetic profile.

THERAPEUTIC APPLICATIONS OF EMULSIONS

This paragraph will first describe the various medical injectable emulsions already on the market as shown in Table 3, a comprehensive description according to therapeutic classes of emulsions in clinical and preclinical stages will then be provided.

I. Marketed Emulsions

Diazemuls® and Diazepam-Lipuro®

Conventional preparations of diazepam for i.v. use contain solvents which cause pain on injection and thrombophlebitis in a high percentage of cases (Von Dardel et al., 1981). However, diazepam can be dissolved with advantage in the oleaginous phase of an oil-in-water emulsion (Diazemuls® and Diazepam-Lipuro®). Diazemuls® is a 0.5% diazepam emulsion. It contains 15% soybean oil, 5% acetylated monoglycerides and 1.2% fractionated egg phospholipids. Glycerol is added as an osmotic agent. Diazemuls® has been given to 9492 patients without serious side-effects. Following i.v. injection, 2435 patients were studied with respect to pain and clinical

Table 3 Marketed emulsion preparations based either on innovative emulsion formulations or commercially available fat emulsion formulations

Emulsion Product	Drug	Company	Indications	Status
Diazemuls®	Diazepam	Kabi-Pharmacia, Dumex, Scandinavia	Status epilepticus, Excitation, Anxiety, Tension, Sedation, Muscle spasm, Convulsions, Tetanus, Delirium treatments	Marketed in Europe, Canada and Australia
Diazepam-Lipuro®	Diazepam	Braun, Germany		
Liple®	Alprostadil (PGE$_1$)	Green Cross, Japan	Peripheral vascular disorders and maintenance of patent ductus arteriosus	Marketed in Japan
Fluosol-DA®	Perfluorodecalin, Perfluorotripropylamine	Green Cross and Alpha Therapeutics	Artificial blood substitutes	Worldwide
Vitalipid®	Vitamins A, D$_2$, E and K$_1$	Kabi-Pharmacia, Sweden	Parenteral nutrition	Marketed in Europe
Diprivan®	Propofol	Zeneca, Pharmaceuticals, U.K.	General anaesthesia	Worldwide
Limethason®	Dexamethasone palmitate	Green Cross, Japan	Chronic rheumatoid arthritis	Marketed in Japan and Germany
Lipo-NSAID® Ropion®	Flurbiprofen axetil	Kaken Pharmaceutical Co., Japan	Post-operative and cancer pain	Japan
Etomidat Lipuro®	Etomidate	Braun, Germany	General anaesthesia	Germany

effect. Only 0.4% experienced pain. The intended clinical effect was recorded in 99% of the patients. I.M. injection of Diazemuls resulted in a significantly smaller frequency of pain in connection with the injection than did the injection of Valium (7% and 43%, respectively). Pharmacokinetic studies have been made after i.v. and i.m. injection of Diazemuls® and Valium®. The distribution and elimination phases after i.v. injection were the same with both forms. Thus the drug probably quickly separated from the oil particles of the emulsion after injection. After i.m. administration, the plasma concentration showed a wide spread with both preparations (Von Dardel *et al.*, 1981).

Liple®

Liple® (5 µg/ml or 10 µg/2ml) is an i.v. injectable prostaglandin E$_1$ (generic name alprostadil) preparation for which lipid droplets are employed as drug carrier. The

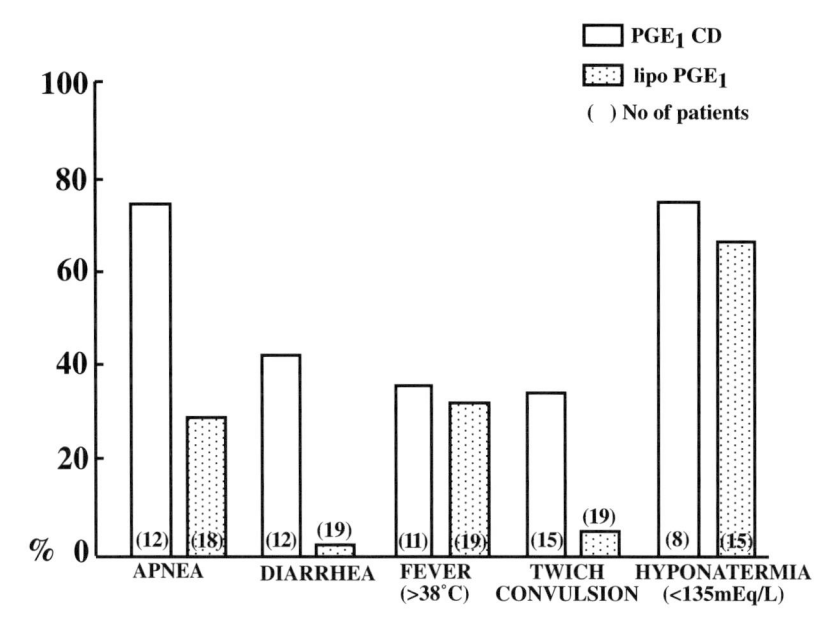

Figure 2 Side effects of PGE$_1$-CD and Lipo-PGE$_1$ in neonates with pulmonary atresia and ductus-dependent pulmonary circulation. According to Momma, 1996.

emulsion contains the active drug (1.8%) and purified soybean oil (10%), high purified yolk lecithin (0.24%), glycerin (2.21%) and water for injection to 100% (Japan Pharmaceutical References). The clinical indications of Liple® are: 1) Buerger's disease and arteriosclerosis obliterans; 2) Improvement of skin ulcers in the following diseases: progressive systemic sclerosis and systemic lupus erythematosus; 3) Improvement of subjective symptoms associated with peripheral vascular disturbances and recovery from peripheral vascular, nervous and kinetic dysfunctions in occupational vibration disease; 4) Patency of ductus arteriosus in ductus dependent congenital heart disease.

Mizushima (1996) claims that Liple® has been widely used in Japan since it was introduced into the Japanese market in 1988 and it is being tested clinically in many countries now.

Momma (1996) treated neonates with critical congenital heart disease and ductus-arteriosus dependent circulation with Lipo-PGE$_1$ emulsion as compared to the conventional PGE marketed product in Japan, PGE$_1$-CD (a cyclodextrin based dosage form from Ono Pharmaceutical, Osaka, Japan). The effective dose was one tenth of the dose of the conventional PGE$_1$ marketed product and the treatment has less side effects such as apnea and diarrhea as shown in Figure 2. Thus Lipo-PGE$_1$ is the first choice for treatment with pulmonary atresia and complete transposition of the great arteries.

Fluosol-DA®

The Fluosol-DA® marketed emulsion and the new generation of perfluorocarbon emulsions are thoroughly discussed in a separate chapter in this book.

Vitalipid®

Vitalipid N Adult and Vitalipid N Infants are mixers of retinol palmitate, ergocaliferol, dl-α-tocopherol and phytomenadione. It has a 2 years shelf life when stored at 2–8°C protected from light.

Diprivan®

Propofol emulsion (Diprivan®, Zeneca, England) is an i.v. injection of 10 mg/ml propofol based on the current commercial Intralipid® emulsion formulation. Propofol has been found useful for three different clinical applications (Deegan, 1992): 1) I.V. bolus for anesthesia induction; 2) I.V. infusion or repeated bolus for maintenance of anesthesia; 3) I.V. infusion or repeated bolus for sedation.

The onset of action is approximately 30 seconds and recovery is usually rapid. The emulsion components are: soybean oil, purified egg phosphatide, NaOH and water.

Deegan (1992) reported that a remarkable feature of propofol is a rapid, smooth recovery which, during administration, allows rapid titration of effect and, after cessation, allows relatively early discharge to the ward or home. Thus, propofol can be expected to facilitate the increasing trend toward day-cease surgery. The apparent safety of propofol in patients with porphyria or malignant hyperthermia susceptibility suggests that propofol may be a valid alternative where barbiturates or inhalational anesthetics are contraindicated. Propofol may also have advantages for ophthalmic and some neurologic surgery. Kirvela et al. (1992) conclude that propofol can be used safely for induction of general anesthesia in uraemic patients. However, cardiovascular and respiratory depression are potentially more serious. Adequate attention to dosage (reduced in elderly), rate of administration of boluses, and concomitant medications (opioids enhance both cardiovascular and respiratory adverse effects) minimize these problems. Pharmacokinetics-based computer-driven infusion regimens allow maintenance of stable hemodynamics and will contribute to the increasing use of propofol. Minor problems of pain on injection and some excitatory phenomena at induction do not significantly limit propofol's use. Doenicke et al. (1996) showed that the cause of pain during the injection is the propofol concentration in the aqueous phase. They suggest to add a fat emulsion to the propofol emulsion before the administration. A higher percentage of water soluble propofol is absorbed by the fat particles reducing the drug concentration in the aqueous phase. Nevertheless, the potential for profound respiratory and cardiovascular depression with propofol requires that its use be largely restricted to situations such as the intensive care unit or operating room where trained personnel and resuscitation equipment are at hand. For these reasons, propofol is not a substitute for the benzodiazepines as an agent of conscious sedation under supervision of the nonanesthesiologist.

Limethason®

Limethason® (4 mg/ml) is an i.v. injectable adrenocorticosteroid preparation that was developed by the Green Cross Corporation. The emulsion formulation is based on the standard marketed fat emulsion formulation in which dexamethasone esterified into more lipid soluble form as dexamethasone palmitate has been incorporated. Dexamethasone palmitate works as a kind of prodrug and in the body it is gradually hydrolized by esterases into its bioactive metabolite, dexamethasone, which demonstrated sustain antiinflammatory effect. Therefore, Limethason® may be used at lower doses than conventional water-soluble dexamethasone drugs and hence this antiinflammatory drug is expected to have reduced risk of steroid-inherent adverse effects. The clinical indication of Limethason® is chronic rheumatoid arthritis (Japan Pharmaceutical Reference).

Limethason® exhibited 2 to 5 times as potent antiinflammatory activity as the water-soluble dexamethasone phosphate on chronic inflammatory disease models (Yokoyama and Watanabe, 1996). The strong anti-inflammatory activity of the drug was primarily based on a high distribution in the inflammatory lesion, a high uptake by macrophages and a suppressive effect on the macrophage function (Yokoyama et al., 1985). A multicenter double-blind comparative clinical trial showed a tendency to a significantly higher rate of improvement with lower frequency of side effects in the Limethason® group than the dexamethasone phosphate group. These results indicate that Limethason® is more useful for rheumatoid arthritis and that the separation of the efficacy and side-effects of steroid could be clinically confirmed to some extent (Yokoyama and Watanabe, 1996).

Lipo-NSAID® — Ropion®

Flurbiprofen axetil, a white emulsion containing 50 mg of flurbiprofen axetil in an ampule (5 ml), was introduced into the Japanese market as an analgesic injection for the treatment of post-operative pain and pain related to various types of cancer in July 1992 (Ohmukai, 1996). Flurbiprofen, a NSAID which strongly inhibits biosynthesis of prostaglandin (Hoshi et al., 1985), the effectiveness (analgesic activity) and safety which have been established, has been extensively used as an oral preparation for clinical practice. However, since the drug is practically insoluble in water like many of the NSAIDs, it is difficult to develop injectable preparations of the drug. Although an injectable flurbiprofen may be prepared using a sodium salt thereof, an injection thus prepared is not suitable for intravenous administration due to irritation at the injection site. Flurbiprofen axetil is a pro-drug prepared by esterification of flurbiprofen which makes the compound lipophilic and soluble in soybean oil within an Intralipid based emulsion formulation. Lipophilic flurbiprofen incorporated into the emulsion can be intravenously administered without irritation. Flurbiprofen axetil is then rapidly hydrolyzed by blood esterase into the active metabolite, flurbiprofen, which makes it possible to secure high blood concentrations and prompt, strong analgesic effects as show in Figure 3 in healthy adult male volunteers. The emulsion exhibits more rapid analgesic effects and less adverse reactions such as gastrointestinal disturbances, than flurbiprofen (Ohmukai, 1996).

Etomidat® — Lipuro

Etomidate is given intravenously for the induction of general anesthesia. One of the major disadvantages of etomidate is the high frequency of pain on injection. A new marketed galenic formulation based on a lipid emulsion for etomidate (Etomidat-Lipuro®, Braun, Melsungen) was compared with the commercial standard (etomidate

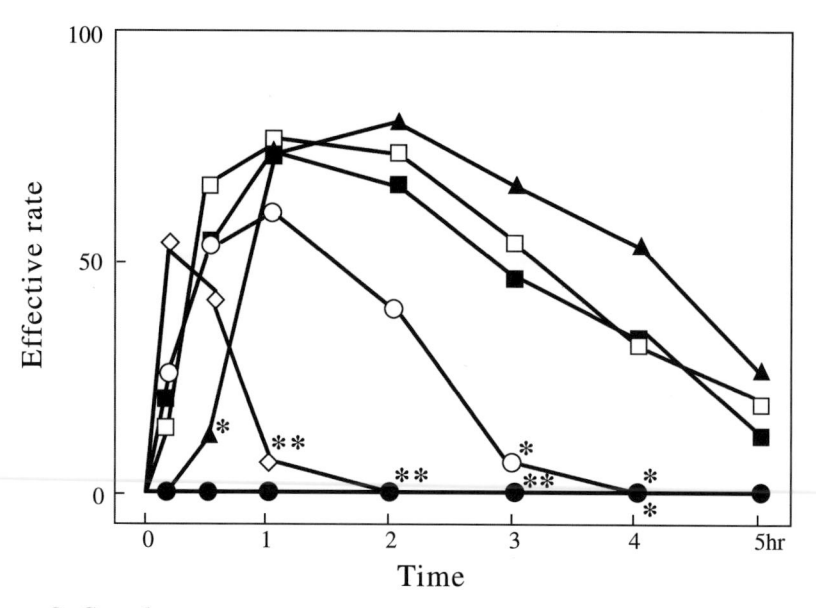

- Control
- Flurbiprofen axetil. 0.5mg/kg (i.v)
- Flurbiprofen. 2mg/kg (p.o.)
- Aspirin-DL-Lysine. 60mg/kg (i.v)
- Ketoprofen. 2mg/kg (i.m.)
- Pentazocine. 3mg/kg (i.m.)

$*p<0.05$. $**P<0.01$: Significant diffrence vs flurbiprofen axetil

Figure 3 Time course of analgesic activities of flurbiprofen axetil and reference compounds on adjuvant induced arthritis pain in rats (n = 10–15). According to Ohumukai, 1996.

in propylene glycol, Hypnomidate, Janssen Pharmaceutica) in a prospective, randomized, double-blind clinical evaluation in 232 patients undergoing elective surgery in general anesthesia (Altmayer et al., 1993). There were marked differences between the two etomidate preparations concerning venous irritation. About 20% of the patients receiving the hypnotic in propylene glycol complained spontaneously of pain on injection, whereas none with the lipid emulsion. No difference was found in the incidence of myoclonic movements. The time interval between the beginning of injection and loss of eyelid closure reflex was about 50 s and not different for the two galenic formulations. Blood pressure during and after induction of anesthesia did not differ. The heart rate in the group of patients with etomidate in lipid emulsion was slightly increased before and immediately after intubation compared to the propylene glycol group. Four percent of the patients in the propylene glycol group suffered from postoperative venous complications as reddening, swelling, induration or pain. These complications could not be seen in the lipid emulsion group.

A second clinical study (Vanacker et al., 1993) was carried out to compare etomidate in a lipid emulsion and in propylene glycol in 90 patients in terms of anesthetic induction characteristics with special reference to injection side effects, haemodynamic changes, and quality of induction. Adrenocortical hormones were determined in 30 patients who received either Etomidat-Lipuro®, Hypnomidate, or propofol (Diprivan®, Zeneca) for induction of anesthesia. It was concluded that local side effects are minimal after the administration of Etomidat-Lipuro® and Hypnomidate. Alfentanil reduces the injection pain of etomidate induction agents. Cortisol and aldosterone are depressed by etomidate as compared to propofol, but the clinical relevance is minimal after a single bolus injection.

II. Emulsion Under Clinical and Preclinical Evaluation

There is no doubt that intensive research efforts have been concentrated on the design of injectable emulsion formulations that led to successful marketed products. Intravenously administered emulsions are excellent carriers for lipophilic drugs which are often difficult to delivery; they are biodegradable, biocompatible, physically stable and relatively easy to produce on large scale. They have been studied widely for parenteral feeding and consequently their preparation, stability and biopharmaceutics are well understood (Mueller and Canham, 1965; Jeppsson, 1972a,b; Kolb and Sailer, 1984; Prankerd and Stella, 1990; Benita and Levy, 1993). In some cases, hydrophobic and amphiphilic drugs can also be incorporated in emulsions provided they can be located at the o/w interface of the dispersed oil droplets. Therefore, numerous potent drugs the formulation of which in conventional aqueous dosage forms is difficult are being investigated while incorporated in a submicron emulsion delivery system. It is not the intention of the present authors to cover all the drugs actually under investigation in an injectable emulsion delivery system but to provide important examples that have been widely reported in the literature in the last few years and to depict them in Table 4. It should be added that the fluorocarbon emulsions will not be discussed in this chapter since they are sufficiently described in another chapter of this book.

Antifungal Agents

Amphotericin B (Am B): Am B is polyene macrocyclic antibiotic derived from *Streptomyces nodosus* which is used for the treatment of fungal infections. Renal disfunction is the best known adverse effect of this drug. Most patients receiving Am B at daily dosage in excess of 0.5mg/kg/day, suffer some degree of kidney damage, often manifested as azotemia and decreased tubular concentrating ability. Am B has high affinity for the fungal membrane sterol-ergosterol, which leads to the antifungal activity. Unfortunately, Am B also binds, though weakly, to mammalian sterols, most probably cholesterol and this is probably the origin of the side effects which can arise when Am B is used clinically. Am B remains the drug of choice for the treatment of a variety of invasive fungal infections. It is active against a broad range of pathogenic fungi and continues to be, after almost 40 years, the standard therapy for the majority of systemic and opportunistic mycoses e.g., Candida spp., Aspergilus spp, Histoplasma capsulatum, Cryptococcus neoformans and Rhizopus spp. all common in patients receiving cytotoxic therapy or immunocompromised patients (Kirsh *et al.*, 1988; Ayestaran *et al.*, 1996; Cleary, 1996; Sorkine *et al.*, 1996). However, the clinical use of Am B is limited by its broad range of potential toxic effects. This drug is highly lipophilic and poorly absorbed orally, thus necessitating

Table 4 Medicated emulsion formulations under preclinical and clinical testing

Drug	Route of Administration	Indication	Clinical Status	Ref.
Amphotericin B	i.v.	Systemic antifungal agent use in neutropenic patients	Phase I	Sorkine et al., 1996
Miconazole	i.v.	Antifungal		Levy et al., 1995
Pregnanolone	i.v.	General anesthesia	Phase I	Gray et al., 1992
Halothane	i.v.	General anesthesia		Johannesson et al., 1984
Isoflurane	i.v.	General anesthesia		Egar and MacLeod, 1995
Palmitoylrhizoxin	i.v.	Cytotoxic, Cancer		Kurihara et al., 1996c
Taxol	i.v.	cytotoxic, cancer		Tarr et al., 1985
Nitrosourea	i.v.	cytotoxic, cancer		Takenaga, 1996
Epirubicin	Transfemoral cannulation or intrahepatic arterial infusion	Chemotherapy, hepatocellular carcinoma	Phase I	Yoshikawa et al., 1994
Penclomedine	i.v.	Cytotoxic, Cancer		Pankerd and Stella, 1988
Cyclosporine	i.v.	Immunosuppressant		Tibell et al., 1995
Isocarbacyclin methyl ester (PGI$_2$)	i.v.	Thrombotic disorders	Phase I	Kurozumi et al., 1996
Perfluorooctyl Bromide, Oxygent®	i.v.	Blood Substitutes	Phase II	Keipert, 1995
Perfluorooctyl Bromide, Imagent®	i.v. and s.c.	Contrast agent	Phase II	Behan et al., 1993

parenteral administration as a mixed micellar dispersion with the surfactant deoxycholate which is often poorly tolerated (Gallis et al., 1990; Caillot et al., 1994; Lance et al., 1995; Cleary, 1996).

The relatively high rate of clinical failures of Am B with the commercial micellar product (Fungizone®) in granulo-cytopenic and other immunocompromised patients could be the result of inadequate local concentrations of the active drug in tissue. Because of its dose-related toxicity the maximal tolerable dose is 0.5 to 1 mg/kg of body weight per day, which may be suboptimal for clinical success (Janknegt et al., 1992).

During the past decade, liposome encapsulation and other colloidal lipid vehicles have been developed to improve the therapeutic index of Am B and reduce its deleterious effects (Gates and Pinney, 1993; Heinemann et al., 1994). A good and comparative description of the various Am B colloidal formulations is provided by Cleary (1996). These colloidal lipid-based delivery systems are reported to reduce the systemic toxicity of Am B and show increased clinical efficacy as compared to the marketed micellar preparation (Janknegt et al., 1992; Heinemann, 1994). Three different colloidal lipid preparations are currently marketed and available in clinical practice as depicted in Table 5. A major drawback is that these new formulations

Table 5 Amphotericin B formulations according to Cleary (1996)

Category	Amphotericin B (Fungizone)	Amphotericin B Lipid Complex (ABLC)	Amphotericin B Colloidal Dispersion (Amphocil)	Liposomal Amphotericin B (AmBisome)	Amphotericin B in Lipid Emulsion (ABLE)
sterol	none	none	cholesterol sulfate	cholesterol sulfate	safflower and soybean oils
phospholipid	none	DMPC and DMPG	none	EPC and DSPG	EPC
Amphotericin B (mole%)	34	33	50	10	variable
Size (nm)	<10	1600–11,000	122 ± 48	80–120	333–500
Manufacturer	Squibb, Lyphomed	Liposome Inc.	Sequus	Nextar	not applicable
Stability	1 wk at 2–8°C or 24 h at 27°C	15 h at 2–8°C or 6 h at 27°C	under investigation	24 h at 2–8°C	months at 4°C
Dosage and rate	0.3–1.0 mg/kg/d	under investigation: 5 mg/kg/d at 2.5 mg/kg/h	under investigation	under investigation: 1–3 mg/kg/d over 30–60 min	investigational: 1.0 mg/kg/d over 1–8 h
Lethal dose 50% (mg/kg)	3.3	10–25	68	175	unknown

DMPC = dimyristoyl phosphatidylcholine; DMPG = dimyristoyl phosphatidylglycerol; DSPG = distearoyl phosphatidylglycerol; EPC = egg phosphatidylcholine.

are very expensive (Pascual *et al.*, 1995; Cleary, 1996). Thus, efforts have been made to develop alternative and less expensive lipid formulations based either on the extemporaneous addition of the drug to commercially available fat emulsions or de novo emulsification as reported by Davis *et al.* (1987).

Kirsh *et al.* (1988) described extemporaneous addition of Am B to Intralipid® 20% (Kabi-Pharmacia). First, the Am B was solubilized in sodium deoxycholate/dimethylacetamide solution and filtered to remove unsolubilized drug. Then, a measured volume was added to a vial containing Intralipid® 20% under aseptic conditions to a final concentration of a 1 mg/ml of Am B. This extemporaneous drug emulsion remains stable for 1 year at 4°C when protected from sunlight. The emulsions formulation exhibits the same MIC for *Candida albicans* as Fungizone® preparation. Numerous studies clearly showed that the Am B fat emulsion combination elicited reduced nephrotoxicity while preserving the antifungal activity of Am B.

An alternative emulsion-based delivery system was developed using "*De novo emulsification*". Davis *et al.* (1985, 1987) described *De novo emulsification* in which the Am B (final concentration 1 or 2 mg/ml) is dissolved in methanol and then mixed with water containing the emulsifier (egg lecithin). After evaporation of the methanol, the oily phase (final volume fraction 20%) was added and the system was emulsified using sonic probe. This emulsion was reported to be stable for 7 months regarding to Am B content and droplet size distribution. *In vivo* experiment in murine candidiasis indicated ED_{50} of 0.78 mg/kg for Fungizone and less than 0.5 mg/kg for the emulsion. Equally important, the reduced toxicity of the emulsion formulation allowed the use of much higher doses of Am B with pronounced therapeutic benefit. The pharmacokinetics of conventional formulations versus fat emulsion formulations of Am B in a group of patients with neutropenia were recently studied (Ayestaran *et al.*, 1996; Villani *et al.*, 1996). The pharmacokinetic behavior was different. In view of the limited toxicity and reduced concentration of the drug in serum with the fat emulsion formulation, it is possible to consider its use in certain clinical situations in which higher doses of Am B are necessary.

Furthermore, Sorkine *et al.* (1996) compared the efficacy and tolerance of Am B administered in 5% dextrose or administered in Intralipid 20% in critically ill patients. The results of the study indicated that Am B in lipid emulsion compared with regular Am B was as effective in eradicating Candida infections; was better tolerated due to the diminished frequency and severity of immediate side effects (hypotension, chills, fever, anaphylaxis); and was causing significantly less renal impairment as clearly evidenced by the results presented in Figure 4.

The conclusion arises from that data is that clinical and renal toxicity of Am B are reduced when the drug is prepared in fat emulsion. Preparation is simple and cost effective. Its efficacy is similar to that of conventional Am B.

Miconazole: Miconazole is a synthetic imidazole with a broad spectrum of antifungal activity. It is poorly absorbed by the oral route and is used primarily as a topical agent for cutaneous mycoses and as an alternative systemic antifungal agent when Am B is either ineffective or contraindicated. The therapeutic use of miconazole yielded encouraging results (Levy *et al.*, 1995), but due to the potential toxicity of the miconazole vehicle excipients rather than to the drug molecule itself, the place of this drug in the therapy of fungal disease remains uncertain since its role has never

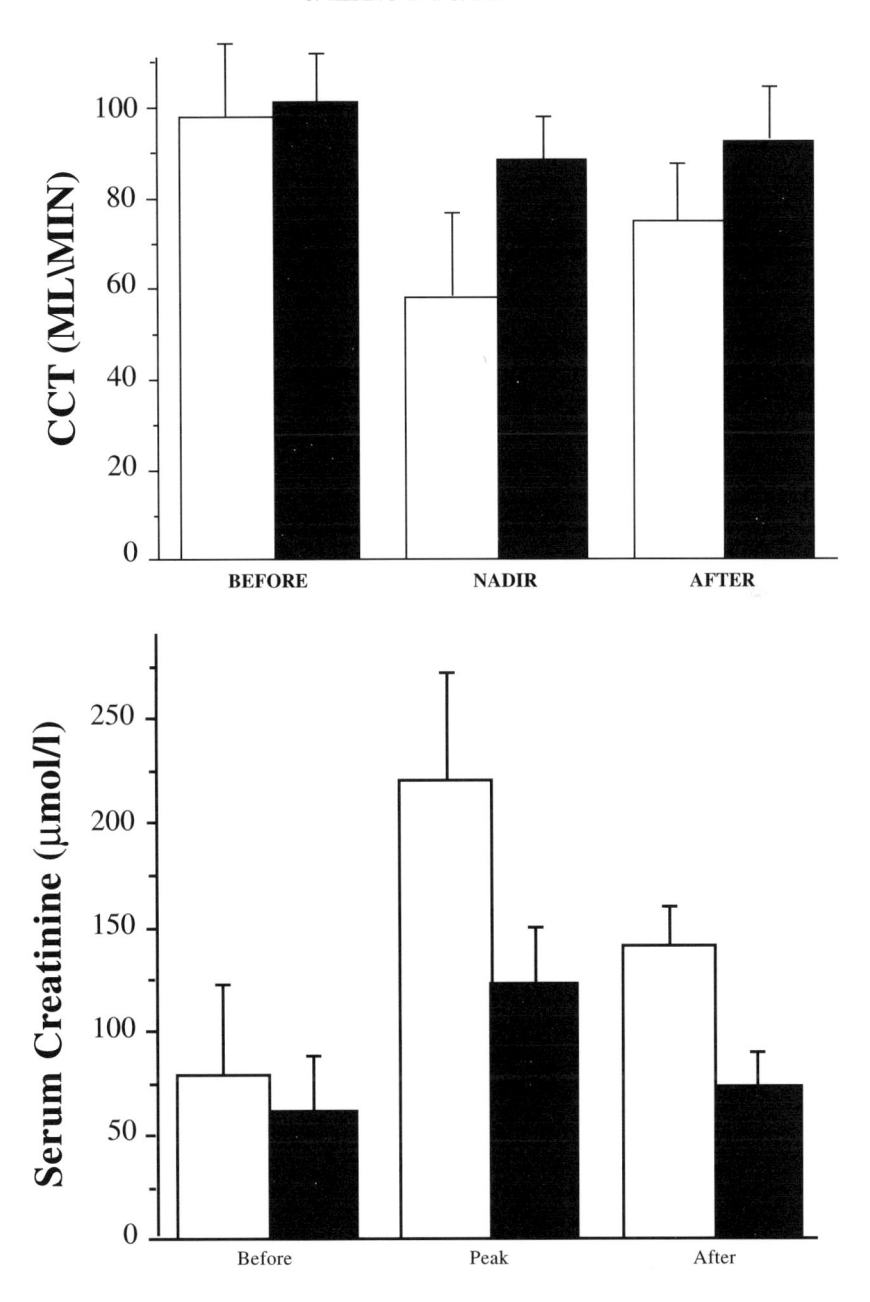

Figure 4 Comparison of the effects on renal function between amphotericin B in 20% lipid emulsion vs. 5% dextrose in water. Values are expressed as mean ± SEM. Group A (solid bars), in which amphotericin B was given in 5% dextrose in water; Group B (open bars) in which amphotericin B was given in a lipid emulsion. *Before,* before amphotericin B therapy; *Nadir,* nadir of creatinine clearance test during amphotericin B therapy; *After,* 1 day after cessation of amphotericin B therapy. *p < 0.05 compared with baseline values. Top graph represents the creatinine clearance test (CCT). Bottom graph represents serum creatinine concentration in the two groups respectively. A decline in renal function was noted in group A, with partial resolution after the cessation of therapy. According to Sorkine *et al.*, 1996.

been defined properly. Severe adverse effect of the marketed aqueous micellar formulations Monistat® or Daktarin® include mainly anaphylaxis, phlebitis and thrombocytosis, especially because of Cremophor EL, a surfactant needed for the micellar solubilization of miconazole (Stevens, 1983).

Levy et al. (1995) demonstrated that miconazole emulsion based on phospholipid, deoxycholic acid, and poloxamer 188 was better tolerated than Daktarin® in the BALB/c mice showing an improved ratio of 1 to 3 in favor of the emulsion. The study also showed that the submicron miconazole emulsion was more effective than Daktarin in the treatment of murine cryptococcosis. They deduced that the emulsion enhanced moderately drug permeation through the blood brain barrier compared to the corresponding micellar solution of miconazole since *Cryptococcus neoformans* is a neutrotropic pathogenic yeast-like fungus which preferentially multiplies in the brain.

Anaesthetic agents

Pregnanolone: Pregnanolone is a naturally occuring metabolite of progesterone with an anaesthetic activity but without endocrine action. The anaesthetic properties of steroids have been appreciated for 50 years (Gray et al., 1992). Seley (1941) found that pregnanedione was the most potent of 75 different steroid preparations studied for their anaeshetic properties. There has been a long delay in the practical development of this knowledge because hormonal effects had to be separated from anaesthetic properties, and these highly lipophilic substances had to be prepared in a formulation suitable for i.v. use.(24). Carl et al. (1990) prepared a "*de novo*" emulsion containing pregnanolone (4mg), soybean oil (200mg), acetyltriglycerides (70mg), egg yolk phosphatides (18mg), glycerol (17mg), and water to 1ml. Kabi 2213 emulsion is a preparation of pregnanolone dissolved in the oil phase of an oil in water emulsion (10% Intralipid®). Gray et al. (1992) reported that pregnanolone emulsion administered to 13 healthy volunteers was found to produce smooth and reliable induction of general anaesthesia with cardiorespiratory effects comparable to those of the i.v. induction agents.

Halothane: The intravenous administration of volatile anaesthetics has many advantages over inhalational delivery. Induction of anaesthesia would be rapid as equilibrium with the anaesthetic circuitry and the lungs functional residual capacity is circumvented. Capital and maintenance cost of anaesthetic equipment could be reduced as the need for an agent specific vaporiser would be eliminated. Halothane and Isoflurane are anaesthetic agents both given by inhalation. Johannesson et al. (1984) investigated the extemporaneous incorporation of liquid halothane into Intralipid® 20% by vigorously shaking. When administered i.v. to rats, this emulsion behaves as a potent preparation with fast recovery. Safety margin between effective dose and lethal dose was narrow for rats. Biber et al. (1982) compared intravenously halothane emulsified in Intralipid and halothane inhalation in dogs. No untoward events were noted nor were any microvascular changes seen. It was concluded that this formulation might prove useful for experimental animals when a short term readily controllable anaesthesia is required.

Isoflurane: Extemporaneous addition of Isoflurane to Intralipid emulsion were prepared by Egar and MacLeod (1995). They calculate the ED_{50} and LD_{50} following single i.v. bolus injection in mice. They concluded that i.v. induction and maintenance with emulsified Isoflurane in Intralipid® can be carried out with safety and reproducibility in the mouse. The only negative effect was local skin ulceration with an inadvertent interstitial injection.

Cytotoxic Agents

This therapeutic class of potent drugs includes many active molecules with different pharmacological mechanisms but most of them are lipophilic and exhibit poor aqueous solubility. Therefore, the potential benefit of incorporating such potent drugs in submicron emulsions which are considered to be adequate vehicles for lipophilic molecules has been extensively investigated. Only part of the published results will be reported herewith.

Rhizoxin: Rhizoxin is a cytotoxic and anti-fungal drug that inhibits tubulin polymerization (Takahashi et al., 1987). The water solubility of rhizoxin is 12 µg/mL while the solubility in soybean oil was found to be 2 mg/mL. Dilution of the reconstituted injection with 10% Intralipid® did not result in precipitation. This approach could therefore be used for slow intravenous infusion of the drug. Rhizoxin is also subject to degradation in aqueous solution, giving a narrow V-shaped pH-rate profile with maximum stability at pH≈5.6. As discussed above, incorporation of a hydrolytically susceptible drug into an emulsion can reduce hydrolysis. However, the aqueous stability of rhizoxin did not seem to improve by dilution with Intralipid® (Prankerd and Stella, 1988). Despite the preferential oil solubility of rhizoxin over the aqueous solubility, part of the rhizoxin still remained localized in the aqueous phase where it could be easily degraded as confirmed by the results previously mentioned. Thus, to favor the localization of this cytotoxic drug in the inner oil phase of an emulsion, a palmitoyl derivative (13-O-palmitoyl-rhizoxin) which is much more lipophilic than rhizoxin was synthesized (log P = 14 instead of log P = 2 for the free drug).

Kurihara et al. (1996a,b) prepared *"de novo"* emulsions containing 13-O-palmitoyl-rhizoxin The formulation contained soybean oil or dioctanoyldecanoylglycerol (as the oily phase), polyoxyethylene-(60)-hydrogenated castor oil (as nonionic surfactant), egg yolk lecithin and water. The emulsification process was done using Microfluidizer resulting in emulsions with droplet size of 208–211nm. The emulsion that contains the non-ionic surfactant and and dioctanoyldecanoylglycerol was tested *in vivo*. Their results indicated that the emulsion are relatively stable to lipolysis by lipoprotein lipase both *in vitro* and *in vivo* compared to the same colloidal solution. In addition, by properly selecting particle size (smaller rather than larger oil droplet size), the emulsions showed high concentration of palmitoyl rhizoxin in tumors of mice bearing the solid tumor M 5076 sarcoma (Kurihara et al., 1996c). The emulsion effectively retarded the tumor growth and increased survival time.

Taxol: Taxol is a poorly water soluble plant product isolated from several species of Western yew. It exhibits excellent antimitotic properties and is presently clinically well accepted for metastatic carcinoma ovary and metastatic breast cancer treatment. Taxol shows confirmed activity against several tumor systems including leukemia, colon, melanoma, and Lewis lung tumor systems. In addition to its antitumor activity, taxol may also be helpful as a tumor cell synchronizing agent. The mechanism of its antimitotic activity appears to be due to its ability to alter normal microtubule assembly and thus cause mitotic arrest (Tarr *et al.*, 1987). Taxol is extremely hydrophobic, therefore the commercially available concentrate for injection is a sterile solution of the drug in Cremophor® EL and dehydrated alcohol (Paclitaxel®, 6 mg/ml Taxol)).

Tarr *et al.* (1997) prepared an emulsion consisting of triacetin, soybean lecithin, pluronic F68, polysorbate 80 and ethyl oleate. Glycerol can be added to the emulsion at a concentration of 10% to prevent creaming. A stable emulsion was found at Taxol concentration of 10 and 15 mg/ml of emulsion. The emulsion gave a 1 μm average diameter droplet with droplet size ranging from 0.5 to 5 μm. The average droplet size grew to 2 μm within 1 week and in 2 month period the mean droplet size increased to 4 μm. Phase separation was observed after 6 months. Comparative hemolysis testing of 10 mg/ml Taxol emulsion proved that it is less hemolytic than 20% Intralipid® emulsion. The acute toxicity of the emulsion excipients alone showed no toxicity when administered at a dose five times greater than that of the concentration in the Taxol emulsion. The acute toxicity of the Taxol emulsion included lethargy, ataxia and respiratory depression.

Penclomedine: Penclomedine is a novel cytotoxic agent which has shown activity in several tumor model systems when screened as an aqueous suspension by the National Cancer Institute. An intravenous formulation of this compound was required for further biological testing, with a drug concentration of 1–5 mg/ml. Penclomedine is extremely insoluble in water and its solubility is low in other hydrogen-bonded co-solvent systems, e.g., 40% propylene glycol/10% ethanol/50% water. However, its solubility is high in hydrocarbon solvents and in vegetable oils, and exceedingly high in polar aprotic solvents, such as DMSO and DMA. The drug is currently under Phase I evaluation (Waud *et al.*, 1997).

Attempts to incorporate penclomedine into Intralipid® using the extemporaneous approach failed. Precipitation of the drug was detected a few hours after dilution in both Intralipid® 10% or 20%. Experiments were therefore performed with the objective of preparing *de novo* emulsions in which penclomedine was pre-dissolved in the oil phase. O/W emulsions were prepared with a formulation similar to that employed for Intralipid® 10% using Polytron® homogenizer and Microfluidizer®. Chemical stability and physical stability were monitored with no significant changes after 12 months. An emulsion containing 4.7 mg/mL of penclomedine was tested for anti-tumor activity in a mouse i.p. tumor model (P388 leukemia). The emulsion formulation was seen to be more active, as judged from median survival times, and less toxic than a suspension of the drug. The emulsion formulation was also active by the i.v. route of administration, suggesting facile transport of penclomedine across biological membranes. This finding encouraged a subsequent evaluation of the emulsion formulation as a means of oral administration of penclomedine (Prankerd and Stella, 1988).

Nitrosourea: Lomustine [1-(2-chloroehtyl)-3-cyclohexyl-1-nitrosourea; CCNU] is a very rapidly hydrolyzed nitrosourea cytotoxic agent. Its *in vivo* distribution pattern in rabbits following intravenous administration as an emulsion formulation was found not to be significantly different from that of aqueous solutions. The formulation was prepared by dilution of an ethanol solution of Lomustine into Intralipid®. However, it was not determined whether or not the emulsion formulation increased the stability of the drug to hydrolysis.

Semustine [1-(2-chlroethyl)-3-(trans-4-methylcyclohexyl-1-nitrosourea (methyl-CCNU] is another unstable cytotoxic nitrosourea which has been formulated in an i.v. emulsion dosage form. It was claimed that the drug was stable for 78 hours at room temperature.

Takenaga (1996) investigated lipid microspheres (lipid emulsion) as a carrier for 1,3-bis (2-chloroethyl)-1-nitrosourea (BCNU). These lipid microspheres showed a significantly enhanced antitumor activity with reduced toxicity in mice with L1210 leukemia when compared to the corresponding dose of free BCNU. The biodistribution of the lipid microspheres with 200 nm size, showed a retention of the microspheres in the tumor up to 0.5 hours after preparation while microspheres with 140 nm size accumulated at tumor sites up to 4 hours after injection.

Lipiodol emulsion containing Epirubicin (4-Epidoxorubicin)

Lipiodol (Lipiodol Ultra-Fluid: Laboratoire Guerbet, France), is a radiologic contrast agent derived by iodinization of poppyseed oil. When administered via the hepatic artery, it is retained by hepatocellular carcinoma for prolonged periods of time. This unusual property of Lipiodol has been exploited therapeutically using the oil as a vehicle for targeted intra-arterial delivery of cytotoxic drugs or radioisotopes to unresectable hepatocellular carcinoma. Drugs that have been conjugated to Lipiodol include doxorubicin, epirubicin, 5-fluorouracil, cisplatin, mitomycin, aclarubicin and maleic acid neocarzinostatin (Nakamura *et al.*, 1990; Konno, 1992; Yoshikawa *et al.*, 1994; de Baere, 1995; Bhattacharya, 1995). Therefore, lipiodol emulsion was mixed with anticancer drugs in an attempt to retain anticancer drugs in the target tumor.

Aoyama *et al.* (1992) compared the survival of patients treated with Lipiodol 4'-epi-doxorubicin emulsion or Lipiodol doxorubicin followed by gelatin sponge to gelatin sponge only. He showed an improvement in the medicated emulsions caused by the direct embolization effect of Lipiodol and the anticancer agent slowly released from it. No significant difference in survival was found between patients treated with Lipiodol containing anticancer drugs. Yoshikawa *et al.* (1994) conducted a prospective randomized trial to evaluate the efficacy of Lipiodol in intrahepatic arterial infusion chemotherapy for patients with hepatocellular carcinoma (HCC). A total of 38 patients with unresectable HCCs and underlying cirrhosis were entered in this trial, and 36 of then were evaluable. Every 4 weeks, 17 patients received 70 mg of 4'-epidoxorubicin (epirubicin) alone (group A), whereas 19 patients received a Lipiodol emulsion containing the same dose of epirubicin (group B) through the hepatic artery. A tumor response (complete and partial) was observed in 12% of group A patients and in 42% of group B patients. The group B patients showed a significantly higher response rate than the group A patients. There was a tendency for an increased duration of survival ($P = 0.09$) in the group B patients. These results suggested that the infusion of the Lipiodol emulsion with epirubicin was more effective than epirubicin alone for the treatment of these patients with HCC.

Other miscellaneous compounds

Cyclosporine A: Cyclosporine A (CyA) is an immunosuppressive agent used in organ transplantation because of its specific mode of action on the T-cells and its lack of myelotoxicity. CyA is a lipophilic drug and its highly bound to body tissues (Shah et al., 1991). The commercially available intravenous preparation of CyA (Sandimmun®), contains Cremophor ® EL which may contribute to the nephrotoxicity observed during i.v. administration. It is also believed to be the cause of anaphylactic reactions reported in connection with Sandimmun® infusions (Besarb et al., 1987). The compatibility of CyA with fat emulsion was studied using 10% or 20% fat emulsion. Jacobson et al. (1993) showed that 0.5 or 2mg/ml of CyA were compatible with 10% or 20% fat emulsion at 23–25°C in glass containers for up to 48 hours. CyA retained more than 96% of its initial concentration in the admixtures, there were no changes in the color or consistency and the pH did not vary by more than 0.11 pH unit. Tibell et al. (1993, 1995) found in a rat model that the administration of CyA incorporated in a soybean oil-based fat emulsion did not influence the glomerular filtration rate, while the infusion of Sandimmun® was associated with an acute decrease in glomerular filtration. The soybean oil carrier did not impair the immunosuppressive effects of CyA when tested in the heterotopic heart transplant model in rats. Pharmacokinetics and tissue distribution were done in several studies. Shah et al. (1991) found in rabbits that co-administration of Intralipid® with CyA decreased both total clearance and volume of distribution in steady state, resulting in a rapid elimination, i.e. decrease in $t_{1/2}$ of CyA from the body. Tissue distribution in rats (Tibell et al., 1995) was not significantly different when comparing Sandimmun® to soybean emulsion, iodized ester of poppy seed oil emulsion and liposomal preparation of CyA. All formulations gave the highest tissue concentrations in the liver followed by the spleen and the kidneys.

Prostacyclin (PGI$_2$): Generation of prostacyclin (PGI$_2$) from endothelial cells is crucial for the maintenance of homeostasis of vasostream, as PGI$_2$ counteracts thromboxane generated from platelets. The sodium salt of PGI$_2$ is formulated in an injectable aqueous solution indicated for dialysis, congestive heart failure and pulmonary hypertension with limited dosage due to side effects such as hypotension, flushing, nausea and so on (Kurozumi et al., 1996). A lipophilic form of prostacyclin, isocarbacyclin methyl ester was incorporated in a lipid emulsion. The methyl ester lipophilic prodrug of isocarbacyclin, a PGI$_2$ agonist was formulated as an emulsion because of 3 hypotheses: 1) the lipid microspheres (oil droplets) would deliver the active drug to the disease area, 2) the drug would be released there gradually from the microspheres (oil droplets) and 3) the isocarbacyclin methyl ester would be hydrolyzed to the isocarbacyclin (active form) by esterase action to exert its pharmacological action. Kurozumi et al. (1996) showed that this formulation increased the vertebral and femoral blood flow in dogs. An anti-platelets effect of this formulation was also observed at a dose less than the dose that elicits hypotensive effect following both bolus i.v. and venous infusion in rabbits. The results indicated that the lipid microspheres possessed both highly potent vasodilative activity and anti-platelets activity like PGI_2. Furthermore, they showed that administration of this formulation resulted in significant improvement in regional cerebral blood supply in stroked rats, and suggested that this preparation would be effective for patients with stroke. Another indication which was tested included therapy of peripheral vascular disorders in rats and the results suggested that this formulation would be very useful clinically for the therapy of peripheral vascular disorders. Phase I studies were carried out on patients with ischemic cerebral disorders such as acute and chronic cerebral thrombosis and patients with peripheral vascular disorders (arteriosclerosis obliterans, thromboangitis obliterans). Patients with cerebral disorders exhibit a significant improvement of observed symptoms and for patients with peripheral vascular disorders there were significant reduction in ulcer area. No serious side effect such as vessel inflammation or hypotension was observed during the therapeutic period. A pilot study of the lipid microspheres on post percutaneous transluminal colonary arterioplasty (PTCA) restenosis was carried out using 37 patients in which the isocarbacyclin lipid microspheres was compared with an aspirin treatment group. Angiographical examinations at 4 months after (PTCA) treatment showed that the isocarbacyclin oil microspheres group had a smaller patient restenosis ratio as well as a lesion restenosis ratio than control (aspirin treated) group (Muramatsu et al., 1991).

REFERENCES

Altmayer, P., Grundmann, U., Ziehmer, M., Larsen, R. (1993) Comparative effectiveness and tolerance study of a new galenic etomidate formula. *Anasthesiol. Intensivmed. Notfallmed. Schmerzther.*, **28**(7), 41–419.

Ammoury, N., Fessi, H., Devissaguet, J.P., Puisieux, F., Benita, S. (1989) Physicochemical characterization of polymeric nanocapsules and *in vitro* release evaluation of indomethacin as a drug model. *S.T.P. Pharma.*, **5**, 647–651.

Ammoury, N., Fessi, H., Devissaguet, J.P., Puisieux, F., Benita, S.J. (1990) *In vitro* release kinetic pattern of indomethacin from poly (d,l-lactide) nanocapsules. *J. Pharm. Sci.*, **79**, 763–767.

Aoyama, K., Tsukishiro, T., Okada, K., Tsuchida, T., Aiba, N., Nambu, S., Miyabayashi, C., Yasuyama, T., Higuchi, K., Watanabe, A. (1992) Evaluation of transcatheter arterial embolization with epirubicin-lipiodol emulsion for hepatocellular carcinoma. *Cancer Chemother. Pharmacol.*, **31**(Suppl I), S35-S59.

Ayestarán, A., López, R.M., Montoro, J.B., Estíbalez, A., Pou, L., Julia, A., López, A., Pascual, B. (1996) Pharmacokinetics of conventional formulation versus fat emulsion formulation of amphotericin B in a group of patients with neutropenia. *Antimicrob. Agents Chemother.*, **40**(3), 609–612.

Bach, A., Guisard, D., Metais, P., Debry, G. (1972) Metabolic effects following a short and medium chain triglycerides load in dogs. I. Infusion of an emulsion of short and medium chain triglycerides. *Arch. Sci. Physiol.*, **26**, 121–129.

Bangham, A.D. (1968) Membrane models with phospholipids. *Prog. Biophys. Mol. Biol.*, **18**, 29–95.

Benita, S., Friedman, D., Weinstock, M. (1986) Physostigmine emulsion: A new injectable controlled release delivery system. *Int. J. Pharm.*, **30**, 47–55.

Benita, S., Friedman, D., Weinstock, M. (1986) Pharmacological evaluation of an injectable prolonged release emulsion of physostigmine in rabbits. *J. Pharm. Pharmacol.*, **38**, 653–658.

Benita, S., Levy, M.Y. (1993) Submicron emulsions as colloidal drug carriers for intravenous administration: comprehensive physicochemical characterization. *J. Pharm. Sci.*, **82**(1), 1069–1079.

Besarab, A., Jarrell, B.E., Hirsch, S., Carabasi, R.A., Cressman, M.D., Green, P. (1987) Use of the isolated perfused kidney model to assess the acute pharmacological effects of cyclosporine and its vehicle Cremophor EL. *Transplantation*, **44**, 195–201.

Bhattacharya, S., Novell, J.R., Dusheiko, G.M., Hilson, A.J., Dick, R., Hobbs, K.E. (1995) Epirubicin-lipiodol chemotherapy versus [131]iodine-lipiodol radiotherapy in the treatment of unresectable hepatocellular carcinoma. *Cancer*, **76**, 2202–2210.

Biber, B., Martner, J., Werner, O. (1982) Halothane by the iv route in experimental animals. *Acta Anaesthesiol. Scand.*, **26**, 658–659.

Boyett, J.B., Davis, C.W. (1989) Injectable emulsions and suspensions. In *Pharmaceutical dosage forms: disperse systems*, edited by H.A. Leiberman, M.M. Rieger, G.S. Banker, vol. 2, pp. 379–416. New York: Marcel Dekker, Inc.

Burnham, W.R., Hansrani, P.K., Knott, C.E., Cook, J.A., Davis, S.S. (1983) Stability of fat emulsion based intravenous feeding mixture. *Int. J. Pharm.*, **13**, 9–22.

Caillot, D., Reny, G., Solary, E., Casasnovas, O., Chavanet, P., Bonnotle, B., *et al.* (1994) A controlled trial of the tolerance of amphotericin B infused in dextrose or in Intralipid in patients with haematological malignancies. *J. Antimicrob. Chemother.*, **33**, 603–613.

Carl, P., Høgskilde, Nielsen, J.W., Sørensen, M.B., Lindholm, M., Karlen, B., Bäckstrøm, T. (1990) Pregnanolone emulsion: a preliminary pharmacokinetic and pharmacodynamic study of a new intravenous anaesthetic agent. *Anaesth.*, **45**, 189–197.

Cleary, J.D. (1996) Amphotericin B formulated in a lipid emulsion. *Ann. Pharmacother.*, **30**, 409–412.

Davis, S.S. (1982) The stability of fat emulsions for intravenous administration. In *Current Perspectives in the Use of Lipid Emulsion*, edited by I.D. Johnston, pp. 35–61. 2nd Int. Sym. Advan. Clin. Nutr., Bermuda. Lancaster, UK: MTP Press.

Davis, S.S., Galloway, M. (1981) Effects of blood plasma components on the properties of intravenous fat emulsion. *J. Pharm. Pharmacol.*, **33** (Suppl.), 88P.

Davis, S.S., Hadgraft, J., Palin, K.J. (1985) Medical and pharmaceutical application of emulsions. In *Encyclopedia of emulsion technology*, edited by P. Becher, vol. 2, pp. 159–238. New York: Marcel Dekker, Inc.

Davis, S.S., Washington, C., West, P., Illum, L. (1987) Lipid emulsions as drug delivery systems. *Ann. N.Y. Acad. Sci.*, **507**, 75–88.

Dawes, W.H., Groves, M.J. (1978) The effect of electrolytes on phospholipid-stabilized soybean oil emulsion. *Int. J. Pharm.*, **1**, 141–150.

de Baere, T., Dufaux, J., Roche, A., Counnord, J.-L., Berthault, M-F., Denys, A., Pappas, P. (1995) Circulatory alterations induced by intra-arterial injection of iodized oil and emulsions of iodized oil and doxorubicin: experimental study. *Radiology*, **194**, 165–170.

Deegan, R.J. (1992) Propofol: A review of the pharmacology and applications of an intravenous anesthetic agent. *Am. J. Med. Sci.*, **304**(1), 45–49.

Doenicke, A.W., Roizen, M.F., Rau, J., Kellermann, W., Babl, J. (1996) Reducing pain during propofol injection: The role of the solvent. *Anesth. Analg.*, **82**, 472–474.

Eger, T.P., MacLeod, B.A. (1995) Anaesthesia by intravenous emulsified isoflurane in mice. *Can. J. Anaesth.*, **42**, 173–176.

Gallis, H.A., Drew, R.H., Packard, W.W. (1990) Amphotericin B: 30 years of clinical experience. *Rev. Infect. Dis.*, **12**, 308–329.

Gates, C., Pinney, R.J. (1993) Amphotericin B and its delivery by liposomal and lipid formulations. *J. Clin. Pharm. Ther.*, **18**, 147–253.

Gershanik, T., Benita, S. (1996) Positively charged self-emulsifying oil formulation for improving oral bioavailability of progesterone. *Pharm. Develop. and Technol.*, **1**(2), 147–157.

Goodman and Gilman (1995) In *The Pharmacological Basis of Therapeutics*, 9th ed., edited by J.G. Hardman, A. Goodman Gilman, L.E. Limbird, pp. 1707–1792. New York: McGraw-Hill.

Gray, H.St.J., Holt, B.L., Whitaker, D.K., Eadsforth, P. (1992) Preliminary study of a pregnanolone emulsion (Kabi 2213) for i.v. induction of general anaesthesia. *Br. J. Anaesth.*, **68**, 272–276.

Guisard, D., Bach, A., Debry, G., Metais, P. (1972) Metabolic effects following a short and medium chain triglycerides load in dogs. II. Influence of the infused fat quantity. *Arch. Sci. Physiol.*, **26**, 195–205.

Hansrani, P.K., Davis, S.S., Groves, M.J. (1983) The preparation and properties of sterile intravenous emulsions. *J. Parenter. Sci. Technol.*, **37**, 145–150.

Hara, T., Liu, F., Liu, D., Huang, L. (1997) Emulsion formulations as a vector for gene delivery *in vitro* and *in vivo*. *Advanced Drug Delivery Reviews*, **24**, 265–274.

Hashida, M., Yoshioka, T., Muranishi, S., Sezaki, H. (1980) Dosage form characteristics of microspheres in oil emulsions. I: Stability and drug release. *Chem Pharm. Bull.*, **28**, 1009–1015.

Heinemann, V., Kähny, B., Debus, A., Wachholz, W., Jehn, U. (1994) Pharmacokinetics of liposomal amphotericin B (Ambisome) vs other lipid based formulations. *Bone Marrow Transplant*, **14**(Suppl 5), S8–S9.

Herman, C.J., Groves, M.J. (1993) The influence of free fatty acid formation on the pH of phospholipid-stabilized triglyceride emulsions. *Pharm. Res.*, **10**(5), 774–776.

Hoshi, K., Mizushima, Y., Shiokawa, Y. (1985) Double-blind study with liposteroid in rheumatoid arthritis. *Drugs Exp. Clin. Res.*, **11**, 621–626.

Hunter, R.J. (1981) Ch. 7. In *Zeta Potential in Colloid Science*, pp. 59–124. London: Academic Press.

Jacobson, P.A., Maksym, C.J., Landvay, A., Weiner, N., Whitmore, R. (1993) Compatability of cyclosporine with fat emulsion. *Am. J. Hosp. Pharm.*, **50**(4), 687–690.

Janknegt, R., De Marie, S., Bakker-Woudenberg, I.A.J.M., Crommelin, D.J.A. (1992) Liposomal and lipid formulations of amphotericin B. *Clin. Pharmacokinet.*, **23**, 279–291.

Japan pharmaceutical reference. Administration and products in Japan (1993) Japan Medical Products International Trade Association, 3rd edition.

Jeppsson, R. (1972a) Effect of barbituric acids using an emulsion form intravenously. *Acta Pharm. Svecica*, **9**, 81–90.

Jeppsson, R. (1972b Effect of barbituric acids using an emulsion form intraperitoneally and subcutaneously *Acta Pharm. Svecica*, **9**, 199–206.

Johanesson G., Biber, A.P., Lennander, O., Werner, O., (1984) Halothane dissolved in fat as in intravenous anaesthesia to rats. *Acta Anaesthesiol. Scand.*, **28**, 381–384.

Kirsh, R., Goldstein, R., Tarloff, J., Parris, D., Hook, J., Bugelski, P., Poste, G. (1988) An emulsion formulation of Amphotericin B improves the therapeutic index when treating systemic Murine Candidiasis. *J. Infect. Dis.*, **158**, 1065–1070.

Kirvelä, Olkkola, K.T., Rosenberg, P.H., Yli-Hankala, A., Salmela, K., Lindgren, L. (1992) Pharmacokinetics of propofol and haemodynamic changes during induction of anaesthesia in uraemic patients. *Br. J. Anaesth.*, **68**, 178–182.

Klang, S.H., Baszkin, A., Benita, S. (1996) The stability of piroxicam incorporated in a positively-charged submicron emulsion for ocular administration. *Int. J. Pharm.*, **132**, 33–44.

Klang, S.H., Frucht-Pery, J., Hoffman, A., Benita, S. (1994) Physicochemical characterization and acute toxicity evaluation of a positively-charged submicron emulsion vehicle. *J. Pharm. Pharmacol.*, **46**, 986–993.

Kolb, S., Sailer, D. (1984) Effect of fat emulsions containing medium-chain triglycerides and glucose on ketone body production and excretion. *J. Parent. Ent. Nutr.*, **8**, 285–289.

Konno, T. (1992) Targeting chemotherapy for hepatoma: arterial administration of anticancer drugs dissolved in Lipoidol. *Eur. J. Cancer*, **28**, 403–409.

Korner, D., Benita, S., Albrecht, G., Baszkin, A. (1994) Surface properties of mixed phospholipid-stearylamine monolayers and their interaction with a non-ionic surfactant (poloxamer). *Colloids and Surfaces B: Biointerfaces*, **3**, 101–109.

Kurihara, A., Shibayama, Y., Mizota, A., Yasuno, A., Ikeda, M., Sasagawa, K., Kobayashi, T., Hisaoka, M. (1996a) Lipid emulsions of palmitoyl rhizoxin: effects of composition on lipolysis and biodistribution. *Biopharm. Drug Disposit.*, **17**, 331–342.

Kurihara, A., Shibayama, Y., Mizota, A., Yasuno, A., Ikeda, M., Hisaoka, M. (1996b) Pharmacokinetics of highly lipophilic antitumor agent palmitoyl rhizoxin incorporated in lipid emulsions in rats. *Biol. Pharm. Bull.*, **19**, 252–258.

Kurihara, A., Shibayama, Y., Mizota, A., Yasuno, A., Ikeda, M., Sasagawa, K., Kobayashi, T., Hisaoka, M. (1996c) Enhanced tumor delivery and antitumor activity of palmitoyl rhizoxin using stable lipid emulsions in mice. *Pharm. Res.*, **13**, 11305–11320.

Kurozumi, S., Araki, H. Tanabe, H., Kiyoki (1996) Lipid microsphere preparation of prostacyclin analogue. *Adv. Drug Del. Rev.*, **20**, 181–187.

Lance, M.R., Washington, C., Davis, S.S. (1995) Structure and toxicity of amphotericin B/triglyceride emulsion formulations. *J. Antimicrob. Chemother.*, **36**, 119–128.

Levene, M.I., Wigglesworth, J.J., Desai, R. (1980) Pulmonary fat accumulation after Intralipid infusion in the preterm infant. *Lancet*, **2**(8199), 815–818.

Levy, M.Y., Benita, S. (1989) Design and characterization of a submicronized O/W emulsion of diazepam for parenteral use. *Int. J. Pharm.*, **54**, 103–112.

Levy, M.Y., Benita, S. (1990) Drug release from submicronized o/w emulsion: a new *in vitro* kinetic evaluation model. *Int. J. Pharm.*, **66**, 29–37.

Levy, M.Y., Benita, S. (1991) Short and long term stability assessment of a new injectable diazepam submicron emulsion. *Parent. Sci. Technol.*, **45**, 101–107.

Levy, M.Y., Benita, S., Baszkin, A. (1991) Interactions of a nonionic surfactant with mixed phospholipid-oleic acid monolayers: Studies under dynamic conditions. *Colloids and Surfaces*, **59**, 225–241.

Levy, M.Y., Polacheck, I., Barenholz, Y., Benita, S. (1990) Submicron emulsion as parenteral carrier of poorly soluble antifungal agents. *AAPS 5th Annual Meeting*, Las Vegas, Nevada, USA, 5–148.

Levy, M.Y., Polacheck, I., Barenholz, Y., Benita, S. (1993) Efficacy evaluation of a novel submicron amphotericin B emulsion in murine candidiasis. *J. Med. Vet. Mycology*, **31**, 207–218.

Levy, Y.M., Polacheck, I., Barenholz, Y., Benita, S. (1995) Efficacy evaluation of a novel submicron miconazole emulsion in a murine cryptococcosis model. *Pharm. Res.*, **12**, 223.

Levy, M.Y., Schutz, W., Fuhrer, C., Benita, S. (1994) Characterization of diazepam submicron emulsion interface. The role of oleic acid. *J. Microencapsulation*, **11**, 79–92.

Liu, F., Yang, J., Huang, L., Liu, D. (1996) Effect of non-ionic surfactants on the formation of DNA/Emulsion complexes and emulsion-mediated gene. *Pharm. Res.*, **13**, 1642–1646.

Magenheim, B., Levy, M.Y., Benita, S. (1993) A new *in vitro* technique for the evaluation of drug release profile for colloidal carriers — ultrafiltration technique at low pressure. *Int. J. Pharm.*, **94**, 115–223.

Manning, R.J., Washington, C. (1992) Chemical stability of total parenteral nutrition mixtures. *Int. J. Pharm.*, **81**, 1–20.

Miyazaki, S., Hashiguchi, N., Hou, W-M., Yokouchi, C. Takada, M. (1986) Preparation and evaluation *in vitro* and *in vivo* of fibrinogen microspheres containing adriamycin. *Chem Pharm. Bull.*, **34**, 3384–3393.

Mizushima, Y. (1996) Lipid microspheres (lipid emulsions) as a drug carrier-An overview. *Adv. Drug Del. Rev.*, **20**, 113–115.

Momma, K. (1996) Lipo-PGE1 treatment of the neonate with critical congenital heart disease and ductus-arteriosus dependent circulation. *Adv. Drug Del. Rev.*, **20**, 177–180.

Muchtar, S., Almog, S., Torracca, M.T., Saettone, M.F., Benita, S. (1992) A submicron emulsion as ocular vehicle for delta-8-tetrahydrocannabinol: effect on intraocular pressure in rabbits. *Ophthalm. Res.*, **24**, 142–149.

Muchtar, S., Levy, M.Y., Sarig, S., Benita, S. (1991) Stability assessment of a fat emulsion prepared with an original mixture of purified phospholipids. *S.T.P. Pharma Sci.*, **1**, 130–136.

Mueller, J.F., Canham, J.E. (1965) Symposium on intravenous fat emulsions. *Am. J. Clin. Nutr.*, **16**, 1–223.

Muramatsu, T., Yabe, Y., Nakano, G., Noike, H., Kanai, M., Saito, T., Ueshima, G. (1991) Concerning the post PTCA restenosis preventive effects of the newly developed lipo-formulated PGI_2 stable derivative TTC-909. *55th Annual Scientific Meeting of the Japanese Circulation Society*, No 276.

Nakamura, H., Hashimoto, T., Oi, H., Swada, S., Furui, S., Mizumoto, S., Monden, M. (1990) Treatment of hepatocellular carcinoma by segmental hepatic artery injection of adriamycin-in-oil emulsion with overflow to segmental portal veins. *Acta Radiol.*, **31**, 347–349.

Ohmukai, O. (1996) Lipo-NSAID preparation. *Adv. Drug Del. Rev.*, **20**, 203–207.

Olson, W.P., Faith, M.R. (1988) Human serum albumin as a cosolvent for parenteral drugs. *J. Parent. Sci. Technol.*, **42**, 82–85.

Pascual, B., Ayestaran, A., Montoro, J., Oliveras, J., Estibalez, A., Julia, A., Lopez, A. (1995) Administration of lipid-emulsion versus conventional amphotericin B in patients with neutropenia. *Ann. Pharmacother.*, **29**, 1197–1201.

Prankerd, R.J., Frank, S.G., Stella, V.J. (1988) Preliminary development and evaluation of a parenteral emulsion formulation of penclomedine (NSC-338720; 3,5-dichloro-2,4-dimethoxy-6-trichloromethyl-pyridine): a novel, practically water insoluble cytotoxic agent. *J. Parenter. Sci. Technol.*, **42**(3), 86–81.

Prankerd, R.J., Stella, V.J. (1990) The use of oil in water emulsions as a vehicle for parenteral drug administration. *J. Parenter. Sci. Technol.*, **44**(3), 139–149.

Rieger, M.R. (1986) In *The Theory and Practice of Industrial Pharmacy*, edited by L. Lachman, H.A. Lieberman, J.L. Konig, 3rd ed., pp. 502–533. Philadelphia, PA: Lea and Febiger.

Rubino, J.T. (1990) The influence of charged lipids on the flocculation and coalescence of oil-in-water emulsions. II: Electrophoretic properties and monolayer film studies. *J. Parent. Sci. Technol.*, **44**, 210–215.

Rydhag, L., Wilton, I. (1981) The function of phospholipids of soybean lecithin in emulsions. *J. Am. Oil Chem. Soc.*, **35**, 830–837.

Santos-Magalhaes, N.S., Benita, S., Baszkin, A. (1991b) Penetration of polyoxyethylene-polyoxypropylene block copolymer surfactant into soya phospholipid monolayers. *Colloids and Surfaces*, **52**, 195–206.

Santos-Magalhaes, N.S., Cave, G., Seiller, M., Benita, S. (1991) The stability and *in vitro* release kinetics of a clofibride emulsion. *Int. J. Pharm.*, **76**, 225–237.

Santos Magalhaes, N.S., Fessi, H., Puisieux, F., Benita, S., Seiller, M. (1995) An *in-vitro* release kinetic examination and comparative evaluation between submicron emulsions and polylactic acid nanocapsules of clofibride. *J. Microencapsulation*, **12**(2), 195–205.

Sasaki, H., Takakura, Y., Hashida, M., Kimura, T., Sezaki, H. (1984) Antitumor activity of lipophilic prodrugs of mitomycin C entrapped in liposome or o/w emulsion. *J. Pharmacobiodyn.*, **7**, 120–130.

Seley, H. (1941) Studies concerning the anaesthetic action of steroid hormones, *J. Pharmacol.*, **73**, 127–141.

Shah, A.K., Sawchuk, R.J. (1991) Effect of co-administration of Intralipid® on the pharmacokinetics of cyclosporine in the rabbit. *Bio. Pharm. Drug Dispos.*, **12**, 457–466.

Shimamoto, T., Ogawa, Y., Ohkura, N. (1973) *Chem. Pharm. Bull.*, **21**, 316–322.

Sorkine, P., Nagar, H., Weinbroum, A., Setton, A., Israitel, E., Scarlatt, A., Silbiger, A., Rudick, V., Kluger, Y., Halpern, P. (1996) Administration of amphotericin B in lipid emulsion decreases nephrotoxicity: Results of a prospective, randomized, controlled study in critically ill patients. *Crit. Care Med.*, **24**(8), 1311–1315.

Stevens, D.A. (1985) Miconazole in the treatment of coccidioidomycosis. *Drugs*, **26**, 347–354.

Takahashi, M., Iwasaki, S., Kobayashi, H., Okuda, S., Murai, T., Sato, Y. (1987) Rhizoxin binding to nibulin at the maytansine-binding site. *Biochim. Biophys. Acta*, **926**, 215–223.

Takenaga, M. (1996) Application of lipid microspheres for the treatment of cancer. *Adv. Drug Del. Rev.*, **20**, 209–219.

Tarr, B.D., Sambandan, T.G., Yalkowsky, S.H. (1987) A new parenteral emulsion for the administration of Taxol. *Pharm. Res.*, **4**, 162–.

Teagarden, D.L., Anderson, B.D., Petre, W. (1988) Determination of the pH-dependent phase distribution of prostaglandin E1 in a lipid emulsion by ultrafiltration. *J. Pharm. Res.*, **5**, 482–487.

Tibell, A., Larson, M., Alvestrand, A. (1993) Dissolving intravenous cyclosporine A in a fat emulsion carrier prevents acute renal side effects in the rat. *Transpl Int.*, **6**, 69–72.

Tibell, A., Lindholm, A., Sawe, J., Norrlind, B. (1995) Cyclosporine A in a fat emulsion carriers: Experimental studies on pharmacokinetics and tissue distribution. *Pharmacol. Toxicol.*, **76**, 115–121.

Turlan, P., Ferre, P., Girard, J.R. (1983) Evidence that medium-chain fatty acid oxidation can support an active gluconeogenesis in the suckling newborn rat. *Biol. Neonate*, **43**, 103–108.

Vanacker, B., Wiebalck, A., Van Aken, H., Sermeus, L., Bouillon, R., Amery, A. (1993) Quality of induction and adrenocortical function. A clinical comparison of Etomidate-Lipuro and Hypnomidate. *Anaesthesist.*, **42**(2), 81–89.

Villani, P., Regazzi, M.B., Maserati, R., Viale, P., Alberici, F., Giacchino, R. (1996) Clinical and pharmacokinetic evaluation of a new lipid-based delivery system of amphotericin B in AIDS patients. *Arzneimittelforschung*, **46**(4), 445–449.

Von Dardel, O., Mebius, D., Svensson, B. (1981) Fat emulsion as a vehicle for diazepam. A study of 9492 patients. *Br. J. Anaesth.*, **55**, 41–47.

Washington, C. (1990) The electrokinetic properties of phospholipid-stabilized fat emulsion. II. Droplets mobility in mixed electrolytes. *Int. J. Pharm.*, **58**, 13–17.

Washington, C. (1990) The electrokinetic properties of phospholipid-stabilized fat emulsions. III. Inter-droplet potentials and stability ratios in monovalent electrolytes. *Int. J. Pharm.*, **64**, 67–73.

Washington, C. Chawla, A. Christy, N., Davis, S.S. (1989) The electrokinetic properties of phospholipid-stabilized fat emulsions. *Int. J. Pharm.*, **54**, 191–197.

Washington, C., Chawla, A., Christy, N., Davis, S.S. (1989) The electrokinetic properties of phospholipid-stabilized fat emulsions. *Int. J. Pharm.*, **58**, 191–197.

Washington, C., Koosha, F. (1990) Drug release from microparticles deconvulsion of measurement errors. *Int. J. Pharm.*, **59**, 79–82.

Waud, W.R., Tiwari, S., Schmid, S.M., Shih, T.W., Strong, J.M., Hartman, N.R., O'Reilly, S., Struck, R.F. (1997) 4-Demethylpenclomedine, an antitumor-active, potentially nonneurotoxic metabolite of penclomedine. *Cancer Research*, **57**(5), 815–817.

Westesen, K., Wehler, T. (1992) Physicochemical characterization of a model intravenous oil in water emulsion. *J. Pharm Sci.*, **81**(8), 777–786.

Westesen, K., Wehler, T. (1993) Characterization of a submicron-sized oil in water emulsion. *Colloids and Surfaces A*, **78**, 115–123.

Wretlind, A.J. (1964) *Acta Chir. Scan. Suppl.*, **325**, 31–42.

Yalabik-Kas, H.S. (1985) Stability assessment of emulsions systems. *S.T.P. Pharma*, **1**, 978–984.

Yokoyama, K., Okamoto, H., Watanabe, M. (1985) Development of a corticosteroid incorporated in lipid microspheres (liposteroid). *Drugs Exp. Clin. Res.*, **11**, 611–620.

Yokoyama, K., Watanabe, M. (1996) Limethason as a lipid microsphere preparation: An overview. *Adv. Drug Del. Rev.*, **20**, 195–201.

Yoshikawa, M., Saicho, H., Ebara, M., Iijima, T., Iwama, S., Endo, F., Kimura, M., Shimamura, Y., Suzuki, Y., Nakano, T., Fukuyama, Y., Fujise, K., Nambu, M., Ohto, M. (1994) A randomized trial of intrahepatic arterial infusion of 4'-epidoxorubicin with lipiodol versus 4'-epidoxorubicin alone in the treatment of hepatocellular carcinoma. *Cancer Chemother. Pharmacol.*, **33**(Suppl), S149–S152.

Zeevi, A., Klang, S., Alard, V., Brossard, F., Benita, S. (1994) The design and characterization of a positively-charged submicron emulsion containing a sunscreen agent. *Int. J. Pharm.*, **108**, 57–68.

6. SUBMICRON EMULSIONS AS DRUG CARRIERS FOR TOPICAL ADMINISTRATION

SHIMON AMSELEM and DORON FRIEDMAN

Pharmos Ltd, Kiryat Weizmann, 76326 Rehovot, Israel

INTRODUCTION

The stratum corneum provides the principal barrier to the percutaneous absorption of topically applied drugs. Attempts have been made to circumvent this barrier both by physical means such as iontophoresis, ultrasound, and electroporation, and by chemical approaches (Chien, 1992). The common methodology applied in order to improve dermal penetration of drugs is the use of chemical penetration enhancers. Examples of skin penetration enhancers are: alcohols (ethanol, dodecanol), glycols, pyrrolidones, dimethylsulfoxide and its derivatives, and hydrophobic compounds that can change the structure of skin lipids and make channels in the skin barrier like Azone® (laurocapram) (see Table 1). However, the inclusion of chemical enhancers, usually organic solvents, is generally associated to some degree with skin irritation, toxicity, and sensitization. Because of the safety issues, only a few chemical enhancers have been used in marketed products and therefore the search for an efficient, safe, and preferably enhancer-free transdermal vehicle continues.

Liposomes have been suggested as therapeutic drug carrier systems for the topical treatment of skin diseases (Braun-Falco *et al.* 1992). Recently it was shown that interaction of phospholipids with the stratum corneum can lead to a structural rearrangement of its lipid layers, followed by hydration. As a result, interlamellar

Table 1 Common chemical skin penetration enhancers

Ethanol
Isopropyl alcohol
Dodecanol
Propyleneglycol
Dimethylsulphoxide (DMSO)
Dimethylformamide (DMF)
Decylmethylsulphoxide (DCMS)
2-Pyrrolidone
N-Methylpyrrolidone (NMP)
Sodium laurylsulphate (SLS)
1-Dodecylazacycloheptane-2-one (laurocapram, Azone®)

attachment can form "holes" in the lipid layers of the hydrated stratum corneum, increasing drug flux through the skin (Blume *et al.* 1993). Polymeric micronsize microspheres have also been used for efficient site-specific topical delivery and controlled release of drugs to treat pathologies associated with pilosebaceous structures (Rolland *et al.* 1993).

Topical application of drugs at the pathological sites offers potential advantages of delivering the drug directly to the site of action and thus producing high tissue concentration of the drug and avoiding unwanted side-effects by other administration routes, like gastric irritation in the case of oral delivery of non-steroidal antiinflammatory drugs. The aim of the present work was to develop a solvent-free topical drug carrier devoid of adverse effects based on drug entrapment in oil-in-water emulsion droplets of submicron size.

SUBMICRON EMULSION (SME) AS TOPICAL DRUG CARRIER

Description

A novel solvent-free colloidal drug delivery technology or lipoidal vehicle consisting of stable, submicron particles of oil-in-water emulsions, termed Sub-Micron Emulsions or SME was developed. The SME droplets are characterized by a mean droplet size of less than one micron (generally in the range of 100–200 nm) uniformly dispersed in an aqueous phase. The droplet size reduction is essential to generate preparations with high stability. The uniqueness of the large internal hydrophobic oil core of the SME droplets provides high solubilization capacity for water insoluble compounds compared to other lipoidal vehicles such as liposomes (Figure 1).

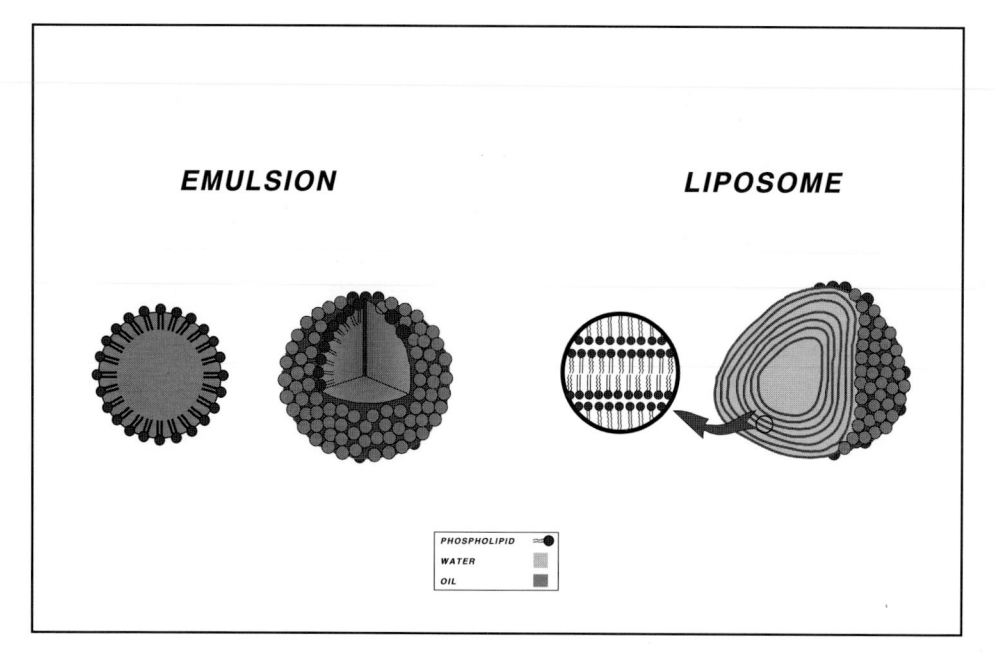

Figure 1 Schematic illustration of the structure of an oil-in-water SME droplet compared to a liposome.

The SME technology has been previously applied succcessfully in the formulation of ocular drugs and Phases I and II clinical trials performed with several ophthalmic drugs formulated using the SME technology have shown improved drug delivery resulting in reduced local irritation and no side effects (Amselem et al., 1993a, 1993b; Garti et al., 1993). In addition, those studies suggest that SME formulations offer sustained drug release allowing the drugs to exert their effects over longer periods of time, thus permitting lower dosage requirements and improving the therapeutic profiles (Bar-Ilan et al., 1993, 1994). The improved ocular delivery of drugs by SME vehicle is probably due to prolonged residence time of the drugs at the administration site with consequent longer contact time resulting in increased corneal penetration and enhanced drug action, as demonstrated using an experimental rabbit model (Beilin et al., 1995; Bar-Ilan et al., 1994). SME formulations have also been used as vehicles for vaccines enhancing the immunogenicity of the incorporated antigens (Kaminski et al., 1996).

SME Composition

The SME contained an oil phase (10–20% w/v) composed of edible natural lipids and oils, mainly oleic acid , MCT oil (medium chain triglycerides), or LCT oil (long-chain triglycerides) and egg-lecithin (0.5–2%), dispersed in a water phase (80–90%) with the aid of a nonionic surfactant (1–2%) such as polysorbates, tyloxapol, poloxamers, or polyoxyethylene castor oil derivatives. The drug is usually dissolved or dispersed in the oil phase. Antioxidants (sodium edetate, tocopherols) and preservatives (parabens) are added to preserve the formulation from microbial contamination or drug degradation. All ingredients used were pharmaceutical grade materials.

SME Preparation Method

The method of SME preparation was described in detail by Friedman and Schwarz (1993) and the general procedure is illustrated in the flow chart depicted in Figure 2. Briefly, the calculated amount of drug is dissolved in the oil phase and mixed thoroughly with the water phase. The mixture is treated with a high shear homogenizer (Polytron K3000, Kinematika, Switzerland) at 15–20,000 rpm for a short time (1–2 min). The coarse oil-in-water emulsion formed is then sized to the submicron range by high pressure homogenization (6 cycles at 800 bar using a Micron Lab 70 homogenizer (APV Gaulin International SA, The Netherlands). The resulting SME preparation is filtered through 0.45 μm Nylon filter (Schleicher & Shuell, Germany). The SME drug content is determined by UV-spectroscopy or HPLC.

Physical Characterization Of SME Droplets

The parameters most frequently used to characterize lipid particles are morphology, particle size and size distribution. Physical characterization of the SME droplets was carried out by Electron Microscopy (EM) and Photon Correlation Spectroscopy (PCS).

```
Preparation of Oil Phase        Preparation of Water Phase
                    ↓         ↓
            Mixing of Oil and Water Phases
                         ↓
        Preparation of Coarse
        Oil-in-Water Emulsion
        by High Shear Homogenization
                         ↓
        High Pressure Homogenization
        (Sizing of emulsion to nanosize range)
                         ↓
                    Filtration
                         ↓
                 Cream Preparation
                         ↓
            pH and Viscosity Adjustment
```

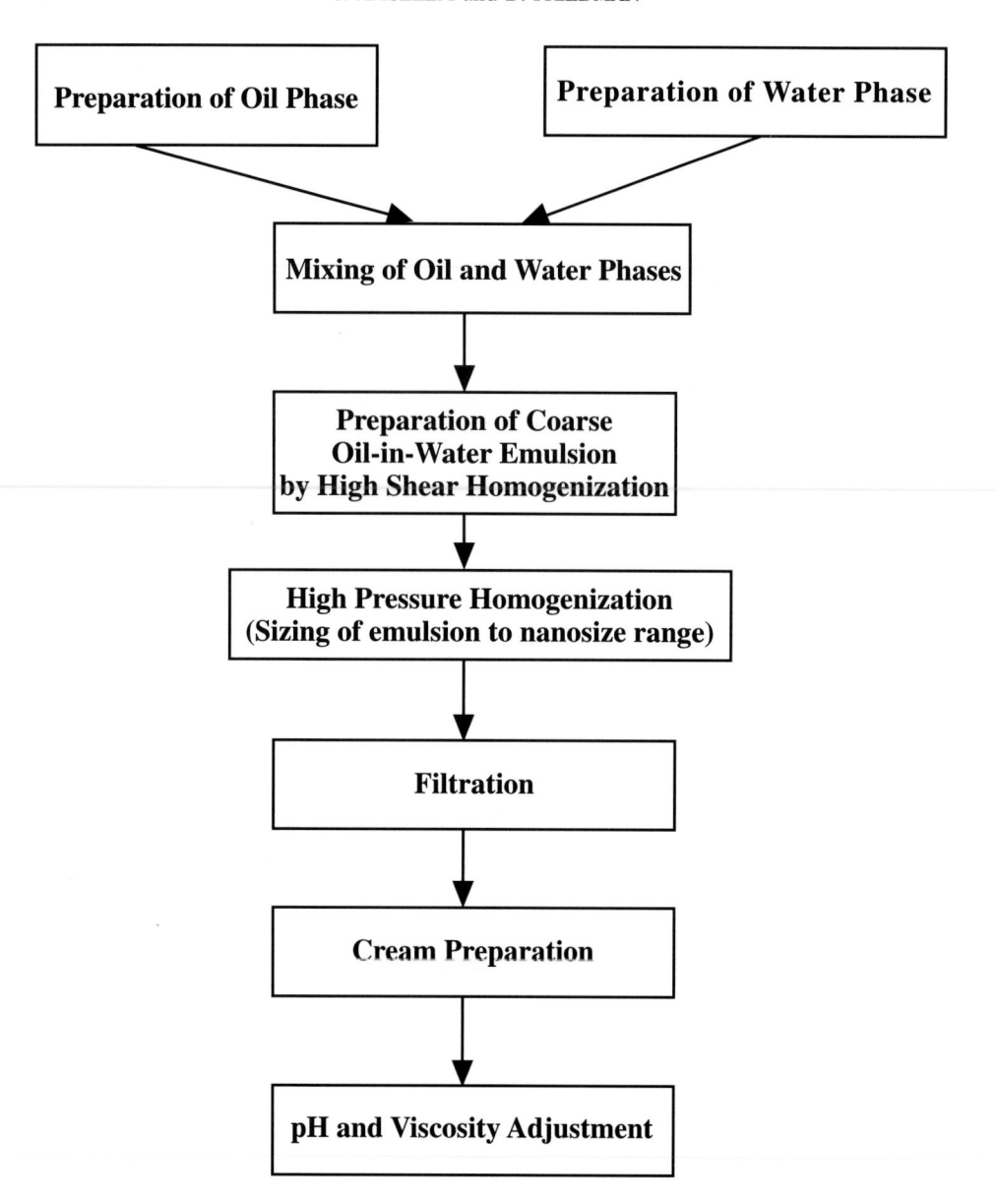

Figure 2 Flow chart describing the manufacture process of SME topical creams.

Morphology

Visualization of SME particles by negative staining electron microscopy shows spheric shape and homogenous and uniform population of oil droplets (Figure 3), having a diameter in the range of 80–130 nm.

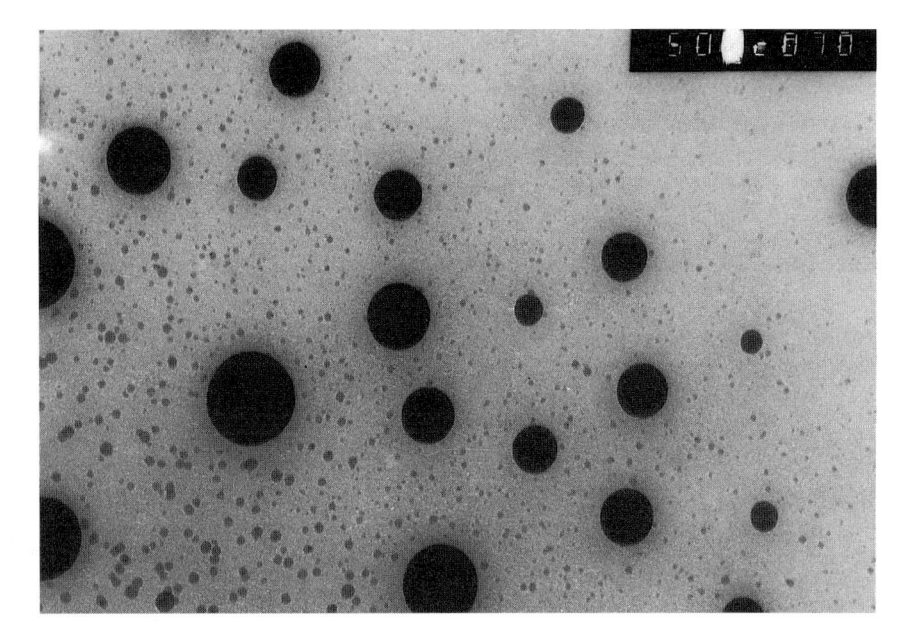

Figure 3 Electron micrograph of SME droplets negatively stained with 1% phosphotungstic acid solution.

Particle size distribution

The narrow size distribution of SME particles was confirmed by laser light scattering data obtained using a Coulter N4MD particle size analyzer (Coulter Electronics, England) (Figure 4). The particle size distribution of SME formulations was determined by photon correlation spectroscopy based on measuring laser scattered-light fluctuations working at the differential weight % operation mode of the instrument (Barenholz and Amselem, 1993). The typical particle size distribution pattern of SME preparations show the existence of single homogeneous populations of SME droplets with a mean particle diameter in the range of 50 to 150 nm and in most cases around 100 nm.

Drug partition in SME

Two ml of SME sample after the high pressure homogenisation step was adjusted to pH 6.0 ± 0.5 (correspondent to SME cream pH value) and placed into an ultrafiltration centrifuge tube (Poretics, USA) with polysulfone membrane (100,000 MW cut-off). The sample was centrifuged at 1,500g for 30–60 minutes until a 250–300 µl of filtrate was obtained. Drug content in the filtrate was determined by UV spectrophotometry and related to the initial total drug content in the SME.

SME Topical Cream Preparation

The use level of SME in finished topical formulations is in the range of 5–20%. Carbopol 940 was used for SME thickening to obtain creams with the desired

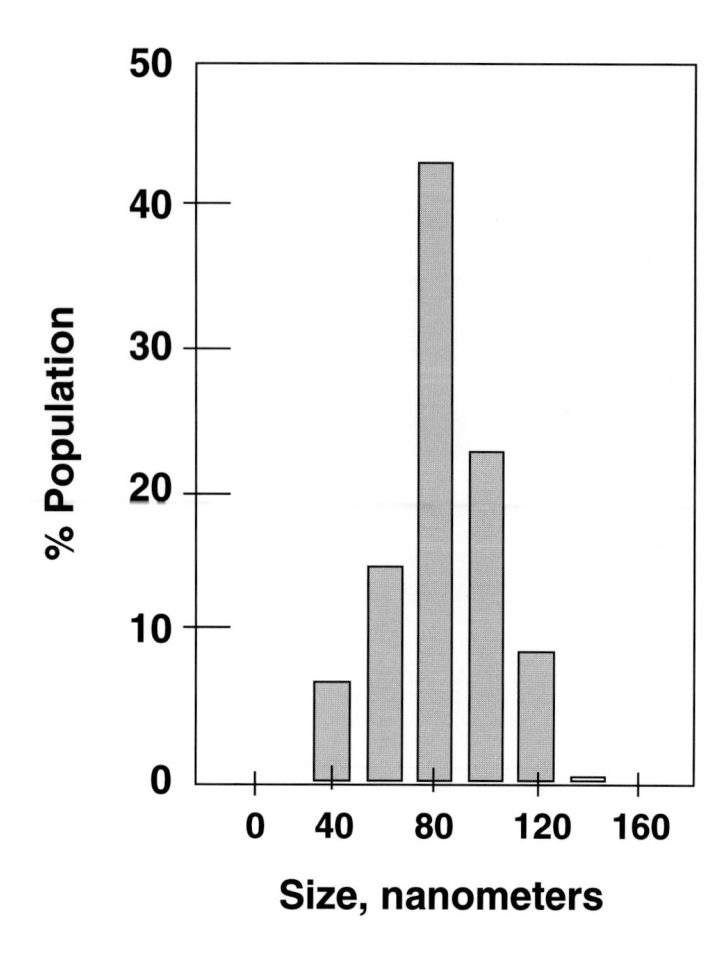

Figure 4 Particle size distribution of typical SME droplets as determined by Photon Correlation Spectroscopy using a Coulter N4MD particle size analyzer.

semisolid consistency. Drug loaded emulsion is mixed with preswollen 10% Carbopol 940/water gel to reach final Carbopol concentration of 0.5–1.0% (w/w), and then mixed with the aid of the high shear homogenizer (10,000 rpm) for 2 minutes. The pH is adjusted to 5.5–8.0 by titration with pure triethanolamine and mixed to obtain a homogenous cream. The product was packed in sealed aluminum tubes. Alternatively, the SME oil phase may be prepared from vegetable jojoba oil instead of fractionated coconut oil.

Stability Of SME Topical Creams

Stability data gathered in follow-up studies indicate that the SME creams are well preserved by parabens and stable for a long time (at least two years at ambient temperature) without any signs of phase separation, oil droplets coalescence, microbial growth or drug degradation.

APPLICATIONS

Drug encapsulation in the oily droplets is required for using the SME technology in topical products. The technology is more recommended for lipophilic or water-insoluble compounds. Good solubility of the drug in the oil phase of the emulsion is a prerequisite for a successful SME formulation.

Recently we demonstrated that submicron emulsions (SME) exhibit enhanced topical delivery of several drugs, incorporated into SME creams, prepared with different types of oil phase components. Drug activity increases from 1.5 to 3-fold were demonstrated for antiinflammatory drugs (steroidal and non-steroidal) (Friedman et al., 1995), diazepam (Schwarz et al., 1995), atropine (Weisspapir et al., 1994) and local anesthetics (Friedman et al., 1993) formulated in SME. The extended drug activity of SME topical creams might be attributed to increased penetration of submicron oil droplets through the stratum corneum of the skin and improved association of the drug with increased surface of the SME particles.

Formulation of NSAID in Topical SME

Topical application of non-steroidal anti-inflammatory (NSAID) drugs is commonly used as anelgetics and in the treatment of different arthropathies. Previous studies have shown the ability of SME to enhance the bioavailability and efficacy of NSAID such as indomethacin applied topically as an ocular pharmaceutical dosage form (Bar-Ilan et al., 1994). The unique penetrative properties of the SME drug delivery technology make it an attractive alternative for formulating NSAIDs in the form of a topical cream. Table 2 shows a list of NSAID which were successfully formulated in topical SME creams. All the drugs tested have a very low water solubility and showed good oil solubility, therefore they are considered as good candidates for SME formulation being entrapped in the hydrophobic core of the oily droplets.

Formulation of diclofenac in SME topical cream

Although the marketed diclofenac topical formulation (Voltaren® Emulgel®, Ciba-Geigy) is an effective treatment for different arthropathies and for local pain relief, a major disadvantage of this preparation is however, the use of organic solvents (propylene glycol and isopropyl alcohol) to improve drug solubility and skin penetration with potential risk of skin irritation or allergic responses.

A new formulation for diclofenac utilizing the SME approach was developed. Diclofenac diethylammonium salt (1.16%, equivalent to 1% diclofenac base) was formulated in SME as a topical cream. The SME contained a 20% oil phase composed of fractionated coconut oil (medium chain triglycerides) and egg-lecithin, dispersed in a water phase with the aid of the nonionic surfactant Cremophor® EL (polyoxyethylene castor oil). The coarse oil-in-water emulsion formed by mixing the oil and water phases was sized to the submicron range (SME) by high pressure homogenization to a final particle size of the SME droplets of 120 ± 40 nm. Antioxidants and preservatives were added and the pH was adjusted to 6.5–7.5 range.

Table 2 Non-steroidal antiinflammatory drugs (NSAID) formulated in SME

Drug	Chemical Structure	Water Solubility
Diclofenac		sparingly soluble
Indomethacin		practically insoluble
Piroxicam		sparingly soluble
Ketoprofen		practically insoluble
Ibuprofen		practically insoluble
Naproxen		practically insoluble

Enhanced antiinflammatory activity of diclofenac in MCT oil SME cream

The efficacy of diclofenac-SME topical cream was evaluated using the Carrageenan-induced rat paw edema model. The antiinflammatory activity of diclofenac-SME creams, applied topically on the inflammation area concomitantly with the Carrageenan injection were compared to the commercial Voltaren® Emulgel® product (Ciba-Geigy, Switzerland). Rats (Wistar, 230–250 g bodyweight, 6 animals in each group, Anilab-Israel, data ± SE) were anesthesized during the experiment by sodium

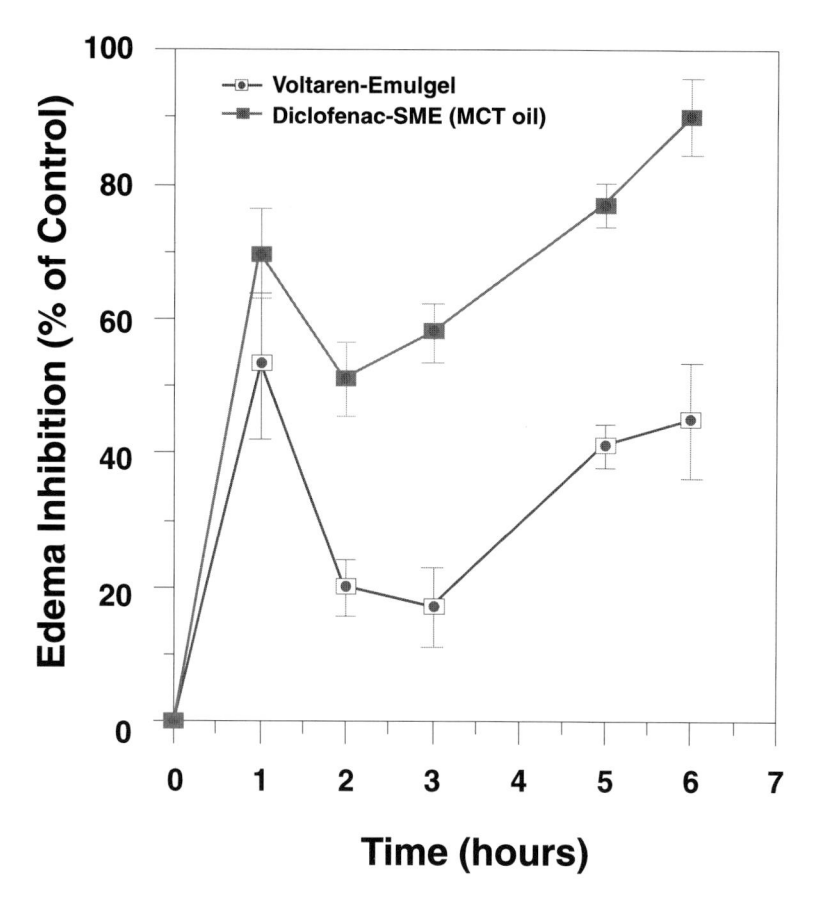

Figure 5 Antiinflammatory activity of diclofenac in SME vehicle (MCT oil phase) compared to Voltaren® Emulgel® following topical delivery in the Carrageenan-induced paw edema model. Rats, n = 6, mean ± SE.

diethylbarbiturate (120 mg/kg S.C., Fluka, Switzerland) and Rompun® (10 mg/kg I.P.) injections. One hundred microliters of 1% iota-Carrageenan (Fluka, Switzerland) solution in saline was injected subplantar into the hind paw of the rat. Sixty µl of the topical preparation containing diclofenac (1.16%, 2.5 mg/kg) were applied at the site of injection and gently rubbed into the skin. The SME cream was absorbed in the skin within 2–3 minutes. The increases in edema volumes (% swelling of the paw) measured by plethysmometry, were compared with the edema volume caused by Carrageenan alone as a control group. The average paw swelling in the groups of the drug treated rats was compared with that of the control rats and the percent inhibition of the edema formation was determined. Edema volume changes were tested at 0, 1, 2, 3, 4, 5, and 6 hours time intervals. No signs of skin irritation were observed during the experiment in any group. Figure 5 shows a significant improvement in reduction of edema volume with diclofenac-SME (MCT oil phase) compared to Voltaren® Emulgel® and the antiinflammatory effect lasted for about 6 hours, returning to the initial edema volume (90 ± 6% inhibition of swelling).

Enhanced antiinflammatory activity of diclofenac in jojoba oil SME cream

Jojoba oil, also known as Jojoba liquid wax, is a a stable highly lipophilic, non-toxic and non-irritative oil, obtained from the desert plant Jojoba (*Simmondsia chinensis*) which is now widely used in cosmetics (Shani, 1983). It is a highly lipophilic compound, consisting almost entirely of wax esters of high molecular weight monounsaturated acids and alcohols, mainly C_{18} — C_{22} (Miwa, 1973). Jojoba oil is stable to oxidation and remains chemically unchanged for years (Miwa, 1973; McKeown, 1983). The skin irritation potential of jojoba oil in different preparation was evaluated by various methods and the material was classified as non-irritating (Johnson, 1992). Acute and sub-chronic toxicity, skin sensitization and mutagenity assessments of jojoba oil also show lack of undesirable effects. Additionally, jojoba oil was found to be non-comedogenic in topical formulations even at high concentrations (Johnson, 1992). The excellent safety profile of Jojoba oil make it a promising component for topical preparations.

The potential use of jojoba oil as excipient for the preparation of pharmaceutical submicron emulsions for topical use was investigated. SME containing 20% jojoba oil and diclofenac diethylammonium (1.16%) was prepared as described previously (Schwarz *et al.*, 1996). The jojoba oil SME formulation containing diclofenac showed a narrow size distribution (156 ± 56 nm), and 100% of the particles were below 215 nm. The viscosity of the jojoba oil SME cream with diclofenac, determined by a Brookfield rotor viscometer DV II+ (spindle LV4, 6 rpm) was about 100,000 cP.

Similarly to MCT oil-SME, diclofenac in jojoba oil-SME vehicle also demonstrated significantly greater antiinflammatory activity than Voltaren® Emulgel® cream in rats (Figure 6). The onset of antiinflammatory activity for diclofenac in jojoba SME vehicle was about 1 hour, and at 3, 4 and 6 hour paw edema volumes were significantly ($p < 0.05$) lower than for Voltaren® Emulgel® with identical drug content. Figure 6 shows that the antiinflammatory effect of diclofenac in jojoba oil-SME, as in the case of MCT oil-SME, lasted for about 6 hours, returning to the initial edema volume (100% inhibition of swelling).

The antiinflammatory activity of diclofenac diethylammonium in SME vehicle, composed of either MCT oil or jojoba oil, was much more pronounced than Voltaren® Emulgel® with identical drug content (1.16% diclofenac DEA, equivalent to 1.0% of diclofenac base). In contrast to the Voltaren® Emulgel® formulation, a fatty emulsion (microsize droplets) in an aqueous gel containing propylene glycol and isopropyl alcohol to improve diclofenac solubility and skin penetration, the solvent-free jojoba oil-SME vehicle (mean droplet size about 100 nm) does not include any organic solvent or other irritative penetration enhancer.

Other NSAID-SME formulations

In addition to diclofenac, other NSAID like indomethacin, naproxen, and piroxicam formulated in topical SME creams were studied. Reference regular creams with drug concentrations equal to those employed in the SME preparations were used for comparison. The composition and preparation of the regular creams were similar to the hydrophilic ointment described in the USP (USP 23-1114) except that propylene glycol was not added. Emulsifying wax was prepared by melting together cetostearyl alcohol and sodium dodecylsulfate (9:1) at 80–90°C. Drug loaded regular

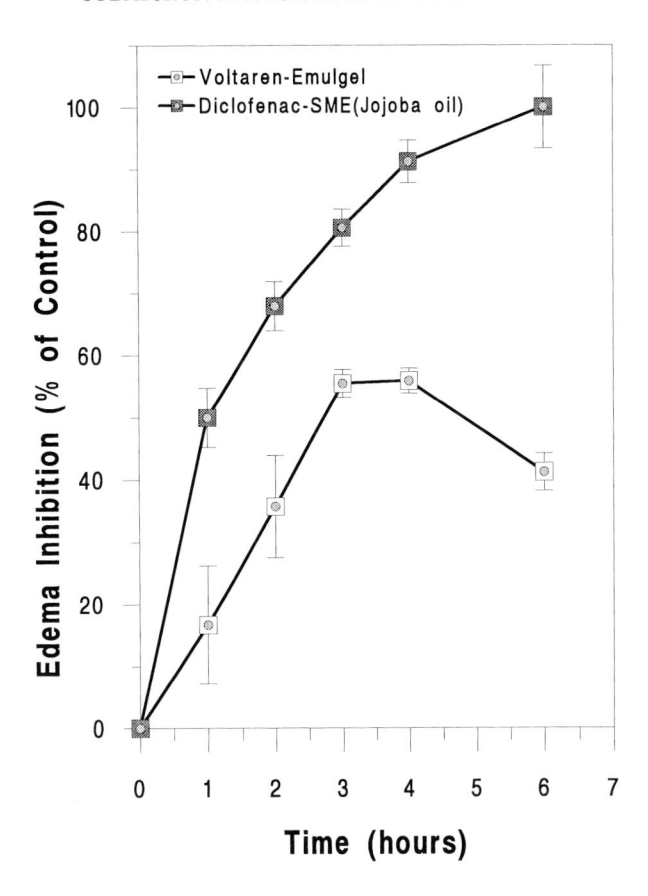

Figure 6 Antiinflammatory activity of diclofenac diethylammonium in jojoba oil SME vehicle and Voltaren® Emulgel® in Carrageenan-induced paw edema model.

cream was obtained by heating simultaneously the active substance, Miglyol (MCT) or paraffin oil and emulsifying wax, followed by addition of boiling water (ratio of water to cetostearyl alcohol 9:1 by weight) and intensive stirring until congealing. After cooling, a soft cream with irregular oil droplets (mean size 10–100 μm) is formed.

Figure 7 shows the antiinflammatory activity of all NSAIDs tested. All the drugs formulated in the topical SME cream showed improvement of efficacy compared to the regular creams containing equivalent amounts of the NSAID.

Drug partition in SME

Partition of entrapped drug between oil and water phases depends on drug lipophilicity and for ionizable drugs on the pH of the preparation. For diclofenac (diethylammonium salt) at pH 6.5, 55 ± 5% of the drug and more than 90% for indomethacin or naproxen at pH 5.5 and piroxicam at pH 6.5 resides inside the oil droplets or is associated at the oil/water interface, as was determined spectrophotometrically after ultrafiltration of the SME.

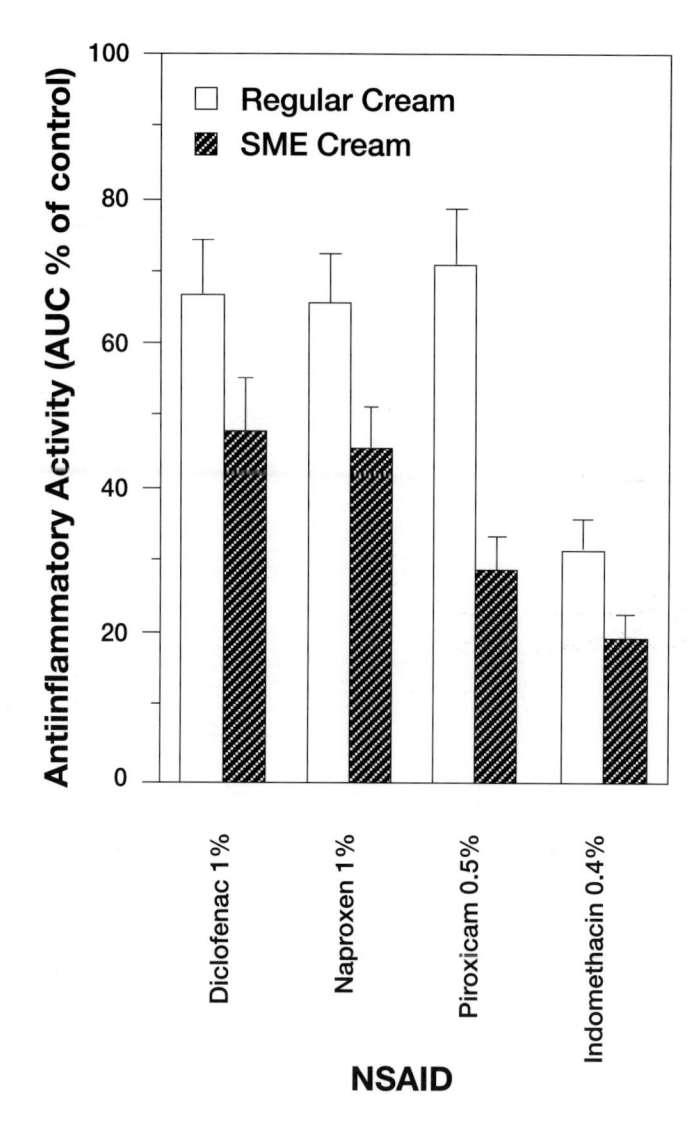

Figure 7 Comparative antiinflammatory activities of NSAIDs formulated either in SME topical creams or regular creams in Carrageenan-induced paw edema model. Percent edema volume reduction was calculated from AUC values compared to control (AUC = 100%) non-treated animals (Rats, n = 6, mean ± SE).

Effect of emulsion droplet size

The effect of SME droplet size on pharmacological activity of encapsulated drug was investigated. The antiinflammatory activities of two diclofenac emulsion formulations having identical composition but differing in droplet sizes, "large droplet emulsion" with droplet size of 10–100 μm and SME prepared by subsequent high pressure homogenization of the initial emulsion to the 0.1–0.2 μm size range, were examined. Figure 8 shows the antiinflammatory activity of diclofenac formu-

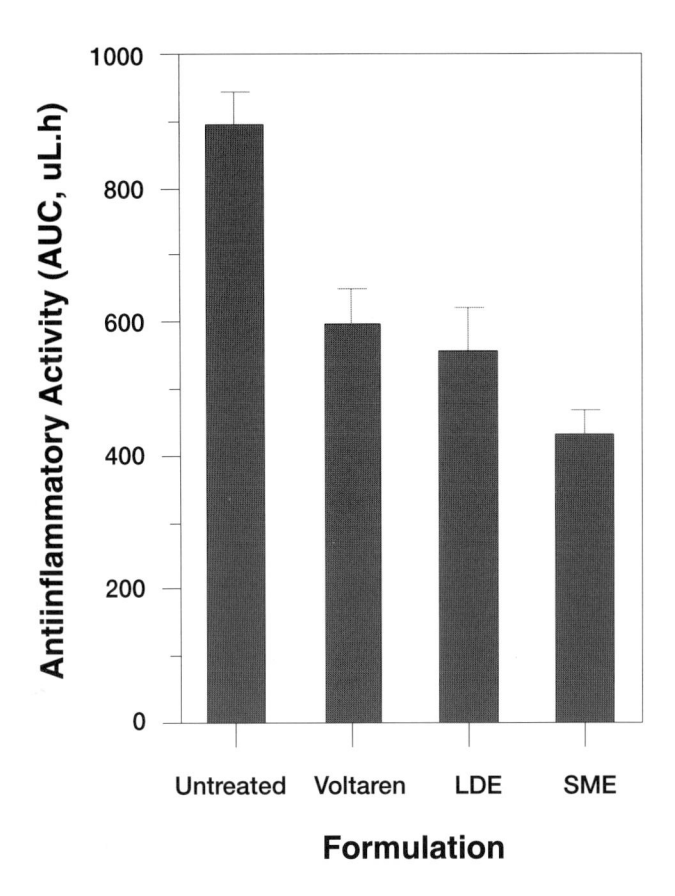

Figure 8 Antiinflammatory activity of diclofenac formulations in large droplet emulsion or SME (MCT oil phase) creams compared to Voltaren® Emulgel® following topical administration in the Carrageenan-induced paw edema model. Wistar rats, Anilab-Israel, 230-250 g bodyweight, 6 animals in each group, data ± SE.

lations expressed in terms of the area under the curve (AUC) for the 6 hours period after carrageenan injection. The large droplet emulsion cream containing diclofenac and Voltaren® Emulgel® (a fatty emulsion of micronsize droplets) were very similar in terms of antiinflammatory activity but less effective compared with the diclofenac-SME formulation. The SME formulation significanly ($p < 0.01$) differed either from the untreated control group and from both compositions.

The dependence of pharmacological activity of topically applied drugs in SME formulations on the particle size of the oily droplets was also demonstrated in a previous work (Shwarz *et al.*, 1995), showing that decrease of particle size to below 0.2 μm has a strong influence enhancing significantly drug penetration.

Effect of SME cream viscosity on drug efficacy

The influence of cream viscosity on the antiinflammatory activity of SME diclofenac creams was studied. Creams with low viscosity (very soft, almost liquid cream or

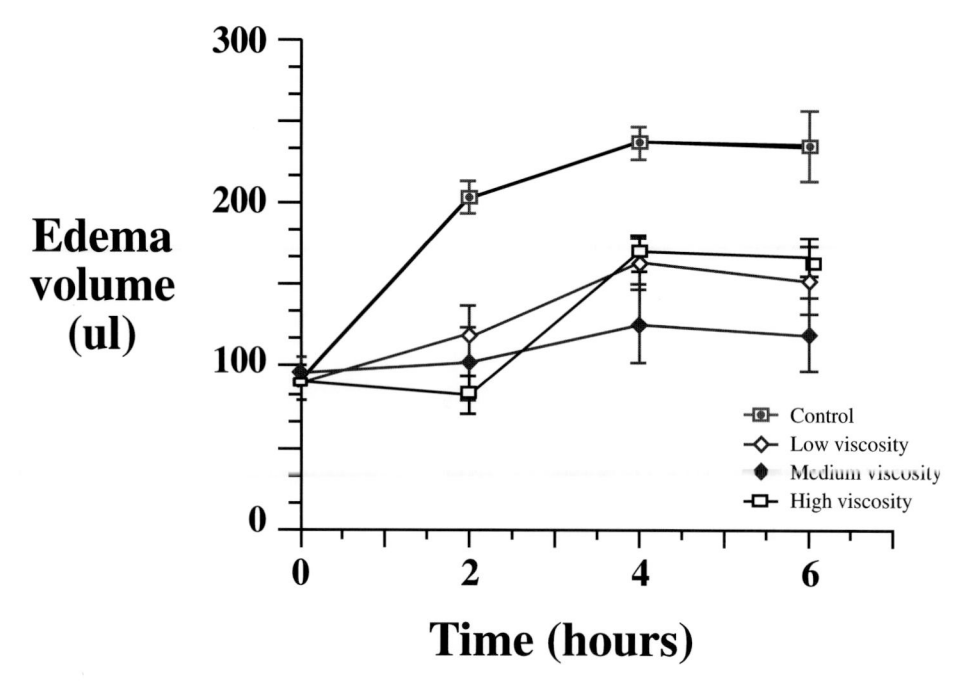

Figure 9 Antiinflammatory activity of diclofenac DEA in SME (MCT oil) vehicles of different viscosities following topical administration in the Carrageenan-induced paw edema model (Rats, n = 6, mean ± SD).

lotion), medium viscosity (normal cream) and high viscosity (rigid gel) were prepared by adding different amounts of Carbopol 940 (thickenig agent, final polymer concentration 0.5%, 1.0% and 1.5% w/w respectively, viscosity values in the range of 50,000 to 120,000 cps). The results in Figure 9 show that changes in viscosities of the SME cream did not affect significantly the antiinflammatory activity of diclofenac included in the formulations.

Formulation of Steroids in Topical SME

Steroid compounds have been successfully incorporated in SME formulations. Steroidal drugs such as dexamethasone, bethamethasone valerate, and bethamethasone dipropionate were dissolved in the oil phase of the SME and incorporated in the hydrophobic oil core of the SME droplet after the high pressure emulsification process.

The steroidal antiinflammatory drugs formulated in SME were tested for pharmacological activity in the Carrageenan-induced inflammation model in rats. Enhanced antiinflammatory efficacy was observed for all the SME formulations, compared with commercial regular semi-solid creams or ointment compositions (Betnovate®, Glaxo; Diprolene®, Schering) containing equivalent drug concentration (Figure 10).

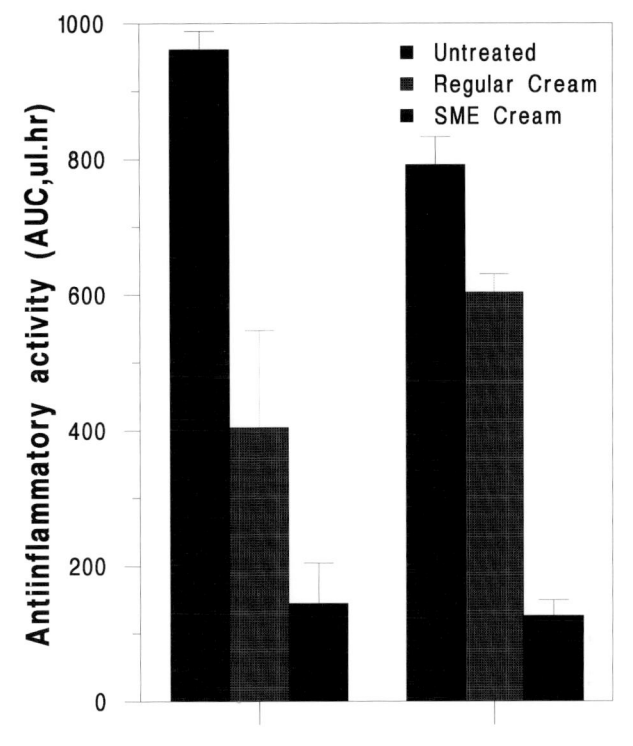

[Figure: Bar chart showing Antiinflammatory activity (AUC, µl·hr) on the y-axis (0 to 1000) for two steroidal drugs — Betham. Valerate (0.1%) and Betham. Dipropionate (0.05%) — comparing Untreated, Regular Cream, and SME Cream.]

Steroidal Drug

Figure 10 Antiinflammatory activity of bethamethasone formulations in SME creams compared to commercial regular semi-solid creams or ointment compositions (Betnovate®, Glaxo; Diprolene®, Schering) containing equivalent drug concentration and following topical administration in the Carrageenan-induced paw edema model (Wistar rats, Anilab-Israel, 230–250 g bodyweight, 6 animals in each group, data ± SE).

Formulation of Local Anesthetics in Topical SME

Local anaethetic have traditionally been viewed as inefective when applied topically to intact skin. Recently, several reports supporting the clinical efficacy of a lidocaine-prilocaine eutectic mixture have appeared in the literature (Maunuksela and Korpela, 1986). Topically induced anaesthesia would be of great value in clinical practice, particularly in pediatric patients. It would enable physicians to perform minor procedures painlessly and without the discomfort and anxiety associated with injection.

The feasibility of incorporation of local anesthetics in SME topical formulations was examined. A 4% lidocaine SME cream containing MCT oil, lecithin, Emulfor EL-620, and Carbopol was prepared according to the general procedure above described. The mean droplet size was 160 nm. For comparison, a conventional 4% lidocaine large droplet emulsion regular cream containing MCT oil, emulsifying

Table 3 Effectiveness of lidocaine and lidocaine/tetracaine eutectic mixture in SME versus regular creams expressed as magnitude of anesthesia (average score) and onset/offset of activity

Formulation	Mean droplet size (μm)	Average Score	Onset min.	Offset min.
Lidocaine in regular cream	10–50	17	60	180
Lidocaine in SME cream	0.25	28	30	270
Lidocaine/tetracaine eutectic mixture in regular cream	20–100	40	30	270
Lidocaine/tetracaine eutectic mixture in SME cream	0.29	58	20	330

wax, and petrolatum jelly was also prepared. The mean droplet size was about 50 μm.

Additionally, a 4% lidocaine/tetracaine eutectic mixture incorporated in SME was prepared and compared versus a lidocaine/tetracaine eutectic mixture in common (regular) cream base. The pH of the lidocaine/tetracaine SME formulation was adjusted to 7.5 and the mean droplet size was about 250 nm. The comparative lidocaine/tetracaine conventional cream prepared in emulsifying wax/petrolatum jelly base had a final droplet size between 20–100 μm.

The local anesthetic effect of topically applied lidocaine and tetracaine creams were investigated and compared. Local anaesthesia was evaluated in humans by applying 0.5g of cream sample over a 4 cm^2 skin area at the forearm of 4 male human volunteers and the degree of local anaesthesia with time was monitored. A gentle touch was made with a sharp needle and the sensitivity of an adjacent (untreated) area was compared to the application site to estimate the anaesthetic effectiveness of the tested preparation. The sensitivity of the site of application was given a score of intensity of 1 to 4 and an average dosage form performance was calculated. Onset and offset of anaesthesia were also recorded. The results are shown in Table 3.

The data obtained show that the lidocaine-SME formulation provided local anesthesia and performed better than the regular cream of larger droplet size. The duration of anaesthetic effect was more prolonged with the lidocaine-SME formulation (90 min longer than the regular cream). The delay in the appearance of anaesthesia after the topical application was also shorter with the lidocaine-SME formulation (time for onset of anaesthesia 30 minutes with lidocaine-SME compared to 60 minutes with the lidocaine regular cream). Similar results were obtained with the lidocaine-tetracaine eutectic mixture, the SME formulation performed better than the regular cream with large droplet size both in terms of onset and duration of anaesthesia (Table 3).

Formulation of Antioxidants and Vitamins in Topical SME

Ubiquinone or Coenzyme Q10, a vitamin K analog is a lipophilic compound with low water solubility and which exhibits low oral absorption. The main function of ubiquinone in biology is to act as redox component of transmembrane electron transport systems, such as the respiratory chain of mitochondria. Another important function exerted by ubiquinone is its action as membrane antioxidant. It has been shown in membrane models that ubiquinone strongly inhibits lipid peroxidation probably by removing free radicals.

A submicron emulsion containing ubiquinone at 5% oil phase was prepared according to the process described in Figure 2. Ubiquinone was dissolved in MCT oil at a concentration of about 60 mg/ml. The oil phase contained additionally lecithin as emulsifier and Tween 80 as nonionic surfactant. The mixture was homogenized by high shear to obtain a coarse oil-in-water emulsion which was then sized to submicron range using a Gaulin MicronLab 70 High Pressure Homogenizer. A single population of droplets with a final particle size of 106 ± 52 nm was obtained as determined using a N4MD Coulter particle size analyzer.

The ubiquinone-SME formulation was shown to be stable at room temperature for the time period tested (6 months), and no change in particle size of droplets was observed. The final ubiquinone concentration in the SME was about 3mg/ml. Ubiquinone-SME was formulated as a topical cream by adding to the SME a carbopol gel and adjusting final pH with triethanolamine. The cream was packaged in aluminum tubes. This ubiquinone-SME formulation may be very useful also in dermatology as an antiaging agent or skin revitalizing product.

Other water-insoluble substances used in personal skin-care products and in OTC preparations as antioxidants and vitamins such as tocopherols (vitamin E), retinoids (vitamin A) have also been successfully incorporated in solvent-free SME formulations in the form of lotions, gels, or creams.

SAFETY OF SME FORMULATIONS

All ingredients used in the preparation of SME formulations are pharmacopeic grade and generally recognized as safe (GRAS) materials. Topical SME formulations defined as solvent-free preparations do not contain penetration enhancers or organic solvents as those listed in Table 1, usually present in commercial topical creams to enhance drug solubility and penetration and reported as potential irritative agents. Topical SME formulations containing different drugs have been tested in animals in preclinical safety and efficacy studies and no adverse effects or skin irritation were reported.

Skin acceptability of topically applied SME placebo cream and diclofenac-SME cream was tested in human volunteers in a irritability test and compared to Voltaren® Emulgel®. A 48 hours human test for primary irritation was performed at the Consumer Product Evaluation Center (Toxicol Laboratories Limited, UK). Twenty-five screened volunteers comprised the test panel. An occlusive patch bearing the test and comparative formulations was applied to the upper outer arm for an initial period of 23 hours. One hour after patch removal, skin sites were assessed for signs of skin irritation, which were rated using a numerical scoring system. Immediately after assessment, an identical fresh patch was applied to the same skin area for a further 23 hour period, and skin sites were again assessed one hour after patch removal. The system of scoring took into account several different conditions of significance depending on the relative severity of the conditions (glazing, wrinkling, dryness, flakiness, erythema, edema, and vesicle formation). In addition, each

Table 4 Human skin irritancy test of diclofenac-SME topical cream*

Cream Sample	Irritation score at 24 Hours (Mean ± SD)	Observations with no irritancy at 24 Hours	Irritation score at 48 Hours (Mean ± SD)	Observations with no irritancy at 48 Hours
Diclofenac SME cream	0.56 ± 1.04	17/25	0.68 ± 1.11	15/25
Voltaren® Emulgel®	0.60 ± 1.32	19/25	1.32 ± 1.52	9/25
Placebo SME cream	0.92 ± 1.29	15/25	0.88 ± 1.42	11/25

* conducted in 25 volunteers for 48 h

condition was scored according to the strength of observed reaction: 0 = no visible reaction; 1 = reaction just present; 2 = slight reaction; 3 = moderate reaction; 4 = severe reaction. To obtain a numerical value for the total reaction at each site, the score for strength of reaction was multiplied by the corresponding condition rating and the resulting values were summed to provide a global score for the degree of irritation. For example, the total score for a site assessed as having slight erythema, moderate wrinkling, and severe dryness would be $(2 \times 3) + (3 \times 1) + (4 \times 1) = 13$. The irritation scores for the tested samples were compared statistically with a Friedman nonparametric ANOVA to analyze both 24 and 48 hour results.

The results obtained in this human study showed (Table 4) that patient compliance with diclofenac-SME was excellent with values equal to or better than Voltaren® Emulgel®. Under the conditions of the irritancy test used, the diclofenac-SME cream as well as the placebo SME cream scored lower than Voltaren® Emulgel® (0.68, 0.88 and 1.32 at 48 hours, respectively); however, there was no statistical significance (see Table 4). Friedman nonparametric ANOVA indicates that there was no significant difference between the three products tested at either assessment (p = 0.14 at 24 hours, p = 0.12 at 48 hours) demonstrating no irritability and very good compliance.

PROPOSED MECHANISM FOR THE ENHANCED DRUG PENETRATION BY SME VEHICLE

Enhanced topical delivery of several lipophilic drugs included into SME-cream formulations has been demonstrated. Drug activity was increased 1.5 to 3-fold for antiinflammatory drugs (steroidal and non-steroidal). Although the exact mechanism is not known yet, the topical activity of the drugs examined increased with the reduction of particle size of the SME droplets. Therefore the extended drug activity might be attributed to increased penetration of submicron oil droplets through the stratum corneum of the skin.

The observed improved efficacy of the SME formulation could be explained based on skin structure. The skin barrier, which prevents penetration of external substances, is localized in the outer horny layer (stratum corneum). It consists of several layers of dead epithelial cells and the intracellular space which is filled with non-polar lipids. These lamellar lipid layers are assumed to be a primary obstacle against penetration of exogenous compounds. The use of phospholipid and oils in SME may suggest similar penetration enhancement mechanisms to those postulated

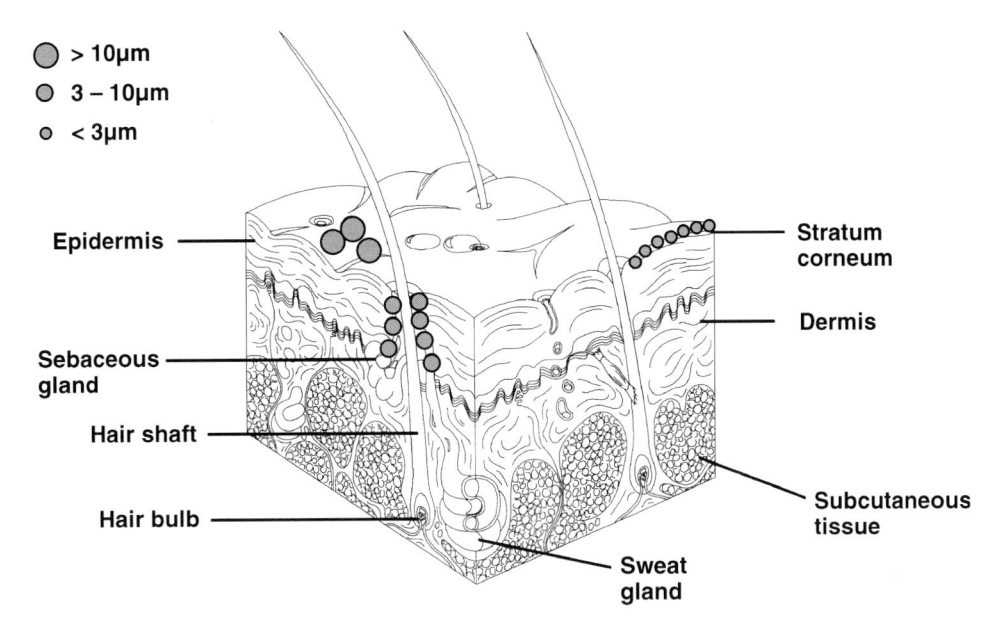

Figure 11 Illustration of the proposed influence of particle size on cutaneous penetration pathways (adapted from the theory suggested by Rolland et al., 1993).

for liposomes (Blume et al., 1993). Since the principal difference between SME cream and the commercial formulations is the small droplet size, it could be hypothesized that oily droplets with a mean particle size of < 1 μm would possibly penetrate the skin more efficiently.

Recently Rolland et al. (1993) observed direct influence of the particle size on its penetration into the skin. It was found that the percutaneous penetration pathway of polymeric microspheres is size dependent. Particles below 3 μm were randomly distributed into the stratum corneum and hair follicles. The main penetration pathway of these microspheres was the transepidermal route since the outer surface of the follicular orifice is only 0.1% of the total skin surface area. The largest microparticles (>10–20 μm) did not penetrate the skin and remained on the stratum corneum outer surface (Figure 11).

Penetration of submicron lipid particles, particularly those containing phospholipids, into the lipid layers of the stratum corneum may lead to change of the structure and composition of the lipid barrier. Its fluidity can increase, and disorder and disruptions of the continuity of the barrier may occur. Formation of gaps and perforations, followed by significant hydratation might then permit the penetration of SME particles through the stratum corneum. It is also possible that under these circumstances other pathways like hair follicles, sebaceous channels, pores, or paracellular ways are enhanced likewise.

CONCLUSIONS

A solvent-free topical vehicle based on drug entrapment in oil-in-water emulsion droplets of submicron size was developed. The uniqueness of the large internal hydrophobic oil core of the SME droplets provides high solubilization capacity for water-insoluble compounds. The SME formulations are prepared by high pressure homogenization of the ingredients resulting in stable solvent-free water-based products which can be applied topically as a lotion or cream. Taken together, our studies demonstrate that SME formulations are safe, resulting in an enhanced efficacy and longer duration of action of the formulated drugs as compared with conventional formulations. An SME-based product has been tested in a human trial and very low irritancy and excellent human acceptance were reported. No skin irritation or allergic responses were observed after topical application in healthy volunteers. The improved skin penetrative properties of the SME delivery technology for lipophilic drugs, its low irritancy, and excellent human acceptance make this novel topical vehicle very promising to achieve increased transcutaneous drug penetration and efficacy.

REFERENCES

Amselem, S., Schwarz, Y., Cohen, A., Wellner, E., Neumann, R., Beilin, M., Garty, N., Friedman, D. (1993a) Submicron emulsion as ocular delivery system for adaprolol maleate, a soft beta blocker. *Pharmac. Res.*, **10**, S205.

Amselem, S., Schwarz, Y., Cohen, A., Wellner, E., Baru, H., Beilin, M., Bar-Ilan, A., Neumann, R., Friedman, D. (1993b) Formulation in Submicron emulsion of HU-211, a novel non-psychotropic cannabinoid with ocular hypotensive activity. *Pharmac. Res.*, **10**, S236.

Barenholz, Y., Amselem, S. (1993) Quality control assays in the development and clinical use of liposome-based formulations. In *Liposome Technology*, edited by G. Gregoriadis, Vol. 1, pp. 527–616. Boca Raton, Florida: CRC press.

Bar-Ilan, A., Aviv, H., Friedman, D., Vered, M., Belkin, M., Amselem, S., Baru, H., Wellner, E., Wolf, Schwarz, Y.J., Neumann, R. (1993) Improved performance of ocular drugs formulated in submicron emulsions, *Invest. Ophthalmol. Vis. Sci.*, **34**, 1488.

Bar-Ilan, A., Baru, H., Beilin, M., Friedman, D., Amselem, S., Neumann, R. (1994) Extended activity and increased bioavailability of indomethacin formulated in submicron emulsion compared to commercially available formulation, *Reg. Immunol.*, **6**, 166–168.

Beilin, M., Bar-Ilan, A., Amselem, S., Schwarz, J., Yogev, A., Neumann, R. (1995) Ocular retention time of submicron emulsion (SME) and the miotic response to pilocarpine delivered in SME. *Invest. Ophthalmol. Vis. Sci.*, **36**, S166.

Blume A., Jansen M., Ghyczy M. and Gareiss J. (1993) Interaction of phospholipid liposomes with lipid model mixtures for stratum corneum lipids. *Int. J. Pharmac.*, **99**, 219–228.

Braun-Falco, O., Korting, H.C., Maibach, H.I. (eds.) (1992) *Liposome Dermatics*. Berlin: Springer-Verlag.

Chien, Y.W. (1992) Transdermal drug delivery and delivery systems. In *Novel Drug Delivery Systems*, edited by Y.W. Chien, pp. 301–380. New York: Marcel Dekker.

Friedman, D., Schwarz, J. (1993) Patent Application PCT/US93/02800, Publication number WO 93/18752 .

Friedman, D., Weisspapir, M., Schwarz, J. (1993) Evaluation of novel transdermal delivery system: SubMicron Emulsion. In *Methods to overcome Biological Barriers in Drug Delivery*, p. 75. Kuopio, Finland: Symposium Proceedings.

Friedman, D., Schwarz, J. and Weisspapir, M. (1995) SubMicron Emulsion Vehicle for enhanced transdermal delivery of Steroidal and non-steroidal antiinflammatory drugs. *J. Pharm. Sci.*, **84**, 324–329.

Garti, N., Melamed, S., Kurtz, S., Greenbaum, A., Amselem, S., Neumann, R. (1993) Adaprolol maleate in submicron emulsion: A novel soft-beta blocking agent is safe and effective in human studies, *Amer. Acad. Ophthalmol. Ann. Meet.*

Johnson W. (1992) Final report on the Safety Assessment of Jojoba oil and Jojoba wax. *J. Am. College of Toxicol.*, **11**, 57–71

Kaminski, R., Loomis, L., Levi, M., Amselem, S., Kersey, K., Vancott, T., Yogev, A., Friedman, D., Smith, G., Wahren, B., Redfield, R., Birx, D., Lowell, G. (1996) HIV peptide and protein antibody responses elicited by immunization with rgp 160 formulated with proteosomes, alum, and/or submicron emulsions, *Vaccine Res.*, **4**, 189–206.

Maunuksela, E.L., Korpela, R. (1986) *Br. J. Anaesthesia*, **58**, 1242–1245.

McKeown, EC. (1983) Jojoba: a botanical with proven functionality. *Cosmet.Toilet.*, **95**, 81–83.

Miwa, T.K. (1973) Chemical aspects of jojoba oil. *Cosmet. Perfum.*, **88**, 39–41.

Rollland, A., Wagner, N., Chatelus, A., Shroot, B., Schaefer, H. (1993) Site-specific drug delivery to pilosebaceous structures using polymeric microspheres. *Pharm. Res.*, **10**, 1738–1744.

Schwarz, J.S., Weisspapir, M.R., Friedman, D.I. (1995) Enhanced transdermal delivery of diazepam by submicron emulsion (SME) creams, *Pharmac. Res.*, **12**, 687–692.

Schwarz, J.S., Weisspapir, M.R., Shani, A., Amselem, S. (1996) Enhanced antiinflammatory activity of diclofenac in jojoba oil submicron emulsion cream, *J. Appl. Cosmetol.*, **14**, 19-24.

Shani A. (1983) Jojoba oil and some of its derivatives in cosmetic and health products. *Soap Cosmet. Chem. Spec.*, **59**, 42–44.

Weisspapir, M., Friedman, D. and Schwarz, J. (1994) SubMicron Emulsion as a Vehicle for improved atropine transdermal delivery. *Pharm. Res.*, **11**, S-183.

7. EMULSIONS OF SUPERCOOLED MELTS — A NOVEL DRUG DELIVERY SYSTEM

HEIKE BUNJES[1], BRITTA SIEKMANN[2] and KIRSTEN WESTESEN[1]

[1]*Institute of Pharmaceutical Technology, Friedrich Schiller University Jena, 07743 Jena, Germany*
[2]*Astra Pain Control AB, Department of Pharmaceutics, 151 85 Södertälje, Sweden*

INTRODUCTION: OBSERVATION OF SUPERCOOLING IN MELT-HOMOGENIZED COLLOIDAL LIPID DISPERSIONS

During the last decades much effort has been focused on the development of colloidal drug carriers, such as polymeric nanoparticles (Allémann *et al.*, 1993), liposomes (Lasic, 1993) and lipid emulsions (Collins-Gold *et al.*, 1990), for the parenteral delivery of poorly water soluble drugs and for drug targeting, i.e. drug delivery to site-specific targets. One of the approaches investigated during recent years is the development of solid lipid nanoparticles (Lucks *et al.*, 1992; Siekmann and Westesen, 1992). Solid lipid nanoparticles represent colloidal dispersions of non-polar lipids such as triglycerides. The idea behind the use of solid lipids is to combine the superiorities of colloidal lipid carriers, such as the biodegradability and biocompatibility of the carrier material as well as the ease of manufacture, with the advantages of the solid physical state of polymeric nanoparticles with respect to size stability, drug leakage and sustained drug release. In the solid lipid matrix the mobility of incorporated drugs is drastically reduced.

Solid lipid nanoparticles with mean particle sizes typically between 50 and 200 nm can be prepared by a melt-homogenization process in which the molten lipids are dispersed in an aqueous phase containing physiologically compatible emulsifiers such as phospholipids, bile salts and poloxamers by the use of high pressure homogenization (Siekmann and Westesen, 1992). An intermediate melt-in-water emulsion is obtained which turns into a suspension upon crystallization of the lipid melt thereby creating the solid matrix.

Although solid-lipid based carrier systems are produced from crystalline raw materials, it has to be considered that crystallization from the dispersed lipid melt might be different from that of the bulk phase due to the high dispersity, the small particle size, the presence of emulsifying agents and drugs as well as the high surface-to-volume ratio. This may lead to differences in the crystallization behavior, the degree of crystallinity, and the polymorphism of the nanoparticulate lipids compared to the bulk materials. Indeed, thermoanalytical investigations of glycerides indicate that polymorphic transitions proceed faster in the dispersed state than in the bulk (Siekmann and Westesen, 1994). Moreover, it has been observed that the melting temperature and the recrystallization temperature of dispersed triglycerides is decreased compared with the bulk material (Siekmann and Westesen, 1994; Westesen and Bunjes, 1995; Bunjes *et al.*, 1996a). Thus, recrystallization of dispersed triglycerides requires significantly more supercooling than in the bulk. As a result of the higher supercooling required for nucleation, recrystallization of melt-homogenized triglycerides may be considerably retarded or even prevented at a given temperature. Westesen and Bunjes (1995) found that nanoparticles prepared from triglycerides solid at room temperature do not necessarily recrystallize on cooling to common storage temperatures. Thus, melt-homogenized dispersions of trilaurin remain in the state of a supercooled emulsion at refrigerator temperatures over several months. A similar effect has also been observed for melt-homogenized dispersions of the lipophilic bioactive substance ubidecarenone (Siekmann and Westesen, 1995).

The aim of this chapter is to draw the reader's attention to the phenomenon of supercooling in dispersed systems which has often been neglected in the past with respect to pharmaceutical applications. As will be demonstrated below, a number of pharmaceutically relevant physicochemical properties of melt-homogenized colloidal dispersions can be explained by effects resulting from supercooling. The drawbacks and potential of supercooled emulsions for use in drug delivery will be discussed.

EMULSIONS AND THE PHENOMENON OF SUPERCOOLING

In the following a short overview on the phenomenon of supercooling, especially with respect to emulsion systems, will be given. For more detailed information, the reader is referred to the more specialized literature (e.g. Turnbull, 1952, Clausse, 1985).

According to the IUPAC definition an emulsion consists of liquid droplets and/or liquid crystals dispersed in a liquid (Everett, 1972). Although an emulsion is metastable with regard to the dispersity of its droplets, the dispersed phase itself is usually in a thermodynamically stable liquid state. If such emulsions are cooled down below the melting temperature of the dispersed material, the droplets fail to crystallize within a certain temperature range below their melting temperature until a critical crystallization temperature is reached. In the temperature range between melting and crystallization temperature the dispersed liquid is called supercooled. In this region, the emulsion is not only metastable with regard to its dispersity but also concerning the physical state of the droplets. Although supercooling is not constricted to dispersed material but is also frequently observed in bulk phases, the temperature range of supercooling in emulsions is usually much larger than in the bulk.

Generally, the limits of supercooling are given on the one hand by the melting temperature of the substance and on the other hand by its crystallization temperature. Crystal growth can only occur after an initial nucleation step in which atomic or molecular aggregates are formed in the liquid. Since the negative free energy of condensation of the molecules is counteracted by the positive free energy due to the creation of a new liquid-solid interface, the aggregates are not stable until they have reached a critical size. The activation energy required for the formation of these critical nuclei is supplied by fluctuations within the liquid. Beside spontaneous nucleation within a liquid volume (homogenous nucleation) nucleation may also be initiated at the interface between the liquid and a foreign substrate e.g. the surface of particulate impurities, an emulsifier layer or the container walls (heterogenous nucleation). The theory of homogenous and heterogenous nucleation in condensed systems developed by Turnbull and Fisher (1949, 1952) describes the random process of nucleation by means of a nucleation rate J. J is the number of nuclei formed per unit time and unit volume (homogenous nucleation) or unit area of favorable nucleation site (heterogeneous nucleation). The nucleation rate is given by (Turnbull and Fisher, 1949; Turnbull, 1952; Walstra and van Beresteyn, 1975):

$$J \cong n \frac{k \cdot T}{h} \exp\left[-\frac{\Delta F_A}{k \cdot T}\right] \exp\left[-\frac{\Delta F_c}{k \cdot T}\right]$$

with

$$\Delta F_c = \varphi \cdot a \cdot \gamma^3 \left(\frac{T_m}{\lambda \cdot (T_m - T)}\right)^2$$

J: nucleation rate
n: number of atoms or molecules per unit volume of liquid
k: Boltzman's constant
T: actual absolute temperature
h: Planck's constant
ΔF_A: free energy of activation per atom/molecule for transport across the liquid-crystal interface
ΔF_c: free energy of formation of a nucleus of critical size
φ: size factor
a: factor determined by the shape of the nucleus; for spherical nuclei $a = \frac{16\pi}{3}$
γ: interfacial free energy between crystal nucleus and liquid
λ: heat of fusion per unit volume
T_m: absolute melting temperature

The factor φ which is 1 for homogenous nucleation processes becomes <1 for heterogenous nucleation (Walstra and van Beresteyn 1975, Clausse et al. 1987) since the potential barrier for nucleus formation is lower and J is consequently higher than in case of homogenous nucleation.

The nucleation rate J strongly depends on temperature. With increasing supercooling the critical radius becomes smaller and the energy of nucleus formation is lowered enhancing nucleation. On cooling a liquid below its melting temperature the nucleation rate is almost zero until a certain critical supercooling is reached where the nucleation rate increases sharply.

Cooling melts of bulk material below their melting point usually results in considerably higher crystallization temperatures than predicted by homogenous nucleation theory, *i.e.* heterogenous nucleation has to be assumed. This behavior is attributed to the presence of particulate impurities within the melt acting as nucleation centers. If the liquid volume is divided into small droplets, the catalytic influence of a given number of particulate impurities is limited to a few individual droplets. For this reason, supercooling observed in emulsions is usually much larger than bulk supercooling.

The appearance of a nucleus in an emulsion droplet can only be described with a certain probability (Turnbull, 1952). For homogenous nucleation, the nucleation frequency k_D for a droplet of diameter D is proportional to its volume v_D indicating that the lifetime of a droplet increases with decreasing particle size:

$$k_D = J \cdot v_D$$

In case of heterogenous nucleation, k_D is proportional to the area of the nucleation site S, e.g. a surface film (Turnbull, 1952):

$$k_D = J_S \cdot S$$

Due to the random phenomenon of nucleation the crystallization temperature of emulsion droplets always scatters around a mean value. Literature data on crystallization temperatures are, e.g. defined as the temperature where the nucleation rate starts to increase considerably (Uhlmann et al., 1975; MacFarlane and Angell, 1982; Cordiez et al., 1982; Labes-Carrier et al., 1995) or as a most probable crystallization temperature, e.g. given as peak temperature of a DSC curve (Clausse, 1985; Bunjes et al., 1996a; Westesen et al., 1997).

Emulsions are favorable systems to study the phenomena of supercooling and nucleation as well as the properties of supercooled materials: Advantageous (e.g. Turnbull, 1952; Cordiez et al., 1982; Clausse, 1991) is the limited nucleation influence of foreign substrates such as bulk impurities or container walls making the study of homogenous nucleation possible. In emulsions, a large number of droplets are automatically studied at the same time allowing a good statistical evaluation. Moreover, very poor heat conducting materials (e.g. organic substances) can be studied more conveniently in a well heat-conducting continuous phase. A review on nucleation and supercooling studies utilizing emulsions, including theoretical models, a survey of measurement techniques, data treatment and determination of characteristic nucleation values is given by Clausse (1985). In special cases, the large supercooling obtained in emulsions may lead to special phenomena such as vitrification or formation of special polymorphic forms (MacFarlane and Angell, 1982; Dumas et al., 1987).

Studies on supercooling in emulsions

The droplet or emulsion technique for supercooling studies was introduced by Vonnegut (1948) and has since then been frequently utilized by researchers from many fields to study nucleation and supercooling phenomena. Metals were the first materials to be investigated in dispersion (Vonnegut, 1948; Turnbull, 1952). Much work has also been performed on water which is very important from the viewpoint of life sciences and meteorology (Clausse, 1985). In the following, the focus will be mainly on emulsion studies of supercooled organic matter since they are of major importance from the pharmaceutical point of view. The values in Table 1 and 2 give an impression of supercooling values obtained with organic substances. A direct comparison of data from different sources can be difficult since the degree of supercooling may depend on parameters concerning the emulsion itself (e.g. particle size or emulsifier, see below), the experimental setup used as well as on the definition of the crystallization temperature. Regarding the investigation of organic material, quite a lot of data can be found on crystallization of alkanes which are of interest

Table 1 Examples for supercooling of organic substances

Substance	T_{melt} (C)	T_{cryst} (°C) in dispersion	Supercooling in dispersion (°C)[a]	(Mean) particle size range	Reference
Stearic acid	68[b]		14.5–20.5[d]	0.5 μm	Grange et al., 1986
Laurone	69[b]		15°C+	5 μm+	Grange et al. 1986
			37°C	0.5 μm	
CCl₄	−23.5[c]		53.5	<1 μm	MacFarlane and Angell, 1982
Benzene	5	−77	71	1 μm	Dumas et al., 1987
Nitrobenzene	5	−66	109	1 μm	Dumas et al., 1987
n-Hexane	−95.5[c]	−104	33.5	1 μm	Uhlmann et al., 1975
n-Octane	−57[c]		24	1 μm	Uhlmann et al., 1975
n-Decane	−29.9[c]		24	1 μm	Uhlmann et al., 1975
n-Dodecane	−9.8[c]		22	1 μm	Uhlmann et al., 1975
n-Hexadecane	18[c]		15.2	1 μm	Uhlmann et al., 1975
n-Octadecane	27.8[c]		12.9	1 μm	Uhlmann et al., 1975
n-Docosane	44.2[α,b], 42.8[β,b]	ca. 34.5°C	9.7[α]/8.3[β]	1–20 μm	Phipps, 1964[e]
n-Hexacosane	56.2[α,b], 49[β,b]	ca. 44°C	12.9[α]/5[β]	1–20 μm	Phipps, 1964[e]
n-Triacontane	65.4[α,b], 57.9[β,b]	ca. 50°C	15.4[α]/7.9[β]	1–20 μm	Phipps, 1964[e]
Polyethylene (linear)	143		55	1.5–2 μm	Koutsky et al., 1967
Isotactic polypropylene	186		101	1.5–2 μm	Koutsky et al., 1967

[a] In general, highest supercooling is presented in table. If possible, data refers to the melting point in dispersion.
[b] Bulk
[c] Dispersion
[d] Depending on emulsifier
[e] Some data was extracted from measurement curves or diagrams published in this reference. Values given should be taken as approximate.
[α] related to the α-Form
[β] related to the β-Form

Table 2 Supercooling data for triglycerides

Triglyceride	T_{melt} (°C) Dispersion	T_{melt} (°C) Bulk	T_{cryst} (°C) Dispersion	T_{cryst} (°C) Bulk	Supercooling in dispersion (°C)[a]	Triglyceride concentration/(mean) particle size range	Experimental method	Reference
Trilaurin			7.5°C	ca. 21°C		30–40%/?	DSC (1.25, 2.5°C/min.)	Zhao and Reid, 1994[b]
Trilaurin			−2	7		40%/?	DSC (10°C/min.)	Simoneau et al., 1993
Trilaurin		14.8$^\alpha$, 46$^\beta$	ca. −4.5°C		19.3$^\alpha$, 50.5$^\beta$	2–3%/1–20 μm	Microscopy (1°C/min.)	Phipps, 1964[b]
Trilaurin	43$^\beta$	46$^\beta$	−8	11	51$^\beta$	10%/0.1 μm	DSC (5°C/min.)	Bunjes et al., 1996a
Trimyristin			10	25		40%/?	DSC (10°C/min.)	Simoneau et al., 1993
Trimyristin		31.8$^\alpha$, 56.3$^\beta$	ca. 12°C		19.8$^\alpha$, 44.3$^\beta$	2–3%/1–20 μm	Microscopy (1°C/min.)	Phipps, 1964[b]
Trimyristin	53$^\beta$	56$^\beta$	8–9	28	44–45$^\beta$	10%/0.1	DSC (5°C/min.)	Bunjes et al., 1996a
Tripalmitin			ca. 37°C	ca. 42°C		30–40%/?	DSC (1.25, 2.5°C/min.)	Zhao and Reid, 1994
Tripalmitin		44.5$^\alpha$, 64.9$^\beta$	ca. 23°C		21.5$^\alpha$, 41.9$^\beta$	2–3%/1–20 μm	Microscopy (1°C/min.)	Phipps, 1964[b]
Tripalmitin	44$^\alpha$, 60$^\beta$	46$^\alpha$, 64$^\beta$	21	42	23$^\alpha$, 39$^\beta$	10%/0.1	DSC (5°C/min.)	Bunjes et al., 1996a
Tristearin			ca. 47°C	ca. 47°C		30–40 %/?	DSC (1.25, 2.5°C/min.)	Zhao and Reid, 1994[b]
Tristearin		54.0$^\alpha$, 71.3$^\beta$	ca. 28°C		26$^\alpha$, 43.3$^\beta$	2–3%/1–20 μm	Microscopy (1°C/min.)	Phipps, 1964[b]
Tristearin	54$^\alpha$, 68$^\beta$	55$^\alpha$, 73$^\beta$	30	51	24$^\alpha$, 38$^\beta$	10%/0.1	DSC (5°C/min.)	Bunjes et al., 1996a

[a] In general, highest supercooling is presented in table. If possible, data refers to the melting point in dispersion.
[b] Some data was extracted measurement curves or diagrams published in this reference. Values given should be taken as approximate.

α related to the α-Form
β related to the β-Form

from a theoretical point of view as well as as model systems in food science (Turnbull and Cormia, 1961; Phipps, 1964; Uhlmann *et al.*, 1975; Dickinson *et al.*, 1991, 1993; Coupland *et al.*, 1993). Other lipidic systems such as triglycerides (Phipps, 1964; Walstra and van Beresteyn, 1975; Simoneau *et al.*, 1993; Zhao and Reid, 1994; Bunjes *et al.*, 1996a; Westesen *et al.*, 1997), and fatty acids (Cordiez *et al.*, 1982; Grange *et al.*, 1986) have also been studied. Also the nucleation behavior of polymers has been investigated in emulsion systems (Cormia *et al.* 1962; Koutsky *et al.*, 1967) as well as a variety of different other organic substances (e.g. Dumas *et al.*, 1987).

Dilatometry (Vonnegut, 1948; Turnbull, 1952) and microscopy (Cormia *et al.*, 1962; Phipps, 1964) were the first methods to study supercooling in emulsions. Today, calorimetric methods are most widely used (Bunjes *et al.*, 1996a; Clausse, 1985; Dumas *et al.*, 1994; Grange *et al.*, 1986; Labes-Carrier *et al.*, 1995; MacFarlane and Angell, 1982; Siekmann and Westesen, 1994; Simoneau *et al.*, 1993). The use of ultrasound velocity and attenuation measurements (Coupland *et al.*, 1993; Dickinson *et al.*, 1991, 1993), NMR spectroscopy and imaging (McClements *et al.*, 1994; Simoneau *et al.*, 1991, 1993; Walstra and van Beresteyn, 1975; Westesen and Siekmann, 1995; Westesen *et al.*, 1997), X-ray diffraction (Bunjes *et al.*, 1996a; Söderberg *et al.*, 1989; Walstra and van Beresteyn, 1975; Westesen *et al.*, 1997) and transmission electron microscopy (Söderberg *et al.*, 1989) has also been described in connection with supercooling studies.

EMULSIONS OF SUPERCOOLED LIPIDS AS POTENTIAL DRUG CARRIER SYSTEMS

Submicron-sized triglyceride emulsions are commonly used as a high-calorie source in parenteral nutrition and may also serve as drug carrier systems for the parenteral, even the intravenous administration of lipophilic drugs (Collins-Gold *et al.*, 1990; Prankerd and Stella, 1990). The low viscosity of the liquid oil droplets is, however, a major drawback with respect to sustained release or drug targeting as the drug can diffuse rapidly out of the droplets upon administration (Washington and Evans, 1995). These difficulties may be overcome by replacing the liquid emulsion droplets by solid colloidal triglyceride particles, a concept that has been realized a few years ago (Lucks *et al.*, 1992; Siekmann and Westesen, 1992). Solid lipid particle systems are supposed to be non-toxic, biodegradable, stable against coalescence and drug leakage and to have a matrix controlled drug delivery.

They are preferably produced by high-pressure homogenization of the molten lipid in a hot aqueous phase and can be stabilized by nonionic or ionic surfactants and their mixtures with phospholipids. Although solid triglycerides are used as matrix materials crystallization of the lipid particles upon cooling of the hot colloidal dispersion below the melting temperature of the lipid does not lead to instantaneous crystallization. Already in an early stage of investigation it became obvious that a considerable amount of supercooling is required to solidify melt-homogenized lipid nanoparticles (Westesen *et al.*, 1993; Siekmann and Westesen, 1994). Hence, systematic studies on dispersions of simple saturated monoacid triglycerides (even-numbered chains from C12 (trilaurin) to C18 (tristearin)) as well as on suppository hard fat masses consisting of low-melting mixed-chain triglycerides were initiated (Westesen and Bunjes, 1995; Bunjes *et al.*, 1996a, Westesen *et al.*, 1997). Nanodispersions were

Table 3 Composition of glyceride dispersions and physical state of the droplets

Matrix lipid (10%)	Emulsifier blend	Droplet state after three months of storage at 20–25°C	4–8°C
D 112	PL/NaGCa, PL/NaGCb, PL/Tyl	liquid[a]	liquid[b]
D 114	PL/NaGCa, PL/NaGCb, PL/Tyl	liquid[c]	solid
D 116	PL/NaGCa, PL/Tyl	solid	solid
D 118	PL/NaGCa, PL/Tyl	solid	solid
E 85	PL/Tyl	liquid	solid
H 42	PL/Tyl, PL/NaGCb	liquid	solid
H 35	PL/Tyl, PL/NaGCa	liquid[a]	solid (or (partially) liquid)

[a] no crystalline material detected after more than 2 years of storage

[b] in bile salt stabilized dispersions about 2 % of the triglyceride crystallizes within more than 2 years of storage

[c] in bile salt stabilized dispersions no or less than 0,5 % of the triglyceride crystallizes within more than 2 years of storage

Matrix lipids: D 112, D 114, D 116, D 118: Dynasan 112 (trilaurin), 114 (trimyristin), 116 (tripalmitin), 118 (tristearin); E 85, H 35, H 42: Hard fats Witepsol E 85, H 35, H 42

Stabilizer compositions: PL/NaGCa: 1.6% Lipoid S100, 0.4% sodium glycocholate; PL/NaGCb: 2.4% Lipoid S100, 0,6% sodium glycocholate; PL/Tyl: 2% Lipoid S100, 2% tyloxapol.

High–pressure homogenization (Micron Lab 40, APV Gaulin) was performed at elevated temperature using 5 cycles at 800 bar. The aqueous phase contained 2,25% glycerol and 0,01% thiomersal.

prepared by high-pressure melt-homogenization of the lipids in an aqueous phase and stabilized by mixtures of phospholipid with the bile salt sodium glycocholate or the nonionic surfactant tyloxapol (Table 3). Approximated mean PCS particle sizes by number were typically in the range between 60 and 150 nm.

According to DSC and X-ray studies (Figure 1) on the physical state of the particle matrix colloidally dispersed shorter-chain triglycerides do not crystallize at room temperature (trimyristin, various hard fats) or at refrigerator temperatures (trilaurin) during several months or even years of storage (Table 3). These X-ray and DSC data are, however, not sufficient to exclude a solid (amorphous) state of the dispersed phase. X-ray diffraction allows only to differentiate between crystalline and amorphous material. DSC, which can in principle be used to differentiate between amorphous solids and liquids, may not be sensitive enough to detect a glass transition of colloidally dispersed material. Additional investigations on the physical state of colloidal trimyristin by ^{1}H NMR spectroscopy indicate a high mobility of the triglyceride molecules in a dispersion stored at room temperature in contrast to that of a cold stored dispersion (Figure 2). This result confirms that the dispersed triglyceride remains in fact liquid and does not form a solid amorphous phase if the dispersion is never allowed to cool down below its critical crystallization temperature. The conclusion is supported by the fact that crystallization of the droplets can be induced by cooling below a critical temperature which would be atypical of a glassy state. In all cases much higher supercooling is necessary to

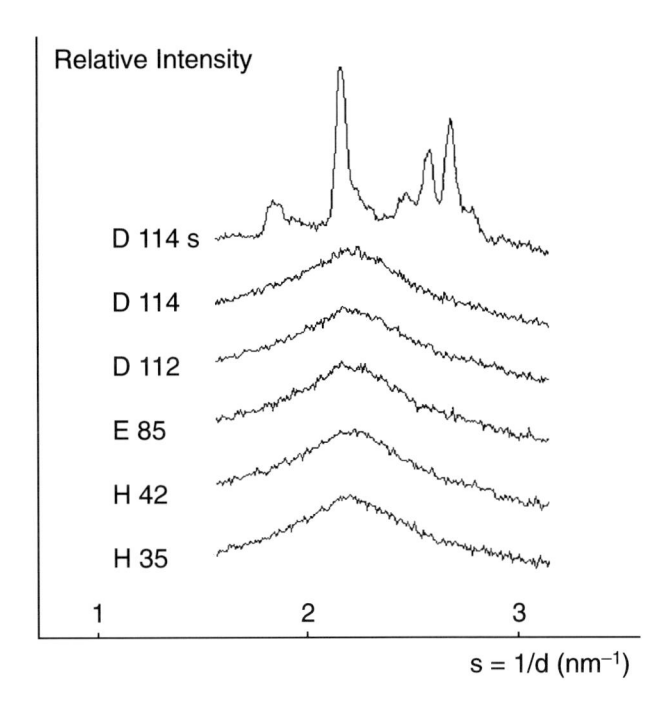

Figure 1 Wide angle X-ray diffractograms of supercooled triglyceride dispersions (D 114, 112: Dynasan 114 (trimyristin) and Dynasan 112 (trilaurin), E 85, H 42, H 35: Witepsol E 85, H 42, and H 35). A trimyristin suspension (D 114 s) is shown for comparison.

crystallize the colloidal triglycerides than the bulk materials. Crystallization in dispersions of simple saturated triglycerides occurs at temperatures about 20°C lower than in the bulk (Table 2, Bunjes et al., 1996a). The highest degree of supercooling was observed with simple saturated monoacid triglycerides for which the difference between final melting and crystallization temperature increases with decreasing chain length of the triglyceride (Figure 3). Although dispersions of liquid hard fat droplets could be easily obtained and stored at room temperature for a considerable period of time the amount of supercooling is much lower for these complex triglyceride mixtures. This effect most probably results from the presence of longer-chain fatty acid groups in the mixed triglycerides. Longer chains may act as nucleation center and induce the crystallization of the fat. A similar effect has been observed in nanoparticles prepared by melt-emulsification of mixtures of simple monoacid triglycerides: Admixture of increasing amounts of tristearin to trimyristin or to trilaurin increases the crystallization temperature of the dispersed phase (Bunjes et al., 1996a).

In conclusion, the dispersions containing liquid droplets at temperatures far below the melting temperature of the matrix lipid have to be regarded as emulsions of supercooled melts which are stable for a pharmaceutically relevant period of time. Since the properties of such emulsions of supercooled melts are expected to be different from ordinary vegetable oil-in-water emulsions with respect to drug release and delivery they may be utilized as a new type of drug carrier system.

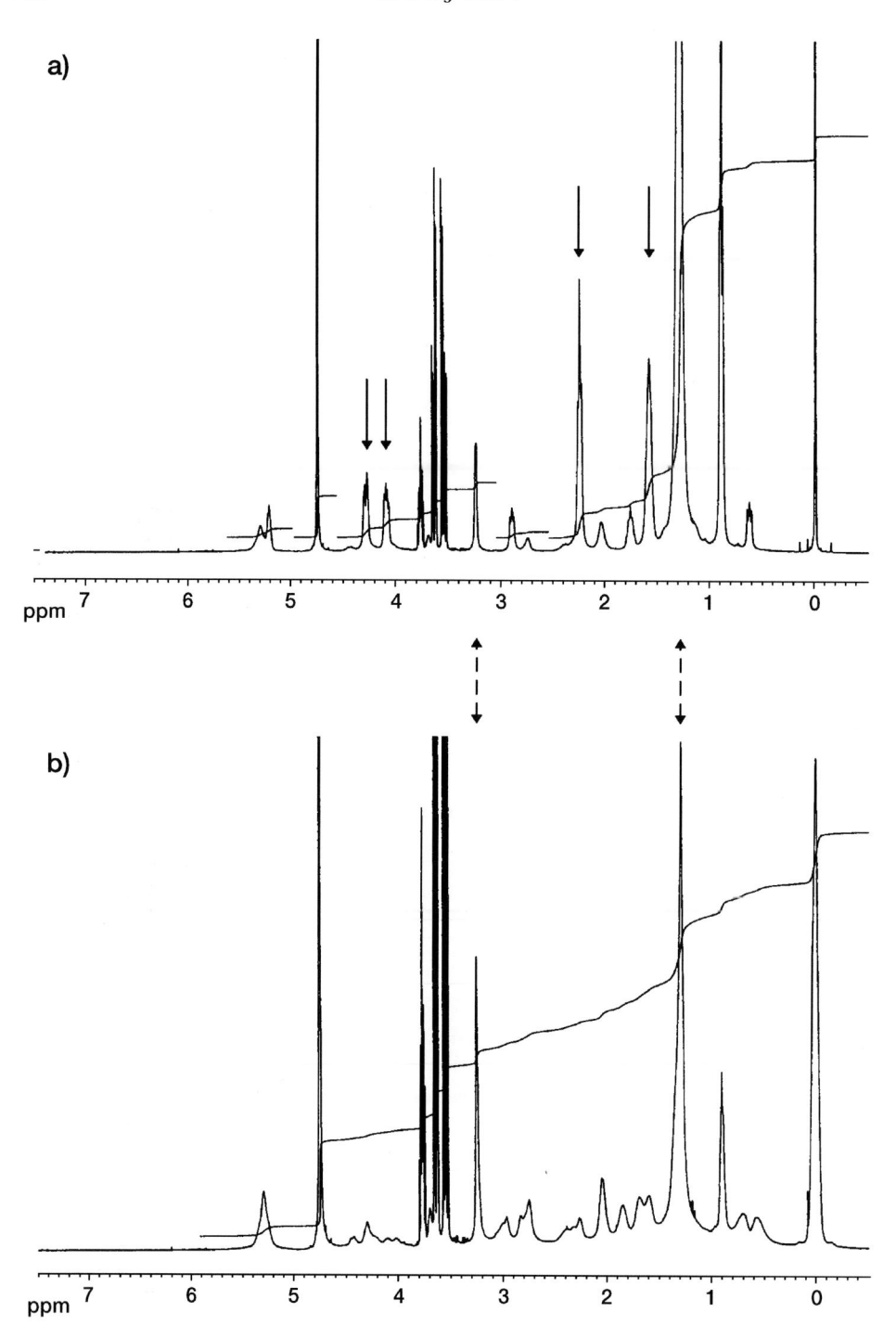

Figure 2 ^{1}H NMR spectra of a trimyristin dispersion stored for one day at room (a) or refrigerator temperature (b). Note the additional signals (marked with arrows) in spectrum a) and the different ratio of areas of the signals marked by broken arrows.

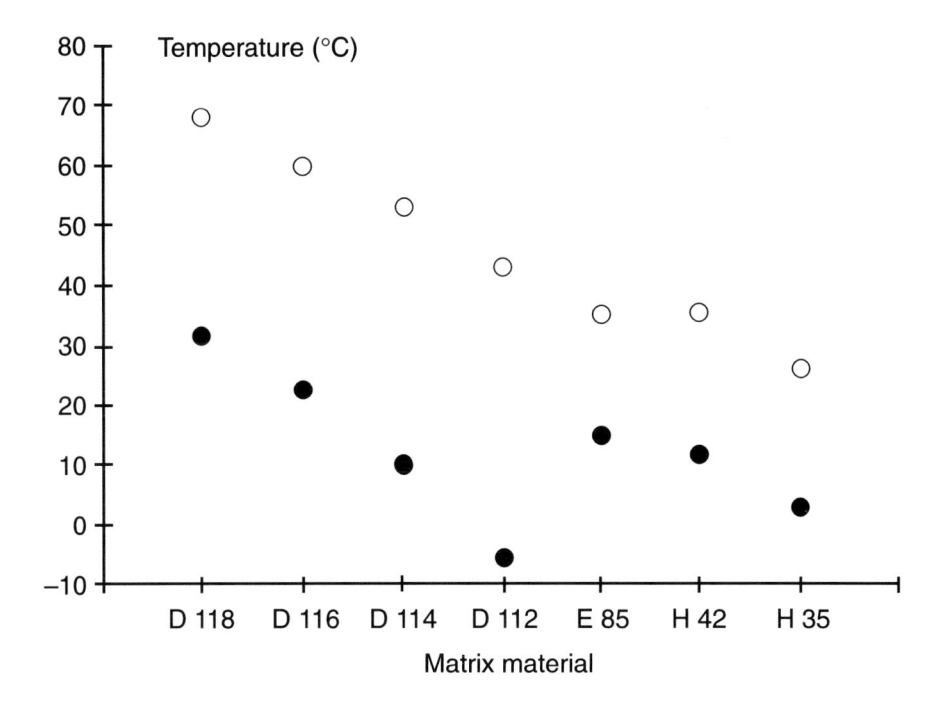

Figure 3 Melting (open circles) and crystallization temperatures (filled circles) of different dispersed triglycerides stabilized with a phospholipid/tyloxapol blend (DSC scanning rate: 5°C/min, crystallization temperatures are given as onset temperatures of the crystallization exotherm).

Especially an increased viscosity of the supercooled droplets compared to ordinary triglyceride oils would be favorable with respect to drug release. Extrapolation of viscosity data for supercooled bulk triglycerides (Phipps, 1962) down to the temperature range in which colloidal emulsions of supercooled triglycerides can exist leads to viscosity values similar to those of soy bean oil used e.g. in parenteral nutrition or as drug carriers (Table 4). Compared to medium chain glycerides which

Table 4 Calculated and extrapolated viscosity of supercooled triglycerides (following Phipps (1962)) in comparison to liquid oils

Triglyceride	Extrapolated viscosity (mPa s) at					
	40°C	37°C	30°C	20°C	10°C	5°C
Tristearin	50	56				
Tripalmitin	42	47	63			
Trimyristin	32	36	48	74		
Trilaurin	24	27	35	55	90	118
Soy bean oil[a]	29				100	
Medium chain triglycerides[a]				27–30		

[a] Wade and Weller 1994

are comparable to the monoacid long chain saturated triglycerides with respect to stability, the viscosity of supercooled long chain triglycerides at 20°C is twice (trilaurin) or three times (trimyristin) as high. It is, however, not clear if such extrapolation is valid for submicron emulsion particles the properties of which may be changed distinctly compared to those of the bulk. Moreover, it cannot be excluded that discontinuities in viscosity values similar to those found in the region of the β-melting point (Phipps, 1962) may occur also at much higher supercooling e.g. in the region of the α-melting point. These questions can only be answered by studies on the viscosity of supercooled colloidal emulsion droplets *in situ* (e.g. by NMR).

Trimyristin and hard fat dispersions which can be obtained as emulsions or suspensions depending on the preparation parameters under convenient laboratory conditions are very interesting model systems to study the effect of the physical state on pharmaceutically relevant particle properties such as their drug incorporation capacity. Incorporation studies indicate that the drug loading capacity of emulsions of supercooled melts may be considerably higher than that of solid lipid nanoparticles (Bunjes *et al.*, 1996a; Westesen *et al.*, 1997).

The supercooling and crystallization behavior of dispersed triglycerides is not only of interest from the pharmaceutical point of view but is also of high importance in food science. A higher supercooling of dispersed triglycerides compared to bulk material has long been known from investigations on milk fat (Mulder, 1953; Walstra and van Beresteyn, 1975; Söderberg *et al.*, 1989). A detailed analysis of this phenomenon was given by Walstra and van Beresteyn (1975) who *inter alia* demonstrated the particle size dependence of the supercooling tendency of the dispersed fat. Phipps (1964) has reported minimum crystallization temperatures of dispersed simple monoacid triglycerides which are similar to the values observed for colloidally dispersed triglycerides (Table 2). Phipps' investigations were performed on micrometer-sized particles in which crystallization was also observed at considerably higher temperatures due to their large size. In contrast, crystallization at higher temperatures was not observed in the colloidal triglyceride dispersions described above. Simoneau *et al.* (1991, 1993) also found an increased supercooling tendency of emulsified trimyristin and trilaurin compared to bulk material. The emulsions under investigation were of comparatively high concentration, presumably had a quite large particle size and were unstable during thermal cycling. In spite of this, the supercooling values from constant cooling experiments (Table 2) approach those for colloidal pharmaceutical emulsions and those given as maximum supercooling by Phipps (1964). Upon isothermal storage, however, the droplets crystallize within minutes at refrigerator temperatures (trilaurin) or around 20°C (trimyristin). In contrast, colloidal droplets can be stored in the liquid state for months at these temperatures (Table 3). The comparatively high crystallization temperatures for triglycerides and milk fat dispersions reported by Zhao and Reid (1994) may also be due to quite large particle size and high concentration of the dispersed phase in combination with a low cooling rate. These results indicate that preparation of stable dispersions of supercooled melts is much facilitated in the colloidal size range with no micrometer-size particles present.

It is obvious from the preceding data that the formation of supercooled melts is a common phenomenon following the emulsification of molten triglycerides. Surprisingly, it is little discussed in the pharmaceutical literature with respect to colloidal systems based on melt-emulsified triglycerides which have received much interest as potential drug carrier systems in the recent years. Sakaeda and Hirano (1995) report on *in vivo* release studies from the hard fats Witepsol E 75 and E 85 (bulk melting points 38.0°C and 43.5°C, respectively) colloidally dispersed with the aid of phospholipids. The authors consider these dispersions as classical emulsions and do not discuss the fact of supercooling at room temperature. Recalling the fact that crystallization of colloidal trilaurin particles requires subzero temperatures (Figure 3), data on optimization of production parameters for solid lipid nanoparticles (SLN) obtained on melt-homogenized trilaurin dispersions (Schwarz *et al.*, 1994) has to be reconsidered. In agreement with our own observations Schwarz (1995) states that trilaurin nanoparticles do not crystallize within one year of storage at 4°C. Studies on serum-degradation of trilaurin SLN (Müller *et al.*, 1995) were probably also performed on supercooled, liquid nanoparticles. It is also doubtful that drug incorporation studies in nanoparticles prepared from trilaurin (Heiati *et al.*, 1997) or the even lower melting triglyceride tricaprin (Domb *et al.*, 1996) were really performed on solid particles as claimed in the literature. In these studies no experimental evidence is given for the solid state of the nanoparticles assumed by the authors. Nor do recent studies describing surface modification/coating of melt-homogenized "solid" trilaurin lipid nanoparticles (Akbarieh *et al.*, 1994; Heiati *et al.*, 1996) consider the possibility of emulsion formation although a spherical particle shape and flotation of the particles upon ultracentrifugation point to the presence of a liquid fat phase.

The question if solid or lipid nanoparticles are obtained by melt-emulsification of triglycerides is not only of interest regarding their drug incorporation and drug release properties. Severe instability phenomena have been reported for nanoparticle systems which were stabilized with phospholipids only analogously to parenteral emulsion formulations. These effects have been attributed *inter alia* to the inability of phospholipids to sufficiently stabilize the new surfaces created by crystallization (Siekmann and Westesen, 1992; Westesen and Siekmann, 1997). Reports on stable phospholipid-stabilized nanoparticle dispersions based on solid triglycerides (e.g. Schwarz *et al.*, 1994; Heiati *et al.*, 1996, 1997; Domb *et al.*, 1996) may have to be reconsidered taking the high supercooling tendency of the matrix lipids (trilaurin, tricaprin) into account which may lead to the formation of emulsion particles instead of lipid suspensions.

EMULSIONS OF SUPERCOOLED DRUGS IN DRUG DELIVERY

The development of solid lipid nanoparticles revealed the possibility to prepare submicron-sized particles from crystalline material by the melt-homogenization process (Siekmann and Westesen, 1992). Although this production method has basically been applied to prepare lipidic drug carriers it is conceivable to employ the same procedure for the comminution of lipophilic drugs.

Numerous poorly water-soluble drugs are commonly available as crystalline bulk materials at room temperature, primarily in the form of poorly wettable powders with grain sizes in the millimeter- and micrometer range which are generated by milling or grinding. A further decrease in particle size by these conventional techniques is expensive, ineffective or even impossible. Additionally, the reduction of solids to submicron-sized powders can bring about heavy difficulties in handling of these dry products such as an increased risk of dust explosions and cross-contamination problems in a factory environment. Moreover, such systems present a risk to health for persons exposed to the possible inhalation and absorption of potent bioactive materials.

For many applications there is, however, an obvious need to reduce the particle size down to the nanometer range. Particle size is an important factor with respect to the parenteral, in particular intravenous administration of drugs. Many lipophilic drugs cannot be formulated as aqueous solutions due to their low aqueous solubility. Intravenous administration of suspensions of sparingly soluble substances in water bears the risk of capillary blockage and embolism since the suspended particles are generally larger than the smallest blood vessels.

Enteral administration of these lipophilic drugs does often lead to bioavailability problems, particularly upon peroral administration, due to low absorption from the gastrointestinal tract (GIT). The low absorption rate of poorly water-soluble, in particular lipophilic substances, from the GIT is generally attributed to the poor solubility of these substances and to their poor wettability in gastrointestinal fluids. The dissolution process of the substance can become the rate limiting step in absorption and might thus lead to a poor bioavailability.

The dissolution rate of a substance is affected *inter alia* by its particle size, its wettability and with crystalline substances also by the energy required to overcome lattice forces. It can therefore be deduced that the bioavailability of poorly water-soluble bioactive agents can in principle be enhanced by the following three technological manipulations:

- reduction of particle size,
- hydrophilization of particle surfaces, and
- reduction of the crystallinity of the substance.

Particle size is interrelated to the dissolution rate, since in diffusion controlled dissolution of sparingly soluble drugs the diffusional distance decreases substantially with particle size (Bisrat *et al.*, 1992). Moreover, reduction in particle size leads to an increase in the specific interfacial surface area (Florence and Atwood, 1981). For example, improvement of the bioavailability after peroral administration due to enhancement of the rate of dissolution by micronization has been described for digoxin (Shaw *et al.*, 1974) and griseofulvin (Atkinson *et al.*, 1962). Micronized substances can, however, exhibit wettability problems, e.g. due to aerophilization during the milling process. The reduced wettability counteracts to the increased dissolution rate achievable by micronization as a result of the reduced particle size and can therefore lead to a reduced dissolution rate. The dissolution process is thus closely related to wettability. Since apolar surfaces are only poorly wetted in aqueous media, the dissolution rate of sparingly water-soluble substances can be increased by hydrophilization of particle surfaces to improve the wettability in aqueous media.

Apart from reduction of particle size and improvement of wettability, the peroral bioavailability of a poorly water-soluble drug can be enhanced if the drug is not present in a crystalline but in an amorphous physical state. In general, amorphous forms of a substance exhibit a higher apparent solubility and a faster dissolution than their crystal forms since the dissolution of amorphous substances does not require lattice energy. It is known, for example, that the antibiotic agent novobiocin can only be absorbed from the intestine after administration of the amorphous

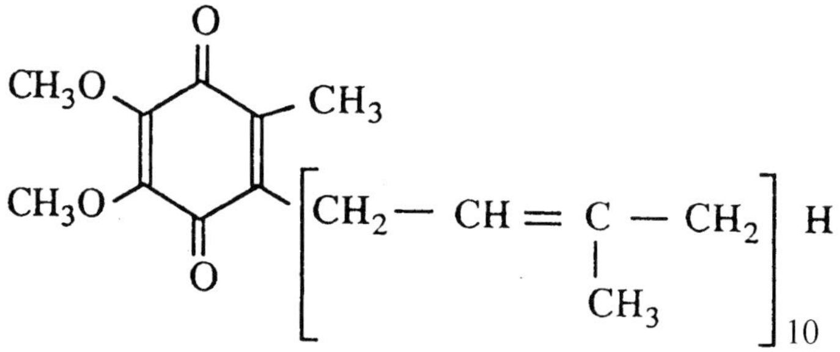

$$\text{CH}_3\text{O}\underset{\underset{\text{O}}{\|}}{\overset{\overset{\text{O}}{\|}}{\bigcirc}}\overset{\text{CH}_3}{\underset{}{}}\left[\text{CH}_2-\text{CH}=\underset{\underset{\text{CH}_3}{|}}{\text{C}}-\text{CH}_2\right]_{10}\text{H}$$

Figure 4 Structure formula of ubidecarenone.

substance which has a solubility ten times higher than the crystalline agent (Mullins and Macek, 1960).

The melt-homogenization process employed for the preparation of colloidal glyceride dispersions (Siekmann and Westesen, 1992) provides a method to reduce the particle size of drug substances which can be melted at temperatures below about 100°C to the nanometer size range. Due to the presence of emulsifying agents/surfactants the resulting nanoparticles are surrounded by one or several layers of amphiphilic molecules which are arranged in such a way that the hydrophobic part of the molecule protrudes into the lipophilic core of the particle whereas the hydrophilic moiety of the surfactant molecule is oriented towards the aqueous phase. Consequently, the particle surface is hydrophilic and should thus exhibit a good wettability. In case that the melt-homogenized drug substance remains in the state of a supercooled melt, as has been found for a number of lipidic materials (see above), the particles are non-crystalline. Their dissolution does thus not require lattice energy. Considering these aspects, submicron-sized particles of supercooled melts should represent a promising formulation approach for sparingly soluble drug substances with poor bioavailability. Therefore, the preparation of melt-homogenized dispersions of the lipophilic model drug substance ubidecarenone (coenzyme Q_{10}) was investigated in detail by Siekmann and Westesen (1995).

Preparation of Melt-Emulsified Ubidecarenone Nanoparticles

Ubidecarenone (Figure 4) is an endogenous quinone and is an essential component of the electron transport chain of oxidative phosphorylation. The substance is therapeutically used *inter alia* in cardiomyopathia, coronary diseases and for the prophylaxis of heart attack (Folkers *et al.*, 1991). The bioavailability of ubidecarenone is generally low due to the poor solubility in gastrointestinal fluids causing a low gastrointestinal absorption of the substance. Kishi *et al.* (1984) observed that the peroral bioavailability of ubidecarenone from solid dosage forms such as tablets and granules is related to the dissolution rate of the preparations.

Ubidecarenone is crystalline at room temperature and has a melting point of 49°C (Ramasarma, 1968). The substance is commercially available as an orange-colored, strongly adhesive powder consisting of crystal agglomerates in the micrometer to millimeter size range. Due to its long isoprenoid side chain the molecule

Table 5 Composition and PCS mean diameter of selected ubidecarenone dispersions prepared by melt-emulsification

Ubidecarenone in% (w/w)	Emulsifier composition in% (w/w)	Mean diameter (PCS) in nm	Preparation
3.0	2.0% Tyl	67	ML
3.0	1.8% SPC	103	MF
3.0	1.8% SPC, 0.4% NaGC	70	MF
5.0	0.9% SPC, 0.4% NaGC	178	PS
10.0	6% SPC, 1.25% NaGC	144	ML
10.0	1.2% SPC, 0.4% NaGC	259	ML

Abbreviations: ML, Micron Lab 40 (APV Gaulin); MF, Microfluidizer 120 E (Microfluidics Inc.); NaGC, sodium glycocholate; PS, probe sonication (MSE Soniprep); SPC, soya phosphatidylcholine.

is extremely lipophilic and the substance is practically insoluble in water. In DSC, recrystallization of bulk ubidecarenone from the melt starts only at 7°C upon slow cooling (cooling rate: 1 K/min.). Hence, already the bulk material displays a high degree of supercooling.

Ubidecarenone nanoparticles can be prepared by melt-emulsification using different types and amounts of emulsifying agents. In the manufacturing process ubidecarenone is melted at approximately 10–20°C above its melting temperature. If phospholipids are used, they are dispersed in the melt, e.g. by sonication. Water soluble surfactants are dissolved in the aqueous phase which is heated and added to the melt. A crude dispersion is produced which is then homogenized by common dispersion techniques, preferably by high pressure homogenization or microfluidization.

By this procedure aqueous dispersions with a ubidecarenone content between 1 and 10% (w/w) have been prepared (Siekmann and Westesen, 1995). Depending on homogenization parameters and composition, approximated mean particle diameters between about 50 and 300 nm can be found employing photon correlation spectroscopy (PCS). Typically, phospholipids, sodium glycocholate and the nonionic surfactant tyloxapol were used as emulsifying agents. The composition and particle size of selected dispersions is summarized in Table 5. Dispersions with a mean particle diameter in the lower nanometer range generally displayed a narrow and monomodal size distribution (Figure 5). Size measurements by laser diffractometry did not reveal the presence of particles above 1 μm (Figure 6). As judged from macroscopic observation and PCS measurements, the ubidecarenone nanoparticle dispersions remain stable on storage at 4°C. No pronounced particle growth or phase separation could be detected over the monitored period of up to 30 months.

Ubidecarenone nanoparticles can also serve as an alternative carrier system for lipophilic drugs. The solubility of drugs in ubidecarenone is expected to be different from that in triglycerides due to different chemical properties of these solvents. The drug carrier properties of emulsion droplets of supercooled ubidecarenone have been demonstrated by incorporating retinyl alcohol and menadione into the particles. Precipitation of the model drugs from the ubidecarenone carrier matrix could not be detected over the monitored period of 12 months. The formulations can thus be stored over pharmaceutically relevant periods of time.

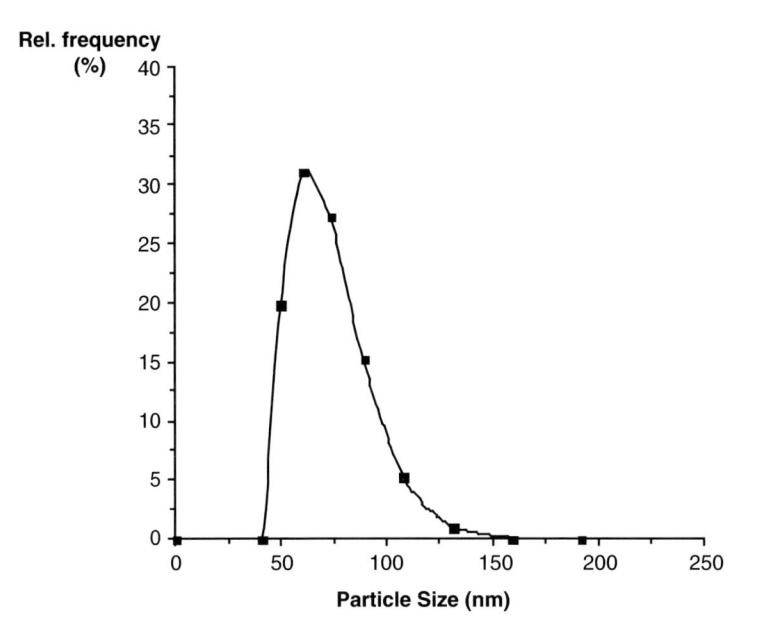

Figure 5 PCS particle size distribution (by number) of a melt-homogenized dispersion of 3% (w/w) ubidecarenone emulsified by 1.8% (w/w) phospholipids and 0.4% (w/w) sodium glycocholate.

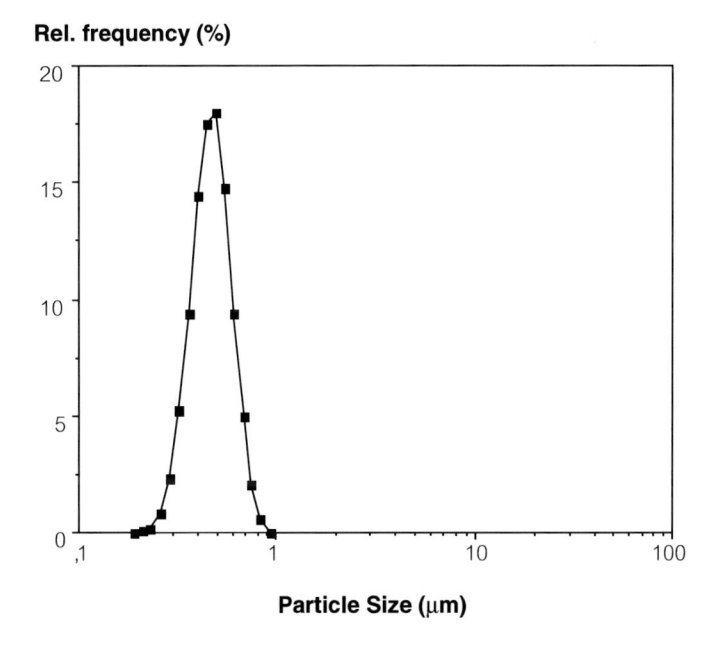

Figure 6 Particle size distribution of a melt-sonicated dispersion of 5% (w/w) ubidecarenone emulsified by 0.9% (w/w) phospholipids and 0.4% (w/w) sodium glycocholate determined by laser diffraction.

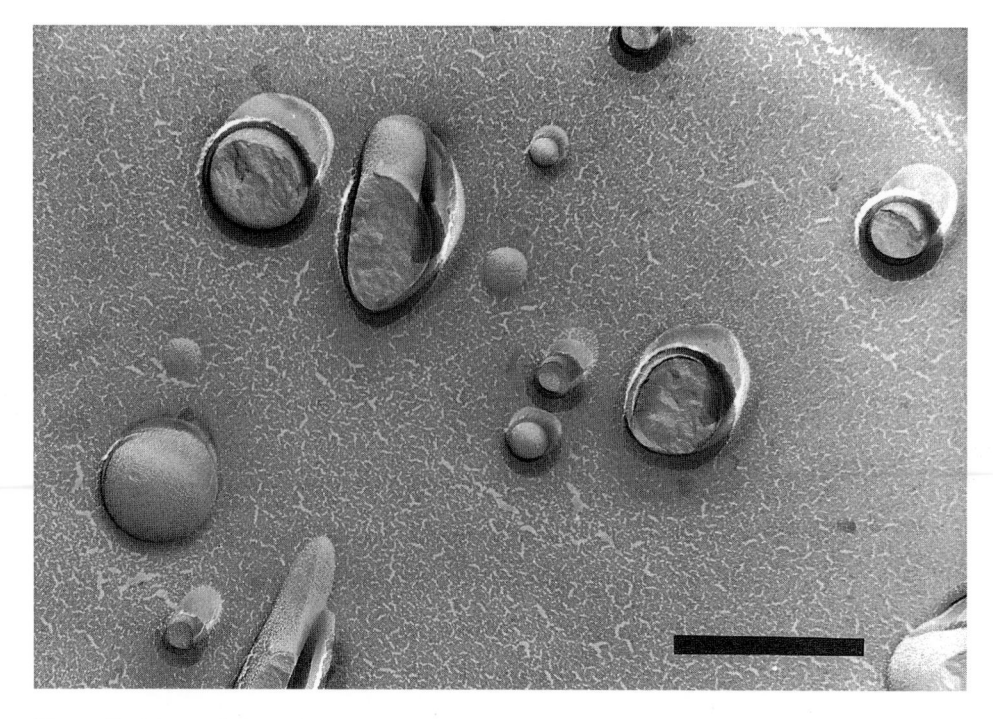

Figure 7 Transmission electron micrograph of a freeze-fractured specimen of a melt-sonicated dispersion of 5% (w/w) ubidecarenone emulsified by 0.9% (w/w) phospholipids and 0.4% (w/w) sodium glycocholate. The bar corresponds to approximately 400 nm.

Physicochemical Characterization of Melt-Emulsified Ubidecarenone Nanoparticles

The structure of phospholipid stabilized ubidecarenone nanoparticle dispersions prepared by melt-homogenization was investigated by transmission electron microscopy of freeze-fractured replica (FF-TEM) and by cryo-electron microscopy of frozen-hydrated specimen (cryo-TEM) (Siekmann and Westesen, 1995). FF-TEM micrographs display spherical particles with a non-structured core (Figure 7) which seem to be surrounded by a phospholipid monolayer. The shape of the particles and the non-structured particle core point to the presence of amorphous ubidecarenone. In contrast, crystalline particles tend to form anisometrical particle shapes and usually display a structured particle core as was demonstrated for tripalmitin nanoparticles (Siekmann and Westesen, 1992, 1997). The cryo-TEM studies confirmed the presence of predominantly spherical particles. Furthermore, the cryo-electron microscopic investigations allowed the detection of phospholipid vesicles in lecithin stabilized ubidecarenone dispersions indicating that the excess of phospholipids forms primarily small unilamellar vesicles (SUVs) in the continuous phase as has been observed earlier for colloidal phospholipid stabilized oil-in-water emulsions (Westesen and Wehler, 1992). Moreover, large numbers of extremely tiny ubidecarenone particles with diameters below about 30 nm were detected by cryo-TEM beside SUVs with diameters in the same size range (Siekmann and Westesen, 1995).

DSC thermograms of freshly prepared as well as stored (at 4°C) melt-homogenized ubidecarenone nanoparticle dispersions did not reveal any transition peak or glass transition in the temperature range from 20 to 80°C. Some of the investigated dispersions had been stored at 4°C for up to 30 months. From DSC thermograms of differently concentrated suspensions of crystalline ubidecarenone in water (concentration range: 0.2 to 10 w%) which demonstrated that concentrations of crystalline ubidecarenone as small as 0.2% could still be detected by DSC, it could be excluded that the absence of transition peaks was related to the relatively low concentration of ubidecarenone in the nanoparticle dispersions. It was not possible to crystallize the colloidal ubidecarenone particles by cooling the dispersions to temperatures far below 0°C in the DSC calorimeter. The DSC studies thus indicated that colloidally dispersed ubidecarenone did not recrystallize upon cooling after melt-homogenization and prolonged storage at 4°C. Further evidence for the absence of recrystallization was obtained by X-ray diffraction studies. For the ubidecarenone nanoparticle dispersions no diffraction peaks could be detected by small and wide angle X-ray diffraction using synchrotron radiation (Siekmann and Westesen, 1995). As with TEM and DSC, these results clearly point to the conclusion that ubidecarenone is in a non-crystalline, amorphous state in the melt-homogenized colloidal particles. Since these methods can, however, not unambiguously differentiate between the amorphous solid and liquid state, additional investigations were performed by ^{1}H NMR spectroscopy which allows to distinguish between solid and liquid materials due to differences in the mobility of hydrogen nuclei (Proctor, 1971).

^{1}H NMR spectra of a crude suspension of crystalline ubidecarenone powder in deuterium oxide (D_2O) stabilized by sodium glycocholate did not show any signals which could be assigned to the drug substance. Upon heating of the crude dispersion to approximately 65°C for about 1 min., which results in melting of the substance, the ^{1}H NMR spectrum reveals signals at approximately 1.6 ppm, 2.0 ppm, 3.1 ppm, 3.8 ppm and 5.1 ppm which could be distinctly assigned to liquid ubidecarenone (Figure 8a). The observed line broadening of the peaks can be attributed to particle size and viscosity effects. A colloidal ubidecarenone dispersion with a mean PCS particle diameter of 144 nm was prepared by probe sonication in D_2O. The ^{1}H NMR spectrum of this dispersion (Figure 8b) also displays signals at 1.6 ppm, 2.0 ppm, 3.1 ppm, 3.8 ppm and 5.1 ppm of liquid ubidecarenone. The (semi-)quantitative analysis of the peak areas of the ubidecarenone signal at 5.1 ppm which corresponds to the (—CH=C) protons of the 10 isoprenoid units as compared with the proton signal of an internal reference substance at 0.0 ppm (3-(trimethylsilyl)-propanesulfonic acid sodium salt, DSS) revealed that most of the ubidecarenone molecules in the comparably crude D_2O dispersion were still in a liquid state after more than 20 months of storage at 4°C.

From the results of the physicochemical characterization it can thus be concluded that melt-homogenized ubidecarenone does not recrystallize at temperatures of 4°C and above when colloidally dispersed, and that the nanoparticles are in the liquid physical state. They thus represent a supercooled melt, and the formulations can be regarded as O/W emulsions according to the IUPAC definition (Everett, 1972). The degree of supercooling amounts to far more than 45°C. Recrystallization of dispersed ubidecarenone could not be observed over the monitored period of up to 30 months.

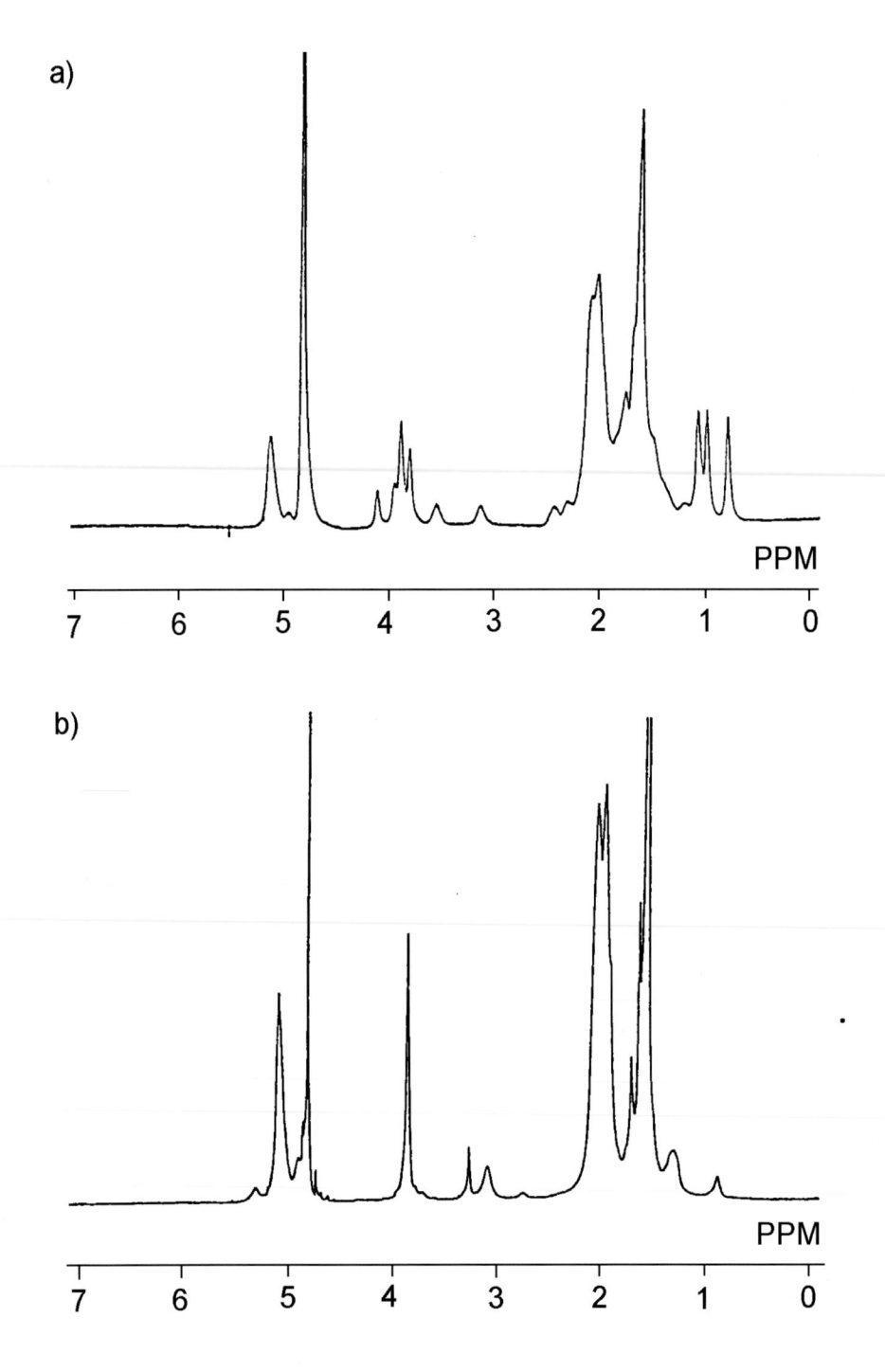

Figure 8 ¹H NMR spectra of a) melted ubidecarenone dispersed in a solution of sodium glycocholate in D$_2$O, and b) a melt-sonicated dispersion of 3% (w/w) ubidecarenone, 1.8% (w/w) phospholipids and 0.4% (w/w) sodium glycocholate in D$_2$O. Spectra were obtained on a Bruker AM-300 NMR spectrometer operating at 300 MHz.

In contrast to our findings, Handa *et al.* (1991) describe the formation of submicron-sized particles with a *solid* core of ubidecarenone surrounded by a phospholipid monolayer when mixtures of ubidecarenone and egg yolk phosphatidylcholine were co-sonicated. The particles are referred to as emulsion particles, but the use of the term "emulsion" is obviously not in accordance with the IUPAC definition (Everett, 1972) according to which an emulsion is a dispersion of two immiscible liquids. The ubidecarenone particles were characterized by transmission electron microscopy of negatively stained preparations as predominantly spherical particles with a diameter of 65 to 75 nm. The coexistence of ubidecarenone particles with a phospholipid monolayer and phospholipid bilayer vesicles was demonstrated by trapped volume determination, proton NMR spectroscopy using a paramagnetic shift reagent, and measurement of collapse and spreading pressures. No direct evidence of the solid nature of ubidecarenone in the particles was provided. The authors mentioned that the presence of solid ubidecarenone in both sonicated and vortexed ubidecarenone/phospholipid dispersions was detected by X-ray small angle scattering measurements. Data was, however, not shown, neither were the experimental conditions for these X-ray measurements described. Considering the manufacturing procedure of the ubidecarenone particles, i.e. co-sonication with phospholipids for 40 min. at 70°C which is above the melting point of ubidecarenone, it may be doubted that the melted ubidecarenone will recrystallize in the colloidal particles in view of our own results on melt-dispersed ubidecarenone presented above.

Due to ubidecarenone's essential role in electron transport of oxidative phosphorylation, there is a number of reports in the literature investigating the mobility, location and association of ubidecarenone in artificial phospholipid membranes prepared by codispersion of phospholipids and ubidecarenone. Although there is still controversy with respect to the precise location of ubidecarenone in phospholipid bilayers, there seems to be general agreement that above a certain mole fraction ubidecarenone forms a separate phase located outside the bilayers. Evidence for the presence of ubidecarenone in the aqueous phase has been obtained by a number of different analytical techniques, but the structure of these non-membrane associated ubidecarenone "aggregates" has not yet been clearly elucidated. Degli Esposti *et al.* (1980) found by EPR spin label studies that the physical state of ubidecarenone in the aqueous phase, i.e. outside phospholipid vesicles, is nonmonomeric, and the organized state is referred to as "micellar". Kingsley and Feigenson (1981) observed two distinct OCH_3 proton resonances in ubidecarenone/dimyristoylphosphatidylcholine (DMPC) vesicles by NMR spectroscopy, which were assigned to ubidecarenone dispersed in the phospholipid bilayer and a separate ubidecarenone-rich phase. Both populations were found to be of similar size by size exclusion chromatography. They could, however, be separated on the basis of density into two fractions with very different ubidecarenone:phospholipid ratios. The ubidecarenone molecules in the ubidecarenone-rich phase seemed to have a greater local motion than those in the bilayer. More evidence that ubidecarenone forms a separate phase in codispersions with phospholipids was presented by Ondorroa and Quinn using infrared spectroscopy (Ondorroa and Quinn, 1986a) and proton NMR (Ondorroa and Quinn, 1986b). The authors suggested some sort of aggregated or micellar form of ubidecarenone, the precise size, structure or location of which in the dispersion was unknown.

These earlier findings on the location of ubidecarenone in codispersions of ubidecarenone and phospholipids, which postulated the existence of a ubidecarenone-rich phase or ubidecarenone aggregates in the aqueous phase without giving a satisfactory explanation of their possible structure, might be reinterpreted in light of the results on aqueous dispersions of melt-emulsified ubidecarenone presented above. In particular when considering that the sample preparation in these earlier studies included heat treatment or, respectively, the use of equipment which locally creates heat, such as sonicators, the presence of a ubidecarenone-rich phase in the aqueous phase might be explained by the formation of submicron-sized emulsion droplets of supercooled ubidecarenone surrounded by a phospholipid monolayer. In fact, Stidham et al. (1984) reported the detection of both solid and supercooled ubidecarenone in crude phospholipid/ubidecarenone dispersions prepared by vortexing at elevated temperatures. Using light microscopy yellow-colored isotropic liquid droplets characteristic of melted ubidecarenone were found beside birefringent lamellar phases and solid ubidecarenone. Complementary studies by ^{13}C-NMR, X-ray diffraction and freeze-fracture electron microscopy pointed to that an appreciable fraction of ubidecarenone formed a separate phase located outside the phospholipid bilayer whereas ubidecarenone which does partition into the bilayer is not localized preferentially between the monolayers. The presence of melted ubidecarenone droplets at room temperature was assumed to be related to the partitioning of phospholipids into the ubidecarenone-rich droplets. In contrast, Ondarroa and Quinn (1986b) did not find any evidence for yellow particles that could be an unincorporated ubidecarenone fraction in ubidecarenone/dipalmitoyl phosphatidylcholine (DPPC) dispersions with low molar fraction of ubidecarenone (below 20 mole%). At higher mole fractions (50 mole%) such particles were, however, clearly visible. Proton NMR investigations of ubidecarenone/phospholipid dispersions using lanthanide shift reagents suggested that ubidecarenone was present in a hydrophobic environment remote from the aqueous phase (Ondarroa and Quinn 1986b). The OCH$_3$ shift observed in proton NMR indicated that the benzoquinone rings were in close proximity. The proton resonances of ubidecarenone resolved in the mixed dispersion were corresponding to those of melted ubidecarenone. On the basis of the chosen experimental conditions according to which ubidecarenone and the phospholipids were codispersed at 60 °C and then cooled for 1 h in an ice bath, the authors argued that ubidecarenone not incorporated into the bilayer would undergo crystallization and thus not contribute to the proton resonances. Ondarroa and Quinn (1986b) suggested that aggregates or micelles of ubidecarenone with a diameter similar to that of the phospholipid bilayer thickness may be formed which could rotate isotropically within the bilayer. In view of our results which demonstrated that colloidal particles of supercooled ubidecarenone cannot be crystallized by storage in a refrigerator for considerably long periods of time, the data presented by Ondarroa and Quinn (1986b) is also consistent with the presence of supercooled ubidecarenone in colloidal particles surrounded by a phospholipid monolayer. Ondarroa and Quinn (1986b) claimed that they could not find evidence from ^{31}P-NMR studies of phospholipid in other than a bilayer arrangement. In our opinion, the ^{31}P-NMR spectra reported are, however, also consistent with the coexistence of phospholipid monolayers, since Ondarroa and Quinn did not use paramagnetic shift reagents to distinguish between monolayer and bilayer arrangements.

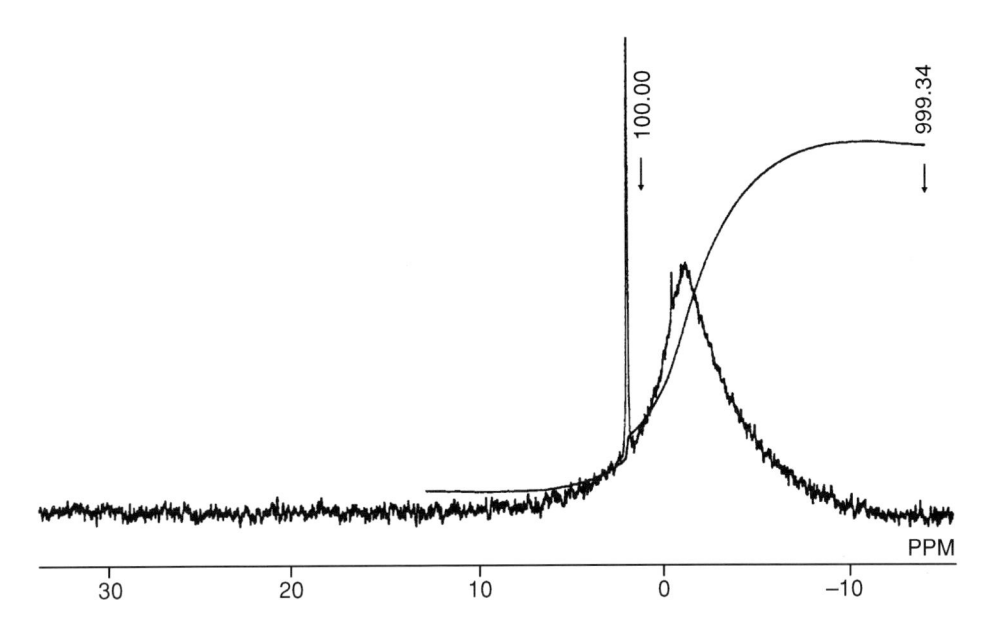

Figure 9 ^{31}P NMR spectrum of a melt-homogenized dispersion of 3% (w/w) ubidecarenone and 1.8% (w/w) phospholipids obtained on a Jeol GX-400 NMR spectrometer.

Our own ^{31}P-NMR studies on melt-homogenized phospholipid stabilized ubidecarenone nanoparticle dispersions according to a method described by Westesen and Wehler (1992, 1993) revealed relatively narrow symmetrical signals (Figure 9) characteristic of phospholipids bound to particles smaller than about 100 nm. By the use of the paramagnetic shift reagent praseodymium (III)-nitrate it could be shown that the predominant part of the phospholipids was present in monolayer arrangements.

A possible relevance of supercooled emulsion droplets of ubidecarenone in electron transport of the respiratory chain can only be speculative and was not an object of the present study. The supercooled state of colloidal ubidecarenone may, on the other hand, have considerable relevance in drug delivery. The possibility to colloidally disperse high concentrations of a poorly water-soluble drug in an aqueous phase without the use of a carrier device is highly interesting for parenteral drug administration. As a consequence of the liquid physical state of the ubidecarenone nanoparticles, it can be deduced that their biopharmaceutical behavior may be significantly different from that of the solid drug substance. As outlined in the beginning of this chapter, the peroral bioavailability of such nanoparticles is expected to be increased, since the dissolution of liquid substances does not require crystal lattice energy. An increase in peroral bioavailability can also be deduced from the increased dissolution rate as compared to conventional formulations owing to the colloidal particle size which leads to an increased interfacial area and a concomitant decreased diffusional distance, as well as from the hydrophilic surfaces which provide for good wettability.

PARAMETERS INFLUENCING THE SUPERCOOLING TENDENCY

For the development of stable pharmaceutical formulations based on emulsions of supercooled melts it is important to know the factors that may influence the degree of supercooling and the stability of the supercooled emulsion droplets. Quite a lot of information on this subject is present in the literature although not all questions concerning certain phenomena (as e.g. surface nucleation) have been answered yet.

The nature of the dispersed material is the main factor determining the supercooling ability. E.g. triglycerides and paraffins of equal chain length or comparable melting point display quite different amounts of supercooling (Tables 1 and 2). In homologous series of triglycerides and n-alkanes an increased difference between crystallization and final melting temperature with decreasing chain length has been found (Phipps, 1964; Uhlmann et al., 1975; Bunjes et al., 1996a). Changes in the composition of the dispersed phase may increase or decrease the amount of supercooling: Admixture of longer-chain triglycerides to triglycerides with a low crystallization temperature or the use of mixed chain triglycerides decreases the amount of supercooling (Bunjes et al., 1996a; Westesen et al., 1997). The same does apply for the presence of partial glycerides, especially monoglycerides, in emulsified triglyerides (Walstra and van Beresteyn, 1975). Admixture of lower melting triglycerides (Bunjes et al., 1996a; Simoneau et al., 1993) or addition of a low crystallizing drug substance (Bunjes et al., 1996b) further reduces the crystallization tendency.

The type of emulsifier may have a pronounced influence on supercooling phenomena (Table 1, Turbull, 1952) which is, however, not yet well understood (Clausse, 1985). The surfactant phenomena are usually attributed to heterogenous nucleation due to interactions with the surfactant film (Turnbull, 1952; Cordiez et al., 1982; Grange et al., 1986). Although interactions with the emulsifier layer usually decrease the amount of supercooling specific interactions between emulsifier and dispersed phase seem to increase supercooling at least at the droplet surface in some cases (Barfod and Krog, 1987).

Particle size is also an important factor. Larger droplets show less supercooling and crystallize more rapidly at a given temperature than smaller ones (Phipps, 1964; Walstra and van Beresteyn, 1975; Clausse, 1985; Grange et al., 1986; Dickinson et al., 1991; McClements et al., 1994). A certain effect of droplet size can be derived from homogenous nucleation theory predicting that the crystallization probability increases with droplet volume. For μm-sized dispersions of triglycerides and paraffins a linear relation between the logarithm of the drop diameter and the mean freezing temperature has been described. In that case, the higher crystallization temperature of the larger droplets was explained by the higher probability for larger droplets to contain nucleating particulate impurities, i.e. by heterogenous nucleation. Only at the temperature of maximum supercooling almost no influence of particle size was found which was attributed to homogenous nucleation at this temperature (Phipps, 1964).

The presence of solid material within in the emulsions, either in form of solidified droplets or as a bulk phase of the dispersed material seems to destabilize the supercooled state of the remaining liquid droplets. The crystallization rate of the supercooled material increases considerably in the presence of solid material (Coupland et al., 1993; Dickinson et al., 1993, 1996; McClements et al., 1994; Labes-

Carrier *et al.*, 1995). Mainly two effects are discussed to explain this phenomenon. On the one hand, crystallization of the supercooled droplets may be induced by collision with crystalline droplets, the so called interdroplet heterogenous nucleation mechanism (Dickinson *et al.*, 1993; McClements *et al.*, 1994) which is similar to the phenomenon of partial coalescence well known from food emulsions (Walstra, 1996). The instability of higher concentrated emulsions of supercooled trilaurin has also been explained by this type of interaction (Coupland *et al.*, 1993). On the other hand, there is also some evidence that transport of molecules from supercooled to already crystalline droplets may be the reason for the increase of the amount of crystalline material in dispersions containing solid and liquid, supercooled droplets (Dickinson *et al.*, 1996). The driving force for this transport would be the lower vapor pressure in solid material compared to supercooled material. Such mass transport was observed between a hexadecane bulk and a dispersed phase as well as between the continuous and the dispersed water phase of W/O/W emulsions (Labes-Carrier *et al.*, 1995; Potier *et al.*, 1992). With increasing concentration of the dispersed phase, the probability of contacts between droplets increases enhancing contact nucleation (Clausse 1985).

The amount of supercooling may also depend on the thermal pretreatment of the emulsion. The occurrence of such memory effects has been attributed to the formation of ordered structures within the emulsifier layer which induce nucleation at higher temperatures. A more intense thermal pretreatment leads to higher supercooling in these cases (Phipps, 1964; Clausse *et al.*, 1987).

Concerning the formulation of stable pharmaceutical emulsions of supercooled melts the following conclusions may be drawn: Only materials with considerable supercooling tendency can be regarded as promising candidates for the formulation of dispersions of supercooled melts as they may display an appropriate storage stability in the supercooled dispersed state. The chosen material should be dispersed as finely and uniformly as possible and appropriate since crystallization is less probable for smaller droplets. The presence of crystalline material (e.g. due to crystallization of larger droplets) should be carefully excluded to avoid further crystallization of the dispersed phase induced by a sort of autocatalytic mechanism. For the same reason, high concentrations of dispersed material seem unfavorable. Possible influences of the type of emulsifier on the degree of supercooling and the stability of the supercooled dispersed phase have to be checked carefully.

Dispersions prepared for the study of nucleation and supercooling phenomena are usually intended for short-time laboratory use and long-term stability data is, therefore, seldom reported. In some cases, information on stability can be extracted from the experimental results of nucleation experiments. Reports on water and organic material indicate that the droplets can be preserved in the highly supercooled state for days or weeks, in some cases even at temperatures close to the critical supercooling (Taborek, 1985; Dickinson *et al.*, 1993; McClements *et al.*, 1994; Clausse *et al.*, 1987). Evidence on the long-term stability of emulsions of supercooled triglycerides and ubidecarenone is given in reports on pharmaceutical formulations as this parameter is crucial for the use as drug carriers (Siekmann and Westesen, 1995; Bunjes *et al.*, 1996a; Westesen *et al.*, 1997).

For the development of pharmaceutical formulations it would be interesting to predict a theoretical stability of the supercooled state of the droplets in a colloidal dispersion at a given storage temperature. As proposed by Walstra and van Beresteyn

(1975) for triglycerides an estimation of the supercooling and crystallization behavior of dispersed materials in dependence on time and temperature might be possible via determination of the nucleation rate J. While a theoretical evaluation of J from physicochemical parameters does not appear very promising from the practical point of view, determination of J from experimental data derived from the systems of interest might be a useful approach to predict the stability of supercooled emulsion droplets at least if homogenous nucleation can be assumed. The nucleation rate J can be derived from isothermal or constant cooling experiments (Clausse, 1985). Such stability predictions may, however, be of restricted validity since they cannot consider physical "side reactions" which may occur upon storage. Deviations may appear due to an increase in particle size or the enhanced nucleation that has been described for supercooled droplets in the presence of crystallized droplets (Coupland et al., 1993; Dickinson et al., 1993, 1996; McClements et al., 1994; Labes-Carrier et al., 1995). Partial crystallization of the droplets may lead to further instability phenomena such as changes in particle size distribution or gelation due to insufficient stabilization of the crystallized droplets (Siekmann and Westesen, 1997). Prediction of stability may be particularly problematic if heterogenous nucleation takes place since the activity of nucleation catalysts can be temperature dependent (Walstra and van Beresteyn, 1975) and may at storage temperature differ from the value derived under the conditions of the experiment in which J had been determined. The possibility to estimate the stability of colloidal supercooled emulsion droplets is currently under investigation in our laboratory.

SUMMARY AND FUTURE PROSPECTS

Colloidal dispersions of melt-homogenized lipophilic substances can display pronounced supercooling which is much higher than in the bulk and may differ considerably from that of microsized emulsions. Despite its practical relevance e.g. concerning biopharmaceutical properties the phenomenon of supercooling has yet received little attention with respect to colloidal pharmaceutical dispersions.

Disadvantages of conventional drug carrier systems such as low payload of the carrier or toxicological side effects which are related to the carrier particles themselves can be circumvented with particles of supercooled melts formulated from pure drug. On the other hand, formulation of colloidal dispersions of supercooled melts allows the direct parenteral — in particular intravenous — administration of practically water insoluble substances without risk of embolism, which is not possible for the crystalline bulk substance suspended in an aqueous medium. Particle sizes below 150 nm which corresponds to the diameter of the fenestrations of the endothelial wall of blood vessels (Wisse et al., 1985) permit extravasation of the particles through these fenestrations to extravascular targets such as the bone marrow or tumor tissues. The surface characteristics of the supercooled particles can be modified e.g. by the choice of stabilizing agents, by the adsorption of polymers or by the attachment of homing devices. By these means it may be possible to modify the bioavailability and the biodistribution with respect to the rate and extent of absorption, the circulation time in the vascular compartment, the transport to the site of action and the organ distribution.

Particles of supercooled melts can be obtained in size ranges which can generally not be achieved by conventional comminution techniques such as milling, grinding or micronization. The small particle size results in a tremendous increase of the specific surface area and consequently of the dissolution rate. Additionally, in diffusion controlled dissolution of sparingly soluble drugs the diffusional distance decreases substantially with particle size which also contributes to an increased dissolution rate (Bisrat et al., 1992). Hence, the bioavailability of bioactive agents formulated as colloidal particles of supercooled melts can be improved. Since such particles are covered by stabilizing agents, they have hydrophilic surfaces and a good wettability facilitating the dissolution of the substance e.g. in the gastro-intestinal tract. As the drug within a supercooled particle is in the liquid state, dissolution of the substance does not require lattice energy. The dissolution rate of the particles is therefore increased resulting in an enhanced bioavailability compared to the crystalline drug substance.

Stable colloidal dispersions of supercooled melts cannot only be formulated from bioactive substances as such but also from pharmacologically inactive materials for use as (colloidal) carrier systems for lipophilic drugs. Since particles of supercooled melts are still at an early stage of investigation, possible advantages of supercooled triglyceride nanoparticles as drug carriers compared to conventional triglyceride emulsions — especially a slower drug release due to an increased viscosity — yet still have to be verified. Additionally, other physiologically inactive and well-tolerated materials with high viscosity in the supercooled state may serve as matrix for drug carrier systems based on dispersions of supercooled melts.

It has to be kept in mind, however, that dispersions of supercooled melts are metastable formulations not only with respect to their dispersity but also concerning the physical state of the dispersed phase. For pharmaceutical applications, the formulations have to be stable during storage, transport and administration. It is therefore necessary to choose compositions which provide sufficient supercooling to guarantee preservation of the supercooled state under these conditions. Ubidecarenone seems to be a suitable material to fulfill these requirements.

REFERENCES

Akbarieh, M., Heiati, H., Tawashi, R. (1994) Coated solid lipid nanoparticles, a new strategy in drug delivery and targeting. *Proceed. Intern. Symp. Control. Rel. Bioact. Mater.*, **21**, 218–219.

Allémann, E., Gurny, R., Doelker, E. (1993) Drug-loaded nanoparticles — preparation methods and drug targeting issues. *Eur. J. Pharm. Biopharm.*, **39**, 173–191.

Atkinson, R.M., Bedford, C., Child, K.J., Tomich, E.G. (1962) Effect of particle size on blood griseofulvin-levels in man. *Nature*, **193**, 588–589.

Barfod, N.M., Krog, N. (1987) Destabilization and fat crystallization of whippable emulsions (toppings) studied by pulsed NMR. *J. Am. Oil Chem. Soc.*, **64**, 112–119.

Bisrat, M., Anderberg, E.K., Barnett, M.I., Nyström, C. (1992) Physicochemical aspects of drug release. XV. Investigation of diffusional transport in dissolution of suspended, sparingly soluble drugs. *Int. J. Pharm.*, **80**, 191–201.

Bunjes, H., Westesen, K., Koch, M.H.J. (1996a) Crystallization tendency and polymorphic transitions in triglyceride nanoparticles. *Int. J. Pharm.*, **129**, 159–173.

Bunjes, H., Westesen, K., Koch, M.H.J (1996b) Incorporation of a model drug into lipid nanoparticle dispersions. *Eur. J. Pharm. Biopharm.*, **42**, 33S.

Clausse, D. (1985) Research techniques utilizing emulsions. In *Encyclopedia of Emulsion Technology, Vol. III*, edited by P. Becher, pp. 77–157. New York: Marcel Dekker.

Clausse, D. (1991) Nucleation and crystallization phenomena hosted in emulsions. Application to microparticle formation. In *Adv. Meas. Control. Colloidal Processes*, edited by R.A. Williams and N.C. de Jaeger, pp. 163–171. Oxford, U.K.: Butterworth-Heinemann.

Clausse, D., Dumas, J.P., Meijer, P.H.E., Broto, F. (1987) Phase transformation in emulsions: Part I: Effects of thermal pretreatments on nucleation phenomena: Experiments and model. *J. Dispersion Science and Technology*, **8**, 1–28.

Collins-Gold, L.C., Lyons, R.T., Bartholow, L.C. (1990) Parenteral emulsions for drug delivery. *Adv. Drug Deliv. Rev.*, **5**, 189–208.

Cordiez, J.P., Grange, G., Mutaftschiev, B. (1982) Droplet freezing experiments in stearic acid-water emulsions. Role of the droplet-medium interface. *J. Colloid Interface Sci.*, **85**, 431–441.

Cormia, R.L., Price, F.P., Turnbull, D. (1962) Kinetics of crystal nucleation in polyethylene. *J. Chem. Phys.*, **37**, 1333–1340.

Coupland, J., Dickinson, E., McClements, D.J., Povey, M, de Rancourt de Mimmerand, C. (1993) Crystallization in simple paraffins and monoacid saturated triacylglycerols dispersed in water, *Spec. Pub.-R. Soc. Chem. 113 (Food Colloids and Polymers Stability and Mechanical Properties)*, 243–49.

Degli Esposti, M., Bertoli E., Parenti-Castelli, G., Fato, R., Mascarello, S., Lenaz, G. (1980) Incorporation of ubiquinone homologues into lipid vesicles and mitochondrial membranes. *Arch. Biochem. Biophys.*, **210**, 21–32.

Dickinson, E., Kruizenga, F.-J., Povey, M.J.W., van der Molen, M. (1993) Crystallization in oil-in-water emulsions containing liquid and solid droplets, *Colloids and Surfaces A*, **81**, 273–279.

Dickinson, E., Ma, J., Povey, M.J.W. (1996) Crystallization kinetics in oil-in-water emulsions containing a mixture of solid and liquid droplets, *J. Chem. Soc. Faraday Trans.*, **92**, 1213–1217.

Dickinson, E., McClements, D.J., Povey M.J.W. (1991) Ultrasonic investigation of the particle size dependence of crystallization in n-Hexadecane-in-water emulsions, *J. Colloid Interface Sci.*, **142**, 103–110.

Domb, A.J., Bergelson, L., Amselem, S. (1996) Lipospheres for controlled drug delivery of substances. In *Microencapsulation*, edited by S. Benita. New York: Marcel Dekker.

Dumas J.P., Zeraouli Y., Strub M. (1994) Heat transfer inside emulsions. Determination of the DSC thermograms. Part 1: Crystallization of the undercooled droplets. *Thermochim. Acta*, **236**, 227–237.

Dumas, J.P., Tounsi, F., Babin, L. (1987) Phase transformations in emulsions: Part II: Polymorphism for organic substances. *J. Dispersion Science and Technology*, **8**, 29–54.

Everett, D.H. (1972) Report of the Commission on Colloid and Surface Chemistry of the Physical Chemistry Devision. *Pure Appl. Chem.*, **31**, 577–638.

Florence, A.T., Attwood, D. (1981) *Physicochemical Principles of Pharmacy*, Macmillan, London.

Folkers K., Littaru G.P., Yamagami T. (1991) *Biomedical and Clinical Aspects of Coenzyme Q, Vol. 6.* Amsterdam: Elsevier.

Grange, G., Lévis, A. Mutaftschiev, B. (1986) Solidification of stearic acid-water and laurone-water emulsions: Role of the droplet-medium interface on nucleation kinetics, *J. Colloid Interface Sci.*, **109**, 542–551.

Handa, T., Asai, Y., Miyajima, K., Kawashima, Y., Kayano, M., Ida, K., Ikeuchi, T. (1991) Formation and Structure of Stably Dispersed Small Particles Composed of Phosphatidylcholine and Ubiquinone-10: Coexistence of Emulsion Particles with Bilayer Vesicles. *J. Colloid Interface Sci.*, **143**, 205–213.

Heiati, H., Phillips, N.C., Tawashi, R. (1996) Evidence for phospholipid bilayer formation in solid lipid nanoparticles formulated with phospholipid and triglyceride, *Pharm. Res.*, **13**, 1406–1410.

Heiati, H., Tawashi, R., Shivers, R.R., Phillips, N.C.(1997) Solid lipid nanoparticles as drug carriers. I. Incorporation and retention of the lipophilic prodrug 3′-azido-3′-deoxythymidine palmitate *Int. J. Pharm.* **146**, 1997, 123–132.

Kingsley, P.B., Feigenson, G.W. (1981) ^{1}H-NMR Study of the Location and Motion of Ubiquinones in Predeuterated Phosphatidylcholine Bilayers. *Biochim. Biophys. Acta.*, **635**, 602–608.

Kishi, H., Kanamori, N., Nishii, S., Hiraoka, E., Okamoto, T., Kishi, T. (1984) Metabolism of exogenous coenzyme Q10 *in vivo* and the bioavailability of coenzyme Q10 preparations in Japan. In *Biomedical and Clinical Aspects of Coenzyme Q, Vol. 4*, edited by K. Folkers, Y. Yamamura, pp. 131–142. Amsterdam: Elsevier.

Koutsky, J.A., Walton, A.G., Baer, E. (1967) Nucleation of polymer droplets. *J. Appl. Phys.*, **38**, 1832–1839.

Labes-Carrier, C., Dumas, J.P., Mendibourne, B., Lachaise, J. (1995) DSC as a tool to predict emulsion stability, *J. Dispersion Science and Technology*, **16**, 607–631.

Lasic, D.D. (1993) *Liposomes: From Physics to Applications.* Amsterdam: Elsevier.

Lucks, J.S., Müller R.H., König, B. (1992) Solid lipid nanoparticles (SLN) — an alternative parenteral drug carrier system. *Eur. J. Pharm. Biopharm.*, **38**, 33S.

MacFarlane, D.R., Angell, C.A. (1982) An emulsion technique for the study of marginal glass formation in molecular liquids, *J. Phys. Chem.*, 86, 1927–1930.

McClements, D.J., Han, S.-W., Dungan, S.R. (1994) Interdroplet heterogenous nucleation of supercooled liquid droplets by solid droplets in oil-in-water emulsions. *J. Am. Oil Chem. Soc.*, **71**, 1385–1389.

Mulder, H. (1953) Melting and solidification of milk fat. *Neth. Milk Dairy J.*, **7**, 149–174.

Müller, R.H., Mehnert, W., Lucks, J.-S., Schwarz, C., zur Mühlen, A., Weyhers, H., Freitas, C., Rühl, D. (1995) Solid Lipid Nanoparticles (SLN) — An alternative colloidal drug delivery system for controlled drug delivery. *Eur. J. Pharm. Biopharm.*, **41**, 62–69.

Mullins, J.D., Macek, T.J. (1960) Some pharmaceutical properties of novobiocin. *J. Am. Pharm. Assoc., Sci. Ed.*, **49**, 245–248.

Ondarroa, M., Quinn, P.J. (1986a) A difference infrared-spectroscopic study of the interaction of ubiquinone-10 with phospholipid bilayers. *Biochem. J.*, **240**, 325–331.

Ondarroa, M., Quinn, P.J. (1986b) Proton magnetic resonance spectroscopy studies of the interaction of ubiquinone-10 with phospholipid model membranes. *Eur. J. Biochem.*, **155**, 353–361.

Phipps, L.W. (1962) Dependence on temperature of the viscosity and density of supercooled triglycerides. *Nature*, **193**, 541–542.

Phipps, L.W. (1964) Heterogenous and homogenous nucleation in supercooled triglycerides and n-paraffins. *Trans. Faraday Soc.*, **60**, 1873–1883.

Potier, L., Raynal, S., Seiller, M., Grossiord, J.-P., Clausse, D. (1992) Study of state transitions within multiple W/O/W emulsions using calorimetry (DSC). *Thermochim. Acta*, **204**, 145–155.

Prankerd, R.J., Stella, V.J. (1990) The use of oil-in-water emulsions as a vehicle for parenteral drug administration, *J. Parenteral Science Technol.*, **44**, 139–149.

Proctor, W.G. (1971) An introduction to NMR. *J. Am. Oil Chem. Soc.*, **48**, 1–3.

Ramasarma, T. (1968) Lipid Quinones. *Adv. Lipid Res.*, **6**, 107–180.

Sakaeda, T., Hirano, K. (1995) O/W lipid emulsions for parenteral drug delivery. II. Effect of composition on pharmacokinetics of incorporated drug. *Journal of drug targeting*, **3**, 221–230.

Schwarz, C. (1995) *Feste Lipidnanopartikel: Herstellung, Charakterisierung, Arzneistoffinkorporation und -freisetzung, Sterilisation und Lyophilisation*, Thesis, Free University of Berlin, Verlag Shaker, Aachen.

Schwarz, C., Mehnert, W., Lucks, J.S., Müller, R.H. (1994) Solid lipid nanoparticles (SLN) for controlled drug delivery. I. Production, characterization and sterilization. *J. Controlled Release*, **30**, 83–96.

Shaw, T.R.D., Carless, J.E. (1974) The Effect of Particle Size on the Absorption of Digoxin. *Europ. J. Clin. Pharmacol.*, **7**, 269–273.

Siekmann, B., Westesen, K. (1992) Submicron-sized parenteral carrier systems based on solid lipids. *Pharm. Pharmacol. Lett.*, **1**, 123–126.

Siekmann, B., Westesen, K. (1994) Thermoanalysis of the recrystallization process of melt-homogenized glyceride nanoparticles. *Colloids Surfaces B: Biointerfaces*, **3**, 159–175.

Siekmann, B., Westesen, K. (1995) Preparation and physicochemical characterization of aqueous dispersions of coenzyme Q10 nanoparticles. *Pharm. Res.*, **12**, 201–208.

Simoneau, C., McCarthy, M.J., Kauten, R.J., German, J.B. (1991) Crystallization dynamics in model emulsions from magnetic resonance imaging. *J. Am. Oil. Chem. Soc.*, **68**, 481–487.

Simoneau, C., McCarthy, M.J., Reid, D.S., German, J.B. (1993) Influence of triglyceride composition on crystallization kinetics of model emulsions. *J. Food. Eng.*, **19**, 365–387.

Söderberg, I., Hernqvist, L., Buchheim, W. (1989) Milk fat crystallization in natural milk globules. *Milchwissenschaft*, 44, 403–406.

Stidham, M.A., McIntosh, T.J., Siedow, J.N. (1984) On the location of ubiquinone in phosphatidylcholine bilayers. *Biochim. Biophys. Acta*, 767, 423–431.

Taborek, P. (1985) Nucleation in supercooled water. *Phys. Rev. B*, **32**, 5902–5906.

Turnbull, D. (1952) Kinetics of solidification of supercooled liquid mercury droplets. *J. Chem. Phys.*, **20**, 411–424.

Turnbull, D., Cormia, R.L. (1961) Kinetics of crystal nucleation in some normal alkane liquids. *J. Chem. Phys.*, **34**, 820–831.

Turnbull, D., Fisher, J.C. (1949) Rate of nucleation in condensed systems. *J. Chem. Phys.*, **17**, 71–73.

Uhlmann, R., Kritchevsky, G., Straff, R., Scherer, G. (1975) Crystal nucleation in normal alkane liquids. *J. Chem. Phys.*, **62**, 4896–4903.

Vonnegut, B. (1948) Variation with temperature of the nucleation rate of supercooled liquid tin and water drops. *J. Colloid Science*, **3**, 563–569.

Wade, A., Weller, P.J. (Eds.) (1994) *Handbook of Pharmaceutical Excipients*. London: The Pharmaceutical Press.

Walstra, P. (1996) Emulsion Stability. In P. Becher, (ed.), *Encyclopedia of emulsion technology*, pp. 1–62.

Walstra, P., van Beresteyn, E.C.H. (1975) Crystallization of milk fat in the emulsified state. *Neth. Milk Dairy J.*, 2935–2965.

Washington, C., Evans, K. (1995) Release rate measurements of model hydrophobic solutes from submicron triglyceride emulsions. *J. Controlled Release*, **33**, 383–390.

Westesen, K., Bunjes, H. (1995) Do nanoparticles prepared from lipids solid at room temperature always possess a solid lipid matrix? *Int. J. Pharm.*, **115**, 129–131.

Westesen, K., Bunjes, H., Koch, M.H.J. (1997) Physicochemical characterization of lipid nanoparticles and evaluation of their drug loading capacity and sustained release potential. *J. Controlled Release*, **48**, 223–236.

Westesen, K., Siekmann, B., Koch, M.H.J. (1993) Investigations on the physical state of lipid nanoparticles by synchrotron radiation X-ray diffraction. *Int. J. Pharm.*, **93**, 189–199.

Westesen, K., Siekmann, B. (1997) Investigation of the gel formation of phospholipid-stabilized solid lipid nanoparticles. *Int. J. Pharm.*, **151**, 35–45.

Westesen, K., Wehler, T. (1992) Physicochemical characterization of a model intravenous emulsion. *J. Pharm. Sci.*, **81**, 777–786.

Westesen, K., Wehler, T. (1993) Investigation of the particle size distribution of a model intravenous emulsion. *J. Pharm. Sci.*, **82**, 1237–1244.

Wisse, E., De Zanger, R.B., Charels, K., Van der Smissen, P., McCuskey, R.S. (1985) The liver sieve: Considerations concerning the structure and function of endothelial fenestrae, the sinusoidal wall and the space of Dissé. *Hepatology*, **5**, 683–692.

Zhao, D., Reid, S. (1994) Thermal studies on the crystallization kinetics of triglycerides and milk fat by DSC. *Thermochim. Acta*, **246**, 405–416.

8. SUBMICRON LIPID SUSPENSIONS (SOLID LIPID NANOPARTICLES) VERSUS LIPID NANOEMULSIONS: SIMILARITIES AND DIFFERENCES

BRITTA SIEKMANN[1] and KIRSTEN WESTESEN[2]

[1]*Astra Pain Control AB, Department of Pharmaceutics, 151 85 Södertälje, Sweden*
[2]*Institute of Pharmaceutical Technology, Friedrich Schiller University Jena, 07743 Jena, Germany*

INTRODUCTION

Submicron-sized oil-in-water (o/w) emulsions have been clinically used for decades in parenteral nutrition (Wretlind, 1981) and also as colloidal drug carrier systems for poorly water soluble substances (Prankerd and Stella, 1990, Collins-Gold et al., 1990). In parallel to the successful clinical introduction of lipid emulsions, first attempts arose to transfer the concept of these emulsion vehicles to the preparation of colloidal lipid suspensions as an alternative parenteral drug delivery system. A colloidal suspension consists of solid particles of colloidal dimensions dispersed in a liquid continuous medium according to the IUPAC definition (Everett, 1972). Colloidal lipid suspensions thus represent aqueous dispersions of lipids which are solid at room temperature.

Colloidal lipid suspensions can principally be prepared by the same manufacturing techniques as lipid emulsions, such as high pressure homogenization (Siekmann and Westesen, 1992). The solid lipids are first melted, and the lipid melt is emulsified in an aqueous medium. Thus an oil-in-water emulsion is created in the heat which is supposed to transform into an aqueous colloidal suspension by recrystallization of the dispersed lipids forming solid lipid nanoparticles. Due to the obvious similarities with lipid o/w emulsions regarding the chemical composition and the preparation method, these systems have often been regarded as "emulsions with solid fat globules".

A number of advantages — such as enhanced physical stability, reduction of drug leakage, sustained drug release and facilitated surface modification — can be theoretically deduced from the solid state of the dispersed lipid phase compared to the liquid state of lipid emulsions (Table 1). Owing to these potential advantages colloidal lipid suspensions have found interest as an alternative colloidal drug carrier system. The lipid suspension concept could, however, not be realized until very recently due to stability problems (Westesen and Siekmann, 1996). As will be outlined below, phospholipid stabilized tripalmitate suspensions with a composition similar to commercial lipid emulsions for parenteral nutrition tend to form semisolid ointment-like gels. Despite the obvious similarities of colloidal lipid suspensions and o/w emulsions, the instability of colloidal triglyceride suspensions containing the same type and concentration of emulsifiers as comparable o/w emulsions point to basic physicochemical differences between colloidal lipid emulsions and suspensions.

Table 1 Potential advantages of lipid suspensions over lipid emulsions due to solid state properties

Solid state properties	Potential advantages
Solid particle core	No particle coalescence
	Improved physical stability
Strongly reduced mobility of incorporated drug	Reduced drug leakage
	Avoidance of drug protruding into emulsifier film
	Sustained/controlled drug release
Static interface solid/liquid	Facilitated surface modification

COMPARISON OF LIPID EMULSIONS AND SUSPENSIONS OF SIMILAR COMPOSITION

Lipid emulsions used in parenteral nutrition and drug delivery are composed of vegetable oils which are emulsified in an aqueous phase using fractionated egg or soya lecithins as emulsifying agents. Typical compositions are given in Table 2. These emulsions are usually produced by high pressure homogenization, and they consist of submicron-sized oil droplets surrounded by a phospholipid monolayer. Fat emulsions have been used as a calory source in parenteral nutrition for decades (Schuberth and Wretlind, 1961; Wretlind, 1981). They are manufactured in large scale, and they display an acceptable long-term stability. Lipid emulsions of this type have also been extensively investigated as drug carrier systems (Collins-Gold et al., 1990; Prankerd and Stella, 1990). Incorporation of drugs might, however, result in a reduced stability of the product owing to perturbations of the stabilizing emulsifier film by drug crystals or diffusing drug molecules which have a high mobility in the liquid oil phase. These perturbations may induce instabilities of either mechanical nature due to reduction of film elasticity and film ruption, or of electrochemical nature thus influencing the zetapotential. These unwanted effects may cause coalescence, particle growth and drug leakage. The high mobility of incorporated drug molecules also leads to a fast release of drug from the carrier in biological fluids so that it is hardly possible to achieve sustained release by an emulsion formulation (Magenheim et al., 1993).

Table 2 Typical compositions of lipid emulsions used in parenteral nutrition

Compound	Typical concentration (wt. %)
Oil (e.g. soya, safflower, MCT)	10–30%
Phospholipids (egg + soya lecithin)	0.6–1.5%
Isotonicity agent (glycerol, xylitol)	2.2–5%
NaOH to adjust pH	q.s.
Water for injection	to 100%

Suspensions of solid lipid nanoparticles have recently been suggested as an alternative drug delivery system which may circumvent the problems associated with lipid emulsions (Table 1). Due to the solid core the particles cannot coalesce, and they may therefore exhibit a better physical stability than liquid droplets. The mobility of incorporated drug molecules is drastically reduced in a solid phase. Therefore, drug leakage from the carrier and drug protrusion into the emulsifier film would be counteracted. Whereas drug release from an emulsion is a diffusion-controlled process which generally leads to fast release from the carrier upon injection into the blood, drug release from solid lipid particles is matrix-dependent, and the degradation rate of the matrix lipids is assumed to determine drug release. It is therefore possible to control drug release from a solid lipid carrier to a certain extent by the choice of matrix constituents with different biological degradation rates. The presence of a static interface might facilitate a surface modification of the carrier particles after solidification of the lipid matrix, e.g. by subsequent adsorption of nonionic surfactants. The latter might be of relevance to reduce carrier uptake by the reticuloendothelial system (RES) which is known to be related to surface properties.

During the preparation of submicron lipid suspensions by melt homogenization, an emulsion of the lipid melt in the aqueous phase is intermediately created before the lipid droplets solidify to form solid lipid nanoparticles. It is thus not surprising that emulsions of lipid melts behave physicochemically like the vegetable oil emulsions used in parenteral nutrition and drug delivery. However, it has been observed that the preparation of lecithin stabilized triglyceride suspensions with a composition similar to fat emulsions results in the formation of semisolid, ointment-like gels (Siekmann and Westesen, 1992; Freitas et al., 1994) as illustrated in Figure 1. As will

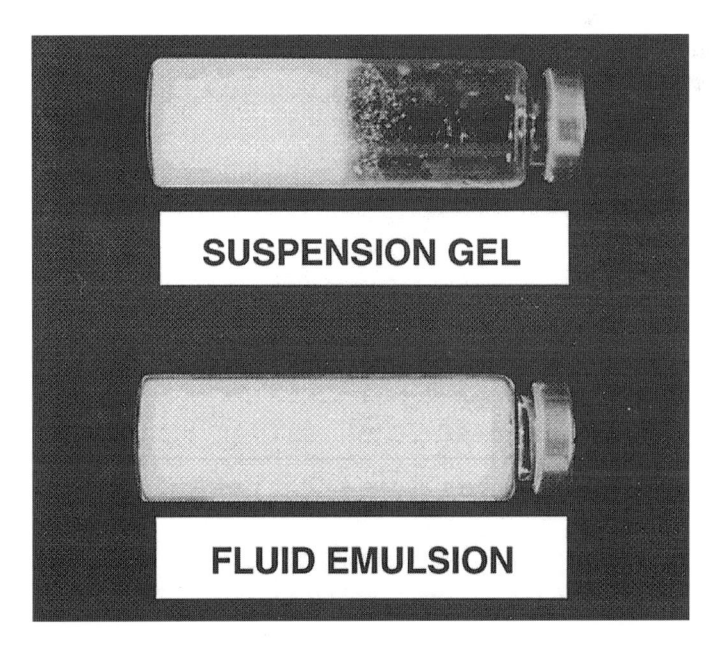

Figure 1 Comparison of similarly composed lipid dispersions: lipid suspension gel (10% tripalmitate, 1.2% S100) and fluid lipid emulsion (10% soya oil, 1.2% S100).

Table 3 Comparison of lipid emulsion and suspension compositions

	Emulsion	Suspension 1	Suspension 2
Stability[1]	stable	gel formation	stable
Oil phase	10% soya oil	10% tripalmitate	10% tripalmitate
Emulsifier	1.2% lecithin	1.2% lecithin	2.4% lecithin
Co-surfactant	–	–	0.4% sodium glycocholate
Isotonicity agent	2.25% glycerol	2.25% glycerol	2.25% glycerol

[1]with respect to storage for a pharmaceutically reasonable time (e.g. more than 6 months).

be outlined below, the gel formation can be avoided by the addition of a co-surfactant. Table 3 compares a typical emulsion composition with two different suspension compositions, one of which is stable on storage and the other tends to form semi-solid gels.

Our results indicate that there are some differences in the kinetics of gel formation depending on the lecithin composition (Siekmann and Westesen, 1997). Melt-homogenized tripalmitate dispersions containing exclusively the phosphatidylcholine rich soya lecithin product Lipoid S100 (S100) as an emulsifier become semisolid immediately on cooling of the hot emulsion whereas dispersions stabilized by the egg lecithin mixture Lipoid E80 (E80) form gels within several hours after preparation. In tripalmitate suspensions stabilized by the cruder soya lecithin Lipoid S75 (S75) the gel formation seems to be retarded, but cannot be completely avoided. The S75 stabilized dispersions usually contain significant concentrations of microscopically and macroscopically observable tripalmitate aggregates directly after cooling and have a poor long term stability. A high tendency to spontaneous gel formation was observed under shear stress such as passage through the needle of a syringe. The less pronounced gelation tendency of the S75 stabilized systems compared to those stabilized by S100 or E80 may be explained by an improved but still not sufficient steric or electrostatic stabilization caused by the minor components of the cruder lecithin mixtures, such as glycolipids. According to the manufacturer of S75, the lecithin may contain up to 15 wt. % glycolipids. In contrast to tripalmitate suspensions, soy bean oil-in-water emulsions stabilized by E80, S75 or S100 did neither exhibit comparably fast particle growth nor gel formation independently of the phospholipid mixture used as emulsifier.

These observations point to basic physicochemical differences between similarly composed lipid emulsions and lipid suspensions. In the following paragraph comprehensive physicochemical investigations will be reported in order to explore the observed differences of these two lipid-based drug carrier systems.

PHYSICOCHEMICAL INVESTIGATION OF THE GEL FORMATION TENDENCY OF CERTAIN LIPID COMPOSITIONS

Comprehensive physicochemical investigations on various phospholipid stabilized triglyceride suspension compositions using tripalmitate as lipid matrix and S100 as emulsifier were initiated to gain information on the gel formation mechanism and to provide a rationale basis for the development of reliable, reproducible and sufficiently stable colloidal lipid suspensions appropriate as potential (intravenously injectable) drug carriers.

An important observation is that gel formation does generally not take place when phospholipid stabilized tripalmitate dispersions are stored at temperatures above the melting temperature of the triglyceride. This indicates that gel formation does not occur as long as the systems exist in the emulsion state. Moreover, gel formation of lecithin stabilized tripalmitate suspensions can be prevented by the use of co-emulsifying agents such as the ionic surfactant glycocholate (Siekmann and Westesen, 1992) and the non-ionic polymer tyloxapol (Siekmann and Westesen, 1994a), or by subsequent adsorption of polyoxyethylene-polyoxypropylene block copolymers of the poloxamer and poloxamine type.

X-ray diffraction studies employing synchrotron radiation indicated that tripalmitate nanoparticles transfer rapidly into the thermodynamically stable β-modification on cooling (Westesen et al.1993; Siekmann and Westesen, 1994b). These findings were confirmed by differential scanning calorimetry (DSC) (Siekmann and Westesen, 1994c). The X-ray and DSC studies revealed that crystallization of the dispersed tripalmitate required an increased degree of supercooling of about 20°C. The melting temperature of the colloidal crystals is significantly decreased compared to the bulk phase. The X-ray and DSC studies did, however, not reveal basic differences between tripalmitate compositions which tended to form gels and those in which gel formation did not occur. The crystalline state of tripalmitate in semisolid systems was comparable to that of tripalmitate in stable colloidal dispersions with respect to the dominating β-modification and the degree of crystallinity. The semisolid systems immobilize, however, the complete aqueous phase of the composition which amounts to almost 90 weight percent water. The immobilization of such a high portion of the aqueous medium points to the existence of a gel structure. The structure of colloidal tripalmitate dispersions and gels was investigated by electron microscopy.

Transmission Electron Microscopy of Colloidal Tripalmite Suspensions

Electron microscopic pictures of freeze fractured replica of tripalmitate dispersions display platelet-like particles independent of the emulsifier composition (Figure 2). Especially larger particles clearly display a layered crystal structure with terraces, steps and kinks. The layers are oriented rectangular to the platelet normal. The thickness of single molecular layers is about 4 nm and corresponds to the β-crystalline modification of tripalmitate. This observation is in accordance with X-ray data which demonstrate that the resolidified tripalmitate particles are in the β-crystalline state (Westesen et al., 1993). Often the platelet-like suspension particles exhibit a thickness of less than 50 nm, that means only several molecular layers. The shape of the nanocrystals resembles melt-crystallized micro- and macroscopic triglyceride crystals of the β-modification (Skoda and van den Tempel, 1967, Skoda et al., 1967). By comparison of the macro- and nanocrystals it is possible to identify the prevailing crystal face of the tripalmitate nanocrystals as the (001)-face.

Based on the observed anisometrical shape of the tripalmitate nanoparticles it can be concluded that the transformation of the spherical emulsion droplets of the tripalmitate melt into solid tripalmitate platelets is accompanied by a significant

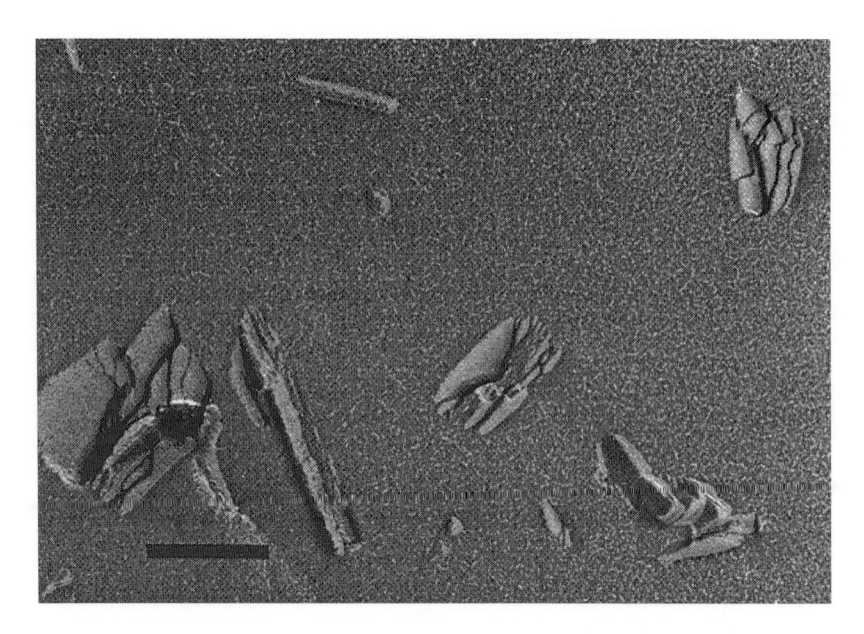

Figure 2 Transmission electron micrograph of a freeze-fractured specimen of a melt-homogenized triglyceride suspension consisting of 10% tripalmitate, 1.2% S100 and 0.4% sodium glycocholate in water. The bar corresponds to approximately 200 nm.

increase in the particle surface area. Further conclusions can be drawn from the preferential occurrence of certain crystal faces such as the (001)-face. As a consequence of the characteristic order of molecules in the crystal lattice, the different crystal faces exhibit different physicochemical properties such as polarity and surface tension. The (001)-face which contains the methyl end groups of the hydrocarbon chains should be nonpolar. Due to its preferential formation in the aqueous medium it can, however, be deduced that the (001)-face of the nanocrystals is hydrophilic. This could be confirmed by decoration of the fractures with water which condenses preferably on the large (001)-face (Figure 3). The detected hydrophilicity of the (001)-face points to the association of surfactant molecules with this nanocrystal face.

In addition to anisometrical crystals, spherical particles can be observed in the dispersions by transmission electron microscopy of freeze-fractured specimen. These were identified as small unilamellar vesicles (SUV) by their low fracture tendency. SUV represent the excess of phospholipids in the system and are generally found in lecithin stabilized lipid emulsions (Westesen and Wehler, 1992). The occurrence of SUV in colloidal tripalmitate suspensions was also verified by cryo-electron microscopy of frozen-hydrated specimen (Figure 4). The phospholipid bilayers of SUV exhibit a high electron density resulting in a high contrast against the aqueous phase. The ring shaped structures in the cryo-preparations reflect the concentric shell structures of phospholipid vesicles. Micrographs taken from cryo-preparations also display the tripalmitate suspension particles. As in freeze-fracture TEM anisometrical shapes with low contrast dominate pointing to the low thickness of the crystals and their platelet-like nature. In addition, needle-like structures can be

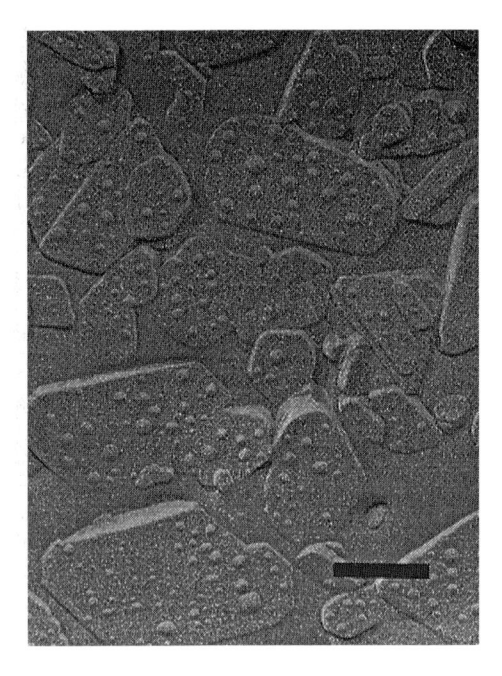

Figure 3 Transmission electron micrograph of a freeze-fractured specimen of a melt-homogenized tripalmitate suspension decorated with condensed water. The bar corresponds to approximately 230 nm.

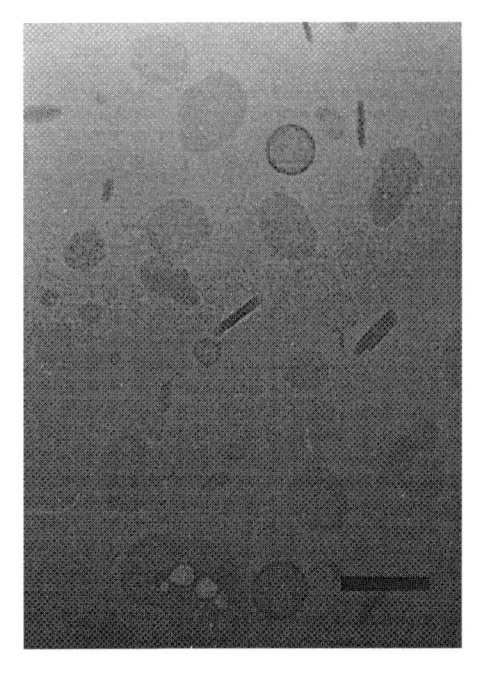

Figure 4 Cryo-electron micrograph of a frozen-hydrated specimen of a triglyceride suspension consisting of 10% tripalmitate, 2.4% S100 and 0.4% sodium glycocholate in water. The bar corresponds to approximately 110 nm.

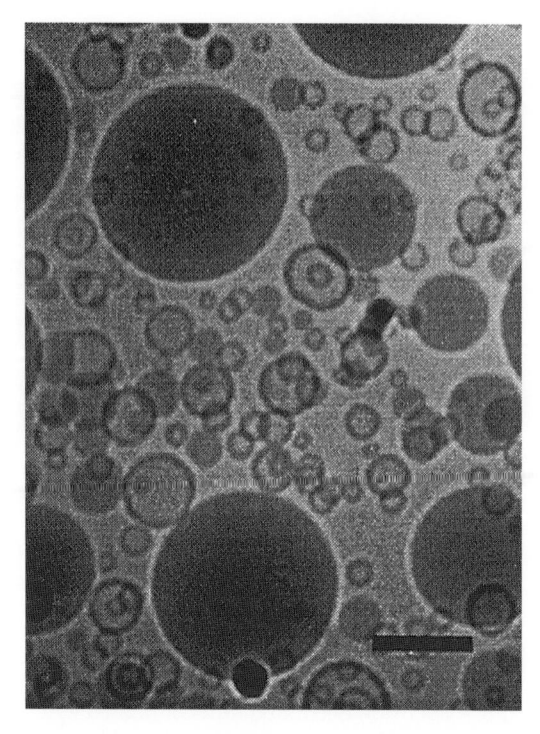

Figure 5 Cryo-electron micrograph of a frozen-hydrated specimen of a triglyceride emulsion consisting of 10% soya oil and 1.2% fractionated egg lecithin in water. The bar corresponds to approximately 110 nm.

observed, and their darkness is in accordance with the expected high contrast of a low contrast platelet viewed perpendicular to the platelet normal. It is noteworthy that the number of SUV in lecithin containing tripalmitate suspensions is considerably lower as in soy bean oil emulsions with lower lecithin content (Figure 5). The excess of emulsifier is thus lower in lipid suspensions compared with lipid emulsions. This is probably a consequence of higher binding of phospholipids to particle surfaces in the suspensions due to the larger specific surface area of the suspension particles. Due to the anisometrical particle shape and the presence of terraces, kinks and steps the surface area of a suspension particle is much larger as that of a spherical emulsion droplet of the same volume.

Transmission Electron Microscopy of Tripalmite Gels

From transmission electron micrographs of freeze-fractured replica of tripalmitate gels, these can be characterized as ultrafine three-dimensional networks formed by individual tripalmitate crystals which have agglomerated to a cardhouse-like structure (Figure 6). The thickness of the cross fractured network is in the order of the thickness of suspension particles. The aqueous phase interpenetrating the network is completely immobilized in these structures. No significant numbers of small vesicles were found in the gels pointing to the contribution of the phospholipids to the network structure and their incorporation into the crystal faces. The network

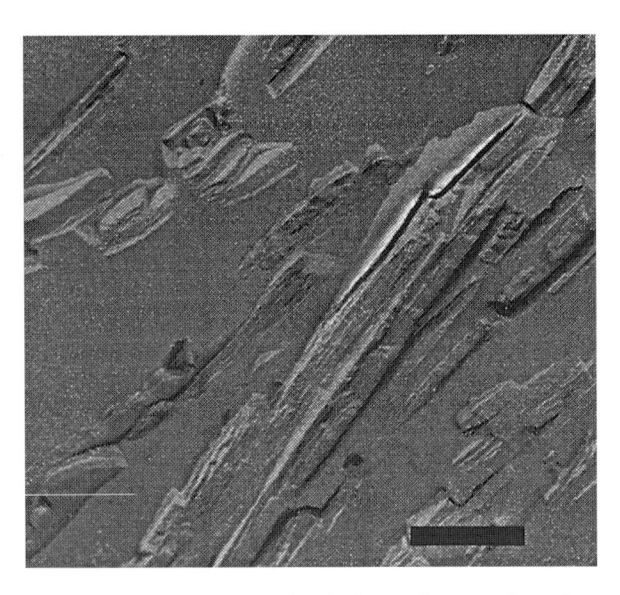

Figure 6 Transmission electron micrograph of a freeze-fractured specimen of a triglyceride gel consisting of 10% tripalmitate and 1.2% S100 in water. The bar corresponds to approximately 250 nm.

seems to consist of sintered particles which have been sintered predominantly via the lateral crystal faces, i.e. the platelet heights. It is striking that aggregation of the platelets occurs via the lateral crystals faces and not via the much larger (001)-face which also represents the prevailing crystal face in the gels. Formation of a network via the platelet heights reduces the number of surfaces from six for the isolated platelets to only two in the network, these being the (001)-faces. It can be deduced from their extremely high specific surface area in combination with a high macroscopic long-term stability of the tripalmitate gels that these network surfaces have extremely low interfacial tensions in contact with the immobilized aqueous media. The hydrophilicity and the low surface tension of the (001)-face points to the association of surfactant molecules with these crystal planes. Obviously, phospholipids are preferably adsorbed or incorporated in these crystal planes resulting in a sufficient stabilization. The phospholipids originate on the one hand from the initial tripalmitate emulsion droplets in the heat, and on the other from the small vesicles representing the excess of emulsifier in the initial emulsion since vesicles could not be detected in the cavities of the three-dimensional networks filled with the immobilized aqueous media.

The gels do not show any significant syneresis on storage for several months, which indicates that they do not contract significantly preserving their initial structure. It is, however, likely that the aggregated crystals sinter together at their contact points. This is indicated by experimental results which demonstrate that newly gelled systems can be redispersed by immediate shaking after gel formation to give colloidal dispersions of approximately the original particle size distribution. Redispersion of stored gels does not yield dispersions of colloidal size but much larger crystals.

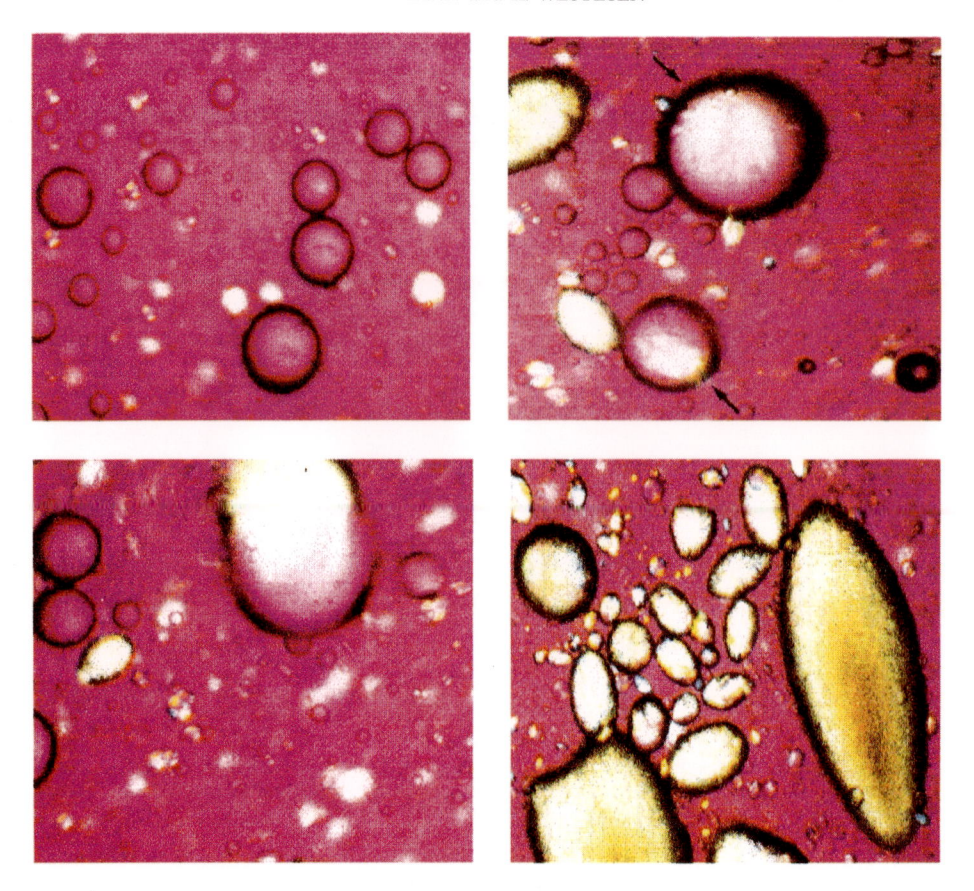

Figure 7 Polarized light microscopy of a crude melt-emulsified dispersion consisting of 10% tripalmitate, 2.4% S100 and 0.4% sodium glycocholate in water. Top left: emulsified melt prior to recrystallization. Top right: the arrows indicate that recrystallization starts at the particle surface. Bottom left: recrystallizing particle. Bottom right: anisometrical suspension particles after recrystallization.

Polarized Microscopy of the Crystallization of Crude Tripalmitate Dispersions

The physicochemical processes of melt-emulsified tripalmitate dispersions during the cooling step can be directly monitored by polarized light microscopy of crude lecithin/sodium glycocholate stabilized tripalmitate dispersions. The dispersed tripalmitate melt forms spherical, isotropic droplets representing the emulsion state of the dispersed lipid melt (Figure 7). The droplets transform into anisometrical, optically anisotropic particles when the melt recrystallizes (Figure 7). Crystallization starts from the particle surface pointing to an epitaxical effect of the emulsifier molecules present at the droplet interface (Figure 7). The anisometrical particles of the crude dispersions have obviously a different particle shape than those viewed by electron microscopy in colloidal dispersions. The different particle shape may tentatively be explained by the formation of crystals of the α-modification or by the formation of polycrystalline particles. The nanoparticles viewed in electron microscopy represent single crystals of the β-modification.

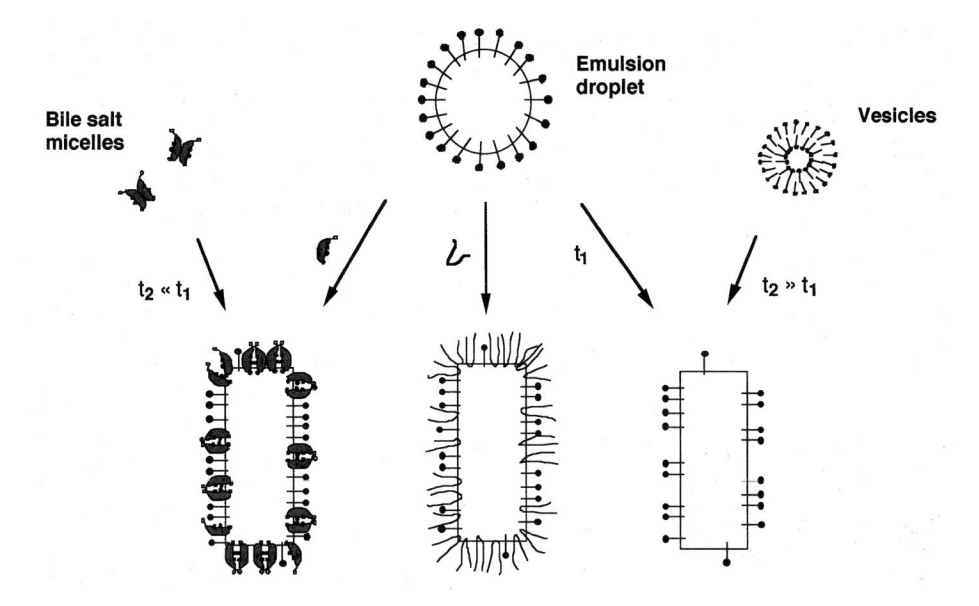

Figure 8 Model of the gel formation mechanism in phospholipid stabilized tripalmitate suspensions (times t_1 = suspension formation; t_2 = surfactant release from micelles/vesicles).

Beside the fat particles, the typical Maltese cross structures representing multilamellar vesicles (MLV) can be observed in the crude tripalmitate dispersions. The MLV correspond to the emulsifier excess analogously to SUV in colloidal dispersions. The high number of MLV indicate that a substantial portion of phospholipids is bound in vesicles.

A MODEL OF THE GEL FORMATION OF PHOSPHOLIPID STABILIZED TRIGLYERIDE COMPOSITIONS

A model based on experimental results and theoretical considerations with respect to crystal structure and molecular mobility has been developed to illustrate the gel formation phenomenon of colloidal tripalmitate suspensions (Figure 8). The electron microscopic investigation of tripalmitate dispersions and gels clearly demonstrated that recrystallization of the colloidally dispersed tripalmitate in the β-modification is accompanied by a tremendous increase in the surface area of the particles due to the formation of platelet-like colloidal crystals with structured surfaces. The change in particle shape during recrystallization results in a sudden local demand for additional emulsifier molecules at the particle surfaces in order to stabilize the freshly created surfaces. Owing to their phase behaviour, phospholipids are not able to immediately cover these newly created interfaces during recrystallization. Phospholipids are insoluble in water, and those phospholipid molecules which do not take part in the stabilization of emulsion droplets during the homogenization of the tripalmitate melt, i.e. the emulsifier excess, form vesicles in the aqueous phase. The mobility of phospholipid molecules bound to vesicles is, however, low. Supposing that t_1 is the time required for the recrystallization the triglyceride and formation of lipid suspension particles and t_2 is the time required for surfactant availability at the newly created surfaces, then the time t_2 which the phospholipid molecules would need to leave the vesicles and diffuse to the surface of the tripalmitate particles is substantially longer than t_1. Since there is no external energy input during the recrystallization process which would promote disruption of the vesicle bilayers and reduction of the diffusional pathways, the low inherent mobility of the phospholipid molecules is not sufficient to counteract the sudden lack of emulsifier that is created locally on the particle surfaces despite an excess of emulsifier in the overall system. From the structure of the tripalmitate gels as revealed by electron microscopy it can be concluded that phospholipid molecules are preferentially adsorbed to, or — due to similarities in molecular geometry — possibly even incorporated into the (001)-face of tripalmitate nanocrystals during recrystallization leaving the lateral crystal faces unprotected. Hence, particle aggregation can proceed via these unprotected lateral faces building up a cardhouse-like gel structure which is able to immobilize the aqueous phase.

In contrast, in dispersions which contain water soluble, highly mobile, micelle-forming co-surfactants, such as bile salts or poloxamers, the time t_2 required for surfactant availability is much shorter than for the phospholipids so that the sudden local lack of stabilizing agents in the surface of recrystallizing tripalmitate particles can immediately be counteracted. Owing to their high mobility these co-surfactants are able to cover the newly created particle surfaces in a time t_2 which is in the order of magnitude of t_1. An additional effect might be that co-surfactants such as glycocholate destabilize the phospholipid vesicles thereby facilitating the disruption of the bilayers and enhancing the surface availability of the phosholipid molecules. The co-surfactants may then form a mixed stabilizer layer at the particle surface together with the originally present phospholipid molecules.

Furthermore, it has to be considered that phospholipids and co-surfactants may adsorb with different preference to different nanocrystal faces. Whereas phospholipid molecules are preferentially adsorbed to or incorporated into the (001)-face, it can be assumed that the lateral faces are covered to a greater extent by the co-surfactants. Particle aggregation and sintering can thus proceed over adsorbed phospholipid molecules due to the similar molecular geometries, but is interrupted where co-surfactants are present at the nanocrystal surfaces.

CONCLUSIONS

Whereas phospholipid stabilized soy bean oil-in-water emulsions generally display a reasonable long-term stability, the corresponding melt-homogenized tripalmitate suspensions tend to form semisolid gels upon cooling of the hot tripalmitate-in-water emulsions. These observations indicate that such colloidal tripalmitate suspensions should not simply be regarded as "lipid emulsions with solidified fat droplets". In fact, complex stability aspects which originate from the crystalline nature, the crystallization kinetics and the polymorphism of the dispersed lipid have to be addressed. It is important to realize that the crystallization of triglyceride nanoparticles may be accompanied by a change of the particle shape from spherical to anisometrical, which leads to a tremendous increase in the specific surface area.

Owing to the underlying kinetics of the suspensions with respect to surface formation and emulsifier mobility, steric and electrostatic stabilization do not give the same stabilizing effects generally obtained with emulsion systems. Sufficiently stable colloidal suspensions can, however, be reproducibly obtained by a proper choice of emulsifier blends. It can be recommended that phospolipids as stabilizers should generally be combined with a micelle forming co-surfactant with high molecular mobility in the aqueous phase.

It has to be considered that the stability of solid lipid based dispersions is closely related to the phase transitions of the dispersed phase, and is thus affected e.g. by the recrystallization tendency of the dispersed lipid. The observed long-term stability of melt-homogenized, phospholipid stabilized trilaurate dispersions recently described by Schwarz et al. (1994) can probably be attributed to the absence of recrystallization. As has been demonstrated by Westesen and Bunjes (1995) melt-homogenized trilaurate dispersions remain in the state of a supercooled melt, even when stored at refrigerator temperature. These systems therefore represent emulsions according to the IUPAC definition (Everett, 1972) and have thus similar physicochemical properties as vegetable oil emulsions with respect to physical stability. These trilaurate emulsions may therefore not exhibit the potential advantages of solid lipid nanoparticles (Table 1).

REFERENCES

Collins-Gold, L.C., Lyons, R.T., Bartholow, L.C. (1990) Parenteral emulsions for drug delivery. *Adv. Drug Deliv. Rev.*, **5**, 189–208.

Everett, D.H. (1972) Report of the Commission on Colloid and Surface Chemistry of the Physical Chemistry Devision. *Pure Appl. Chem.*, **31**, 577–638.

Freitas, C. Lucks, J.S., Müller, R.H. (1994) Effect of storage conditions on long-term stability of "solid lipid nanoparticles" (SLN) in aqueous dispersion. *Eur. J. Pharm. Sci.*, **2**, 178.

Magenheim, B. Levy, M.Y., Benita, S. (1993) A new *in vitro* technique for evaluation of drug release profile from colloidal carriers — ultrafiltration technique at low pressure. *Int. J. Pharm.*, **94**, 115–123.

Prankerd, R.J., Stella, V.J. (1990) The Use of Oil-in-Water Emulsions as a Vehicle for Parenteral Drug Administration. *J. Parent. Sci. Tech.*, **44**, 139–149.

Schuberth, O., Wretlind, A. (1961) Intravenous infusions of fat emulsions, phosphatides and emulsifying agents, *Acta Chir. Scand.*, **278** (Suppl.), 1–20.

Schwarz, C., Mehnert, W., Lucks, J.S., Müller, R.H. (1994) Solid lipid nanoparticles (SLN) for controlled drug delivery. I. Production, characterization and sterilization. *J. Controlled Rel.*, **30**, 83–96.

Siekmann, B., Westesen, K. (1992) Submicron-sized parenteral carrier systems based on solid lipids. *Pharm. Pharmacol. Lett.*, **1**, 123–126.

Siekmann, B., Westesen, K. (1994a) Melt-homogenized solid lipid nanoparticles stabilized by the nonionic surfactant tyloxapol: I. Preparation and particle size determination. *Pharm. Pharmacol. Lett.*, **3**, 194–197.

Siekmann, B., Westesen, K. (1994b) Melt-homogenized solid lipid nanoparticles stabilized by the nonionic surfactant tyloxapol: II. Physicochemical characterization and lyophilisation. *Pharm. Pharmacol. Lett.*, **3**, 225–228.

Siekmann, B., Westesen, K. (1994c) Thermoanalysis of the recrystallization process of melt-homogenized glyceride nanoparticles. *Colloids Surf. B: Biointerfaces*, **3**, 159–175.

Siekmann, B., Westesen, K. (1997) Investigation of the Gel Formation of Phospholipid Stabilized Solid Lipid Nanoparticles. *Int. J. Pharm.*, **151**, 35–45.

Skoda, W., van den Tempel, M. (1967) Growth Kinetics of Triglyceride Crystals. *J. Crystal Growth.*, **1**, 207–217.

Skoda, W., Hoekstra, L.L., van Soest, T.C., Bennema, P., van den Tempel, M. (1967) Structure and Morphology of β Crystals of Glyceryl Tristearate. *Kolloid Zeitschrift & Zeitschrift Polym.*, **219**, 149–156.

Westesen, K., Bunjes, H. (1995) Do nanoparticles prepared from lipids solid at room temperature always possess a solid lipid matrix? *Int. J. Pharm.*, **115**, 129–131.

Westesen, K., Siekmann, B. (1996) Biodegradable Colloidal Drug Carrier Systems Based on Solid Lipids. In *Microencapsulation: Methods and Industrial Applications*, edited by S. Benita, pp. 213–258. New York: Marcel Dekker.

Westesen, K., Wehler, T. (1992) Physicochemical Characterization of a Model Intravenous Oil-in-Water Emulsion. *J. Pharm. Sci.*, **81**, 777–786.

Westesen, K., Siekmann, B., Koch, M.H.J. (1993) Investigations on the Physical State of Lipid Nanoparticles by Synchrotron Radiation X-Ray Diffraction. *Int. J. Pharm.*, **93**, 189–199.

Wretlind, A. (1981) Development of Fat Emulsions. *J. Parent. Enteral Nutr.*, **5**, 230–235.

9. SOLID LIPID NANOPARTICLES (SLN®) FOR CONTROLLED DRUG DELIVERY

R.H. MÜLLER and S.A. RUNGE

Free University (FU) of Berlin, Department of Pharmaceutics, Biopharmaceutics and Biotechnology, Kelchstr. 31, D-12169 Berlin, Germany

DEFINITION OF SLN

General features of parenteral fat emulsions for drug delivery are their good *in vivo* tolerability, i.e. low systemic toxicity and low cytotoxicity, their composition of physiological compounds, the relatively low costs of the excipients and the ease of industrial scale production by high pressure homogenization. Incorporation of drugs can reduce distinctly drug side effects, e.g. thrombophlebitis associated with intravenously injected diazepam or etomidate (Schuhmann, 1996). However, due to the liquid state of the oil droplets, a prolonged drug release cannot be achieved. After intravenous injection, there will be a partitioning of the drug within milliseconds or seconds between the liquid oil phase and the aqueous phase of the blood. Even very lipophilic drugs will exhibit a burst release due to the relatively large volume of the water phase compared to the few ml of the oil phase of the emulsion. A prolonged drug liberation from emulsions obtained in *in vitro* studies can be attributed to the experimental set up used. When applying a dialysis tube or inverted dialysis tube method one measures rather the distribution between the two aqueous phases inside and outside the tube than the release from the oil droplets (Benita *et al.*, 1986). A major disadvantage of emulsions as drug carrier systems is therefore the burst release due to the lack of a solid matrix. Furthermore, emulsions are relatively fast metabolized limiting additionally prolonged drug release.

To overcome the disadvantages associated with the liquid state of the oil droplet, the liquid lipid was replaced by a solid lipid leading to the formation of solid lipid nanoparticles (SLN) (Schwarz, 1995; Müller and Lucks, 1996a). The SLN combine advantages of emulsions — composition of physiological compounds, good tolerability, large scale production by high pressure homogenization — with advantages of solid polymeric particles — solid matrix for controlled drug release, protection of incorporated drugs against chemical degradation, slowlier *in vivo* metabolism. Basic work in the area of solid lipid particles has been performed by Speiser at the beginning of the 80's. He reported about production of lipid microspheres by spray-gelation (Kecht-Wyrsch, 1987) and lipid nanopellets for oral delivery (Speiser, 1990). To produce the lipid nanopellets, the lipids were melted and dispersed in a hot aqueous surfactant solution by steering or ultrasonic treatment. Similar production techniques were used by Domb to produce his system called "lipospheres" (Domb, 1991). Gasco uses microemulsions for the production of solid lipid nanoparticles. The hot microemulsion containing the lipid is poured into water leading to the precipitation of nanoparticles (Gasco, 1993). A different approach is the high pressure homogenization of either melted or even solid lipids (Schwarz, 1995) which is also being used by other research groups, e.g. Westesen and Siekmann. (Westesen and Siekmann, 1994). Advantages of this production by high pressure homogenization are the relatively narrow size distribution of the product (low content of microparticles), the acceptability of the homogenization equipment by the regulatory authorities (even for parenteral products), the avoidance of organic solvents, the ease of scaling up and the availability of homogenization production lines in industry.

The trade products SLN® and Lipopearls® (solid lipid nanoparticles in cosmetic products) are produced by high pressure homogenization. In contrast to emulsions, the particles consist of a solid core made from solid lipids. They are characterized by a mean diameter between approximately 80 nm to 1000 nm at simultaneously very low content of microparticulate contamination (especially important for intravenous administration). SLN in aqueous dispersion are stabilized by surfactants, however, it is also possible to produce surfactant-free SLN by producing them e.g. in PVA solutions. SLN can be lyophilized or spray-dried. Potential formulations in pharmacy and cosmetics utilizing different administration routes are discussed in the section "Possible applications of SLN".

PRODUCTION TECHNIQUES

There are two basic production techniques for SLN, homogenization of melted lipids at elevated temperature (hot homogenization technique) and homogenization of a suspension of solid lipids at room temperature or below (cold homogenization technique).

Hot Homogenization Technique

The lipid matrix material is melted, drug incorporation can be performed by dissolving the drug in the melted lipid. Alternatively, insoluble drugs can be dispersed in the melted lipid in the form of nanocrystals, e.g. magnetite particles (Weyhers, 1995a). In the next production step the drug-containing lipid will be dispersed in its molten state in a hot aqueous surfactant solution possessing a temperature slightly above the melting point of the lipid (Figure 1). Dispersion is performed using a rotor-stator stirrer. The obtained coarse pre-emulsion is then homogenized using a gap homogenizer such as an APV Gaulin LAB 40. The pressures applied range from 100 to 1500 bar. Typically one to three homogenization cycles are sufficient. The obtained product is an oil-in-water emulsion. Cooling down of this emulsion to room temperature (or below) will lead to lipid crystallization and formation of the solid lipid nanoparticles.

The hot homogenization technique can be applied to lipophilic and insoluble drugs. Even many heat-sensitive drugs can be processed because the exposure time to higher temperatures is relatively short. The technique is not suitable for incorporating hydrophilic drugs into SLN. During the homogenization of the melted lipid phase the drug will partition to the water phase resulting in a too low entrapment efficiency.

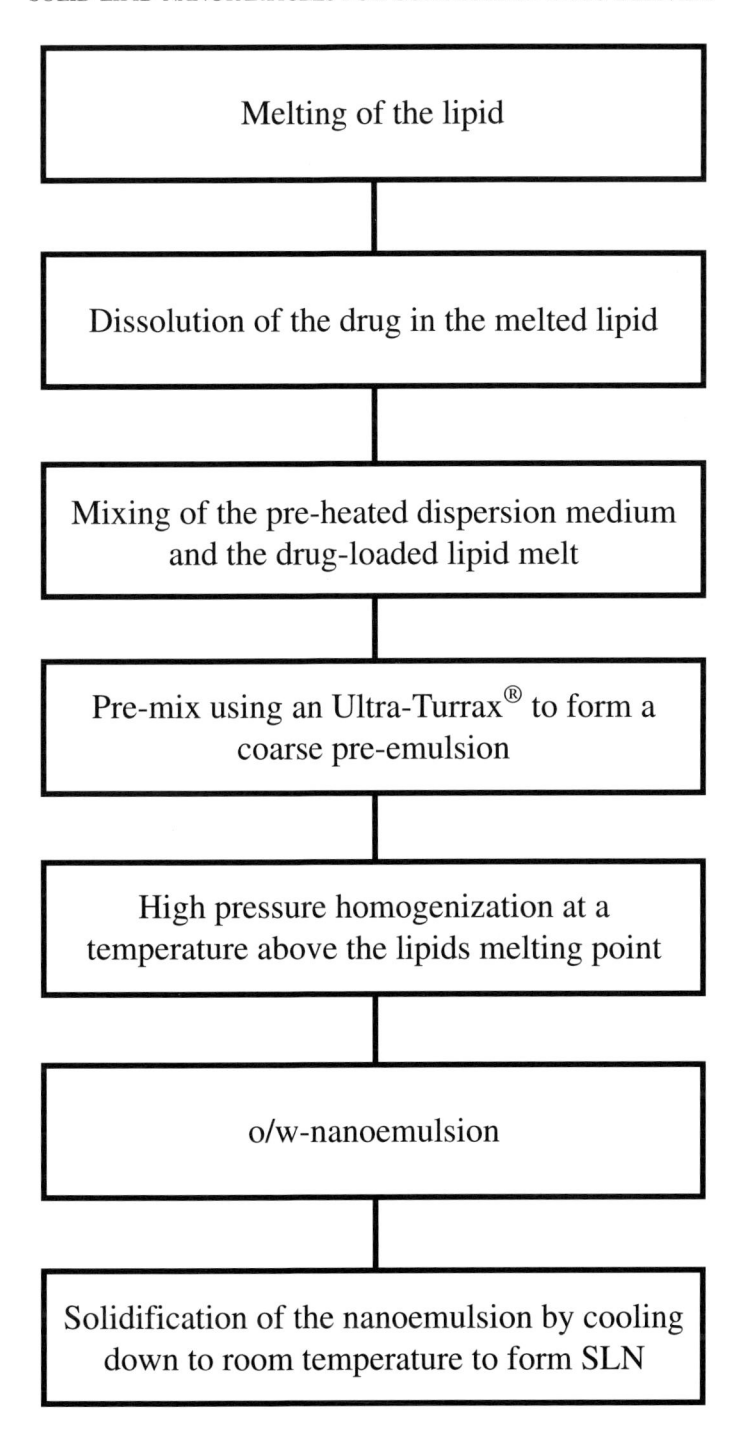

```
┌─────────────────────────────────────────┐
│         Melting of the lipid            │
└─────────────────────────────────────────┘
                    │
┌─────────────────────────────────────────┐
│ Dissolution of the drug in the melted lipid │
└─────────────────────────────────────────┘
                    │
┌─────────────────────────────────────────┐
│ Mixing of the pre-heated dispersion medium │
│      and the drug-loaded lipid melt     │
└─────────────────────────────────────────┘
                    │
┌─────────────────────────────────────────┐
│  Pre-mix using an Ultra-Turrax® to form a │
│          coarse pre-emulsion            │
└─────────────────────────────────────────┘
                    │
┌─────────────────────────────────────────┐
│      High pressure homogenization at a   │
│ temperature above the lipids melting point │
└─────────────────────────────────────────┘
                    │
┌─────────────────────────────────────────┐
│            o/w-nanoemulsion             │
└─────────────────────────────────────────┘
                    │
┌─────────────────────────────────────────┐
│ Solidification of the nanoemulsion by cooling │
│  down to room temperature to form SLN    │
└─────────────────────────────────────────┘
```

Figure 1 SLN® production using the hot homogenization technique.

```
┌─────────────────────────────────────────┐
│         Melting of the lipid            │
└─────────────────────────────────────────┘
                    │
┌─────────────────────────────────────────┐
│  Dissolution/solubilization of the drug │
│           in the melted lipid           │
└─────────────────────────────────────────┘
                    │
┌─────────────────────────────────────────┐
│  Solidification of the drug-loaded lipid│
│        in liquid nitrogen or dry ice    │
└─────────────────────────────────────────┘
                    │
┌─────────────────────────────────────────┐
│        Grinding in a powder mill        │
│          (50–100 μm particles)          │
└─────────────────────────────────────────┘
                    │
┌─────────────────────────────────────────┐
│ Dispersion of the lipid powder in the cold │
│  aqueous dispersion medium (=pre-mix)   │
└─────────────────────────────────────────┘
                    │
┌─────────────────────────────────────────┐
│   Homogenization at room temperature    │
│                or below                 │
└─────────────────────────────────────────┘
                    │
┌─────────────────────────────────────────┐
│         Solid Lipid Nanoparticles       │
└─────────────────────────────────────────┘
```

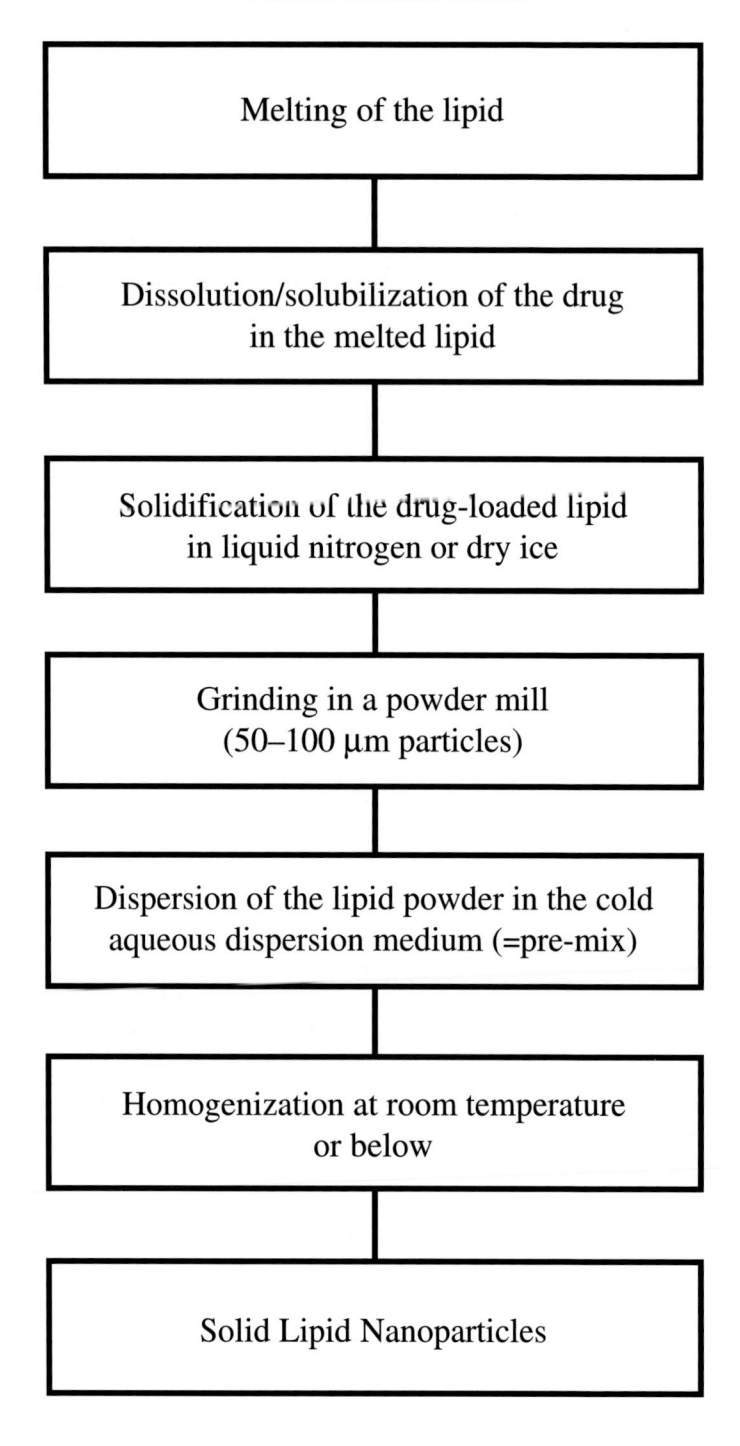

Figure 2 SLN® production using the cold homogenization technique

Cold Homogenization Technique

For a hydrophilic drug the cold homogenization technique is the method of first choice. The hydrophilic drug is dissolved in the melted lipid. In case of a too low solubility of the hydrophilic drug in the lipid, surfactants can be used for solubilization of the drug. In the next production step, the drug-containing melted lipid is solidified in dry ice or liquid nitrogen and milled using e.g. a mortar mill. Dry ice or liquid nitrogen are used to increase the brittleness of the lipid and to ease the milling procedure. The obtained lipid microparticles (appr. 50 to 100 μm) are dispersed in a cold aqueous surfactant solution and this lipid suspension is homogenized at room temperature or below (Figure 2). The cavitation and shear forces in the homogenization gap are sufficiently high to break the microparticles and to yield solid lipid nanoparticles.

This homogenization technique avoids or minimizes melting processes of the lipid. Temperature peaks ocurring inside the homogenizer during the homogenization process obviously do not possess a sufficiently high energy to melt the lipid. In case of an inlet temperature of about 20°C, the outlet temperature of the product will typically be about 40°C. The outlet temperature can be reduced by cooling the homogenization tower. For basic studies, the hydrophilic X-ray contrast agent Iotrolan was incorporated into SLN. Iotrolan is extremely hydrophilic, two parts of Iotrolan can be dissolved in one part of water. About 1% of Iotrolan could be incorporated in the lipid by solubilization (percentage calculated on the basis of the lipid being 100%). After producing SLN applying the cold homogenization technique there were still 0.5% of Iotrolan incorporated in the nanoparticles. A loss of Iotrolan from the lipid particles can be explained by the increase in surface area during the transfer from microparticles to nanoparticles.

SLN produced by the cold homogenization technique possess a slightly higher polydispersity in size distribution compared to particles obtained by hot homogenization, the mean particle sizes are also slightly higher compared to hot processing of the same lipid at identical homgenization parameters (pressure, temperature, number of homogenization cycles). To further reduce the mean particle size and to minimize the polydispersity, a higher number of homogenization cycles can be applied.

Alternatively, the homogenization can be performed slightly below the melting point of the lipid (e.g. 5 to 10°C) which seems to lead to a softening of the lipid during the homogenization process. The softened lipid can be more easily dispersed leading to a more uniform product of smaller mean particle size. The homogenization temperature needs to be carefully selected because otherwise the loss of hydrophilic drugs to the water phase is too high.

DRUG INCORPORATION: PAY LOAD AND ENTRAPMENT EFFICIENCY

The maximum pay load of lipophilic drugs in SLN is determined by their solubility in the melted lipid. It needs also to be considered that during solidification of the lipid an exclusion of the drug from the lipid might occur. For drugs miscible with the melted lipid in any ratio a very high pay load can be achieved. In theory, the pay load might approach 100%. The increase in pay load at a simultaneous reduction

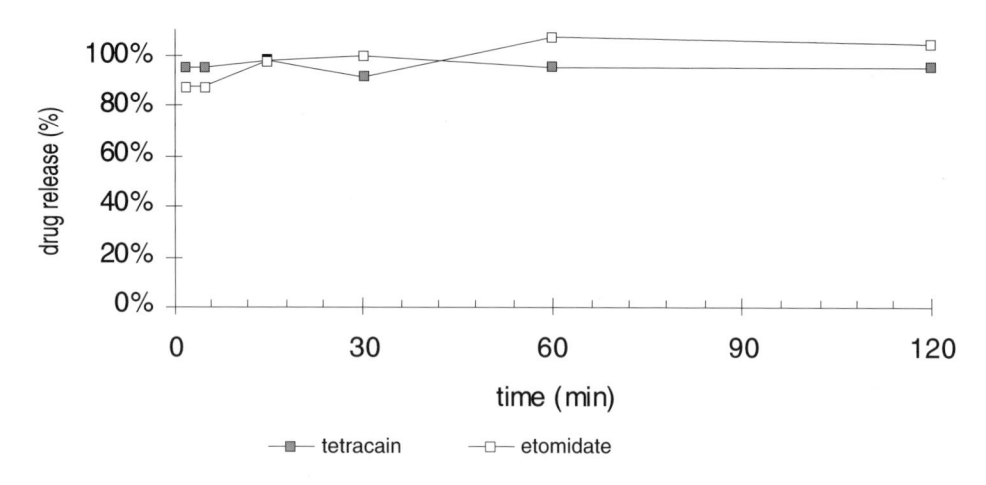

Figure 3 Burst release profiles obtained with tetracaine and etomidate incorporated in SLN as drug carrier (lipid matrix: Compritol) (Schwarz, 1995).

of the matrix material will create a more heterogeneous matrix structure accelerating drug release. That means that the pay load is also limited by the desired duration of drug liberation.

Pay load studies were performed using tetracaine and etomidate as model drugs. Practically, the pay load was limited to 10 up to a maximum of 20% (Schwarz, 1995). Higher pay loads led to the formation of a gel after the homogenization process, particle formation did not take place any more. Possible disturbances of the particle formation process need therefore also to be considered when increasing the pay load.

Entrapment efficiency between 80 and up to 99% were achieved when incorporating the model drugs tetracaine, etomidate and prednisolone in various lipid matrices (Schwarz, 1995; zur Mühlen, 1996). The entrapment efficiency is defined as the percentage of drug which is incorporated in the SLN, the total amount of drug added to the formulation is said to be 100%. The high entrapment efficiencies can be explained by the lipophilic character of the model drugs, only between 1 and a maximum of 20% of the added drug were found in the water phase of the SLN dispersion. The entrapment efficiency remained unchanged during long-term storage of the aqueous SLN dispersions (zur Mühlen, 1996).

DRUG RELEASE PROFILES

To control the drug release and to adjust the release profile in a controlled way it is a prerequisite to understand the drug incorporation mechanism. A basic problem of drug incorporation into SLN was the resulting burst release, e.g. observed with tetracaine and etomidate (Figure 3).

The SLN behaved identically to drug-loaded emulsions. Figure 3 shows as example the release profiles obtained with these two drugs. Differential scanning calorimetry (DSC) and X-ray diffraction studies indicated that the drugs were present in the

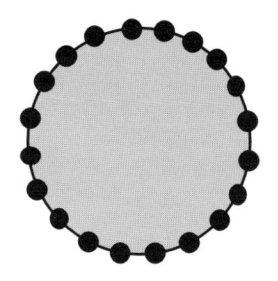

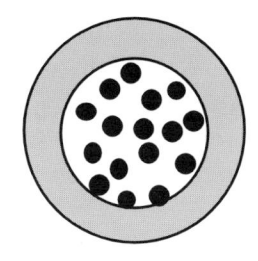

Figure 4 (left) Burst release after enrichment of drug in the outer shell of the nanoparticle (zur Mühlen, 1996); (right) Prolonged release of a drug-rich core and an outer shell of drug-poor or drug free lipid (zur Mühlen, 1996).

form of a solid solution. The existence of pure drug crystals inside the SLN could not be detected. Drug crystals in the water phase of the aqueous SLN dispersion — a reason for fast release — could be excluded (Schwarz, 1995). The solid state of the SLN was verified by DSC measurements. A possible explanation for the observed fast drug release is the enrichment of drug in the outer shell of the nanoparticle (Figure 4, left). Such an enrichment can occur when the hot nanoemulsion obtained in the hot homogenization process cools down. The pure lipid itself might crystallize first forming a core of pure lipid in the centre of the SLN, during continuation of the crystallization process a drug-rich outer lipid shell might be formed. However, a burst release was also observed when applying the cold homogenization technique to produce tetracaine-and etomidate-loaded SLN. Changes in the lipid crystalline structure of the SLN during the homogenization process and after it might lead to some exclusion of drug from the inner lipidic core and a drug enrichment in the outer shell. X-ray studies being performed at present might be able to prove such drug migration effects.

A prolonged *in vitro* drug release was achieved when incorporating prednisolone into SLN. The shape of the release profile could be modified by changing the production technique (hot or cold homogenization) and the formulation composition (e.g. surfactant concentration).

Again, DSC and X-ray data indicated that the drug was present as a solid solution. A possible explanation for the prolonged release is the formation of a drug-rich core and an outer shell of drug-poor or drug-free lipid (Figure 4, right) (zur Mühlen, 1996).

The extent of the burst release during the first minutes can be modified by changing the production temperature and the surfactant content. Changing these parameters is assumed to alter the drug concentration in the outer shell of the SLN. At high surfactant concentration and high temperature (hot homogenization process) the solubility of the drug in the outer aqueous phase is increased during the homogenization process. As a consequence, drug will partition from the lipid phase to the aqueous outer phase. During cooling down of the obtained hot nanoemulsion, the solubility of the drug in the outer phase decreases leading to a migration of drug into the outer shell of the SLN or even onto the particle surface in the surfactant layer (Figure 5) (zur Mühlen, 1996).

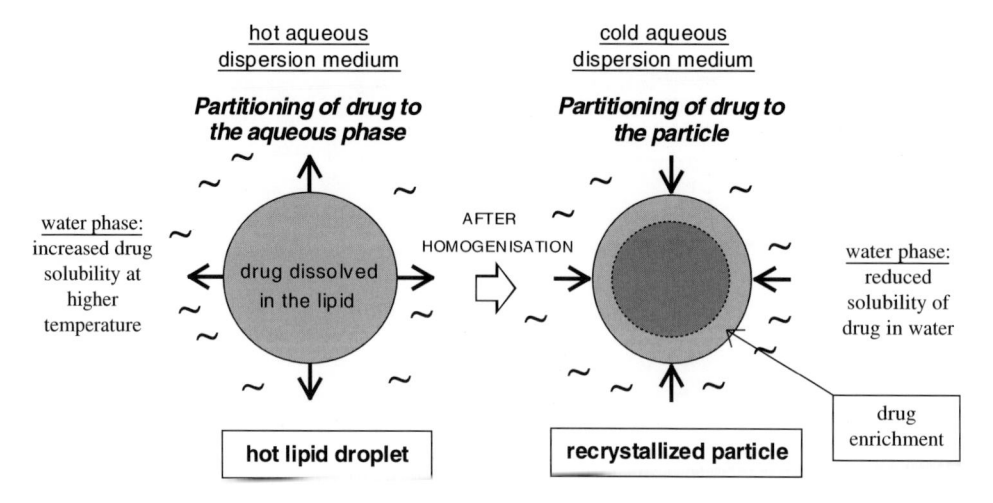

Figure 5 Drug partition from the lipid phase to the aqueous outer phase during cooling down of the obtained hot nanoemulsion using the hot homogenization technique (zur Mühlen, 1996, modified).

The solubility of drugs into the outer aqueous phase can be minimized by using a surfactant concentration as low as possible and homogenization at low temperatures. By varying these parameters, the extent of burst release and the shape of the release profile can be adjusted. If no initial dose is desired, the burst release can be avoided (Figure 6) (zur Mühlen, 1996).

C: Compritol-SLN / cold homogenization
B: Compritol-SLN / hot homogenization (40°C)
A: Cholesterol-SLN / cold homogenization

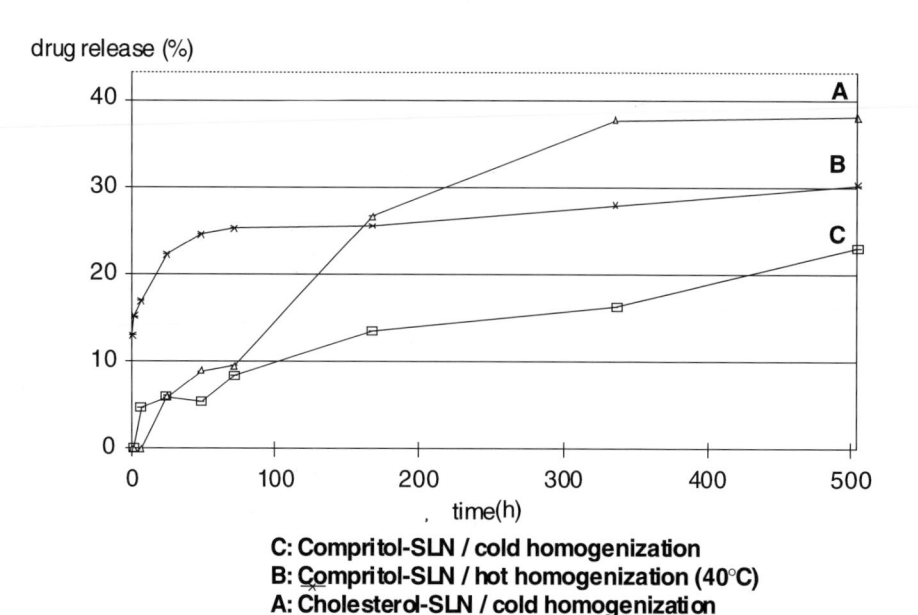

Figure 6 Variation of the extent of burst release and shape of release profile by varying the production method and lipid composition (zur Mühlen, 1996).

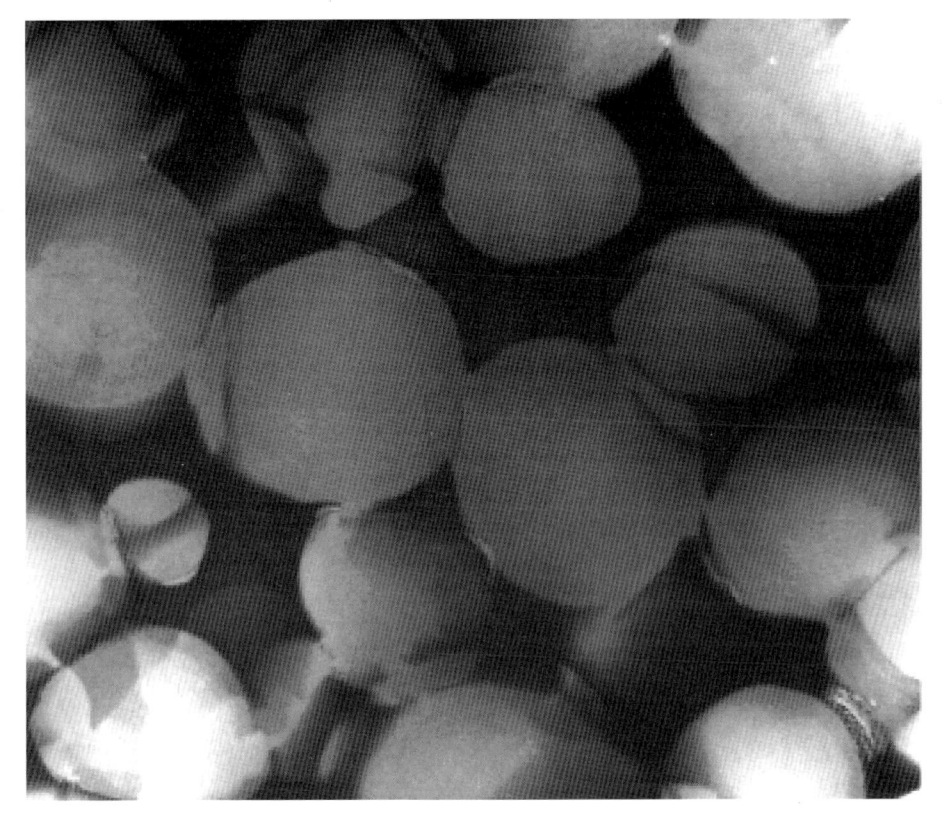

Figure 7 SLN of spherical shape produced by using a lipid and a surfactant from cosmetic products (cetylpalmitate, Plantaren).

The localization of the drug inside the nanoparticles is a determining factor for the drug release behaviour. Based on our X-ray studies two possibilities of drug incorporation are suggested. In the first case, the drug is incorporated in a molecular dispersed form between the lipid layers and lipid nanocrystals. Reorientation of the lipid molecules can lead to an exclusion of the drug from certain lipid areas leading to the second case, the formation of amorphous drug clusters between lipid crystal layers or lipid crystals. The formation of such amorphous drug clusters is favoured the less perfect the lipid crystals are. In case of perfect lipid crystallization, e.g. in case of high purity lipids, the drug will be expelled from the SLN, localized in the outer shell or on the surface and be released in the burst. Chemically polydisperse lipid mixtures form less perfect crystalline structures leaving more space for hosting the drug. To produce SLN for controlled drug release, it appears therefore favourable to use lipid blends instead of perfectly crystallizing lipids consisting of only one compound (e.g. Dynasan).

The composition of the lipid matrix determines not only the drug incorporation properties but also the shape of the nanoparticles. Relatively pure lipids lead to the formation of more cubic or rod-like nanoparticles, in contrast using chemically non-uniformly lipid blends leads to more spherical particles. Especially many lipids used in cosmetics led to the formation of more spherical SLN (Figure 7).

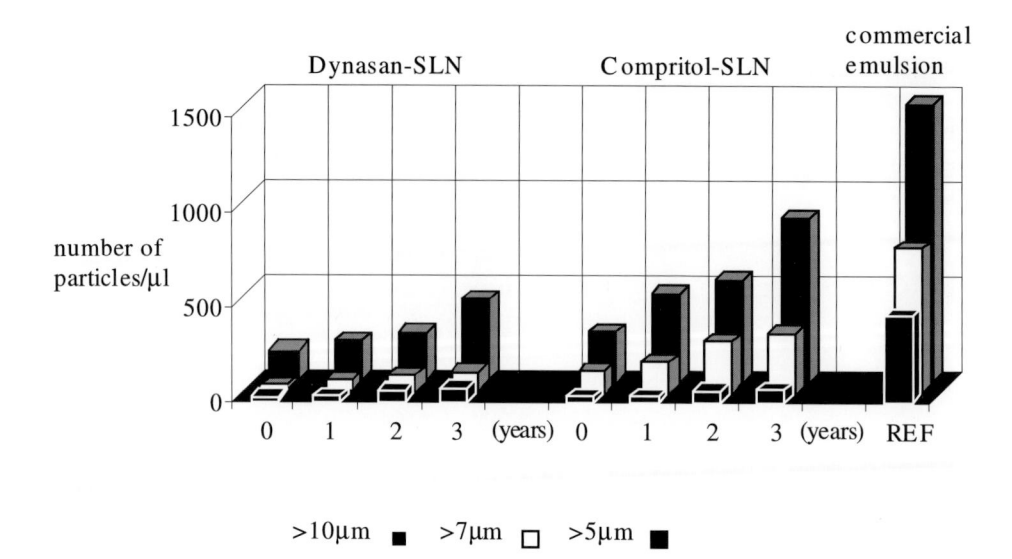

Figure 8 Long term stability of optimized SLN-formulations compared to a commercial emulsion. Number of particles per volume determined by a Coulter counter Multisizer II (REF=reference: particles counted in a commercial fat emulsion (10%) for parenteral nutrition) (Schwarz, 1995, (modified)).

Crystallinity of the spherical particles was assessed by DSC to exclude that the spherical particles are droplets of non-recrystallized lipid.

PHYSICAL LONG-TERM STABILITY

Ideally the SLN should be physically stable as aqueous dispersion. This abandons a reconstitution prior to use. At optimized composition aqueous SLN dispersions proved to be stable for more than 3 years. The mean particle size determined by PCS did not change (Müller et al., 1996b). However, especially for intravenous administration the content of microparticles and its increase during storage is a very crucial parameter. Therefore the PCS measurements alone are meaningless because the measurement range is only 3 nm to approximately 3 μm.

The advantage of using high pressure homogenization is the uniformity of the product and its low content of microparticles. To judge the suitability of SLN dispersions for intravenous injection the content of microparticles was determined by Coulter counter measurements and compared with commercial emulsions for parenteral nutrition (e.g. Lipofundin®, Intralipid®). During long-term storage of the SLN dispersion there should be only a minor increase in the number of microparticles per volume unit of the dispersion. Figure 8 shows that the content of particles larger than 5 μm per volume unit in SLN dispersions directly after production is below the values obtained for emulsions for parenteral nutrition. In contrast to the PCS diameters, the content of microparticles increases slightly during storage of three years. However, it is still below the content present in commercial emulsions (Figure 8).

When judging the suitability for i.v. injection it needs to be considered, that emulsion droplets are flexible and might pass even capillaries smaller than the droplet size. In contrast, SLN are rigid. However, when considering the distinctly lower injection volume of SLN dispersions compared to the administration volume of parenteral emulsions (daily application e.g. 10–20 ml compared to 500 ml and more) an intravenous administration seems feasible. This was confirmed by first *in vivo* studies (Weyhers *et al.*, 1995b).

It might be possible that an SLN formulation appears highly attractive with regard to toxicological aspects, however it proves to be physically unstable during storage as aqueous dispersion. In such cases the SLN dispersion can be transferred to a dry product by lyophilization (Schwarz, 1995) or by spray-drying (Freitas, 1994). The production of dry SLN might also be favourable in case they should be incorporated in hard gelatine capsules or tablets (c.f. section "Possible applications of SLN").

IN VITRO AND *IN VIVO* TOXICITY

The toxicity is the governing factor deciding if a product has the chance to be introduced to the pharmaceutical market. Ideally, the product should contain only excipients which are already accepted in formulations by the regulatory authorities. This is possible when producing SLN for cosmetics or for pharmaceuticals intended for topical, ophthalmic, oral or peroral administration. The materials used are excipients already present in cosmetical or pharmaceutical products accepted by the regulatory authorities, the full range of GRAS substances and substances of recognized GRAS status is available (Food additives, 1994). The list of these substances includes also compounds with surface activity or surfactants suitable for SLN stabilization. To produce SLN for parenteral administration, the full range of lipids can be used which is composed of physiological compounds, e.g. glycerides with C16 to C22 fatty acids (e.g. Compritol — a mixture of glycerides with behenic acid). Egg lecithin, sodium cholate, poloxamer 188 and polysorbate 80 can be used as surfactants because they are accepted in i.v. products.

For parenteral, especially intravenous administration it will be necessary to perform a toxicity study — despite the fact that the lipids are composed of physiological compounds. By now *in vitro* cytotoxicity and preliminary *in vivo* toxicity studies with SLN have been performed (Weyhers, 1995a; Weyhers *et al.*, 1995b). The SLN were compared with other colloidal drug carriers, especially nanoparticles from polylactic acid and polylactic glycolic acid (GA) polymers. These polymeric materials are accepted by the regulatory authorities for implants and parenteral microparticles. However, it needs to be pointed out that there is a difference between the systemic toxicity and the cytotoxicity. A material might be well tolerated systemically, after uptake by the cells in form of nanoparticles it might exhibit cytotoxic effects. Cytotoxicity was assessed by measuring the viability of e.g. human granulocytes after incubation with different colloidal drug carriers. Viability was measured by employing the MTT test (Weyhers, 1995a). Incubation of human granulocytes with 0.5% PLA GA nanoparticles led to total cell death, incubation with 10% SLN, however, reduced a viability only to 80–90% (Rühl, 1997). From this, in our assay the SLN exhibited a 20 times lower cytotoxicity than the polymeric nanoparticles. For a detailed discussion of the cytotoxicity studies we refer to (Weyhers, 1995a; Rühl, 1997; Maaßen *et al.*, 1993).

For the first assessment of *in vivo* toxicity SLN were injected into mice. Multiple high dosed bolus injections were administered into the tail vein every 2 days (3 times, 1.33 gram lipid per kilogram body weight). The lipid matrices injected were cetylpalmitate and Compritol. The injections were well tolerated without any signs of acute toxicity. By the end of the injection period, the animals were sacrificed, the organs weighted and histologically examined. Little change was found for the high dosed cetylpalmitate-SLN. A distinct increase in liver and spleen weight including infiltration of macrophages and the presence of fat was observed with the high dosed Compritol nanoparticles. However, the changes proved to be reversible (Weyhers, 1995a; Weyhers *et al.*, 1995b). This could be explained by the slower *in vivo* degradation of Compritol-SLN compared to cetylpalmitate-SLN (Rühl, 1997). The metabolizing capacity of the body was just not sufficient to cope with the administered high dose of lipid. It should be pointed out, that the injected dose would be equivalent to a bolus injection of 100 g pure lipid in man (75 kg body weight). Reducing the dose of Compritol SLN administered to the mice could avoid these side effects (Weyhers, 1995a).

To sum up, from the *in vitro* cytotoxicity and the *in vivo* toxicity data the SLN appeared to be a very well tolerated drug carrier system. They seemed to be even better tolerated than nanoparticles produced from accepted polymers.

SLN VERSUS OTHER COLLOIDAL DRUG CARRIERS

Principally a drug formulation should be as simple as possible. There is no need to use a more sophisticated drug carrier system if a simple system does the job. This means that there is no need for SLN if a drug can be formulated in a conventional oil-in-water emulsion (e.g. diazepam and etomidate, trade products: Diazepam®-Lipuro and Etomidate®-Lipuro). Emulsions proved to be sufficient to distinctly reduce the risk of thrombophlebitis. However, SLN appear as a very attractive carrier system if a prolonged release or a protection of the drug against chemical degradation is required. Incorporation of the drug into the solid lipid matrix might surely be a better protection than can be achieved in the oily coreinterface of emulsions or in liposomes. There is still easy access for e.g. water to hydrolyze a drug. As discussed above, prolonged release from emulsions does not appear to be feasible. However it should be kept in mind that also SLN exhibiting burst release are a very attractive carrier system (e.g. "Parenteral formulations").

Compared to polymeric nanoparticles, the SLN possess some genuine advantages. Apart from the lower cytotoxicity, due to the absence of solvents in the production process, and the relatively low costs for the excipients it is surely a major advantage that large scale production is possible by the simple process of high pressure homogenization. Such equipment already exists in pharmaceutical industry for the production of emulsions for parenteral nutrition and emulsions as drug carriers.

Compared to liposomes the SLN possess the advantage of better protection of drugs against chemical degradation. There is no or little access of water to the inner core of the lipid particles (prerequisite: lipids without water-solubilizing capacity are used). Depending on the nature of the drug, a higher pay load might be achieved. In addition, the SLN provide more possibilities to modify the drug release profile.

An important issue is the possibility to sterilize dispersions of colloidal drug carriers. Aqueous SLN dispersions can be autoclaved at 120 °C for 15 minutes (Schwarz et al., 1994). SLN stabilized with block copolymers such as poloxamers show some aggregation at this sterilization temperature. This is attributed to the reduced steric stabilization close to the CFT (critical flocculation temperature) of the polymeric stabilizers. Aggregation can be minimized or avoided by reducing the sterilization temperature. During autoclaving the SLN melt and recrystallize again during cooling. Alternatively aqueous SLN dispersions can be sterilized by γ-irradation. This might be necessary as an alternative method in case of heat-sensitive drugs or in case the melting and subsequent recrystallization during autoclaving changes the properties of the lipid matrix and subsequently the release profile of the drug.

POSSIBLE APPLICATIONS OF SLN

In general, SLN can be potentially applied in all drug formulations in which polymeric nanoparticles or colloidal drug carriers are useful. In the sections below potential applications are discussed.

SLN in Cosmetical Formulations

Cosmetic formulations appear especially attractive because the requirements by the regulatory authorities are not (or better: not yet) as tough as for pharmaceutical formulations. The range of possible excipients is much broader than for pharmaceuticals. A possible application is the use of SLN in skin care products. Similar to liposomes they can form a protective film, due to their small size a penetration into gaps between stratum corneum cells might be feasible. Basic studies are being presently undertaken. In addition they can act as carrier for active ingredients which prove to be chemically unstable in aqueous formulations such as creams or lotions.

Topical Pharmaceutical Preparations

The SLN might be used similarly to topical cosmetical products in dermatological pharmaceutical formulations. The SLN can act as a drug reservoir providing controlled drug release. Depending on the penetration of SLN into the skin they might also act as penetration enhancer to increase the drug concentration in the upper skin layer. Possible drugs are antimycotics and corticoids.

Ophthalmic Preparations

Nanoparticles were found to prolong the duration of drugs in the eye (Zimmer et al., 1994). Polymeric particles such as butylcyanoacrylate possess the disadvantage of the release of formaldehyde during their degradation. Gasco could show that drug incorporation into SLN was able to distinctly enhance drug duration times (γ-scintigraphy data, personal communication).

Oral Administration of SLN

Nanoparticles in general possess adhesive properties. This could be exploited to produce formulations with SLN being mucoadhesive in the mouth, e.g. buccal or sublingual. Application could be performed as aqueous dispersion or SLN incorporated in a gel. Due to their small size they might be less irritant than other mucoadhesive oral delivery systems (e.g. patches).

Peroral Formulations

Drugs chemically instable in the fluids of the gastrointestinaltract (GIT) can be incorporated into SLN to enhance their chemical stability, e.g. peptides. Adhesion of the nanoparticles to the walls of the GIT and release of the drug close to the intestinal wall could enhance the bioavailability of drugs (e.g. danazol) (Liversidge, 1996). In addition, application of a drug in form of nanoparticles can lead to a more reproducible bioavailability compared to conventional formulations. This was shown for drug nanoparticles of naproxen (Liversidge, 1996) compared to conventional formulations. Similar bioavailabilities were achieved when administering drug nanoparticles to fasted and to fed patients (Liversidge, 1996). A potential drug candidate for SLN is cyclosporin, a hydrophobic peptide with sufficient solubility in lipids. The erratic bioavailability might be reduced and in general the bioavailability increased.

Parenteral Formulations

Possible ways of administration are intracavital, intramuscular and intravenous injection. Intracavital and intramuscular administration are less critical against the presence of microparticles. A low content of microparticles is required for intravenous preparations to avoid capillary blockade. Targets for SLN formulations might be the reduction of side effects or — on long perspective — the targeting of drugs. A possible drug candidate for SLN is Paclitaxel. At present it is on the market in a formulation containing Cremophor® EL. The Cremophor is being held responsible for side reactions such as anaphylactic shock. Paclitaxel could be incorporated in SLN stabilized with well tolerated egg lecithin. Preliminary investigations show that the incorporation in SLN is possible.

In the case of Paclitaxel the SLN should preferentially show a burst release. A burst release imitates the injection of the commercial solutions, that means no change in pharmacokinetics of the drug is expected. This demonstrates nicely that even SLN with burst release are a very useful and attractive carrier.

A similar job could be done by a Paclitaxel-loaded o/w emulsion. Incorporation of the drug leads however to physical stability problems of the emulsion but not in SLN®.

PERSPECTIVES

Lipopearls® and SLN® are registered as trade marks for the cosmetic and the pharmaceutical marked, respectively. Cosmetic products are in preparation, the first clinical study with SLN is envisaged for, 1997. If SLN are a suitable carrier for cosmetics and pharmaceuticals will be answered by the market, that means the appearance of products.

The solid lipid nanoparticles represent an alternative colloidal carrier system to emulsions, liposomes and polymeric nanoparticles. The increasing number of research groups and pharmaceutical companies working with solid lipid particles is an indicator for their potential. Similary to liposomes the first product is expected to be launched on the cosmetic market. Possible products are skin care lotions containing SLN without any active ingredient. These SLN contain skin lipids or lipids with skin caring effects. Other cosmetic products will contain active ingredients previously unstable in the traditional formulations. In the pharmaceutical sector the first products might be dermatological products or peroral formulations, especially when bearing in mind the regulatory aspects. In contrast to delivery systems made from new polymers the SLN have the distinct advantage that they can be made from excipients of approved status, e.g. GRAS status (Food additives, 1994). At the end of the day the cosmetic and pharmaceutical market will decide about the success of a new delivery system for active ingredients. A delivery system is successful if it leads to products being launched on the markets, however, not only launched but also bringing high sale numbers and a fast cash return flow. The future will show if the delivery system SLN is able to do so.

REFERENCES

Benita, S., Friedmann, D., Weinstock, M. (1986) Pharmacological evaluation of an injectable prolonged release emulsion of physostigmine in rabbits. *Journal of Pharmacy and Pharmacology*, **38**, 653–658.

Domb, A.J. (1991) Liposheres for controlled delivery of substances. PCT WO 91/07171.

Food additives — GRAS substances (1994) *Food Drug Cosmetic Law Reports*, Chicago.

Freitas, C. (1994) Stabilization of solid lipid nanoparticles by spray drying. *European Journal of Biopharmaceutics*, **40** (Suppl.), 29.

Gasco, M.R. (1993) Solid lipid microspheres having a narrow size distribution and method for producing them. European Patent Application 91113152.2.

Kecht-Wyrsch, P. (1987) Hochdisperse Glycerid-Mikropartikel als perorales Arzneiträgersystem. *PhD thesis*, Eidgenössische Technische Hochschule Zürich.

Liversidge, G.G. (1996) Workshop Particulate Drug Delivery Systems. *23nd Intern. Symp. Control. Rel. Bioact. Mater*, Kyoto.

Maaßen, S., Schwarz, C., Mehnert, W., Lucks, J.S., Yunis-Specht, F., Müller, B.W., Müller, R.H. (1993) Comparison of cytotoxicity between polyester nanoparticles and solid lipid nanoparticles (SLN). *Proc. Intern. Symp. Control. Rel. Bioact. Mater*, **20**, 490–491.

Müller, R.H. and Lucks, J.S. (1996a) Arzneistoffträger aus festen Lipidteilchen, Feste Lipidnanosphären (SLN). European Patent No. 0605497.

Müller, R.H., zur Mühlen, Freitas, C., A., Mehnert, W. (1996b) Solid lipid nanoparticles for intravenous drug delivery. *Proc. 23rd Int. Symp. Control. Release Bioact. Mater*, Kyoto.

Rühl, D. (1997) Arzneistoffträgertestung an Zellkulturen. *PhD thesis*, Free University of Berlin.

Schuhmann, R. (1996) Präparate zur parenteralen Ernährung. In *Pharmazeutische Technologie: Moderne Arzneiformen*, edited by R.H. Müller, G.E. Hildebrand, pp. 127–136. Wissenschaftliche Verlagsgesellschaft Stuttgart.

Schwarz, C, Mehnert, W., Lucks, J.S., Müller, R.H. (1994) Solid Lipid Nanoparticles for controlled drug delivery. I: Production, characterization and sterilization. *Journal of Controlled Release*, **30**, 83–96.

Schwarz, C. (1995) Feste Lipid Nanopartikel: Herstellung, Charakterisierung, Arzneistoffinkorporation und -freisetzung, Sterilisation und Lyophilisation. *PhD thesis*, Free University of Berlin.

Speiser, P. (1990) Lipidnanopellets als Trägersystem für Arzneimittel zur peroralen Anwendung. European Patent EP 0167825.

Westesen, K., Siekmann, B. (1994) Solid lipid particles, particles of bioactive agents and methods for the manufacture and the use of thereof. PCT WO 94/20072.

Weyhers, H. (1995a) Feste Lipid Nanopartikel für die gewebsspezifische Arzneistoffapplikation (SLN) — Herstellung, und Charakterisierung oberflächenmodifizierter Formulierungen. *PhD thesis*, Free University of Berlin.

Weyhers, H., Ehlers, S., Mehnert, W., Hahn, H., Müller, R.H. (1995b) Solid lipid nanoparticles — determination of *in vivo* toxicity. *Proc. 1st World Meeting APGI/APV*, Budapest.

Zimmer, A.K., Maincent, P., Thouvenot, P., Kreuter, J. (1994) Hydrocortisone delivery to healthy and inflamed eyes using a micellar polysorbate 80 solution. *International Journal of Pharmaceutics*, **110**, 211–222.

zur Mühlen, A. (1996) Feste Lipid Nanopartikel mit prolongierter Wirkstoffliberation — Herstellung, Langzeitstabilität, Charakterisierung, Freisetzungsverhalten und -mechanismen. *PhD thesis*, Free University of Berlin.

10. THE DESIGN AND ENGINEERING OF OXYGEN-DELIVERING FLUOROCARBON EMULSIONS

MARIE PIERRE KRAFFT[1], JEAN G. RIESS[2,3] and JEFFRY G. WEERS[3]

[1]*Institut Charles Sadron, Strasbourg, France*
[2]*School of Medicine, University of California, San Diego, USA*
[3]*Alliance Pharmaceutical Corp., San Diego, USA*

NEED FOR AND REALITY OF A BLOOD SUBSTITUTE

Many concerns and questions were raised during the eighties about the safety of blood transfusions. They were initiated by the recognition that AIDS and hepatitis could be transmitted by blood. Additional problems, such as the transmission of other infectious agents, allergic reactions and immunosuppression effects, have further contributed to the realization that the administration of donor blood is not totally devoid of risk, and have led to further precautions in the collection, handling and distribution of blood. Even though our blood supply has never been as safe as today, this is not the perception of the public (Newman *et al.*, 1994), and there is a general desire to reduce the transfusion of allogeneic (i.e. homologous, or donor) blood as much as possible.

This situation intensified the interest in transfusion reduction strategies and, obviously, in the development of substitutes for blood and red blood cells. Blood substitutes could also relieve concerns that stem from a projected shortfall in blood supply to meet the needs of the increasingly larger elderly population (Vamvaskas and Taswell, 1994). The following few citations reflect this demand: "Regard elective transfusion with homologous blood as an outcome to be avoided" (The American College of Physicians, 1992); "An effective, safe and sterile oxygen carrier that is stable at room temperature or at refrigerated storage would provide a major advance in transfusion therapy" (H.G. Klein, from the National Institutes of Health, 1994); "A red cell substitute is both needed and feasible" (The US Navy Research Advisory Committee, 1992).

Considerable efforts are now being invested in research and development of such products both in public institutions and in private companies, the goal being to obtain a safe, universal, disease-free, shelf-stable, cost-effective and readily available injectable oxygen carrier. These efforts are illustrated by the abundant literature that is being published, numerous patents that are being filed, and by the frequency of the meetings that are being held on the subject.

Developing a substitute for blood turned out, however, to be a formidable challenge, and none of the products presently under development (whether hemoglobin- or fluorocarbon-based) can truly be considered as a substitute for blood. There are two main reasons for this: First, the only function provided by the present formulations is to carry oxygen and carbon dioxide *in vivo*; none provide the complex regulatory, metabolic, coagulation and host defense functions of natural blood. Second, the intravascular persistence of these preparations is very brief compared to that of red blood cells. Some of them can contribute very effectively to delivering oxygen to tissues, although temporarily, as for the duration of a surgical intervention; none is capable of replacing red blood cell transfusions in cases of chronic anemia. "Blood substitutes" is therefore a misnomer; injectable oxygen carriers or anti-hypoxic agents are more accurate descriptions for these products. Fluorocarbon emulsions are a unique kind of drug delivery system where the active — and vital — drug is actually oxygen.

The above limitations of the fluorocarbon-based oxygen delivery systems must imperatively be taken into account if one wants to identify realistic areas of application, and define conditions of use that optimize their therapeutic benefit. One such application is the reduction in the use of donor blood transfusion when the oxygen carrier is utilized in conjunction with acute normovolemic hemodilution (ANH) (Faithfull, 1994a; Zuck and Riess, 1994; Keipert, 1998; Keipert et al., 1996; Riess, 1998). This is one of the principal targeted indications of *Oxygent*™ (Alliance Pharmaceutical Corp., San Diego, CA, a fluorocarbon emulsion that has now successfully completed Phase II trials for this indication. The use of *Oxygent* is expected to be of benefit to patients by providing increased safety and reduction of donated blood transfusions during surgery, thereby increasing the effectiveness of and helping to promote blood-saving strategies. It should be called to mind in this respect that over 60% of the *ca* 11 million transfusions performed in the US each year are utilized in relation with surgery (Consensus Conference, 1988; Vamvaskas and Taswell, 1994; Wallace et al., 1995). An effective oxygen-carrier would obviously be invaluable in managing elective surgical procedures.

Other applications that appear to be within the reach of the present generation of injectable fluorocarbon-based oxygen carriers include priming of the cardiopulmonary bypass circuit during cardiac surgery (Holman et al., 1995); reduction of myocardial ischemia and stroke (Holman et al., 1994; Kloner and Hale, 1994; Ogilby, 1994); reduction of myocardial ischemia during percutaneous transluminal coronary angioplasty procedures (Kent et al., 1990; Forman et al., 1991; Kerins, 1994); reduction of microemboli associated with cardiopulmonary bypass (Menasché et al., 1992; Spiess et al., 1986); improved organ and tissue preservation (Brasile et al., 1996; Voiglio et al., 1996); sensitization of cancerous cells to radiation and chemotherapy (Evans et al., 1993; Rockwell, 1994; Teicher, 1995; Stern and Guichard, 1996); cell culture (Lowe, 1994b); use as contrast agents for diagnosis (Mattrey, 1994), and drug delivery (Riess, 1994c; Riess et al., 1996; Riess and Krafft, 1997). See also recent reviews by Riess (1992, 1998), Biro (1993), Faithfull (1994a), Lowe (1994), Marchbank (1995), Spiess (1995), Tremper and Wahr (1995), Riess and Weers (1996). Note that red blood cells cannot be used for many of the applications outlined above, thus illustrating another aspect in which fluorocarbon emulsions do not function simply as substitutes for blood.

This Chapter will focus primarily on the design and engineering of injectable submicronic fluorocarbon emulsions designed for *in vivo* oxygen transport. It will therefore briefly review the basic principles that are relevant to this objective, and discuss the selection of component fluorocarbons and emulsifiers, the formulation and preparation of the emulsions, and the properties of typical emulsions, with special emphasis on stability and biocompatibility. Finally, a short section will be devoted to other submicronic emulsion systems that contain a fluorocarbon phase.

Further information on the fluorocarbon approach to *in vivo* oxygen transport and on the status of the diverse applications of injectable fluorocarbon emulsions can be found in the proceedings of the International Symposia on Blood Substitutes, the most recent of which were held in San Diego in 1993 (Chang *et al.*, 1994; Riess, 1994a) and in Montreal in 1996 (Chang *et al.*, 1997), as well as in the papers cited in this review.

The preclinical and clinical safety and efficacy data will not be treated to any significant extent, as they are the subject of other review articles (Keipert, 1998; Riess and Keipert, 1998). Development of a pharmaceutical product involves many more facets and tasks than those treated in this Chapter. These are related to clinical evaluation, regulatory submission, quality assurance and control, process and method validation, and industrial operations such as scale up, engineering and preparation for manufacture.

HISTORICAL PERSPECTIVES

The Early Days

A therapeutically useful "artificial blood" has been on man's wishlist for over a century. A disclosure suggesting that hemoglobin extracted from red blood cells could be injected in the form of a solution was, for example, deposited at the French Academy of Sciences in 1886 (Deschiens, 1886), while in Boston one physician administered milk to his patients (Thomas, 1878) in the expectation that it would relieve their anemic condition. The first documented administration of a hemoglobin solution in humans appears to date back to Sellards and Minot (1916). By 1978 about fifteen other clinical trials had followed, which eventually led to the conclusion that simple solutions of native hemoglobin could not be utilized as such (Winslow, 1992). Numerous avenues were subsequently explored in view of restoring hemoglobin's oxygen-delivery capacity after it has been extracted from the red blood cells, of prolonging its intravascular persistence, of understanding and reducing its side-effects. Although all hurdles have not yet been surmounted, significant progress was achieved and at least seven modified hemoglobin-based products are now in diverse stages of clinical evaluation (Chang *et al.*, 1994; Winslow *et al.*, 1995; Chang, 1997, 1998).

The demonstration by Clark and Gollan (1966) that animals could safely breathe an oxygen-saturated liquid perfluorocarbon (PFC) initiated a totally different, non-biomimetic approach to *in vivo* oxygen delivery. PFC's are excellent solvents of gases, however, because they are virtually insoluble in water, they need to be formulated as emulsions prior to being injected into the circulation. This was achieved by Sloviter and Kamimoto (1967), who were the first to prepare such emulsions; when using them to perfuse isolated rat brains, significant prolongation of the organs' electrical activity was obtained. Geyer *et al.* one year later (1968), replaced close to 100% of the blood of rats by such an emulsion. By 1973 the "bloodless" rats survived the operation (Geyer *et al.*, 1973). Unfortunately, perfluorotributylamine, the PFC which was utilized, was retained in the organs of the reticuloendothelial system (RES) for several years. Had this been a feature common to all fluorocarbons, the PFC approach to injectable O_2-carriers would have been terminated.

Table 1 PFCs most extensively investigated for use as injectable oxygen carriers

Formula	Code (MW)	Preparation (purity)	Boiling pt (°C) vapor pressure (mm Hg 37°)	Solub O$_2$ CO$_2$ (vol%, 37°)	Organ half-life (days)
(perfluorodecalin structure)	FDC (462)	CoF$_3$ (~57%)	142 12.5	42 142	7
(perfluorotripropylamine structure)	FTPA (521)	electrochem (>95%)	131 18.	45 166	65
(FMIQ structure)	FMIQ (495)	electrochem (~95%)		42	11
(FMCP structure)	FMCP (596)	electrochem (~55%)	168 2	40	90
(FDN structure)	FDN (562)	CoF$_3$ (50–55%)		40	~14
(F-44E structure)	F-44E (464)	telomerization (>99%)	12.5	50 247	7
(PFOB structure)	PFOB perflubron (499)	telomerization (>95%)	143 11	50 210	4
(PFDCO structure)	PFDCO (471)	electrochem	155 6	43	7

The Fluosol Era

Fortunately, in 1972, Clark *et al.* (1973) in the US, and Okamoto *et al.* (1973) in Japan found that another PFC, perfluorodecalin (Table 1; actually a mixture of the *cis* and *trans* isomers), was excreted from the body in a matter of weeks, with an organ half-life of about 7 days only. This finding led to the conviction that a

PFC-based blood substitute was feasible, and to considerable investment by the Green Cross Corp. (Osaka, Japan) in the development of a commercial product. The first perfluorodecalin (FDC) emulsion investigated, Fluosol-DC, was too unstable, however, for medical use (Naito and Yokoyama, 1975). Addition of perfluorotripropylamine (FTPA) resulted in some improvement (at the cost, however, of longer organ retention), and the new emulsion, Fluosol-DA (Naito and Yokoyama, 1978, 1981; Yokoyama et al., 1982) later known as Fluosol®, went all the way through animal studies into human clinical trials.

These trials demonstrated that the emulsion delivered the expected amount of oxygen and that this oxygen could have a definite and immediate beneficial impact on the patient's condition; they also confirmed the short iv persistence that had been seen during the animal work. Thus, for example, when a dose of Fluosol amounting to 4 g of PFC/kg body weight was given prior to surgery to oxygen-breathing severely anemic patients, oxygen consumption was seen to increase by 22% and the partial pressure of oxygen in the mixed venous blood (PvO_2) by ca 60%. The fluorocarbon provided $24 \pm 7\%$ of the patients' oxygen consumption while mixed venous hemoglobin saturation reached $90 \pm 6\%$ (Tremper et al., 1982). It was concluded that the amount of oxygen provided by Fluosol was clinically important. The benefit was, however, only temporary since the half-life of the product in the circulation was only about 20 hours. In another study with highly anemic surgical patients it was found that Fluosol's PFC unloaded its oxygen highly effectively ($82 \pm 5\%$) and contributed at least as much to oxygen consumption as the patients' own red blood cells ($28 \pm 7\%$). The outcome for the patients, who refused blood transfusion on religious grounds, could, however, not be improved in view of the product's short intravascular residence (Gould et al., 1986). As a logical result Fluosol was rejected by the US Food and Drug Administration (FDA) when submitted in the early eighties as a treatment for anemia.

The conclusion from these clinical trials should not be that Fluosol was not an effective oxygen-delivery system: it was. The correct conclusion is that treatment of sustained anemia is not a valid indication for such a product.

Fluosol actually gained approval from the FDA a few years later (1989) for use during high-risk percutaneous transluminal coronary angioplasty (PTCA). In this procedure a catheter fitted with a balloon is inserted into a vessel that is partially obstructed by an atheroma plaque; the balloon is then inflated so as to crush the plaque; during this inflation period the myocardium is, however, deprived of oxygen. Oxygenated Fluosol, when administered through a central lumen of the catheter, was shown to significantly reduce tissue ischemia (Kent et al., 1990; Forman et al., 1991; Kerins, 1994). Approval of Fluosol by the FDA means that both efficacy and safety had been demonstrated for this application.

Fluosol, however, did not meet with commercial success. This time the main reason for its failure was not the selection of an inappropriate indication or lack of efficacy, but lack of user-friendliness: the emulsion was so unstable that it had to be shipped and stored in the frozen state. Prior to injection, Fluosol then had to be thawed and reconstituted by admixing two annex solutions; after which it had to be utilized within eight hours or discarded. In addition to going through this cumbersome process, a test-dose had to be given in order to detect those patients who were sensitive to Pluronic® F-68, one of the components of the emulsion that can provoke complement activation. Little wonder that surgeons were not inclined to use this product.

Fluosol was nevertheless an important milestone in the history of fluorocarbon-based O_2-carriers. In spite of Fluosol's imperfections, studies with this product established that considerable amounts of PFC could be administered intravenously without major problems and that PFCs did effectively load and deliver oxygen. It greatly increased our understanding of the *in vivo* behavior and pharmacology of fluorocarbons and fluorocarbon emulsions. It allowed the exploration of a range of new potential applications. Last but not least, the very analysis of its shortcomings (see, for example, Ohyanagi *et al.*, 1990; Riess, 1987, 1991) has inspired and oriented subsequent research, which led to significantly improved products. A range of so-called "second-generation" fluorocarbons were synthesized and screened, and several experimental emulsions were formulated in view of resolving Fluosol's shortcomings; it was crucial, in particular, to find fluorocarbons that were both rapidly excreted and amenable to forming stable emulsions. It is regrettable, though, that certain misinterpretations of early clinical results led to misrepresenting and grossly underrating the potential of fluorocarbon emulsions as oxygen carriers, thus delaying their development.

Meanwhile, two other emulsions rather similar to Fluosol were developed in the former Soviet Union and in China. The first one, Perftoran (Perftoran Co, Pushchino, Russia), previously known as Ftorosan (Beloyartsev *et al.*, 1983; Ivanitsky and Vorobyev, 1993; Vorobyev and Ivanitski, 1994; Obraztsov, 1994) has essentially the same limitations as Fluosol. It nevertheless received approval from the Russian health authorities in 1996 for general use as an antihypoxic agent (Vorobyev, 1996, personal communication). The Chinese product, Emulsion n° II (Institute for Organic Chemistry, Shanghai, China), which appears to be even closer to Fluosol in its design, has been reported in the treatment of war casualties (Chen and Yang, 1989).

Second Generation Products

The post-Fluosol synthesis and evaluation of new fluorocarbons resulted in further improvement of our basic knowledge of fluorocarbon emulsions, but the next significant breakthrough occurred serendipiditiously. Because they wanted to explore the possibility of using PFCs as contrast agents Long, Mattrey and coworkers became interested in brominated PFCs, the bromine atom providing the desired opacity to X-rays (Long *et al.*, 1972; Long *et al.*, 1988; Mattrey, 1994). It turned out that one such compound, perfluorooctyl bromide (PFOB, perflubron) had simultaneously the benefit of a short organ-dwelling time and the capacity to be formulated into stable emulsions. This compound was subsequently selected for developing *Oxygent*™, the ready-for-use injectable oxygen carrier that is now being investigated for alleviating donor blood transfusion during surgery when used in conjunction with ANH (Faithfull, 1994a; Keipert, 1998; Keipert *et al.*, 1996; Zuck and Riess, 1994, Riess and Keipert, 1998). Finally, it was by defining proper indications and strategies of use and by bringing together the appropriate resources and skills, including those that concern the regulatory, manufacturing, marketing and managerial aspects of drug development, that an effective product was made possible.

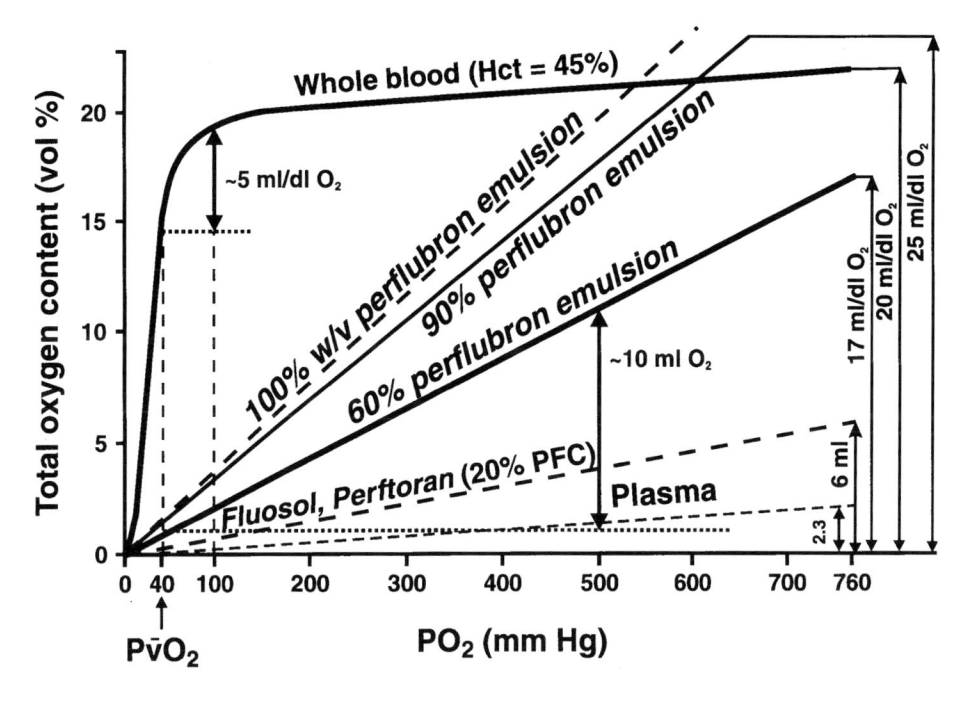

Figure 1 Oxygen content of variously concentrated perfluorocarbon emulsions as compared to whole blood and plasma, as a function of oxygen partial pressure.

FUNDAMENTALS OF FLUOROCARBON-BASED OXYGEN TRANSPORT AND DELIVERY

The basic principles that underlie the use of fluorocarbons and fluorocarbon emulsions as oxygen carriers will be summarized briefly in this Section. Those aspects that need to be taken into account when developing an effective product will be discussed further in later Sections.

The "Physiology" of Fluorocarbon Emulsions

The properties of fluorocarbons that are fundamental for their use as injectable oxygen carriers are their oxygen solubility and chemical and biological inertness. Unlike hemoglobin, PFCs do not bind oxygen chemically, but simply dissolve it physically. The interactions between the PFCs and O_2 molecules are of the van der Waals type and are very weak. As a consequence, oxygen dissolution essentially follows Henry's law: it increases linearly as a function of partial pressure or concentration (Figure 1). The oxygen dissolving capacity of an emulsion depends primarily on its concentration in fluorocarbon and to a lesser extent on the molecular structure of the fluorocarbon, as will be shown later. The amount of oxygen dissolved can be increased five-fold by simply using 100% pure oxygen rather than air. In order to fully exploit this advantage it is therefore beneficial to have patients breathe pure or close to pure oxygen. It should be noted that under these conditions the amount of oxygen dissolved in the plasma compartment of blood, which also follows

Henry's law, is no longer negligible, while the amount of oxygen taken up by hemoglobin is barely improved. There is no saturation phenomenon with fluorocarbons, and oxygen solubility continues to augment when hyperbaric conditions are applied.

Infusing a PFC emulsion can be considered, to a large extent, as equivalent to increasing the oxygen solubility of the plasma compartment of blood. In addition, the very numerous and small PFC droplets are believed to fill in the plasma gaps that develop between red cells in the microcirculation when hemodilution is practised, and to facilitate the diffusion of oxygen between the erythrocytes and tissues (Faithfull, 1992, 1994b; Zaritskii et al., 1993; Ivanitsky and Vorobyev, 1996). Furthermore, and unlike hemoglobin, infusion of fluorocarbon emulsions allows the increase in cardiac output and consequent improvement of oxygen delivery to tissues that normally follows hemodilution. The effectiveness of PFC emulsions in delivering oxygen is thus expected to be greatest in the capillary beds and when red blood cells become scarce, as when the patient is hemodiluted.

Because pO_2 values become and remain high when fluorocarbons are present, an immediate and persistently large oxygen gradient is created between blood and tissues which provides a strong driving force for diffusion of oxygen to the tissues (Faithfull, 1992). Because the PFC-oxygen interactions are weak, oxygen is much more easily released to tissues from fluorocarbons than from hemoglobin. The extraction rates and ratio are consequently much higher with PFCs than with hemoglobin. When both carriers are present simultaneously, fluorocarbons release their oxygen first, while the hemoglobin-bound oxygen remains as a safety reserve.

As noted, fluorocarbons are formulated into emulsions when intravascular administration is intended. The emulsion droplets need to be small, with diameters typically in the 0.1–0.2 μm range, i.e. about 30 to 70 times smaller than for red blood cells. These droplets, however, do not leak out of the vasculature as acellular hemoglobin solutions do. This is of importance since free hemoglobin has been shown to bind and sequester nitric oxide, an important biological mediator, thus causing the vasoconstriction phenomenon usually observed when solutions of hemoglobin-derived oxygen carriers are infused to patients (Chang et al., 1994; Winslow, 1994, Winslow et al., 1995; Hess, 1996). Because of their biochemical inertness, PFCs are also not subject to oxidation, nor do they participate in free-radical reactions, bind carbon monoxide, or show any of the reactivity-related side-effects associated with hemoglobin-based blood substitutes. PFCs are not metabolized, hence do not present any metabolite-derived toxicities. Altogether, the pharmacology and side-effect profile of fluorocarbon emulsions are comparatively much simpler and better understood (Flaim, 1994) than those of hemoglobin solutions.

The fluorocarbon approach to intravascular oxygen delivery and the synthetic nature of the carrier solve, by essence, some otherwise most arduous problems, namely those concerning supply, safety and cost-effectiveness. Another advantage is that production and sterilization of emulsions for parenteral use is well established in the pharmaceutical industry.

The contribution of even small doses of such emulsions to oxygen consumption can be highly significant because of the possibility of increasing oxygen dissolution in PFCs by simply increasing the oxygen fraction in the atmosphere, the much higher extraction ratio (up to 90% compared to ca 20% for hemoglobin), and the significant increase in cardiac output that is observed with hemodiluted patients is preserved when fluorocarbon emulsions are administered.

Because emulsions are particulate matter they are cleared from the circulation at a rate that depends strongly on the size of the emulsion droplets: the larger they are, the faster they are cleared (Okamoto et al., 1973; Yokoyama et al., 1975, 1982; Klein et al., 1994). Clearance also depends on the dose and, to some extent, on the nature of the surfactant system utilized, which constitutes the outer, "visible" coating of the droplets.

An Optimized Target Application: Surgical Hemodilution

Both the specific advantages of fluorocarbon-based oxygen carriers and their limitations must be considered when defining a strategy of use that optimizes benefit for the patient. Clinical regulatory approaches, market size, supply of goods, manufacturing issues, cost of production, distribution strategies, reimbursement policies, also need to be taken into account when developing such a product.

As noted, one advantage of fluorocarbon emulsions lies in the ability of small doses of the drug to immediately and very effectively deliver oxygen to patients with low hemoglobin levels. Their principal limitation is their short persistence in the circulation. While this prevents their use for treating chronic anemia, it does not constitute a limitation when temporary use, as for the duration of a surgical operation, or as a "bridge" to transfusion to stabilize a patient in emergency situations is considered.

Based on these premises a novel strategy for reducing the need for donor blood transfusions has been defined that involves the use of a fluorocarbon emulsion in conjunction with acute normovolemic hemodilution (ANH) (Faithfull, 1994a; Zuck and Riess, 1994; Keipert, 1998; Keipert et al., 1996). A portion of the patient's blood, usually 2-4 units, is collected prior to surgery, set aside, and replaced by a plasma expander to maintain constant circulatory volume. By operating at lower hematocrit, fewer red blood cells are lost during bleeding. An oxygen carrier is used during the surgery to maintain tissue oxygenation in the hemodiluted patient. The stored blood can then be used when needed, during or after the operation, thus reducing the need for donor blood transfusion. This procedure is expected to increase safety, even at lower hemoglobin levels, allowing more profound hemodilution, and eventually to result in further reduction of exposure to allogeneic blood transfusion.

Fluorocarbon emulsions present some definite advantages over hemoglobin solutions for this application, the most important of which being high oxygen consumption *vs* transport ratio, absence of vasoconstrictive effect, and large-scale, cost-effective production capabilities.

Efficacy of Fluorocarbon Emulsions in Delivering Oxygen

The ability of fluorocarbons to carry and deliver the expected amount of oxygen has been demonstrated with the first generation emulsions. Numerous data from animal hemodilution or shock models indicated that *Fluosol* could effectively increase oxygen consumption in animals having an oxygen insufficiency, and significantly improve survival (see, for example, Okada et al., 1975; Ohyanagi and Mitsuno, 1975; Makowski, 1978; Elliot et al., 1989). Clinical trials established that Fluosol made a meaningful contribution to oxygen consumption in severely anemic patients (Tremper et al., 1982; Gould et al., 1986; Mitsuno et al., 1982a; Spence et al., 1994).

Efficacy of Fluosol in reducing ischemia of the myocardium when used in conjunction with PTCA was demonstrated (Kent et al., 1990; Forman et al., 1991), leading to its approval by the FDA.

A computer model has been developed that allows prediction of the mixed venous oxygen tension, PvO$_2$ (an indicator of tissue oxygenation), and other physiological responses to both ANH and surgical blood loss when an oxygen carrier is administered (Faithfull et al., 1994). It shows, for example, that a single dose of 1.35 g/kg body weight of fluorocarbon can maintain global tissue oxygenation (i.e. maintain PvO$_2$ at or above predosing levels) while hemoglobin levels are allowed to fall from 8 to 4 g/dL, which corresponds to the loss of approximately three liters of blood.

The capacity of *Oxygent* to increase oxygen consumption has been thoroughly investigated in a number of models, including a canine model that mimics normovolemic hemodilution and surgical bleeding (Keipert et al., 1994a; Cernaianu et al., 1994; Keipert et al., 1996; see also Flaim, 1997). Cardiac output was seen to rise as expected in response to hemodilution. The observed increase of PvO$_2$ was in agreement with the increase predicted by computer simulation. When 2.7 g PFC/kg was administered to oxygen-breathing dogs the contribution of the PFC to total oxygen delivery was only 8–10%, but, because of high extraction, accounted for 25–30% of the total oxygen consumption. This allowed oxygen consumption to be maintained while hemoglobin levels were decreasing to values as low as 2.0 g/dL. The treated dogs were able to withstand loss of almost 70 mL of blood per kg (about two thirds of their blood), compared to 10 mL/kg in controls, before PvO$_2$ fell below the initial baseline (Keipert et al., 1994, 1996; Cernaianu et al., 1994). Tissue pO$_2$ of skeletal muscle, gut and brain were seen to increase in response to administration of the emulsion (Keipert and Conlan, 1996). Preservation of normal PvO$_2$ was also seen in hemorrhaged dogs receiving *Oxyfluor*, another recently developed PFC emulsion (Hemagen-PFC, St Louis, Mo) (Kaufman, 1994, 1995).

Further recent experimental work that demonstrates the significant contribution to tissue oxygenation provided by small doses of PFCs include efficacy in experimental cardiopulmonary bypass (Holman et al., 1995), which led to commencement of human clinical trials for this application; increase in maximal O$_2$ consumption by a working skeletal muscle in the presence of PFC (Hogan et al., 1992); sustainment of cardiac tissue oxygenation for a 20-30 min period following arrest of coronary perfusion of isolated rat hearts (Zweier et al., 1994); improved myocardial O$_2$ delivery and aerobic metabolism during cold cardioplegic arrest of isolated rabbit heart when the perfusate was enriched by a PFC emulsion (del Balzo et al., 1995); effective cardiac muscle function in a canine model of low-flow coronary ischemia (Ogilby et al., 1992); preservation of brain stem auditory evoked potential following brain stem ischemia in dogs (Guo et al., 1995); significantly increased retinal oxygen tensions in mechanically ventilated anesthetized cats (Braun et al., 1990); enhanced oxygen delivery in capillary tube oxygenators (Vaslef and Goldstick, 1994); significant improvement of systolic function and reduction of myocardial edema and acidosis when standard blood cardioplegia was supplemented with PFC in dogs that underwent experimental myocardial ischemia (Waschke et al., 1994); and additional data showing better tissue oxygenation in hemodiluted dogs receiving a PFC emulsion compared to dogs receiving blood (Habler et al., 1998).

Human trials with Oxygent have confirmed calculations and preclinical animal data. In a pilot Phase II study of *Oxygent*, seven adult patients received a low 0.9 g PFC/kg dose after acute normovolemic hemodilution (Wahr *et al.*, 1996). A significant increase in mixed venous oxygen tension was achieved. As hemoglobin levels decreased due to surgical blood loss, the PvO$_2$ values remained at or above predosing levels, demonstrating that even very small doses of emulsion can translate into measurable improvement of PvO$_2$ during intraoperative ANH.

More recently, multicenter Phase II studies in the US and in Europe involving a large cohort of patients undergoing surgery with ANH showed correction of physiological indicators for transfusion at a 1.8 g/kg dose of *Oxygent*, and substantial delays before transfusion of the stored autologous blood had to be given, thereby reducing the need for donor blood transfusion (Keipert, 1998; Riess and Keipert, 1998). Phase III trials with this product are planned to begin in 1998 for the ANH application.

THE COMPONENTS: SELECTING THE FLUOROCARBON

History has told us that proper selection of the carrier fluorocarbon is vital for designing a beneficial oxygen carrier. Since this fluorocarbon must be administered in the form of an emulsion, an emulsifier needs to be involved; it plays a key role in determining the product's physicochemical and biological characteristics. Selection of the surfactant, and adequate formulation of the emulsion, are therefore also crucial. A few ancillary components, such as salts and antioxidants, are also necessary, but it is noteworthy that product formulations have been becoming more simplified. Finally, all the components, and the formulation, and the characteristics of the emulsion have to comply with severe constraints in order for the product to be therapeutically effective, well tolerated by the patient, approved by the FDA, accepted by the physicians, and commercially successful.

Fluorocarbons for intravascular use need to be pure and well-defined; they should be devoid of toxicity; they must not be degraded during processing and storage and in the conditions of use; they should not be retained in the organism for too long a period of time; they must be amenable to forming stable emulsions that are ready for use and easy to administer; they should have high gas-solubilities; and last but not least, they must be manufacturable on a large scale in a reproducible and cost-effective manner.

General Characteristics of Fluorocarbons

Perfluorocarbons (PFCs), or fluorocarbons, or perfluorochemicals (these denominations are used more or less indistinctively) are a class of chemicals essentially composed of carbon and fluorine instead of carbon and hydrogen as hydrocarbons are. Each organic compound can, in principle, have its perfluorinated analogue (Figure 2).

In practice, the number of commercially available perfluorochemicals is limited. They consist primarily of perfluoroalkanes, halides, ethers, amines and acids. Mixed fluorocarbon-hydrocarbon compounds are also available. Numerous compounds exist that have one fluorocarbon chain grafted onto an otherwise "normal" organic

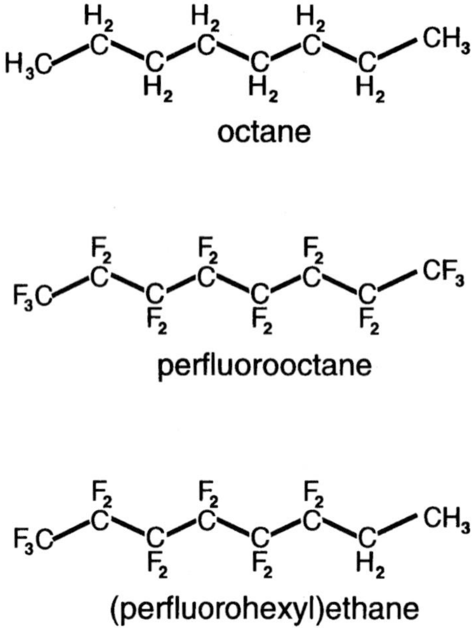

octane

perfluorooctane

(perfluorohexyl)ethane

Figure 2 Molecular structures of octane, perfluorooctane and (perfluorohexyl)ethane. Perfluorooctane, which is lipophobic (as well as hydrophobic), does not mix with octane. (Perfluorohexyl)hexane, which is amphiphilic, is miscible with the two former compounds.

molecule; these compounds often display strong amphiphilic character (Greiner et al., 1993; Riess et al., 1996; Riess and Krafft, 1998).

Highly fluorinated materials have multiple uses in the chemical, electronic, nuclear, magnetic media and aerospace industries (Banks et al., 1970, 1994). These applications take advantage of their outstanding thermal and chemical resistance, non-adherence and antifriction properties, repellence to both water and oil, unique dielectric, rheological and optical characteristics, and excellent gas-dissolving properties.

As noted, the two essential features that are the foundation of the principal applications of fluorocarbons in medicine, intravascular oxygen delivery and liquid ventilation (Faithfull, 1994a; Keipert et al., 1996; Leach et al., 1996; Riess and Le Blanc, 1978, 1988; Riess, 1994a; Weers, 1993; Zuck and Riess, 1994), are their unique gas-dissolving capacities and their exceptional chemical and biological inertness. The first is a consequence of the weakness of the *inter*molecular forces that prevail in liquid fluorocarbons, which facilitate the formation of "holes" that can accomodate gas molecules within the liquid. The second, on the contrary, reflects the strength of the *intra*molecular chemical bonds. The C-F bond is the strongest single bond (~485 kJ mol^{-1}, compared to ~425 kJ mol^{-1} for a standard C-H bond) encountered with carbon in an organic molecule (Banks and Tatlow, 1986), and its strength is further increased when several fluorine atoms are present on the same carbon atom; it was reported to reach 531 kJ mol^{-1} in CF_3 groups as in CF_3CF_3 (Smart, 1983). The C-C backbone itself is strengthened by fluorine substitution; the C-C bonds are, for example, stronger by 34 kJ mol^{-1} in polytetrafluoroethylene (Teflon®) than in polyethylene (Banks, 1970).

The larger size of fluorine atoms (with an estimated van der Waals radius of 147 pm) compared to hydrogen (120 pm) (Bondi, 1964) and their high electron density result in a compact electron shield which provides effective protection of the molecule's backbone. This dense electron coating also exercises some sort of a repellent "scotchguard"-type effect against most reagents (Riess, 1994b). The bonds of perfluoroalkylated moieties to oxygen, nitrogen, chlorine or bromine are also reinforced compared to hydrocarbon analogues and the potentially functional sites inactivated. When chlorine or bromine atoms are present, it is likely that the electronegativity of the fluorocarbon chain counterbalances that of the heavier halogen, which results in reduced bond polarity, polarizability and reactivity. Fluorocarbons are metabolically inert. There is no report either of enzymatic cleavage of a fluorocarbon.

Synthesis

For a long time the question of the purity of the fluorocarbon material investigated in biomedical applications was an important issue. In the early days the material utilized often consisted of complex, ill-defined mixtures with poor batch-to-batch reproducibility. Still in, 1982 one could read the following in the abstracts of an American Chemical Society's Symposium on Organofluorine Compounds in Medicine and Biology (1982): "All were mixtures ... composed of a primary PFC and related isomers and perfluorinated products that co-distill." "All contained partially fluorinated (toxic) compounds which were removed by exhaustive treatment (5 days to 3 weeks) with $KOH/HNEt_2$." "Not a single chemical compound." "They are multiple component mixtures." "Analysis and purity is still a complex issue." "About 10 peaks in vapor phase chromatography (about perfluorotrimethylbicyclononane)." "We still have to learn how to make them ..." No wonder that certain of the well over one hundred, often crude candidate fluorocarbons investigated were found to be toxic and that some of the physicochemical data reported at that time are subject to caution.

Fortunately this situation has changed. The number of fluorocarbons of interest has boiled down to a few, the manufacture of which is generally under good control. Although they are seldom fully disclosed, the procedures utilized for preparing the compounds shown in Table 1 fall into two categories depending on whether the fluorocarbon is produced by substituting fluorine atoms for hydrogen atoms in the parent hydrocarbon analog of the desired compound, or whether it is made up by combining smaller, already-fluorinated building blocks. Electrochemical fluorination, fluorination by high-valency metal fluorides such as cobalt trifluoride, and direct fluorination by elemental fluorine belong to the first category, while telomerization of tetrafluoroethylene or tetrafluoroethylene oxide belong to the second (Figure 3). The preparation of cyclic, polycyclic and branched compounds, of amines and of α,ω-disubstituted compounds relies primarily on the substitution route, while the telomerization approach is particularly well suited for most linear fluorocarbons. All these processes are now amenable to large-scale production.

The telomerization route readily provides well-defined pure fluorocarbons. The substitution processes are more difficult to control, and the results, in terms of product purity and reliability, is highly dependent on individual molecular structures (Riess and Le Blanc, 1988). Replacing one hydrogen by a fluorine atom in a

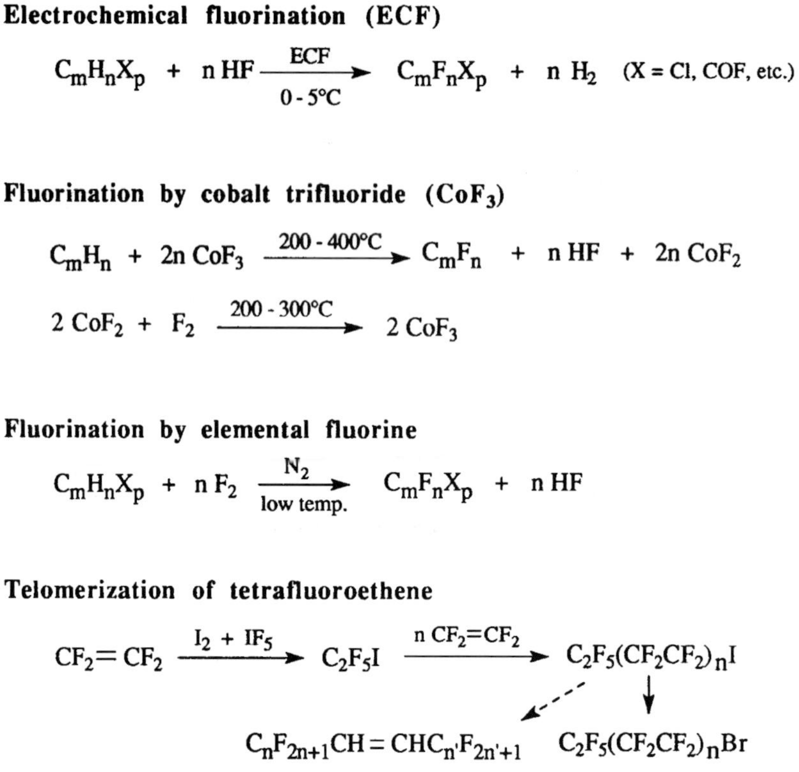

Electrochemical fluorination (ECF)

$$C_mH_nX_p + nHF \xrightarrow[0-5°C]{ECF} C_mF_nX_p + nH_2 \quad (X = Cl, COF, etc.)$$

Fluorination by cobalt trifluoride (CoF$_3$)

$$C_mH_n + 2n\,CoF_3 \xrightarrow{200-400°C} C_mF_n + nHF + 2n\,CoF_2$$

$$2\,CoF_2 + F_2 \xrightarrow{200-300°C} 2\,CoF_3$$

Fluorination by elemental fluorine

$$C_mH_nX_p + nF_2 \xrightarrow[low\ temp.]{N_2} C_mF_nX_p + nHF$$

Telomerization of tetrafluoroethene

$$CF_2{=}CF_2 \xrightarrow{I_2 + IF_5} C_2F_5I \xrightarrow{n\,CF_2{=}CF_2} C_2F_5(CF_2CF_2)_nI$$

$$C_nF_{2n+1}CH{=}CHC_{n'}F_{2n'+1} \quad C_2F_5(CF_2CF_2)_nBr$$

Figure 3 Principal routes for the synthesis of fluorocarbons.

molecule releases about 60 kJ mol^{-1} of energy; when 20 hydrogen atoms are to be replaced, this amounts to about 1200 kJ mol^{-1}. This is an enormous amount of energy which, if the reaction is not properly controlled, easily leads to bond-breaking, elimination of hydrogen fluoride, isomerization, and other structural rearrangements which, in turn, may impose laborious purification/detoxification efforts. More details on the preparation of fluorocarbons and relevant issues can be found in Riess and Le Blanc (1988). The possibility of manufacturing well-defined, very pure fluorocarbons on a large scale in a cost-effective way is a definite advantage of fluorocarbon-based oxygen carriers over hemoglobin-derived products.

Gas Solubilities

The gas-dissolving capacity of fluorocarbons stems essentially from the weakness of the intermolecular cohesion forces in the liquid. There does not appear to be any chemical bonding, coordination or charge-transfer complexes between fluorocarbons and the dissolved gas molecules. The enthalpies and entropies of solution are usually small (Patrick, 1982). The behavior of PFCs appears typical of non-polar, non-associated liquids whose gas-dissolving capacities are essentially determined by the shape of the molecule (Chandler, 1978). Unlike the case of hemoglobin, oxygen loading and unloading by PFCs is not hindered by a decrease in temperature;

oxygen solubility in PFCs actually increases as temperature decreases. For the purpose of interpreting and predicting solubility data a formal dissolution process is generally postulated which consists first in opening a cavity in the solvent large enough to fit the gas, then introducing this solute into the cavity. Two papers suggest, however, on the basis of deviation from Henry's law and lesser diffusivity of oxygen in emulsions at partial pressures lower than *ca* 300 mm Hg, that there exists some interaction between perfluorotributylamine or perfluorobutyltetrahydrofurane (FC-80) and oxygen (Navari *et al.*, 1977; Zander, 1974).

A xenon radioisotope was utilized as a prototype solute to investigate the solubility of a nonpolar gas in perfluoroalkanes and other solvents, and the results were analyzed in terms of thermodynamics, statistical mechanics and solute-solvent interactions (Kennan and Pollack, 1988, Pollack *et al.*, 1989). The chemical potential, enthalpy and entropy associated with the dissolution process were calculated. The excess chemical potential, i.e. work required to insert the solute molecules into the solvent, was found to be much lower (less negative) for fluorocarbons than for hydrocarbons (*ca* −20 *vs* −40 kJ mol^{-1} at 20°C). Likewise the Gibbs free energy for opening a cavity in fluorocarbons is significantly lower than in hydrocarbons, reflecting again the lesser cohesion of the former liquid. The entropy term, on the other hand, was shown to be remarkably independent of solvent. The solubility of xenon and hydrogen in water, blood plasma, perfluorotributylamine (FTBA) and a 20% w/v FTBA emulsion, Oxypherol® (Green Cross Corp., Osaka, Japan), were also measured. Solubilities were about 9% less in plasma than in water, probably as a result of a salting-out effect due to sodium ions in plasma. The solubilities measured for Xe in Oxypherol/plasma mixtures were in good agreement with those calculated by assuming that the gas dissolves independently in each two liquid phases of the mixture (Pollack *et al.*, 1992).

The dissolution of O_2 in various fluorocarbons has been thoroughly investigated using the perturbation induced in the nuclear relaxation of the ^{13}C nuclei of the PFC molecule by the paramagnetic oxygen molecule in solution (Hamza *et al.*, 1981). The results, including the decrease in solubility from aliphatic to cyclic to aromatic structures, were also rationalized on the basis of ease of formation of cavities within the liquid rather than on the occurrence of any specific interaction. The compressibilities of a range of PFCs have been measured and their internal pressures calculated (Serratrice *et al.*, 1982). The former are much higher and the latter lower than those of their hydrocarbon analogs, reflecting again lower intermolecular interactions. Good correlation was found between the isothermal compressibility factor and the solubility of O_2, N_2, He and Ar (but not CO_2) further supporting the view that solubility of gases in liquid PFCs is principally related to the ease of formation of cavities that can accomodate them.

The solubilities of O_2, CO_2 and N_2 in a few typical fluorocarbons and, for comparison, in some other chemicals are collected in Table 2. Further data can be found in a paper by Riess and Le Blanc (1982). Solubility values published by different groups can present serious discrepancies whose origins can arise from differences in experimental methods, lack of standardisation of procedures and uncertainties about the exact constitution of the PFC sample. The methods most frequently utilized are manometric (Gjaldbaek, 1952) or volumetric (Zander, 1974), chromatographic (Navari *et al.*, 1977; Wesseler *et al.*, 1977) or spectroscopic (NMR in the case of O_2) (Hamza *et al.*, 1981).

Table 2 Gas solubilities at 25°C (vol.%) of various perfluorocarbons and related compounds (see also Table 1)

	O_2	CO_2	N_2	CO	H_2
H_2O	3.1	82.8	1.59	2.33	1.91
CCl_4	27.8	243.7	14.9	20.3	7.73
n-C_7H_{16}	15.2 16.7	–	–	26.3	10.4
n-C_7F_{16}	54.8	207.0	38.6	38.6	14.1
n-C_8H_{18}	28.8 28.6	–	18.0	–	9.4
n-$C_{10}F_{18}$	52.1	–	–	–	–
⬡H	20.6 22.5	245.5	11.3	16.9	6.5
⬡F	48.8 46.8	426	34.8	41.1	–
$C_8H_{17}Br$	18.4	–	–	–	–
$C_8F_{17}C_2H_5$	38.9	–	–	–	–
$C_8F_{17}Br$	52.7	–	–	–	–

For the compounds pertinent to intravascular use the oxygen solubilities range from 40 to 50 volume % and those for carbon dioxide from 140 to 240 vol.% (Ricss and Le Blanc, 1982; 1988). They are larger than in water by a factor of 20 or more if expressed in vol.%, or of 200 if expressed in molar fraction, but differ only by about a factor of 2 from those in hydrocarbon analogues. It should be clear that it is water, among liquids, which has an exceptionally low solubility for gases. Within a homologous series, oxygen solubilities increase with decreasing molecular weight and molecular volume, as exemplified by a series of bis(perfluoroalkyl)ethenes (Figure 4) (Riess and Le Blanc, 1988).

For a given molecular weight, differences in structure can translate into differences in oxygen solubilities that can reach 20–25% (Figure 4). Such differences should definitely not be neglected when it comes to selecting a fluorocarbon for iv oxygen delivery. Figure 4 shows that, for a given molecular weight, linear fluorocarbons, including those which have a double bond, an oxygen atom or a terminal bromine atom, have a clear advantage over cyclic or polycyclic ones. The presence of a terminal hydrocarbon fragment results in increased molecular volume, hence reduced gas solubility. Lesser oxygen solubility has also been found for α,ω-dichlorooctane (Kaufman, 1995). The dissolving capacity for various gases decreases in the order: $CO_2 \gg O_2 > CO > N_2 > H_2 >$ He, apparently following the decrease in molecular volume of the solute.

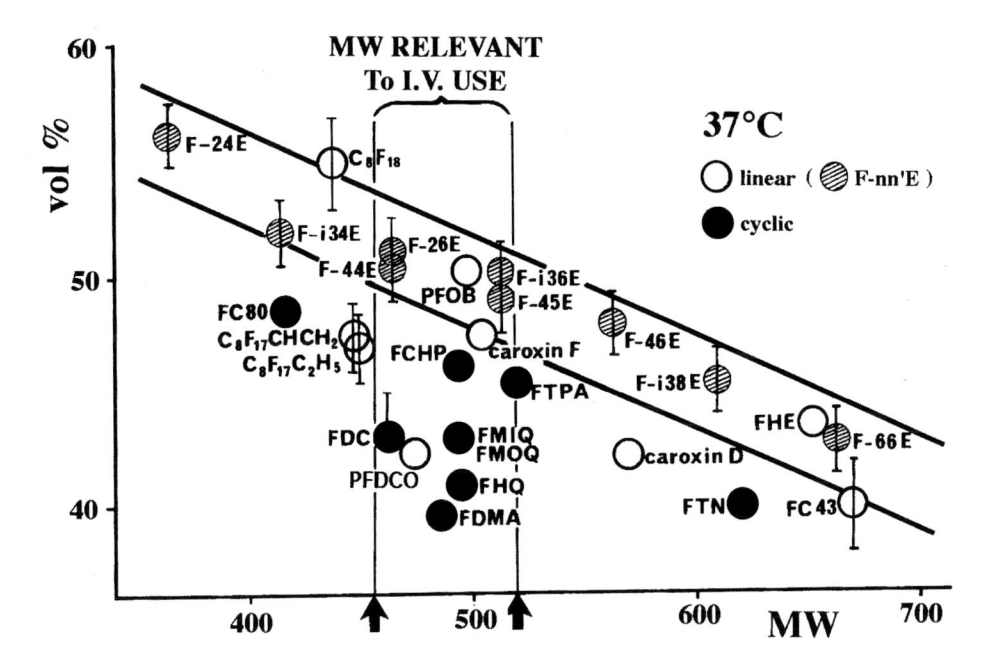

Figure 4 Solubility (vol.%) at 37°C of O_2 in various fluorocarbons as a function of molecular weight. The homologous series of bis(perfluoroalkyl)ethenes (striped dots) illustrates the decrease in O_2-solubility as molecular weight increases. The window of molecular weight acceptable for iv use is outlined. From Riess and Le Blanc (1988), with permission.

Prediction of the dissolving capacities of PFCs are still being made on the basis of Hildebrand's early work and on his solubility parameter $\delta = (\Delta E_v/V_m)^{1/2}$, where ΔE_v is the energy of vaporization and V_m the molar volume of the fluid (Hildebrand and Scott, 1950). In order to be mutually soluble, two fluids must have similar δ values. Those of PFCs are close to 6 hildebrands, as compared to 5.7 for oxygen, 7 to 9 for hydrocarbons, and 23.4 for water.

Semi-empirical approaches to gas solubilities were derived from the scaled particle theory, and express the free energy of solution as the sum of the free energy for formation of cavities in the solvent to host the solute molecules, and of the free energy of interaction between solute and solvent molecules (Pierotti, 1976; Patrick, 1982). Correlations are also predicted between O_2 solubility and surface tension, compressibility (Serratrice et al., 1982) and viscosity (Wesseler et al., 1977) of the solvent, since these are macroscopic manifestations of the degree of internal cohesion of the solvent molecule.

A group additivity system was developed to predict the energy of vaporisation and molar volume of PFC's from their structural formulas. From these two parameters, the vapor pressure and solubility of oxygen were predicted for a range of PFC's using empirical equations (Lawson et al., 1978). The agreement between calculated and experimental oxygen solubilities is rather satisfying.

Gas solubilities in emulsions were measured by chromatographic (Navari et al., 1977) or polarographic (Sharts et al., 1978) methods, as well as by redox titration after oxidation of ferrous thiocyanate by the oxygen present in the emulsion (Watanabe et al., 1975) or by enzymatic determination using glucose oxidase (Ghosh et al., 1970). The experimental gas-dissolving capacities of PFC emulsions are close to those predicted by adding the values obtained for the two phases taken separately. Uptake and release of oxygen by FTBA emulsions were measured by stopped-flow spectrophotometry to be about two times faster than by hemoglobin solutions (Ohyanagi et al., 1977).

Pharmacokinetics and Excretion Mechanisms

PFC emulsion droplets, when injected into the vasculature are opsonized and progressively phagocytized by circulating monocytes and macrophages of the reticuloendothelial system, and cleared from the blood stream. These initial steps are responsible for the limited intravascular persistence of the emulsions. The fluorocarbon component is then temporarily stored in the organs of the RES, primarily the liver, spleen and bone marrow (Miller et al., 1976; Yokoyama et al., 1978; Tsuda et al., 1988; Mitten et al., 1989; Ravis et al., 1991; Obratsov et al., 1992; Flaim, 1994; Ni et al., 1996). The mechanism by which the PFC returns to the circulation and is eventually excreted by the lungs has been progressively elucidated: The PFC is thought to slowly diffuse across cell membranes from the RES organs back into the blood vessels. It is then taken up by lipid carriers at a rate that depends on its degree of lipophilicity and is delivered to the lungs. It is eventually excreted through the alveoli with expired air. Some of the PFC is also deposited into adipose tissue, where its residence time is somewhat longer, before it is excreted by the same pathway as above.

When 20 mL (4g PFC)/kg body weight of Fluosol was administered to rats, the PFC content of liver, spleen and lung was seen to increase rapidly as PFC concentration in blood decreased, and to peak after about one day, whereas PFC in adipose tissues increased more gradually and peaked after ca two weeks (Tsuda et al., 1988). The perfluorodecalin component was shown to be eliminated from the blood, liver, spleen and lung more rapidly than perfluorotripropylamine while its presence in adipose tissues became relatively greater. This was an indication that the fate of individual PFCs depended on their affinity for lipids. Likewise, more FDC than FTPA was found in the milk of sucklings after the mother rat had received Fluosol. Although macrophages having phagocytized PFC droplets were found in alveoli within hours after administration of Fluosol to rats (Tsuda et al., 1989), excretion through a macrophage-related route is considered to be only a secondary mechanism (Tsuda et al., 1988).

The circulatory half-time (the time, $t_{1/2}$, required for the PFC concentration to decrease by half in the circulation) of the PFC is species- and dose-dependent. For Fluosol-DA it was evaluated as 13, 24 and 29 h, respectively, for rat, dog and rabbit. Dose-dependence in humans is illustrated by $t_{1/2}$ values of 7.5 to 22 h for doses of 2 to 6 g PFC/kg (Yokoyama et al., 1981). Another dose-dependence study with Fluosol in rats indicated a counter-intuitive decrease of the estimated half-lives over time. Simultaneously the FTPA fraction of the PFC that remained in blood increased from the initial 30% to about 54% after 96 hr for a higher 10 g PFC/kg dose (Lutz and Stark, 1987). The latter phenomenon may be due to faster removal of the larger droplets which are being selectively enriched in FDC by Ostwald ripening while the remaining smaller droplets are richer in FTPA.

When a perfluoro-*N*-methylisoquinoline (FMIQ)/EYP emulsion was given to rats, and blood plasma was analyzed by HPLC one week later, it was found that most FMIQ was present in the high density lipoprotein (HDL) fraction, while the intact FMIQ emulsion was observed in another fraction (Tsuda *et al.*, 1988). It was suggested that the PFC had moved across cell membranes from the RES organs and returned into the blood where it was taken up by lipoproteins which delivered it to the lungs. The role of lipid carriers in this excretion mechanism was further illustrated by Obraztsov *et al.* (1992) who showed that the rate of excretion of FDC is significantly increased when a lipid emulsion is administered iv after five days. Reduced retention (and three- to four-fold longer intravascular persistence) of FTPA (administered in rats in the form of a FTPA/EYP emulsion) has also been achieved by subsequent daily injections of lecithin; organ half-life of the PFC was reported to be reduced from ca 65 to ca 10 days (Sloviter and Mukerji, 1983). Prolonged intravascular half-life of a FDC/EYP emulsion (from 2h to 5h) was also achieved by this means (Putyativa *et al.*, 1994). It is noteworthy that circulation half-life was not prolonged by injections of EYP dispersions when a poloxamer was used as the initial surfactant.

Using FDC organ distribution data, Tsuda *et al.* (1988) developed a three-compartment pharmacokinetic model which provided good correlation between observed and simulated blood and organ PFC concentration vs time. It was proposed that excretion of PFC as an emulsion and of PFC *per se* had to be distinguished, and that the excretion rate constant was small for the emulsion form. It is somewhat surprising that no adipose tissue compartment was taken into account in this study; it should also be noted that the experimental data covered only a two-week period.

Obraztsov *et al.* (1992) proposed a four-compartment pharmacokinetic model (PFC in blood, PFC in RES, PFC in lipids in blood and PFC in adipose tissues) and established that the rate-determining step is the dissolution of the PFC into the lipid carriers, hence it depended critically on the solubility of the PFC in lipids.

A further study of the pharmacokinetics of fluorocarbons concerns perfluorooctyl bromide (perflubron). Ni *et al.* (1996) evaluated six possible pharmacokinetic compartment models by nonlinear regression analysis with expiration data over a 28-day period from rats after i.v. administration of a 3 mL (2.7g PFC)/kg dose of a 90% w/v concentrated perflubron emulsion. One of these models (Figure 5) with four compartments (PFC emulsion in blood, PFC in RES tissues, PFC in non-RES tissues, PFC dissolved in blood via lipoproteins) approximates the experimental data rather well. It correlates the expiration data (Figure 6) with tissue distribution data, and in particular with the 2–3 day peak in PFC concentration found in the RES organs. Physiologically-based models were also investigated. Some uncertainty remains as to the existence of direct transfer of the PFC from the emulsion into adipose tissues.

Fluorocarbon Excretion Rate vs Molecular Structure

It is essential that fluorocarbons for intravascular use be excreted rapidly from the organs *and* also be formulated into stable emulsions. Emulsions have to be stable enough to allow convenient storage, transportation and implementation, if possible at room temperature. On this depends their usefulness, convenience and commercial

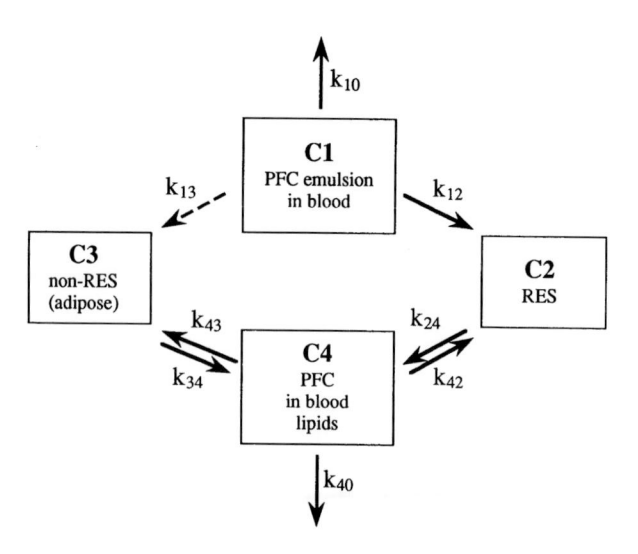

Figure 5 Pharmacokinetic compartment model for PFC emulsions. A first-order output from each compartment is assumed; k_{ij} represents the first-order rate constant from compartment Ci to compartment Cj; k_{i0} represents the expiration rate constant from compartment Ci to the air; the PFC dose is administered into compartment C1. Adapted from Ni *et al.* (1996), with permission.

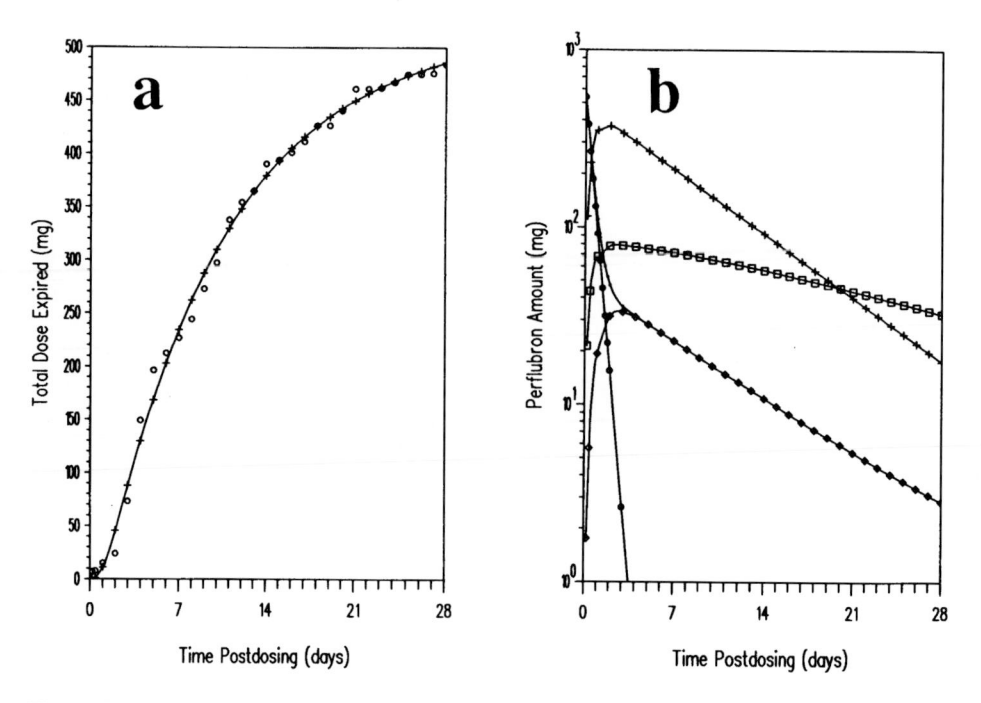

Figure 6 a) Cumulative amount of perflubron expired in the air as a function of time: (O) experimentally determined; (+) predicted on the basis of the model depicted on Figure 5. b) Semi-log plot of the predicted PFC amounts present in each compartment (C1: O; C2: +; C3: □; C4: ◇), as well as of the sum of PFC in C1 and C4 (●), vs time. The simulated PFC amount in C2 peaks at about 2–3 days, which is in agreement with experimental tissue analysis of perflubron in the RES organs. From Ni *et al.* (1996), with permission.

value. At the same time the PFC should not be retained in the organism too long after it has fulfilled its mission.

It was soon discovered, however, that there exists an inverse relationship between these two characteristics. Those PFCs that are excreted rapidly usually give unstable emulsions, and vice-versa. Thus, perfluorotributylamine provides very stable and fine emulsions even with a relatively poor emulsifier such as Pluronic F-68, but it was disqualified for use in humans because of its several-year-long retention in the RES. Perfluorodecalin on the other hand has an organ half-life of only 6–7 days, but attempts to formulate it into a stable emulsion have failed (Naito and Yokoyama, 1978, 1981; Yokoyama et al., 1982).

These early observations nonetheless oriented for over a decade the intense research efforts that were devoted to finding PFCs that would satisfy both requirements simultaneously. Because FTBA contains a heteroatom (Table 1), nitrogen, the idea developed that heteroatoms favored emulsion stability, at the expense, however, of excretion rate. Likewise, FDC, because it is bicyclic, led to the belief that cyclization facilitated excretion, albeit at the expense of emulsion stability. The observation that, for a same number of carbon atoms, excretion rates increased rapidly when the number of cycles present in the structure increased, reinforced this belief (Moore and Clark, 1982, 1985). So did the fact that organ retention increased when heteroatoms (oxygen or nitrogen) were *added* to a given structure.

The Green Cross Corp. "solved" the excretion rate vs emulsion dilemma by mixing perfluorodecalin with perfluorotripropylamine, a lower molecular weight homolog of perfluorotributylamine. Such was the conceptual basis for Fluosol-DA (Naito and Yokoyama, 1978; Yokoyama et al., 1982). FTPA indeed improved emulsion stability, although not sufficiently to ensure practicality as it turned out, and at the expense of a 65-day-long organ half-life. The heteroatom-plus-cycle approach was also the basis for the synthesis and evaluation of FMIQ and similar compounds as the Green Cross's second generation fluorocarbons (Ohyanagi et al., 1990). FMIQ (Table 1) consists indeed of a bicyclic compound (like FDC) that contains a nitrogen atom within its structure (like FTPA).

During the same period intense efforts by several groups were devoted to the synthesis of a variety of new fluorocarbons with cycles, branches, double bonds and heteroatoms present within their molecular structure (Clark et al., 1974; Geyer, 1979; Le Blanc and Riess, 1982; Moore and Clark, 1982; Jeanneaux et al., 1984; Yokoyama et al., 1984). Precise comparison of data resulting from their evaluation is not always easy, as each research group had its own protocol for measuring excretion rates and an often subjective way of assessing emulsion stability. Only those data originating from the same team can be meaningfully compared. Particularly valuable in this respect are the papers by researchers of the Green Cross Corp (Yokoyama et al., 1983, 1984; Yamanouchi et al., 1985) which report on no less than 53 PFCs.

Analysis of these data showed that excretion rates actually depended simply, but exponentially, on the fluorocarbon's molecular weight (Figure 7) (Riess, 1984). Neither the presence of cycles *per se*, nor the presence of heteroatoms *per se* had any significant influence on the PFC's excretion rate. These structural features were shown to influence organ retention only in as much as their introduction changes the compound's molecular weight.

Thus, for example, perfluorodecalin ($C_{10}F_{18}$, MW = 462; bicyclic) has, within experimental error, the same excretion rate, 6-7 days, as bis(F-butyl)ethene ($C_{10}F_{18}H_2$,

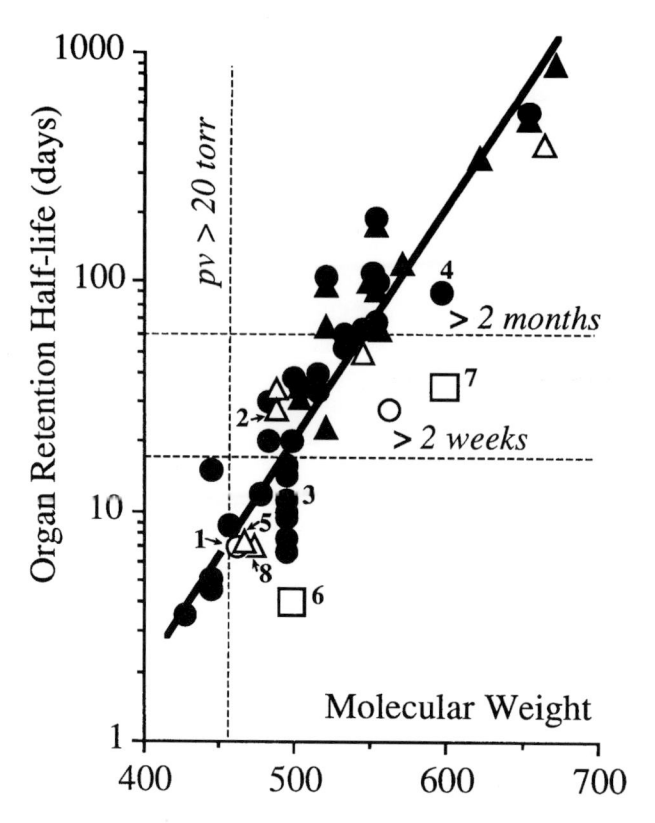

Figure 7 Semilogarithmic plot of organ retention half-times for PFCs as a function of their molecular weight. △ linear, ○ cyclic, ▲ linear with heteroatom, ● cyclic with heteroatom). An exponential variation is found. The two most deviant points (□) correspond to lipophilic brominated fluorocarbons which are excreted significantly faster than standard, non-lipophilic fluorocarbons. **1**: perfluorodecalin, **2**: perfluorotripropylamine (both in Fluosol); **3**: perfluoro-*N*-methyldecahydroisoquinoline; **4**: perfluoro-*N*-methylcyclohexylpiperidine (in Perftoran along with **1**); **5**: bis(perfluorobutyl)ethene (in Therox); **6**: perfluorooctyl bromide, **7**: perfluorodecyl bromide (both in Oxygent); **8**: perfluorodichlorooctane (in Oxyfluor). Data from Table 1 and from Yamanouchi *et al.* (1985). Adapted from Riess (1984), with permission.

MW = 464, non-cyclic). The addition of a nitrogen atom (and consequently of a fluorine atom), as in FMIQ ($C_{10}NF_{19}$, MW = 495), slows down excretion ($t_{1/2}$ = 11 days), while the replacement of a carbon atom by a nitrogen, as in F⎔FN— ($C_9F_{17}N$, MW = 445) accelerates excretion ($t_{1/2}$ ≈ 5 days), in line with the respective increase or decrease in molecular weight.

The dependence of excretion rate on molecular weight is consistent with the fact that rapid excretion requires a certain degree of solubility of the PFC in lipids, a characteristic which decreases rapidly with increasing molecular weight (Le *et al.*, 1996). Both FDC and FTPA were shown by ^{19}F NMR studies to be partly soluble in the bilayer of phosphatidylcholine vesicles, while FTBA was not (Kong *et al.*, 1985). Likewise the increase in emulsion stability with increasing molecular weight is logical now that the mechanism of particle growth has been elucidated (see Section on emulsion stability p. 286).

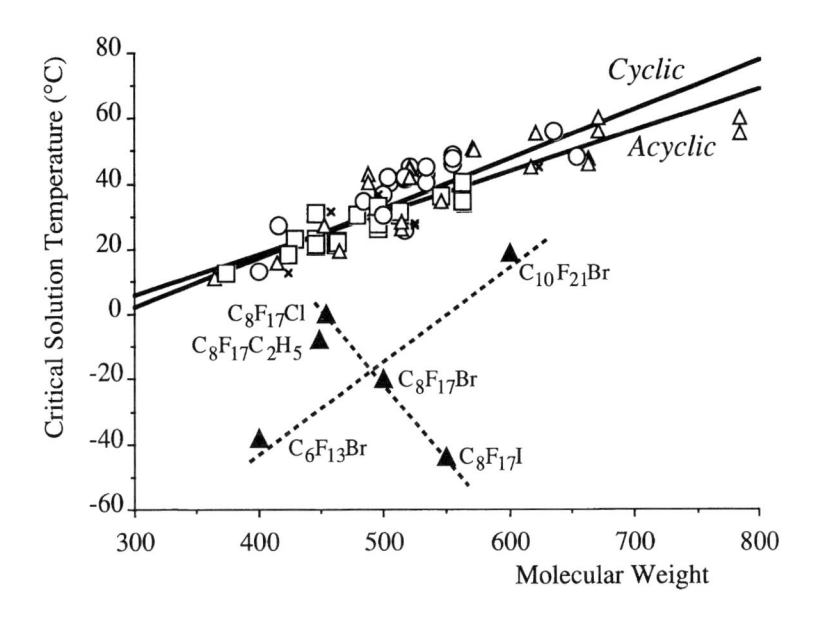

Figure 8 Critical solution temperatures (CSTs) of perfluorocarbons in hexane (as a mesure of their lipophilic character) vs molecular weight (MW): △, acyclic; ○, monocyclic; □, bicyclic; ×, tricyclic; ▲, lipophilic. The larger, filled triangles correspond to exceptions to the linear CST vs MW relationship. Adapted from Grec et al. (1985), and incorporating data from Yamanouchi et al. (1985).

The steepness of the increase in organ-retention time with increasing molecular weight is remarkable. Small variations in molecular weight provoke considerable changes in both the organ dwell time and emulsion stability. PFCs with low molecular weights and vapor pressures above ca 20 mm Hg are inacceptable since they cause lung emphysema and other pulmonary complications (Clark et al., 1975; Okamoto et al., 1975), thus placing a lower limit to the acceptable range of molecular weights. The range of molecular weights acceptable was eventually proposed to be from ca 460 to ca 520 (Riess, 1984). This leaves a rather narrow window of possibilities since it represents less than the molecular weight of one single CF_3 group!

It was proposed rather early on that the critical solubility temperature (CST) of a PFC in hexane, which reflects the fluorocarbon's lipophilicity, be a means of selecting excretable PFCs (Moore and Clark, 1982, 1985). The decrease of CST that was observed when, for a given number of carbon atoms, the number of cycles increased, led again to the belief that cyclizations favor excretion, overlooking the fact that each cyclization reduces molecular weight by 38 (two fluorine atoms being expelled). Yamamouchi et al. (1985) found that neither the connectivity (cyclization and ramifications) nor the presence of heteroatoms had significant effects on organ retention, thus basically confirming our views. They proposed that the best correlation for retention times was with a linear combination of CST and vapor pressure. Vapor pressure alone, however, is a poor indicator of excretion potential. Thus, for example, FDC, with a vapor pressure of 12 mm Hg, has an organ half-life of about seven days, while FTPA, with a vapor pressure of 20 mm Hg, has a half-life of ca 65 days. For the series of fluorocarbons investigated in these studies, the CST correlated closely with the molecular weight (Figure 8; correlation factor 0.84), showing once again the excretion rate of fluorocarbons to be independent of the presence of cycles or heteroatoms *per se* for these series of compounds (Grec et al., 1985).

Faster Excretion Rates: Lipophilic PFCs

At the time when the above analysis was made (1983) the excretion rate *vs* molecular weight dependence was without exception, but for one compound, perfluorooctyl bromide (perflubron, Table 1), which was to become the keystone of the present generation of emulsions.

As noted, perfluorooctyl bromide was initially selected (Long et al., 1972; Long et al., 1988) for use as a contrast agent for diagnosis. This is the reason for the radiopaque bromine atom. For about the same molecular weight as FMIQ (499 vs 495) perflubron's organ half-life is less than half of that of FMIQ (4 vs 11 days). It turned out that perflubron also tended to give rather stable emulsions, especially when emulsified with egg yolk phospholipids. The superiority of this fluorocarbon vis-a-vis the excretion rate/emulsion stability dilemma was soon assigned to the lipophilic character induced by its well exposed terminally located bromine atom, which was confirmed by the much lower CST of this compound in hexane (Riess, 1987) or octane (Weers, 1993) as compared to other fluorocarbons with similar molecular weights. The bromine atom of perflubron is inactivated owing to the presence of the electronegative fluorocarbon chain, and no evidence of metabolism has been found (Flaim, 1994). These unique characteristics, plus the fact that perflubron can easily be manufactured on a large scale in a high state of purity by the well-established telomerization route, and that it ranks among the fluorocarbons that have the highest O_2 and CO_2 dissolving capacities, made it eminently eligible for further development.

The benefit of introducing lipophilic termini such as a bromine or chlorine atom or a short hydrocarbon segment into fluorocarbons was confirmed with other compounds (Figure 8). A method for assessing the lipophilicity of the more lipophilic fluorocarbons has recently been devised by Le *et al.* (1996). It uses n-bromohexane as a reference compound and has the merit of moving the CST for such fluorocarbons into a conveniently measurable temperature range. A group additivity scheme for predicting the new CST_{BrHex} values was proposed. These values also correlate well with the olive oil solubilities of the PFCs (Figure 9). It is noteworthy that the influence of one bromine atom on CST is essentially equivalent to that of two chlorine atoms and almost comparable to that of a C_2H_5 group.

Various fluorocarbons terminated by one or two chlorine or bromine atoms have been synthesized (Kabalnov et al., 1992). More recently α,ω-dichloroperfluorooctane has been selected for development of the concentrated fluorocarbon emulsion *Oxyfluor*® (HemaGen/PFC, St Louis, Mo, USA) (Kaufman, 1994, 1995).

Toxicity of Fluorocarbons

No toxicity, carcinogenic, mutagenic or teratogenic effects, nor immunological reactions, have ever been reported for fluorocarbons when pure and chosen within the appropriate molecular weight range. When toxicity is observed in an individual sample this sample should first be suspected of containing some toxic by-product or impurity. It is generally found that such toxicity can be removed by appropriate

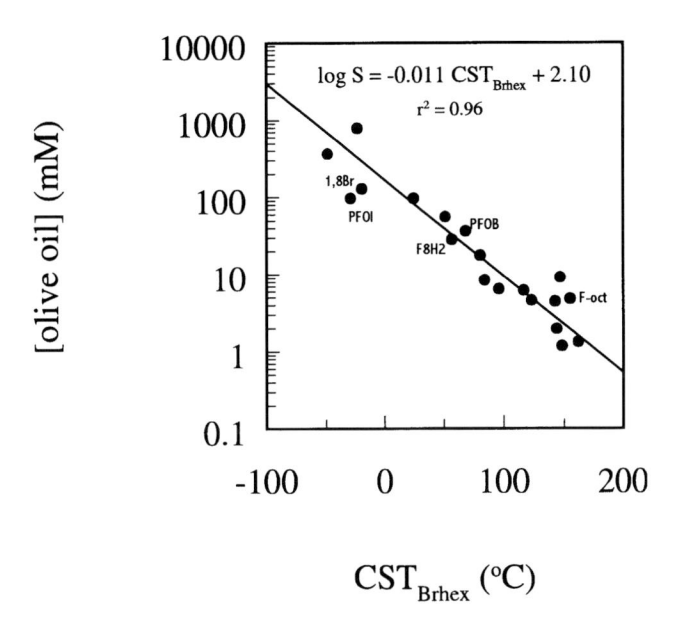

Figure 9 Correlation between the olive oil solubility and CST_{Brhex} value for various fluorocarbons. Taken from Le et al. (1996), with permission.

treatment. Distillation, repeated washing with a KOH solution, and/or filtration over alumina suffice in most cases. Cell cultures provide a sensitive test for assessing such impurity-related toxicity and for monitoring purification (Geyer, 1973; Le Blanc et al., 1985; Lowe, 1994).

There is no evidence of metabolism for fluorocarbons and in particular for any of the fluorocarbons selected for *in vivo* oxygen delivery. There is no sound evidence either that the presence of isolated hydrogen, chlorine, bromine, secondary oxygen or tertiary nitrogen atoms, or of a double bond in the fluorocarbon induces any toxicity or favors enzymatic attack or metabolism. No reactivity was found for these elements in the conditions of processing and use involved in the applications considered here.

Concerns about a possible toxic effect of certain PFCs in the lungs proved unfounded. Such concerns resulted from the observation that the lungs of rabbits given Fluosol or emulsions of certain PFCs such as perfluorodecalin, did not deflate normally at autopsy (Clark et al., 1992). This phenomenon, which was called lung hyperinflation or, more accurately, an increased pulmonary residual volume (IPRV) effect, is due to retention of air in the alveoli, and was subsequently shown to be highly species-dependent. Sensitive species include rabbit, swine and macaque monkey, while the phenomenon was not observed in mouse, dog or human (Leakakos et al., 1994). No such effects were ever reported for Fluosol and other perfluorodecalin-based emulsions in humans, although they have been administered to several thousands of patients. Pulmonary function was carefully monitored for patients receiving Oxygent and no effect was seen there either (Wahr et al., 1996; Keipert, 1995b). The mechanism of IPRV has nevertheless been thoroughly investigated. It was shown that the air bubbles that normally and continuously form in the alveoli are osmotically stabilized when fluorocarbon vapor is present (Schutt et al., 1994). High transpulmonary pressures (which lead to bubble breakage), large airway dimensions, and low perflubron vapor concentration in the lung (i.e., low capacity to stabilize the bubbles) ensure that the phenomenon is not operative in humans. As noted above, even Fluosol, which contains a PFC with higher vapor pressure than the present generation of emulsions, does not cause any such lung effect in humans.

The Fluorocarbons of Choice

Most of the over one hundred fluorochemicals that were screened in the seventies and eighties for use as injectable oxygen carriers did not meet the criteria set at the beginning of this section; they were however of paramount importance for our understanding of structure/properties relationships and for refining our selection criteria.

As indicated, among the initially selected "second-generation" products that emerged, most were polycyclic and many were designed to combine the structural characteristics of perfluorodecalin (the cycles, which were thought to facilitate excretion) and of perfluorotripropylamine (the heteroatom, which was thought to improve emulsion stability). None, however, provided a solution to the stability vs excretion problem, while in many cases the preparation, purity and reliability issues were worsened because of increased molecular complexity. The latter issue was not encountered with the bis(perfluoroalkyl)ethenes which can be produced in pure form by telomerization; they also have larger O_2-dissolving capacities and give more stable emulsions than perfluorodecalin (Riess and Le Blanc, 1988). An emulsion of bis(perfluorobutyl)ethene (F-44E) was developed for experimental research in the 80s by Dupont (Wilmington, DE) under the trade-name Therox®. A rather ill-defined, complex mixture of polycyclic compounds, including principally perfluorodimethylbicyclononane, resulting from the fluorination of methyladamantane by CoF_3, was selected by Adamantech (Marcus Hook, PA) for the development of Addox (Moore, 1989).

It was eventually the lipophilic fluorocarbons that have proved to be superior in terms of meeting the selection criteria required for i.v. use, and which were consequently elected for developing the emulsions now in clinical trials.

Perfluorooctyl bromide (perflubron) stands out among PFCs since, its molecular weight being taken into account, it has an exceptionally fast excretion rate (three days half-life in the RES for a 2.7 g/kg dose in humans), and forms emulsions with superior stability when EYP is utilized as the surfactant. Perflubron also ranks among the PFCs that have the highest O_2 and CO_2 dissolving capacities (50 and 210 vol% at 37°C) and it can be manufactured in better than 99% pure form on a large scale. Existing production capacity is already at the 100 ton/year level, and can be scaled higher without difficulty. In addition, perflubron being radiopaque has potential in diagnosis (Mattrey, 1994), and in liquid ventilation (Faithfull, 1994a; Leach et al., 1996), where its very low surface tension and positive spreading coefficient are advantageous. The principal physicochemical characteristics of perflubron are collected in Table 3.

α,ω-Dichloroperfluorooctane, PFDCO, another lipophilic fluorocarbon, has recently also been proposed as a candidate oxygen carrier, in spite of its somewhat

Table 3 Physical properties of perflubron

Property	Symbol	Data
molecular formula		$C_8F_{17}Br$
molecular weight	M_W	499 g mol^{-1}
molar volume	V_m	261.3 cm^3 mol^{-1}
molecular volume	V	432 Å^3
density	ρ	1.918 g cm^{-3} (25°C)
melting point	T_m	7.5°C
boiling point	T_b	143°C
vapor pressure	P_v	5.015 torr (25°C) 10.503 torr (37°C)
heat of vaporization	ΔH_v	4.83 kJ mol^{-1}
energy of vaporization	ΔE_v	4.58 kJ mol^{-1}
entropy of vaporization	ΔS_v	162 J mol^{-1} K^{-1}
solubility parameter	δ	27.1 J cm^{-3}
refractive index	n_D	1.30 (25°C)
kinematic viscosity	v	1.0 centistokes (25°C)
surface tension	γ	18.0 mN m^{-1}
interfacial tension vs. saline	σ^i	51.3 mN m^{-1}
spreading coefficient	S (o/w)	+2.7 mN m^{-1}
oxygen solubility	[O_2]	50 vol.% (25°C)
carbon dioxide solubility	[CO_2]	210 vol.% (25°C)
compressibility coefficient	k	1.3434 × 10^{10} cm s^2 g^{-1}
critical solution temperature	CST	−20°C (n-hexane) 4°C (n-octane)
solubility in olive oil	[PFOB]	0.037 mol L^{-1}
organ retention time	$T_{1/2}$	3 days (2.7 g kg^{-1} dose, rats)

longer organ half-life (about eight days for a 4 mL/kg dose) and lower oxygen solubility (42 vol% at 37°C) compared to perflubron (Kaufman, 1995). The claim that it has a decreased aptitude to increase pulmonary residual volume in baboons than perfluorodecalin appears irrelevant since this particular effect is not observed in humans.

THE COMPONENTS: SELECTING THE EMULSIFIER

One key function of the surfactant is to reduce the large tension which, at the interface between the fluorocarbon and aqueous phases, opposes the dispersion of the former phase in the latter one. Another function is to stabilize the emulsion once it is formed. To be acceptable for i.v. use, surfactants must be devoid of toxicity and other non-desirable physiologic effects. They should also be readily available and, if possible, already listed in the pharmacopea.

Except for a range of new fluorinated surfactants, much less effort has been devoted to synthesizing and assessing emulsifiers suitable for emulsifying fluorocarbons than to synthesizing and assessing new fluorocarbons. This may *a priori* seem surprising, since the surfactant not only plays a crucial role in preparing and stabilizing the emusions, but also can affect and help control the recognition and phagocytosis, hence the intravascular persistence of the emulsion particles and, possibly, the subsequent organ distribution of the fluorocarbon. This situation probably results not from lack of interest, but from the cost and delays involved in determining the pharmacology and toxicology of a new surfactant and having it accepted by the regulatory authorities. Surfactants are amphiphilic molecules that tend to adsorb at interfaces, including on biological membranes. Such surface-active components can hardly be expected to be totally devoid of biological activity. Many indeed are hemolytic and display other forms of toxicity that are not compatible with intravascular use (Attwood and Florence, 1983).

As a result of such considerations, only two surfactants have been utilized to a substantial extent in the formulation of injectable fluorocarbon emulsions: poloxamer 188 (also known under the trade-names Pluronic F-68® and Proxanol-188®) and egg-yolk phospholipids (Table 4).

A range of fluorinated surfactants, i.e. surfactants with hydrophobic tails consisting of a fluorocarbon chain, have also been investigated as emulsifiers for fluorocarbon emulsions. Such surfactants display a high affinity for the fluorocarbon phase and very low fluorocarbon/water interfacial tensions. Clark *et al.* (1983) pursued an industrial grade fluorinated amine oxide, XMO-10. Several terminally perfluoroalkylated polyoxyethylene oxide or poloxamer derivatives were synthesized (Selve and Castro, 1983; Fung *et al.*, 1989; Meinert *et al.*, 1992). The synthesis of series of highly pure fluorinated surfactants with a modular design destined for biomedical use was undertaken (Riess *et al.*, 1989, 1992b; Greiner *et al.*, 1993; Riess and Krafft, 1998). These surfactants combine fluorinated segments of various chainlengths coupled with chain promulgating hydrocarbon segments. The hydrophobic groups were then linked through a variety of junction groups to a range of hydrophilic polar headgroups derived from biocompatible natural products including polyols, sugars, amino acids, phosphocholine, phosphatidylcholine and trishydroxymethyl-amino methane. As a class, the fluorinated surfactants (relative to their hydrogenated counterparts) were found to be significantly less hemolytic in spite of their higher surface activity. Interfacial tensions at the PFC/water interface are on the order of 1–10 mN m^{-1}. Although such surfactants were often very effective in stabilizing fluorocarbon emulsions, their development still suffers from poor knowledge and understanding of their toxicity and pharmacodynamics.

Poloxamers

Poloxamers are neutral block copolymers constituted of two terminal polyoxyethylene (POE) blocks flanking a central polyoxypropylene (POP) block (Table 4). When used to emulsify an oil in water, the latter segment, which is essentially hydrophobic,

Table 4 Principal emulsifiers and co-emulsifiers investigated for preparing fluorocarbon emulsions

Egg yolk phospholipids

$R = CH_2CH_2\overset{+}{N}(CH_3)_3$ (PC)
$CH_2CH_2NH_2$ (PE)

Poloxamers   Potassium oleate

$HO(CH_2CH_2O)_n(CHCH_2O)_p(CH_2CH_2O)_{n'}H$ $cis\text{-}CH_3(CH_2)_7CH=CH(CH_2)_7COO^-\ K^+$
    |
    CH_3

Fluorinated surfactants

$(CF_3)_2CFO(CF_2)_3\ C(O)NH(CH_2)_3N(O)(CH_2)_3$ (XMO-10)

(F8CHCO-trehalose)   (F8AXY-1)

Fluorocarbon/Hydrocarbon diblocks

$C_nF_{2n+1}C_mH_{2m+1}$ $C_nF_{2n+1}CH=CHC_mH_{2m+1}$

(FnHm)   (FnHmE)

---

will adhere onto the surface of the oil droplets, while the two hydrophilic POE chains extend as a brush into the aqueous phase (Figure 10). The POE chains are substantially hydrated due to hydrogen bonding between water molecules and the ether oxygens of the POE chains.

Poloxamers are low-cost synthetic materials that are produced in large tonnages and have found countless industrial applications in the food, cosmetic and pharmaceutical industries, where they are used as emulsifiers, solubilizers, dispersing agents and drug delivery systems (Schmolka, 1977, 1992, 1994; Stolnik et al., 1995; Reeve, 1997). The conventional nomenclature for poloxamers comprises a three-digit number. The first two digits refer to the molecular weight of the POP block, while the last digit indicates the percentage of ethylene oxide in the polymer when multiplied by 100 and 10, respectively. Thus in poloxamer 188 the central POP block has an average molecular weight of ca 1800, while the POE chains represent about 80% of the total molecule and have molecular weights of approximately 3600 each. Poloxamers do not consist of single molecules but rather in a more or less stochastic distribution of molecules over a broad molecular weight range. When analyzed by gel permeation chromatography, commercial poloxamer 188 actually shows a bimodal distribution, with a major peak (about 95% of the mass) having a molecular weight

Egg yolk phospholipids

~~~~~COO⎤
~~~~~COO⎦
           O⁻
           |
           OPOR
           ‖
           O
←— ca 5 nm —→

R = PC, PE, etc.
C12 - C18 saturated/unsaturated chains

Poloxamers
(polydisperse block polymers)

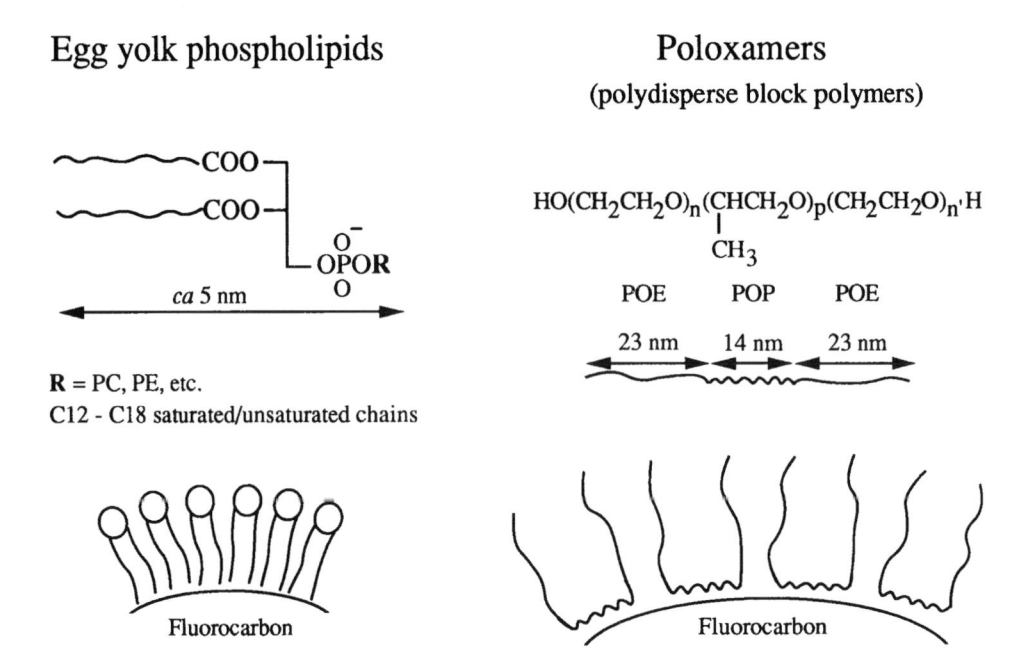

$HO(CH_2CH_2O)_n(CHCH_2O)_p(CH_2CH_2O)_{n'}H$
                    |
                    CH_3

  POE   POP   POE

  23 nm   14 nm   23 nm

Figure 10 Molecular structure of the two emulsifiers used in commercially developed perfluorocarbon emulsions and schematic representation of their configuration at the water/fluorocarbon interface.

ranging from about 6,000 to 13,000 and a minor peak between 3,000 and 5,000 (Reeve, 1997) (Figure 11). Various impurities are found in most commercial products. They include traces of acetaldehyde, propionaldehyde, formic and acetic acids, etc. Some unsaturated reaction products may also be present. An antioxidant such as O,O-ditertiobutylcresol is usually added for preservation. Standard commercial

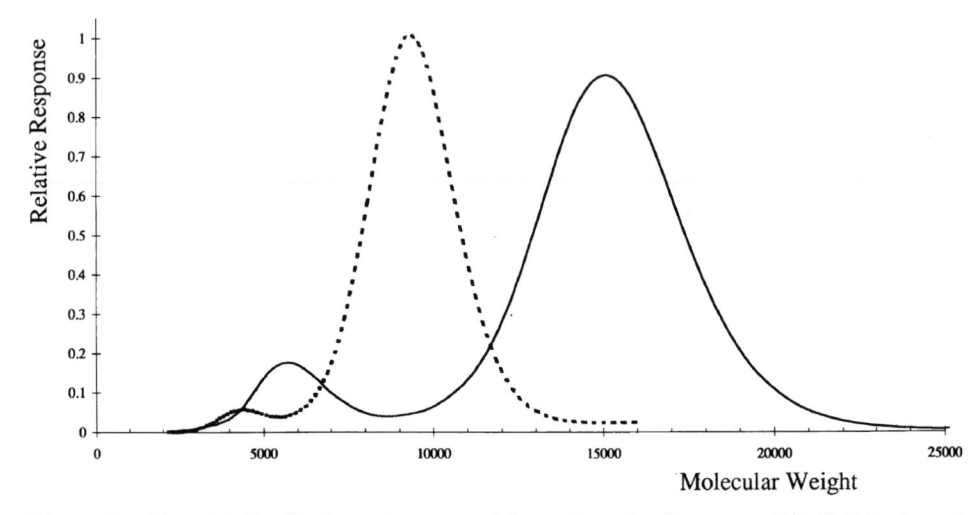

Figure 11 Bimodal distribution of commercial samples of poloxamers 407 (full line) and 188 (doted line), as analyzed by gel permeation chromatography and refractive index detection. From Reeve (1997), with permission.

grade poloxamers are obviously not intended for intravascular use. Moreover, the POE/POP ratio, as well as the molecular weight distribution and the nature and amount of the impurities and side-products present, can vary significantly among suppliers and lots. Purification can be achieved by treatment with ion exchangers, fractionating crystallization, and other procedures (Bentley, 1989; Lane and Krukonis, 1988).

Poloxamer 188 has been utilized as the emulsifier in all first generation, Fluosol-type injectable fluorocarbon emulsions. In addition to providing a steric barrier against coalescence (see Section VIII), the hydrophilic EO coat that extends into the continuous water phase also alters the opsonization and uptake of emulsion droplets by the reticuloendothelial system (Davis and Illum, 1995; Stolnik et al., 1995). Differences in the hydrophilic/lipophilic balance of the polymer may also alter the ultimate disposition of the particle. For example, particles coated with poloxamine 908, another block copolymer with POE chains, were rapidly cleared by the liver, while poloxamer 407-coated particles were largely taken up by the bone marrow (Davis and Illum, 1995; Moghimi et al., 1993; Porter et al., 1992). Poloxamers can therefore play a significant role in surface engineering of injectable particulates.

The use of poloxamer 188, however, raises several problems. The first stems from its relatively poor surface activity and low affinity for fluorocarbons. For example, the interfacial tension between FDC and water is only reduced from 56 to ca 30 mN m^{-1}, compared to about 1–5 mN m^{-1} when phosphatidylcholines are utilized. Another problem comes from the low state of purity and variability of the commercially available products. Still another difficulty is encountered when heat sterilization is contemplated. This arises from the fact that poloxamer 188 has a cloud point at about 110°C, i.e. below the standard sterilization temperature of 121°C, where dehydration of the surfactant layer suddenly occurs with consequent breakdown of the emulsion. A further problem is due to the fact that poloxamers tend to form gels at room temperature (Wanka et al., 1990; Nakashima et al., 1994; Schmolka, 1994). This severely limits the fluorocarbon concentration in submicronic emulsions, as higher concentrations require larger amounts of surfactant while the volume of the continuous aqueous phase becomes smaller. Viscosity thus increases rapidly when the fluorocarbon content is larger than about 30 v/v%. Finally, a number of side-effects that were observed upon administration of Pluronic-stabilized fluorocarbon emulsions have been attributed to the surfactant, which eventually led to its replacement by phospholipids.

Poloxamer 188 when administered intravascularly is not metabolized. Excretion occurs in the urine (Naito and Yokoyama, 1981). The acute toxicity of Pluronic F-68 was shown to be very low, with LD$_{50}$ values that can reach 8g/kg body weight when given intravenously to rats (Yokoyama et al., 1983). Pluronic F-68, however, has been found responsible for the unpredictable anaphylactic reaction observed in some patients in response to the injection of Fluosol-DA (Tremper et al., 1984; Hammerschmidt and Vercelotti, 1989). Dogs were seen to experience an abrupt drop in arterial pressure when infused a FTBA/Pluronic F-68 emulsion (Clark et al., 1972), in contradiction to another report according to which dogs tolerated continuous infusion of 500 mg/kg/hr of the product for three days (Justicz et al., 1991). Pluronic F-68 was also reported to cause an impairment of phospholipase A$_2$ activity and to have an *in vitro* inhibitory effect on the chemotactic, phagocytic and metabolic functions of human neutrophils (Shakir and Williams, 1982; Lane and Lampkin,

1984, 1986; Virmani et al., 1983, 1984; Williams et al., 1988) accompanied by an impairment of host resistance to bacterial infection (Lane and Lampkin, 1986). Other studies suggest that the Pluronic-containing emulsions Fluosol-DA and Fluosol-43 activate monocyte procoagulent generation, although no significant cytotoxicity was observed, and may impair normal monocyte oxidative metabolism (Janco et al., 1985). Inhibition by Fluosol-DA of the growth of cultured human embryonic lung cells (Wake et al., 1985) and of macrophages obtained from peritoneal exudates of mice (Bucala et al., 1983) could also be due to this surfactant. Contradictory reports have appeared on the influence of fluorocarbon emulsions on platelet aggregation and coagulation (Kitazawa and Ohnishi, 1982; Colman et al., 1980; Mitsuno et al., 1982b); when observed, these effects were also attributed to the surfactant. Thus, no effects on platelets were noted when lecithins were used as the surfactant instead of Pluronic F-68 (Sloviter and Mukherji, 1983). It should furthermore be noted that Pluronic F-68 fractions purified by Amberlite resin filtration (Bentley et al., 1989) or supercritical fluid fractionation (Lane and Krukonis, 1988) showed markedly reduced toxicity.

On the other hand, some of the physiological effects of Pluronic F-68 may have therapeutic utility. Thus, poloxamer 188 has been under investigation for treatment of circulatory pathologies, including for inhibition of thrombosis following myocardial infarction (Justicz et al., 1991, Schaer et al., 1994), improvement of blood flow and perfusion of damaged tissues (Mayer et al., 1994; Colbassani et al., 1989, Hunter et al., 1990), and reduction in clot formation time (Carr et al., 1995). Pluronic F-68 has also been used to reduce fat embolism (Adams et al., 1959), and as a protective agent against hemolysis during extracorporeal circulation (Miyauchi et al., 1966). Poloxamer 407 is presently being investigated for prevention of post-surgical adhesions (Reeve, 1997).

Phospholipids

Egg yolk phospholipid has been selected as the emulsifier in the presently developed fluorocarbon emulsions for a number of reasons. Significant improvements in PFC emulsion stability with EYP vs Pluronic was reported (see, for example, Sloviter and Mukherji, 1983; Varescon et al., 1989). The excellent match between the hydrophilic-lipophilic balance of EYP and perflubron was emphasized (Weers, 1993). It results in improved cohesiveness between EYP's hydrophobic fatty acid chains and perflubron, as compared to other PFCs. Phospholipids have a long history of use in pharmaceuticals; they are well documented, and there exist reliable commercial sources of pharmaceutical grade egg yolk phospholipids (March, 1987; Cevc, 1993). EYPs are, however complex, sensitive, oxidizable materials, whose preparation, analysis, quality control, handling and implementation require specific expertise.

Phospholipids are of universal occurence in living organisms. They are the main constituents of the membranes that surround the cell and compartmentalize it into zones across which only specific exchanges can occur. Thus they play the role of selective barriers and are the support of membrane proteins. Phospholipids are amphiphilic molecules constituted of a polar (or charged) zone which has a strong affinity for water, and of an apolar zone constituted by fatty acid chains which is hydrophobic. This amphipathic structure leads to specific properties including a strong tendency to form bilayers and liposomes when dispersed in water, and

Table 5 A typical EYP composition including fatty acid composition (Wendel, 1995)[a]

Phospholipids	w%	Fatty Acids	w%
phosphatidylcholine	65–70	palmitic	37.0
phosphatidylethanolamine	9–13	stearic	9.0
lysophosphatidylcholine	2–4	oleic	32.3
lysophosphatidylethanolamine	2–4	linoleic	16.7
sphingomyelin	2–3	arachidonic	5.0
free fatty acids	≤1		
mono-, diglycerides	traces		
triglycerides	10–15		
water	≤1.5		

[a] Egg yolk phospholipids often also contain small amounts of cholesterol, phosphatidylinositol, N-methylphosphatidylethanolamine, phosphatidic acid, etc.

monolayers in oil-in-water emulsions. In the latter case the fatty acid moiety of the phospholipids faces the oil phase while the head group faces the aqueous phase.

Natural phospholipids consist in crude mixtures made of phosphatidylcholine (PC), phosphatidylethanolamine (PE), phosphatidylinositol (PI) (Table 4), other phospholipids and a variety of other compounds such as fatty acids, triglycerides, sterols, carbohydrates and glycolipids. They are obtained by solvent extraction from the natural source followed by various purification steps including recrystallization and/or column chromatography (Wendel, 1995). The main sources of phospholipids include vegetable oils from soy bean, cottonseed, corn, sunflower, rapeseed, and animal tissues (egg yolk and bovine brain). Egg and soy phospholipids are by far the most important in terms of amounts produced. A typical composition of egg yolk phospholipids is given in Table 5.

Phospholipids are excellent wetting and emulsifying agents whose properties have been exploited in the food and cosmetics industry, in paints and petroleum products and numerous other applications. Phospholipids are used as a dietetic source of phosphatidylcholine. Phospholipids have been in use for many years in intravenous injectable lipid emulsions for parenteral nutrition. The best known of these emulsions, Intralipid™ (Pharmacia, Stockholm, Sweden), consists of soybean oil droplets dispersed in water and is stabilized by egg yolk phospholipids (Rotenberg et al., 1991; Westesen and Wehler, 1993). The rationale behind its use is that the small phospholipid-coated oil droplets can mimic chilomicrons, i. e. the natural blood fat particles produced by the mucosal cells of the small intestine (Wretlind, 1977). Only few side effects with no clinical consequences were observed with such products and these side effects appear to relate to the particulate nature of the emulsion rather than to the presence of phospholipids (see p. 277).

It was shown that phospholipid composition (minor components and fatty acid composition) and the level of fatty acid unsaturation (as determined by iodine value) may have an effect on the oxidative and particle size stability, and the viscosity of perflubron emulsions (Pelura et al., 1992; Yoon and Burgers, 1996), as well as on lipid emulsions (Washington, 1996).

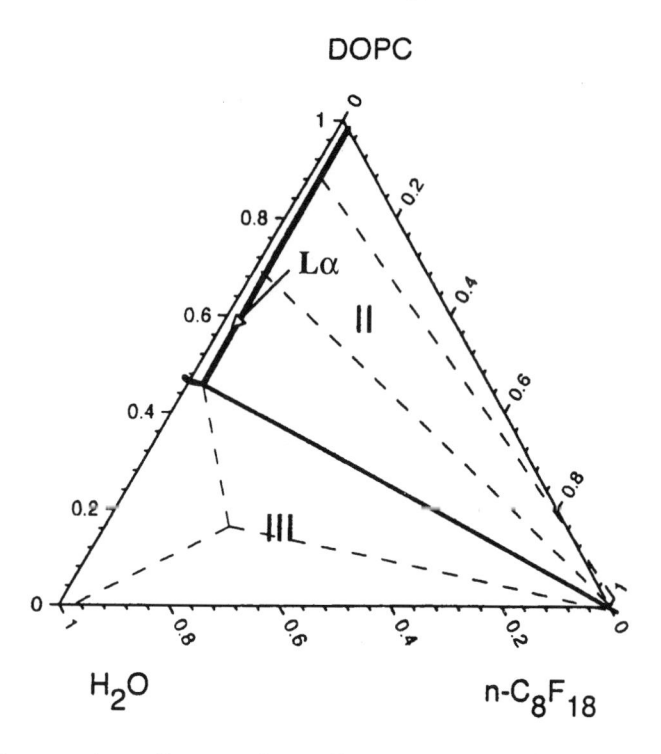

Figure 12 Ternary phase diagram of n-perfluorooctane-water-dioleylphosphatidylcholine (DOPC) at $22 \pm 2°C$. The horizontal dimension of the L_α region is not to scale; the actual C_8F_{18}/DOPC ratio is ca 5.10^{-4} (w/w). Composition ranges above 20% w/w DOPC were not studied. From Kabalnov *et al.* (1996), with permission.

Phase behaviour and complex fluids found in the ternary fluorocarbon/water/phospholipid system

The phase equilibria of unsaturated phosphatidylcholines in water (e.g. dioleylphosphatidylcholine, DOPC) are characterized by the coexistence of a lamellar liquid crystalline phase (L_α) in excess water (Sjölund *et al.*, 1987). The addition of a fluorocarbon oil does little to alter the phase behavior due to effective demixing between the phospholipid acyl chains and the PFC (Kabalnov *et al.*, 1996). Thus, ternary mixtures are characterized by a Winsor III equilibrium of a lamellar liquid crystalline phase in excess water and PFC (Figure 12). The results obtained are actually similar to those found in soybean oil/water/egg yolk phospholipid mixtures (Rydhag and Wilton, 1981).

Friberg *et al.* (1976) have suggested that oil-in-water (O/W) emulsions prepared within such three phase regions may exhibit enhanced stability due to the formation of a lamellar mesomorphic phase at the oil/water interface. Although such stabilization may occur in large emulsion droplets prepared without high pressure homogenization procedures, submicron emulsion droplets are stabilized primarily by a single monomolecular layer of phospholipid, with remaining phospholipid present in the form of small unilamellar vesicles (SUVs) (Groves *et al.*, 1985; Handa *et al.*, 1990; Rotenberg *et al.*, 1991; Postel *et al.*, 1991; Habif *et al.*, 1992; Westesen and Wehler, 1993; Weers *et al.*, 1994b; Meinert *et al.*, 1994). Where PFC emulsions

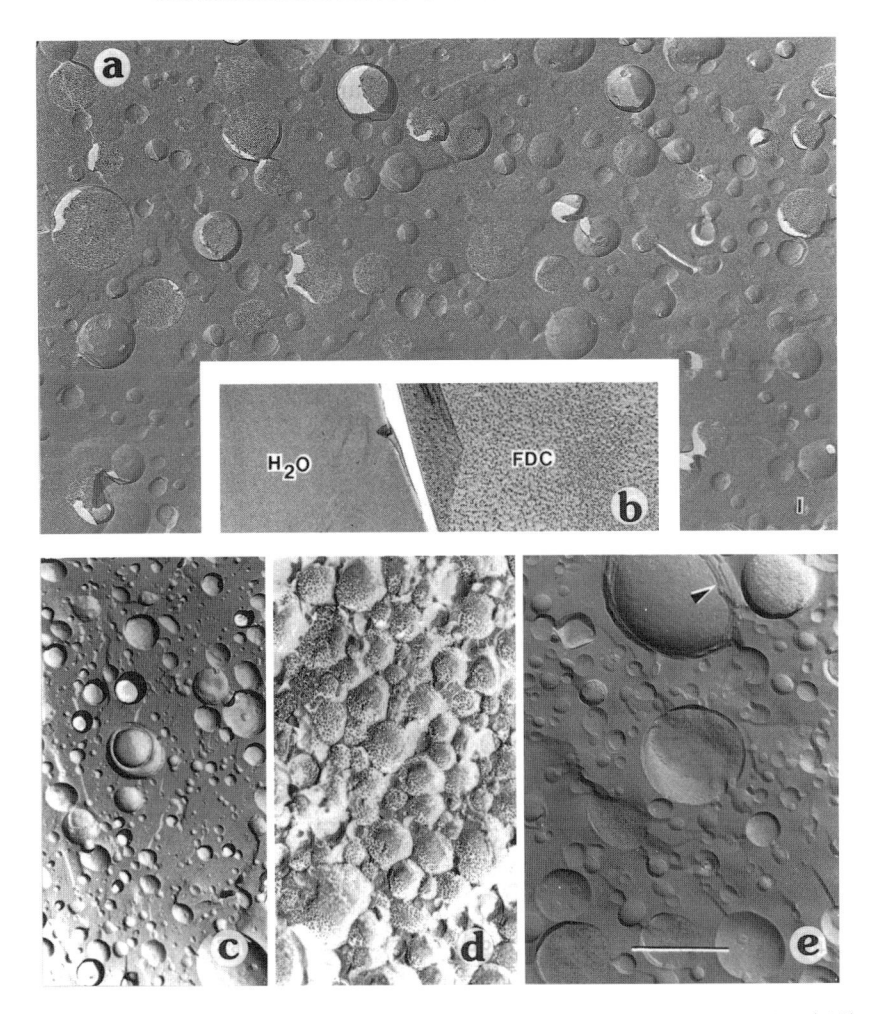

Figure 13 Freeze-fracture transmission electron micrographs (FF-TEM) of a 70% w/v perfluorodecalin (FDC) emulsion stabilized by 8% w/v egg yolk phospholipid. a) FF-TEM of entire dispersion; b) FF-TEM of simultaneously frozen droplets of water (on the left) and FDC (on the right); c) FF-TEM of the supernatant taken after centrifugation of the 70/8 FDC/EYP dispersion; d) FF-TEM of the infranatant taken after centrifugation of the 70/8 FDC/EYP dispersion; e) FF-TEM micrograph of the 70/8 FDC-EYP dispersion showing rare multilamellar ordering on droplets. The bar represents 0.2 μm. From Postel *et al.* (1991), with permission.

are concerned, it has been shown that the amount of phospholipid involved in such free vesicles increases sharply when the EYP/PFC ratio increases (Krafft *et al.*, 1991).

The coexistence of emulsion droplets and SUVs in perfluorocarbon emulsions has been confirmed by a number of independent techniques. Photomicrographs obtained via freeze-fracture transmission electron microscopy (FF-TEM) for a 70% w/v dispersion of perfluorodecalin in water are shown in Figure 13 (Postel *et al.*, 1991). The dispersion is stabilized by 8% w/v EYP. The emulsion particles are clearly distinguishable from the SUVs by their characteristic granular appearance following cross-fracture. Due to large differences in density between the emulsion droplets

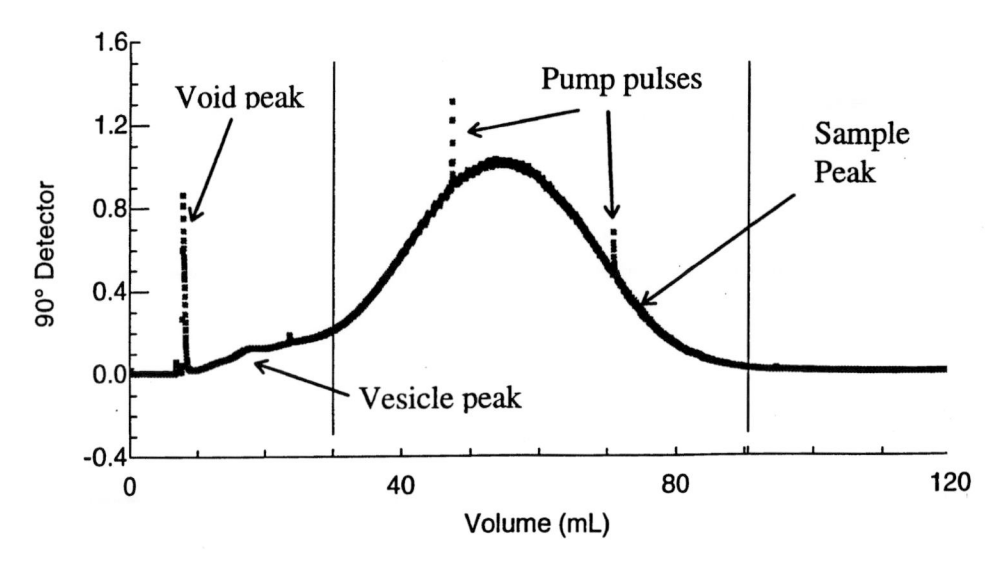

Figure 14 FlFFF/MALLS fractogram obtained for a 60% w/v dispersion of perflubron stabilized by EYP (Oxygent™, Alliance Pharmaceutical Corp., Formula AF0144). Distinct populations of emulsion droplets and vesicles are noted.

and SUVs, these particles may be fractionated via centrifugation. The supernatant containing the SUVs was found to contain no PFC by ^{19}F nuclear magnetic resonance spectroscopy. Partitioning of the electron spin resonance probe TEMPO was also found to be consistent with the presence of SUVs in the supernatant phase. Analysis of the fractionated phases by FF-TEM revealed the SUV's to be in the supernatant and the dense PFC-containing droplets (with characteristic granular appearance) in the infranatant.

Emulsion droplets and SUVs can also be fractionated via cross-flow field-flow fractionation with multiangle laser light scattering detection (FlFFF/MALLS). Figure 14 shows a fractogram obtained for the *Oxygent*™ (Formula AF0144) emulsion (Weers, 1996, unpublished). The broad peak eluting between roughly 30 and 80 mL contains the polydisperse emulsion droplets, while the shoulder eluting between ca. 10–20 mL contains the SUVs. The emulsion droplet size (root mean square radius, rms) ranges from roughly 0.04 to 0.160 µm with a peak at 0.060–0.065 µm. This corresponds to a hydrodynamic median diameter of ca. 0.155–0.168 µm. The population of SUVs has a rms radius of roughly 0.025–0.030 µm, corresponding to a hydrodynamic diameter of 0.05–0.06 µm.

The partitioning of EYP between emulsion droplets and SUVs was also examined in fractionated 90% w/v perflubron dispersions (Weers *et al.*, 1994). Concentrations of EYP in the supernatant and infranatant were determined by high performance liquid chromatography (HPLC). By knowing the median particle size and assuming a monolayer coverage the authors determined the percentage of EYP bound to the emulsion droplets. These results are shown in Table 6. A large decrease in binding efficiency was noted with increasing EYP concentration. Above a certain limiting concentration or surface coverage, additional EYP did little to reduce droplet size. Instead, the additional surfactant partitioned into the SUV particles. It is interesting

Table 6 The effect of EYP concentration on binding efficiency to perflubron emulsions as determined by HPLC (taken from Weers et al. (1994b), with permission)

[EYP] (%w/v)	[PFC]/[EYP]	Median Diameter (μm)	Efficiency (% EYP Bound)	Area/Molecule (Å^2)
2	45	0.38	72	67
4	22.5	0.22	70	63
6	15	0.18	53	63
9	10	0.17	38	63

to note that the area/molecule for EYP remained constant on the emulsion droplets and was independent of droplet size. The value obtained agreed well with the 60–65 Å^2 molecule^{-1} obtained by Rosenberg (1971) for condensed dipalmitoylphosphatidylcholine (DPPC) monolayers at FTBA/water interfaces.

Chemical stability of phospholipids in PFC emulsions

Due to the presence of labile ester linkages and unsaturated fatty acids, chemical hydrolysis and oxidation of EYP are of concern. Hydrolytic decomposition of EYP occurs primarily via classical acid/base catalyzed reactions resulting in the formation of one molecule of a free fatty acid (FFA) and one of lysophospholipid (LPL). Parameters which affect hydrolysis include: temperature, pH, ionic strength, phospholipid headgroup, and fatty acid groups. Intravenous administration of LPL's or FFA's have been shown to have negative effects biologically (e.g. cell lysis, arrhythmia, enzyme inhibition) (Teelman et al., 1984). As a result, the formation of hydrolysis products can limit the shelf-life of PFC emulsions. Song et al. (1994) studied the effect of pH and buffer concentration on the hydrolysis of EYP-stabilized PFC emulsions. Minimum levels of FFA generation were found at a pH of 6.0. Increases in droplet growth with decreasing pH, presumably due to a decrease in the zeta potential as the pKa of free fatty acids is approached, were also reported.

Oxidative decomposition in EYP can occur in unsaturated acyl chains and cholesterol. The measurement of oxidative degradation products in PFC emulsions is a difficult task because of the numerous different products which form. Major degradation products include fatty acid hydroperoxides, aldehydes, endoperoxides, malonic dialdehyde, hydrocarbons, and aldol condensation products. Tarara et al. (1994) showed that the phospholipid composition, degree of unsaturation, PFC purity, and the presence of oxygen and trace metals all have a significant effect on phospholipid oxidative decomposition. Oxidation in PFC emulsions is minimized by the inclusion of metal chelators (e.g. EDTA), and antioxidants (e.g. α-tocopherol) into the formulation.

Alkylglycerophosphorylcholine surfactants have also been reported as stabilizers of FC emulsions (Kaufman and Richard, 1995). These surfactants contain an ether linkage instead of the ester linkage found in natural phospholipids. As such, they are less susceptible to hydrolytic decomposition. The authors claim that these surfactants improve the stability to oxidative decomposition as well. Little is known about the pharmacology of these surfactants, however.

EMULSION FORMULATION

The early fluorocarbon emulsions were often crude and uncontrolled. Inappropriate particle sizes, osmotic pressure, etc., led to toxicities that had nothing to do with the fluorocarbon, although the latter was often blamed for them (Riess, 1990). These emulsions will not be reviewed here. The first emulsion that was developed on a rational basis and in a well-controlled industrial environment was Fluosol.

Evolution of emulsion formulation since the inception of Fluosol is characterized by no less than six significant mutations: 1) the selection as the oxygen carrier of a fluorocarbon having some lipophilic character; 2) the replacement of the poloxamers initially utilized as emulsifiers by phospholipids; 3) a several-fold increase in fluorocarbon concentration; 4) a simplification of the overall formulation; 5) a significant increase in stability, and 6) a far superior ease of use.

The composition of the emulsions that reached some degree of commercial development is seldom fully disclosed. Some of the information available on such emulsions is collected in Table 7.

First Generation Emulsions — Fluosol

Fluosol came as three separate preparations, a stem emulsion and two annex solutions, that had to be combined prior to use (Naito and Yokoyama, 1981; Fluosol, 1990). The composition of these preparations and that of the reconstituted emulsion are given in Table 8.

As indicated above, the choice of perfluorodecalin and perfluorotripropylamine as the fluorocarbons in Fluosol-DA resulted from a compromise between emulsion stability and organ retention of the PFC. The low fluorocarbon concentration was dictated by the desire to maintain proper emulsion fluidity, a characteristic that is no longer preserved at higher concentrations when poloxamers are utilized as surfactant.

Fluosol actually utilizes a three-component surfactant system, consisting primarily of poloxamer-188 accompanied by small amounts of EYP and potassium oleate (Table 8). The poloxamer provides steric stabilization and a strongly hydrophilic coating that may play a role in prolonging intravascular persistence. The anionic potassium oleate introduces negative charges on the droplets, which hinders the flocculation process. The pH is adjusted to physiological values using a carbonate buffer. Proper osmolarity is provided by the mineral salts, glycerol and dextrose.

The formulations of the other first-generation emulsions destined for therapeutic use, Perftoran and Emulsion n° II, are closely related to that of Fluosol. Both are diluted 20 w/v% (ca 11 v/v%) emulsions, with FDC as the principal fluorocarbon. In Perftoran FTPA is, however, replaced by perfluoromethylcyclohexylpiperidine (FMCP) as a stabilizer (Beloyartsev et al., 1983; Ivanitski and Vorobiev, 1993). In view of its molecular weight and absence of lipophilic element FMCP is predicted to have an organ half-life well above 100 days; a half-life of 90 days has been reported (Vorobiev and Ivanitski, 1994). Perftoran uses a purified poloxamer as the sole surfactant and is terminally filter-sterilized. It is only stable for ca one month at 4°C and requires freezing for longer storage.

The 20% w/v perfluorotributylamine/Pluronic F-68 emulsion, Fluosol 43 (Naito and Yokoyama, 1981), later renamed Oxypherol, has been commercially available

Table 7 Fluorocarbon emulsions having reached some stage of development

Trade Name	PFC[a]	Concentration v/v (w/v)	Surfactant(s)	Company	Observations	Status (march 1997)
Fluosol®	FDC/FTPA 7:3	11% (20%)	poloxamer EYP[b] potassium oleate	Green Cross Corp. (Japan)	frozen stem emulsion + 2 annex solutions	approved in US for PTCA dec. 89; discontinued
Perftoran	FDC/FMCP 7:3	11% (20%)	poloxamer EYP	Perftoran Co. (Russia)	high organ retention of FMCP	approved in Russia 1996
Emulsion n°I	FDC/FTPA	11% (20%)	EYP poloxamer	Inst. Org. Chem. (China)	sterile filtered	
Oxypherol®	FTBA	11% (20%)	poloxamer	Green Cross Corp. (Japan)	high organ retention,	for experimental use only; discontinued
FMIQ emulsion	FMIQ	13% (25%)	EYP K oleate	Green Cross Corp. (Japan)		abandoned
Addox®	"FMA"[c] FDN	21% (40%)	EYP	Adamantech (USA)	low PFC definition	abandoned
Therox® **B(40)**	F-44E	40% (78%)	EYP	DuPont (USA)	for research only	discontinued
Oxyfluor®	PFDCO	40% (78%)	EYP	HemaGen (USA)	stabilized with triglycerides	Phase I clinical trials
Oxygent® **(AF0144)**	PFOB (perflubron)	32% (60%)	EYP	Alliance Pharm. Corp. (USA)	stabilized with PFDB[d]	completed Phase II clinical trials

[a] see Table 1 for abreviations; [b]EYP = egg yolk phospholipids; [c]"FMA" perfluoromethyladamantane; [d]perfluorodecyl bromide

Table 8 Composition of Fluosol (Green Cross Corp. Product Information, 1990)

Stem emulsion (w/v%) (frozen)		Final emulsion after reconstitution (w/v%)*		
Perfluorodecalin	17.5	80 mL Stem emulsion		
Perfluorotripropylamine	7.5	+ 6 mL Annex solution C		
Pluronic F-68	3.4	+ 14 mL Annex solution H		
Yolk phospholipids	0.5			
Potassium oleate	0.04			
Glycerol	1.0			
Annex solution C (w/v%)		**Composition**		**Function**
KCl	0.56	Perfluorodecalin	14.0	O$_2$-carriers
NaHCO$_3$	3.5	Perfluorotripropylamine	6.0	
		Pluronic F-68	2.7	
		Yolk phospholipids	0.4	surfactants
		Potassium oleate	0.03	
Annex solution H (w/v%)		Glycerol	0.8	cryoprotector
NaCl	4.29	NaCl	0.60	
CaCl$_2$, 2H$_2$O	0.254	KCl	0.034	
MgCl$_2$, 6H$_2$O	0.305	MgCl$_2$	0.020	ionic balance
Dextrose	1.29	CaCl$_2$	0.028	pH and osmotic pressure control
		NaHCO$_3$	0.210	
all in pyrogen-free distilled water		Dextrose	0.180	

*The earlier Fluosol-DA formulation contained 3% hydroxylethyl starch which came in Annex solution H, and glucose instead of dextrose.

for many years for experimental use. This emulsion is very stable, but its use in humans could of course not be considered in view of the several-year-long organ-dwelling time of FTBA.

Second Generation Formulations — Oxygent

The change from poloxamer-188 to egg-yolk phospholipids led to significantly more stable emulsions. It was also dictated by the better side-effect profile of phospholipids and by the fact that the latter have been in medical practice for parenteral use for some 25 years. Furthermore, the use of phospholipids allowed the preparation of significantly more concentrated yet nevertheless fluid emulsions. The amount of EYP utilized determines to a large extent the size of the emulsion droplets. It is difficult, however, to obtain droplet diameters lower than ca 0.08 μm, and an excess of EYP eventually becomes detrimental to emulsion stability (Krafft et al., 1991). For its second-generation emulsion the Green Cross Corp. substituted EYP for the poloxamer, and utilized FMIQ as the fluorocarbon (Ohyanagi et al., 1990) but did not increase concentration to a significant extent. The new emulsion could, however, be stored in normal refrigerated conditions and was ready for use.

The low fluorocarbon content of Fluosol was regarded as one of the serious limitations of the product. Fluosol contained only about 11% fluorocarbon by volume. The subsequent second-generation emulsions were all three to five times more concentrated (Table 7). The first highly concentrated emulsion was a 100% w/v (52% v/v) perflubron emulsion developed by Long et al. (1989) for both

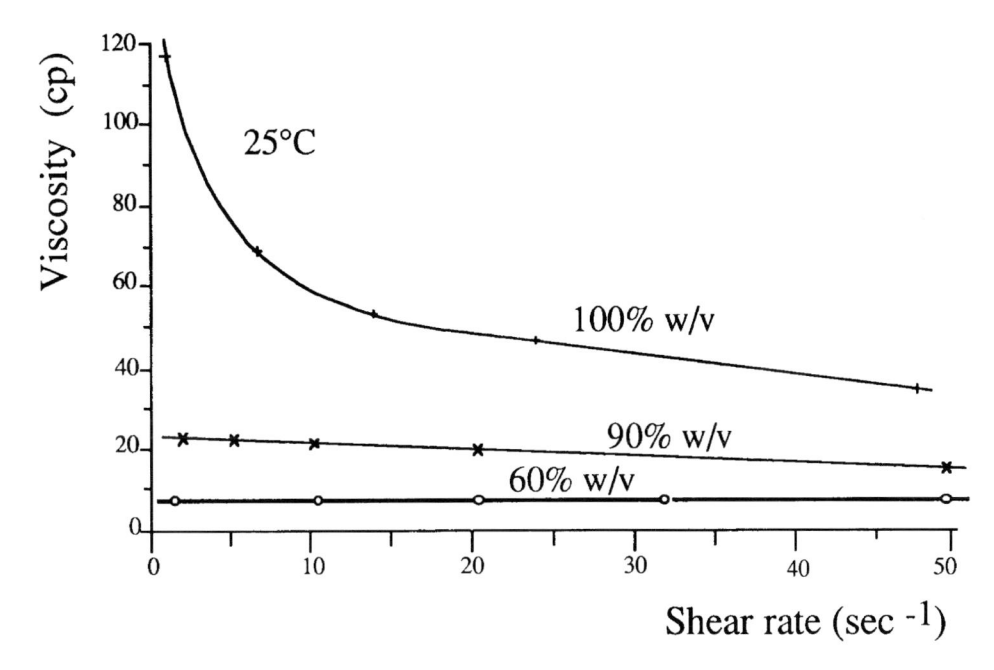

Figure 15 Viscosity at 25°C of variously concentrated perflubron/EYP emulsions, as a function of shear rate. From Riess et al. (1992a), with permission.

diagnosis and oxygen transport applications. It was subsequently shown that a slight decrease in concentration to 90% w/v (47% v/v) led to significantly improved rheologic characteristics (Figure 15) (Riess et al., 1992a). Lesser viscosity is indeed desirable, especially at the low shear rates that are relevant to capillary beds. The rheological profile of the 90% w/v emulsion was close to Newtonian. In addition, it was found that the physical characteristics of such emulsions also depend far less on processing parameters (which facilitates lot-to-lot consistency), that they are easier to sterilize, and that they display better resistance to mechanical stress.

Optimal emulsion concentration depends on the intended use. Some applications may require maximally concentrated emulsions, for example 90% w/v of PFC, to be practical; this is the case for diagnostic applications for which rapid injection of significant amounts of the product is often needed. Military exigencies also favor high oxygen carrying capacity per volume ratios for logistic reasons. For use in perioperative hemodilution, on the other hand, the preparations do not need to be as concentrated. Emulsions with a fluorocarbon concentration around 60% w/v appear to be ideal for this purpose, as they are easy to infuse and still offer greater versatility than the more dilute emulsions. Emulsion viscosity should be low for easy infusion; it is no longer an issue once the emulsion is injected into the circulation, where fluid balance is rapidly reequilibrated.

Oxygent, whose first target application is use in conjunction with surgical hemodilution, is a 60% w/v (32% v/v) concentrated emulsion of lipophilic perfluoroalkyl bromides (Section IV). The principal fluorocarbon is perfluorooctyl bromide (perflubron, PFOB). A small percentage of its higher homologue, perfluorodecyl bromide, is added for stabilization against molecular diffusion (see p. 295 and 302).

pH is controlled through a phosphate buffer, and osmolarity is adjusted using sodium chloride. Minute amounts of an antioxidant, tocopherol, and of a chelating agent, EDTA, are added to protect the EYP against oxidation. EDTA's role is to sequester any transition metal ion that would be present and could catalyse the oxidation process.

Oxygent's formulation is significantly simpler than that of Fluosol. Fluosol-DA contained some low molecular weight hydroxyethylstarch (HES) to support oncotic (colloid osmotic) pressure. Such an agent, which may be needed when exchange-perfusion of animals is practised, does not seem necessary in any of the realistic clinical applications that have been explored so far. HES was actually removed from Fluosol's formulation in, 1984 when the principal target application was changed from whole-blood replacement to PTCA. Glycerin, which was required for cryoprotection since the stem emulsion had to be frozen for storage, is no longer needed in the present emulsions for which this constraint has been removed. The divalent cations, in the form of $MgCl_2$ and $CaCl_2$, present in Fluosol also tend to be omitted in the newer formulations.

HemaGen/PFC added some triglycerides to its formulation for the purpose of improving emulsion stability. An initial attempt to develop a concentrated FDC emulsion using this procedure was, however, abandoned. The lipophilic fluorocarbon α,ω-dichlorooctane was subsequently selected to prepare Oxyfluor, which is now in Phase I clinical trials (Kaufman, 1995).

Several other post-Fluosol formulations have been reported, some of which were available in the 80s for research purposes. Both Therox and Addox were lecithin-based and concentrated. Both emulsions were reported to be shelf-stable for over one year at 4°C. Both products are now abandoned. Lowe et al. prepared a new PFD/poloxamer emulsion that was stabilized by addition of a polycyclic high-molecular-weight fluorocarbon, perfluoroperhydrofluoranthene (Sharma et al., 1989; Lowe, 1994). An experimental emulsion of a radiopaque mixed fluorocarbon-hydrocarbon compound with an internal iodine atom, $C_6F_{13}CH=CIC_6H_{13}$, was reported that has enhanced radiopacity for use as an X-ray contrast agent (Sanchez et al., 1994). A novel perfluorooctyl bromide/EYP formulation stabilized by a fluorocarbon-hydrocarbon diblock (see p. 304) has been elaborated (Riess et al., 1992c; Riess et al., 1994) that is being investigated as a medium for normovolemic organ preservation (Voiglio et al., 1996; Mathy-Hartert et al., 1997). A similar emulsion has been reported but with a poloxamer as the emulsifier (Meinert et al., 1992).

Exploratory work with fluorinated surfactants is briefly reviewed in a later Section for their ability to strongly stabilize fluorocarbon emulsions.

Clinical Side-effect Profile

Concerns about side-effects of the Fluosol-type emulsions were largely dominated by the complement-activation-related reactions attributed to the poloxamer (p. 265). These reactions are no longer observed with the EYP-based emulsions (Hammer-schmidt and Vercelotti, 1989 ; Flaim, 1994).

As indicated, the fate of the fluorocarbon droplets present in the circulation is, as for other particulate matter, to undergo opsonization (i.e. binding of plasma proteins that promote recognition) and be subsequently phagocytized by macrophages (Miller et al., 1976; Yokoyama et al., 1978; Lutz, 1985), which accounts for the relatively short circulation half-life of the emulsion. Most of the fluorocarbon is then distributed in the liver, spleen and bone marrow. Large or repeated doses may lead to hepato- and splenomegaly, and saturation of the RES's clearance capacity (Castro *et al.*, 1984; Lutz, 1985). Similar effects on the RES were observed with other particulates, including certain lipid emulsions (e.g. Schubert and Wretlind, 1987; Fischer *et al.*, 1980; Castro *et al.*, 1984) and liposomes (Beach *et al.*, 1992; Storm *et al.*, 1993; Rudolph, 1994). Although these effects were shown to be reversible and did not cause any permanent tissue alteration in animals even at high doses, they may prevent use of large doses or closely repeated dosing in humans.

Clinical trials with second-generation emulsions have shown a side-effect profile comprised of an immediate and a delayed response, both referred to as mild but rather frequent. The immediate response consisted of skin flushing and occasional lower back pain that occurred during or shortly after infusion, and dissipated shortly afterwards. The delayed response (2–12 h) was described as a flu-like syndrome with fever and occasional chills and nausea (Bruneton *et al.*, 1989; Behan *et al.*, 1993; Flaim, 1994; Kaufman, 1994, 1995). All the symptoms resolved usually within 12 hours. Again, comparable reactions have been described with certain injectable lipid emulsions, especially in the earlier times (Schubert and Wretlind, 1961; Castro *et al.*, 1984) and liposomes (Beach *et al.*, 1992; Rudolph, 1994).

The mechanism of these effects was thoroughly investigated and shown indeed to be related to normal phagocytic removal of the emulsion droplets from circulation (Flaim, 1994). This mechanism is characterized by a dose-dependent stimulation of the macrophages which, during the phagocytic process, release metabolites of the arachidonic acid cascade such as thromboxanes, prostaglandins and interleukins. Both the immediate and the delayed effects could be blocked prophylactically by cyclooxygenase inhibitors or corticosteroids (Flaim, 1994; Kaufman, 1994). A decrease in platelet count was also observed during the early clinical trials (Kaufman, 1994; Keipert, 1995a). All these reactions were transient and fully reversible, and none was considered as posing a toxicologic risk.

These side-effects were significantly reduced with the newer Oxygent formulation AF0144. Fevers became infrequent and did not exceed 1°C, and antiinflammatory prophylactic treatment became unnecessary. Platelet counts also remained within the normal range (Keipert, 1995b, 1997). A Phase I trial in healthy volunteers that was specifically devoted to assessing coagulation/hemostasis and immune function showed no impairment of these functions.

Extensive preclinical safety pharmacology investigations of Oxygent revealed no complement activation, plasma contact system activation, immunogenic or allergic reactions, no platelet or leucocyte activation, no vasoconstrictive or microcirculatory disturbances, and no abnormal effect on liver or lung function (Keipert, 1995b, 1997).

PROCESSING

Preparation of fluorocarbon emulsions involves the dispersion of the fluorocarbon into submicron droplets in a continuous saline phase in the presence of the surfactant. The surfactant is now most generally egg yolk phospholipids. Details on the processing equipment and conditions utilized for producing fluorocarbon emulsions industrially are usually not disclosed. Even information originating from academic laboratories is scarce.

The free energy of emulsion formation, ΔG_{form}, is given by the relation $\Delta G_{form} = \Delta A \sigma^i - T \Delta S_{config}$, where ΔA is the variation in total interfacial area, σ^i the interfacial tension between the two liquids and $T \Delta S_{config}$ is a configurational entropic term that, for a macroemulsion, is negligible when compared to $\Delta A \sigma^i$ (Tadros and Vincent, 1983). Therefore, in most cases, ΔG_{form} is large and positive, which means that it is necessary to supply energy for the emulsion to form and that when it is formed it is thermodynamically unstable or metastable. This is the case for the injectable fluorocarbon emulsions. As a consequence, the characteristics of these emulsions, including those which have an impact on biological tolerance, such as particle size and size distribution, presence of unemulsified fluorocarbon, viscosity, etc., and their stability depend on processing conditions and not only on formulation. Further parameters such as lysolecithin and free fatty acid content and pH can also be affected by processing.

The preparation of fine, narrowly dispersed and stable fluorocarbon emulsions requires emulsification procedures that provide a high energy density, as we have seen that small droplets have longer intravascular persistence and lesser side-effects, and facilitate oxygen diffusion. The impact of various process parameters (temperature, pressure, recycling, preparation and structure of the phospholipid dispersion, sterilization parameters, etc.) on both initial droplet size and size stability need to be determined and controlled. Computer-assisted experimental design, which allows simultaneous assessment of the effect of several parameters, has been utilized for process optimization.

Small particle size fluorocarbon emulsions are now being produced on an industrial scale in compliance with good manufacturing practices. Extensive quality control is required to ensure meeting the specifications set for such products, including batch-to-batch and vial-to-vial consistency. This supposes specific equipment, know-how and professional handling difficult to achieve in non-specialized laboratories.

Emulsification Procedures

Emulsification is usually achieved by applying mechanical energy; sonication is sometimes used for preparing small laboratory samples. First, the interface between the two immiscible phases is deformed to such an extent that droplets form. These droplets are then broken up into smaller ones. The amount of energy that is involved is higher by three or four orders of magnitude than the thermodynamical energy ΔG_{form}. This comes from the fact that the deformation and disruption of droplets require an increase in their surface's curvature (local increase of the Laplace pressure) according to the equation $\Delta P = 2\sigma/R$ (Walstra, 1983). Although an appropriate surfactant can considerably reduce the energy required to obtain a certain droplet size, it is likely that the energy needed to form a fluorocarbon emulsion is higher than in the case of a hydrocarbon emulsion, because of the higher interfacial tension that exist between fluorocarbons and water. Lipophilic fluorocarbons such as perfluoroctyl bromide or perfluorooctylethane are easier to emulsify than perfluorodecalin, for example, perhaps as a consequense of lower interfacial tension. Other important factors affecting the formation of submicronic emulsion droplets include continuous phase viscosity, prevention of recoalescence and Ostwald ripening, and the rate of surfactant adsorption to the interface.

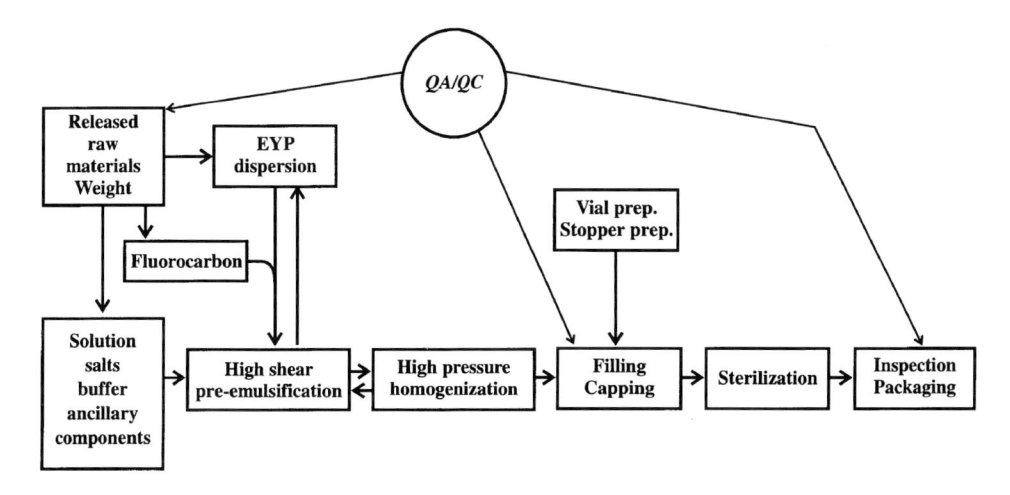

Figure 16 A production flow diagram for fluorocarbon emulsions.

For the presently developed, phospholipid-based fluorocarbon emulsion the first step of the process involves the dispersion of the water-insoluble egg yolk phospholipids in an aqueous phase using a high shear rotor-stator type homogenizer (e.g. Ultra-Turrax) (Figure 16). The fluorocarbon is then injected under stirring in the continuous saline phase, where it is broken down into fairly large droplets. This pre-emulsification step can also be achieved with an Ultra-Turrax mixer, leading to a crude premix with an average particle size of ca 5 μm. Final emulsification is achieved preferably by using a high pressure mechanical procedure (Gaulin-type homogenization, or microfluidization; see below). Subsequent steps involve bottling, capping and terminal heat sterilization. Until the product is bottled, these operations must be performed in a clean room under oxygen exclusion.

Fluorocarbon emulsions destined for biomedical uses have essentially been obtained by sonication, high pressure homogenization and microfluidization. Sonication is based on cavitation, which is the rapid and repeated formation and implosion of microbubbles in a liquid, resulting in the propagation of microscopic shock waves (Basedow and Ebert, 1977). Sonication presents the advantage of allowing the preparation of very small, mL-size batches, which can be of value for research purposes when only small samples of experimental fluorocarbons or surfactants are available. Sonication, however, tends to yield rather wide particle size distributions, and suffers from poor reproducibility since the results depend on such evasive parameters as size and shape of the ultrasonic probe, size, shape and filling of the vessel that contains the emulsion, position of the sonic probe in the liquid, etc. It also often requires subsequent prolonged low-temperature centrifugation to eliminate large fluorocarbon droplets (Sloviter, 1985) and titanium dust released from the sonicator probe (Clark, 1970; Huang et al., 1987). Furthermore, sonication was shown to provoke the release of fluorine as fluoride ions (Clark et al., 1975; Sharma et al., 1988), which means that some degradation of the fluorocarbon occurs during the process. The formation of fluoride ions can, however, be almost supressed if sonication is performed under an atmosphere of carbon dioxide (Geyer, 1975). Degradation of the EYP can also occur. Finally, sonication has little large-scale feasibility. For these various reasons mechanical procedures such as microfluidization or high pressure homogenization are preferable for emulsifying fluorocarbons.

Microfluidization has been introduced as a method for preparing parenteral emulsions in the, 1980's, i. e. relatively recently (Korstvedt, 1984; Lidgate *et al.*, 1989) A flow of crude premix is divided into two separate streams funneled through precisely defined microchannels and these streams are forced to impinge on each other under high velocities in an interaction chamber. The Microfluidizer (Microfluidics, Newton, MA) operates at pressures up to 20,000 psi using a pump operating with a 100 psi air supply. The emulsion is circulated through a cooling coil between passes through the interaction chamber. Microfluidization allows preparation of laboratory-size samples of *ca* 50 mL-up, as well as medium- and large-scale production.

Originally designed for preparing dairy products, the Gaulin-type high pressure homogenization process was invented in the 1890's. The premix enters a valve seat from the pump cylinder at low velocity but under high pressure. This pressure is generated by a positive-displacement pump, and the restriction to flow is caused by the valve being forced toward the seat by an actuating force. The pump provides a constant rate of flow and therefore generates the required pressure as the restricted area between the valve and seat is increased or decreased. (Pandolfe, 1983). A large variety of valves can be used. High pressure homogenizers are easy to control, give narrow particle size distributions and can be operated on very large scales. Small size equipment is now available (Rannie MiniLab, APV Gaulin, Everett, MA) that allows 100 mL- and liter-size laboratory sample production.

High pressure homogenization is the procedure of choice for manufacturing fluorocarbon emulsions on a large scale. Advantages of this technology include GMP compliance design, continuous process, scale-up, recycling and clean-in-place capabilities.

An industrial emulsion production flow-chart is schematically depicted on Figure 16. Consistency in particle size and particle size distribution is achieved through continuous automatic control of temperatures, pressures and mass flows. Nitrogen sparging and blanketing is used throughout the process to minimize exposure to oxygen. Emulsion production is achieved in class 100.000 environment and filling is performed under a class 100 laminar flow hood. High efficiency (99.99%) particle HEPA filters are utilized to remove particulates and microorganisms. Pyrogen-free, automatically monitored, continuously recirculating water-for-injection is used. The product is terminally steam sterilized in a rotary autoclave. Sixty percent w/v concentrated perflubron emulsions are currently being produced in a commercial scale facility. Product consistency is extremely reproducible, resulting in average particle diameters of 0.16 ± 0.01 μm (Chapman *et al.*, 1996).

Recently a novel high pressure homogenizer with small capacity (0.5–20 mL, pressure up to 30000 psi) has become available (EmulsiFlex™ B Class, Avestin, Canada). The sample is introduced through the plug seat and placed under high pressure by a pump activated by a 100 psi air supply. A valve is opened and the sample is pushed through the homogenizing gap at a set pressure which is controlled by a regulator. The reproducibility achieved with this device is much superior than with sonication. It is therefore very useful in the laboratory, in particular to screen new compounds or to perform studies requiring the preparation of a large number of samples. It was also utilized to produce reverse water-in-fluorocarbon emulsions (Sadtler *et al.*, 1995).

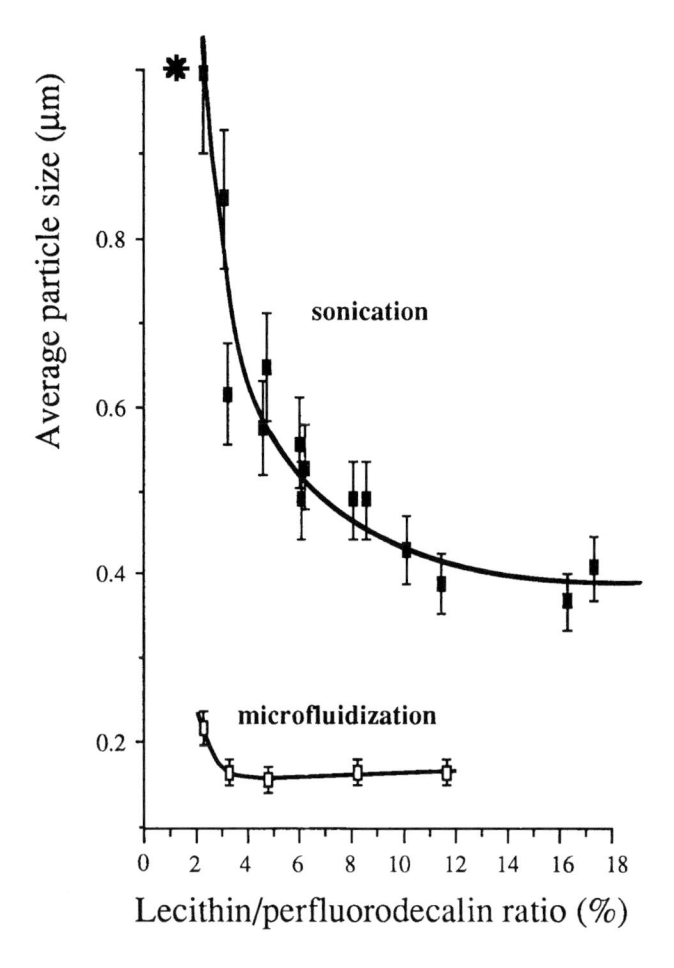

Figure 17 Impact of the emulsification process — sonication vs microfluidization — on particle size of a FDC/EYP emulsion as a function of the EYP/FDC ratio (* only stable for one hour). From Riess and Krafft (1992), with permission.

As noted, detailed information on emulsification conditions are scarce but there exist a few reports in the literature. In one such study, a series of emulsions with a phospholipid/perfluorodecalin (EYP/FDC) ratio varying from 2 to 18 were prepared by sonication or by microfluidization and droplet size was monitored over time (Riess and Krafft, 1992). As shown in Figure 17, for every EYP/FDC ratio, the microfluidized emulsions were consistently finer, more narrowly dispersed, resisted better to heat sterilization, and displayed higher shelf-stability than those obtained by sonication. The superiority of the mechanical procedure over sonication was most pronounced for the lower EYP/FDC ratios. Another study compared, for a given emulsion formulation, the results obtained using sonication, a hydroshear process and high pressure homogenization (Riess, 1990). The finest emulsions and narrowest particle size distributions were obtained by high pressure homogenization. The hydroshear device (Peczeli, 1975) yielded somewhat larger average particle sizes and left more large-size particles. Sonication led to much wider particle size distribution and was poorly reproducible.

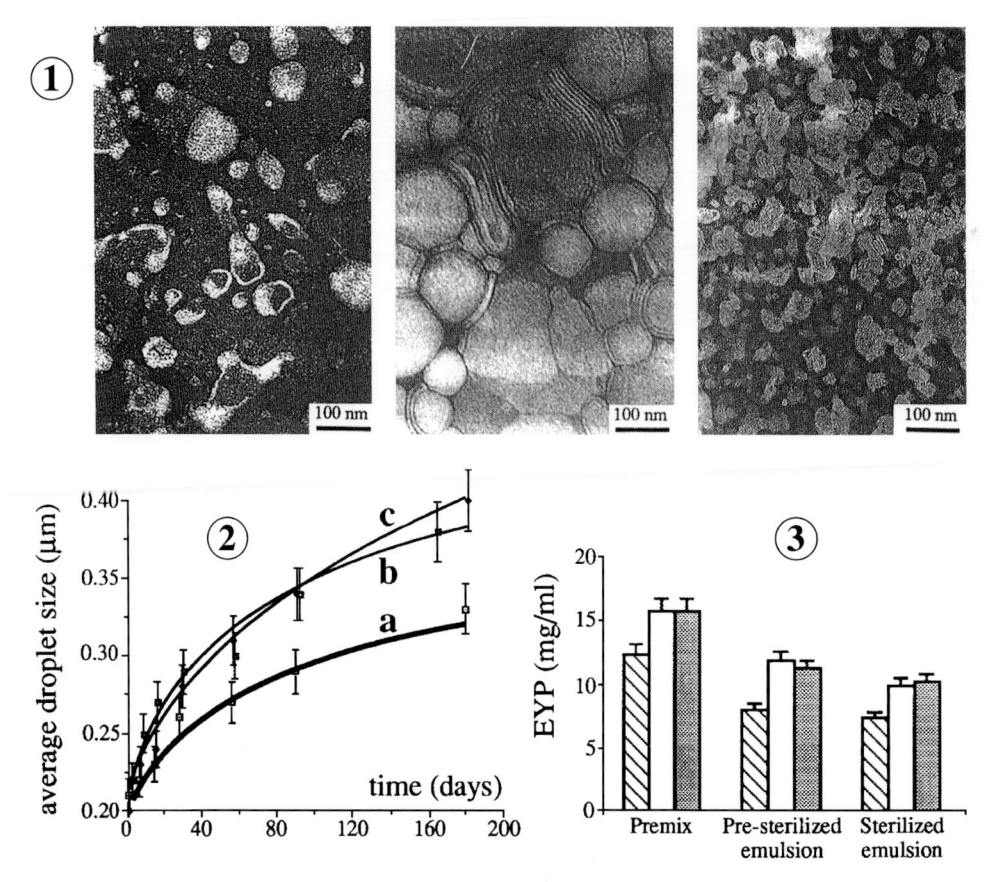

Figure 18 1) Negative staining transmission electron micrographs (TEM) of phospholipid dispersions obtained : (a) by Ultra-Turrax mixing for 1 min at 8000 rev min^{-1}; (b) by Ultra-Turrax mixing for 10 min at 8000 rev min^{-1}; (c) by microfluidization for 15 min at 1000 bars. Sheet-like non-closed layers ("pre-liposomes") can be seen in (a), while there are mainly MLVs in (b) and mainly SUVs in c). 2) Variation at 25°C of the average particle size of fluorocarbon droplets as a function of time in perflubron-phospholipid (90/4% w/v) emulsions prepared from : (a) "pre-liposomes", (b) MLVs and (c) SUVs. 3) Quantitative determination of free phospholipid present in the supernatant of the emulsions. The emulsions prepared from "pre-liposomes" (striped) MLVs (open) and SUVs (grey) were analyzed at each step of their preparation (premix, pre-sterilization and post-sterilization). From Cornélus et al. (1993a), with permission.

Impact of Process Parameters on Drop Size and Size Stability

Structure of the phospholipid dispersion

The structure of the phospholipid dispersion which is prepared at the very first step of the process was shown to have significant impact on emulsion stability (Cornélus et al., 1993a) (Figure 18). Depending on the procedure used and energy applied, the dispersions of phospholipids (4% w/v) can consist of poorly organized non-closed "pre-liposomes", of multilamellar vesicles (MLVs), or of small unilamellar vesicles (SUVs). The perfluorooctyl bromide (90% w/v) emulsion prepared from

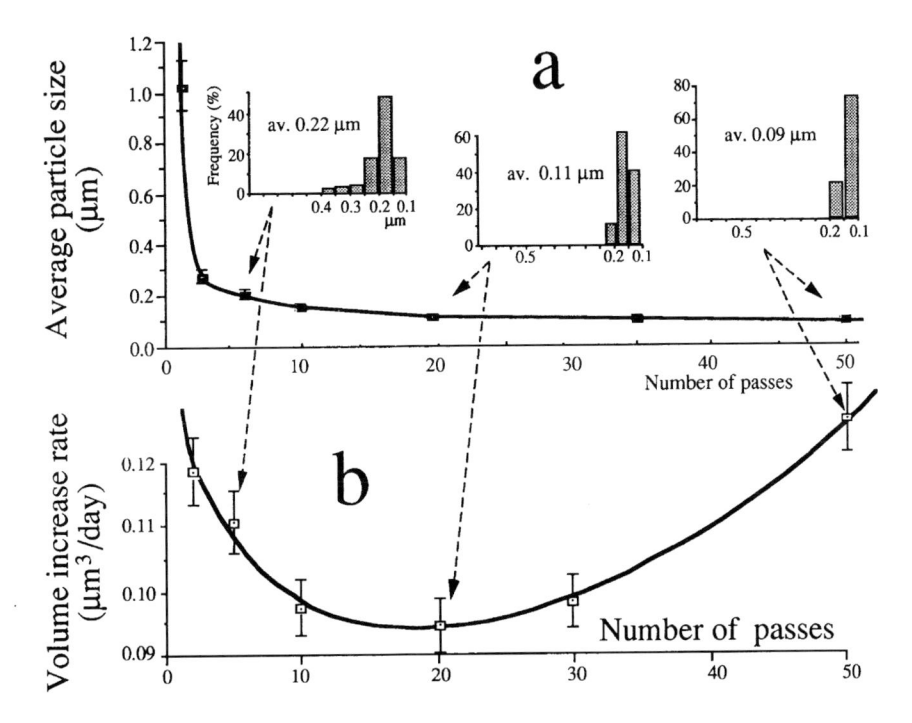

Figure 19 Influence of the number of passes (a) on the average particle size of a perflubron/phospholipid emulsion (90/4% w/v), when measured immediately after preparation, and (b) on particle size increase upon aging showing "overworking" as the number of passes becomes larger than ca 20. From Riess and Krafft (1992), with permission.

"pre-liposomes" was significantly more stable than those prepared from either MLVs or SUVs. The former emulsion was shown to contain less fluorocarbon-free phospholipid vesicles than the other two. These results support previous observations concerning the detrimental effect of free vesicles on the stability of concentrated fluorocarbon emulsions (Krafft et al., 1991).

Number of passes

A series of 90% w/v concentrated perfluorooctyl bromide emulsions with natural phospholipids as the emulsifier (4% w/v) were prepared by microfluidization (Cornélus and Krafft, 1992, unpublished, reviewed in Riess and Krafft, 1992). The number of passes of the emulsion through the interaction chamber ranged from 1 to 50. Emulsion stability was observed to go through a maximum for 15–25 passes (Figure 19). While multiple passes are necessary to obtain a fine and stable emulsion, significant destabilization was observed when the number of passes was larger than 30–40. A lower amount of phospholipid was then present at the surface of the fluorocarbon droplets and there was, correlatively, a larger amount of fluorocarbon-free liposomes. This indicates that excess energy leads to stripping the phospholipid layers from the fluorocarbon droplets. The stripped lipids then readily reorganize into liposomes whose presence has a negative impact on emulsion stability.

Process optimization

Optimization studies were designed to identify the process variables that influence the characteristics of interest, i. e. droplet size and distribution, viscosity, percent of unemulsified perflubron and large droplets, possible formation of breakdown products, etc. They were also intended to determine relationships between process variables and responses. The objective was not to optimize each process variable separately, but to find an adequate compromise under a given set of restrictions. It was also important to reduce the number of experiments needed to achieve this goal, as compared to the approach which consists in changing one variable at a time. Response surface methodology was applied to process optimization of a 90% w/v emulsion of perflubron (Hanna et al., 1992). The E-Chip™ computer program (E-Chip Inc., Delaware) was used to design and analyze the experiments. Process variables were pre-emulsification temperature and mixing time, mixer type and speed, rate of fluorocarbon addition, emulsification temperature, pressure and number of passes. Median diameter seem to be affected significantly by emulsification temperature and pressure, and only marginally by the rate of addition of the fluorocarbon. The percent unemulsified perflubron depended sligthly on the number of passes.

Likewise, Ni et al. (1994) investigated the effects of processing on initial droplet size and droplet growth of 90% w/v concentrated perflubron emulsions. The independent variables examined (and their range) were emulsification temperature (30–60°C), pressure (3000–9000 psi), perflubron concentration (40–90% w/v), fluorocarbon/EYP ratio (22.5–30) and number of passes (4–10). The responses, i. e. initial droplet diameters and droplet growth rates at 40°C, were fitted with a quadratic model of the above five independent variables using E-Chip. The droplet growth rate was seen to decrease appreciably with decreasing pressure. A similar trend was observed for 100% w/v perflubron emulsions (Ni et al., 1992). It was also shown that growth rate varied more or less quadratically with temperature. An optimal balance between number of passes and pressure was determined (Figure 20). To maintain optimal process energy and avoid overprocessing, increase of one of the energy variables requires reduction of the other. Temperature and pressure were shown to have only slight effects on initial particle size; the smallest average initial droplet size was obtained for the higher pressures and lower temperatures.

The effect of processing conditions (temperature, pressure and number of passes) on viscosity of 100% w/v perflubron emulsions was also investigated (Ni et al., 1992). Results show that processing has a large influence on drop size and drop deformability, hence on the viscosity.

Sterilization

Terminal heat sterilization is required for parenteral emulsions to be licensed. Appropriate technology has been established for the lipid emulsions utilized for parenteral nutrition (Figure 21). Detailed sterilization conditions are not publicized by companies who develop fluorocarbon emulsions. A report on the sterilization of 100% w/v concentrated perflubron emulsions shows that standard sterilization is ineffective in providing the required probability of less than one non-sterile unit in 10^6 while maintaining emulsion quality (Dalfors and Espinosa, 1992). Innovative

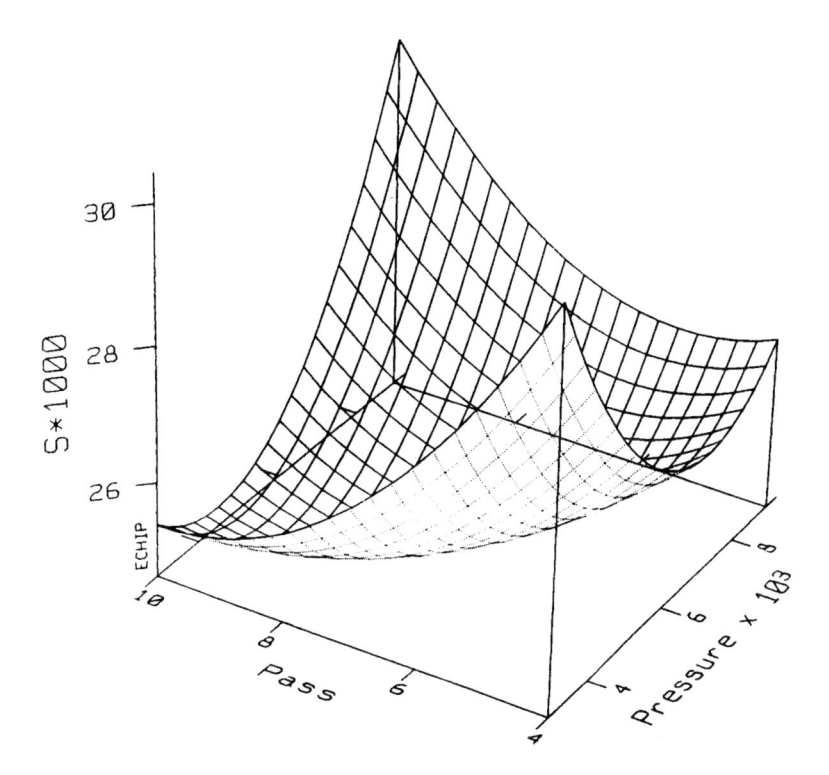

Figure 20 Example of process parameter optimization using response surface methodology (E-Chip). The figure represents the droplet growth for the following conditions : perflubron% = 60 ; perflubron/EYP = 24 and T = 30°C and indicates the optimal conditions in terms of number of passes and pressure. In order to avoid "overworking", i. e. degradation of the emulsion due to excess energy, increase of one of the energy variables requires reduction of the other. From Ni et al. (1994), with permission.

heat sterilization procedures and means of demonstrating sterility have been designed to meet the challenge encountered with concentrated emulsions where uniform heat penetration becomes difficult to achieve. Heat sterilization of an emulsion is a complex technical operation, which requires careful control and validation.

Heat sterilization parameters must also take into consideration the fragility of EYP which is subject to hydrolysis, leading to the formation of by-products when heated in an aqueous medium especially at high or low pH. Some of these by-products, such as lysolecithins, can be toxic. Heat sterilization also has an effect on the emulsion's physicochemical characteristics. For example, the average particle size was reported to increase from 0.12 μm to 0.20 μm for a 90% w/v fluorocarbon emulsion containing 4% of phospholipids, and the distribution of droplet size to undergo significant broadening (Cornélus et al., 1993a). Emulsions stabilized by perfluorodecyl bromide were, however, found to resist better to heat sterilization, and a post-sterilization diameter of only 0.12 μm could be achieved (Weers et al., 1994b).

Such parameters as head space and head space pressure in the bottles, which are often overlooked in research laboratories, also play a significant role, especially on the amount of free fluorocarbon present and on emulsion stability.

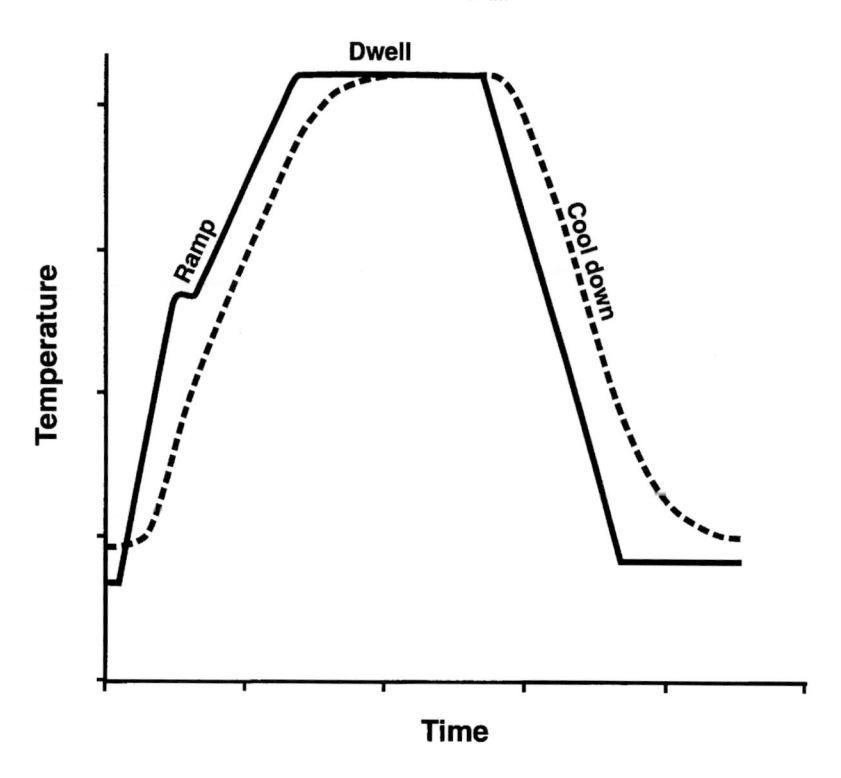

Figure 21 Schematic representation of the sterilization process of an industrially developed fluorocarbon emulsion. Detailed conditions are not publicized. From Chapman et al. (1996), with permission.

Low-pressure filtration (*ca* 0.5 bar) on a 0.22 µm sterilizing PVDF membrane has been examined as an alternative to heat sterilization (Cornélus et al., 1993b). After one year at 40°C the filtered emulsions presented the same average particle sizes than the heat-sterilized ones; they were however significantly more fluid.

EMULSION STABILITY

Instability in PFC emulsions is governed by four mechanisms: Ostwald ripening, coalescence, flocculation, and sedimentation. Of the four, Ostwald ripening is the dominant mechanism leading to irreversible droplet growth during storage. Coalescence governs instability to mechanical stress (often incurred during product shipping), and high temperatures (found during terminal sterilization). Flocculation is generally not problematic unless saturated phospholipid emulsifiers or large excesses of polymeric surfactants are used. Sedimentation resulting from the large differences in density between the dispersed PFC particles and the continuous phase is fully reversible and is not considered problematic. It will not be considered within this chapter. It must be emphasized that as formulators tackle the problems of emulsion instability they must always be cognizant of the biological implications of the formulation changes they make (Postel et al., 1994).

Coalescence

The role of monolayer spontaneous curvature

Emulsion type and stability for nonpolymeric surfactants is controlled to a large extent by the properties of the monolayer separating oil and water domains. Surfactant monolayers are not constrained to a planar geometry but can acquire any curvature or topology which is energetically favored. They also are considered to be "topologically ordered", in that the hydrophilic portion of the surfactant lies on one side of the surfactant film and the hydrophobic portion on the other. Every point on the surface of the film can be explicitly defined by its mean curvature H and Gaussian curvature K. These are related to the principal radii of curvature R_1 and R_2 by equations 1 and 2:

$$H = \tfrac{1}{2}(1/R_1 + 1/R_2) \tag{1}$$

$$K = 1/(R_1 R_2) \tag{2}$$

For spherical emulsion droplets $R_1 = R_2 = R$, and $H = 1/R$, $\kappa = 1/R^2$.

Introducing bends within the monolayer causes the hydrophobic portions of surfactant molecules to either squeeze together (if the monolayer is bending towards the oil phase) or be pushed farther apart (if the monolayer bends towards the water phase). Helfrich (1973) realized the importance of the bending energy E in determining the thermodynamic properties of surfactant films, and derived equation 3:

$$E = 2\kappa(H - H_0)^2 + \bar{\kappa}K \tag{3}$$

where κ and $\bar{\kappa}$ are the bending and saddle splay moduli, and H_0 is the spontaneous curvature. κ and $\bar{\kappa}$ are expressed in units of energy, with typical values for flexible monolayers of approximately 1 kT. For rigid monolayers as found in phospholipid based systems ca 10–100 kT. H_0 depends both on the nature of the surfactant, and on the composition of the aqueous and oil phases it separates. By convention, H_0 is considered positive if the monolayer bends towards the oil (O/W emulsions) and negative if it bends towards the aqueous phase (W/O emulsions).

Monolayer bending properties contribute to droplet coalescence by affecting the thermally activated rupture of emulsion films (Kabalnov and Wennerström, 1996). On a molecular scale the surface of even submicron emulsion droplets is virtually flat. This led to the incorrect conclusion that monolayer curvature does not contribute to emulsion stability. Kabalnov and Wennerström (1996) hypothesized that although emulsion droplets are not highly curved, the monolayer at the edge of a nucleation hole is. According to their model, the film lifetime τ is determined by the activation energy W^* for creating a critical hole in an emulsion film.

$$\tau = f \exp\left(\frac{W^*}{kT}\right) \tag{4}$$

where the preexponent f is a constant. The bending energy penalty involved leads to a strong dependence of the coalescence barrier on the sign and absolute value

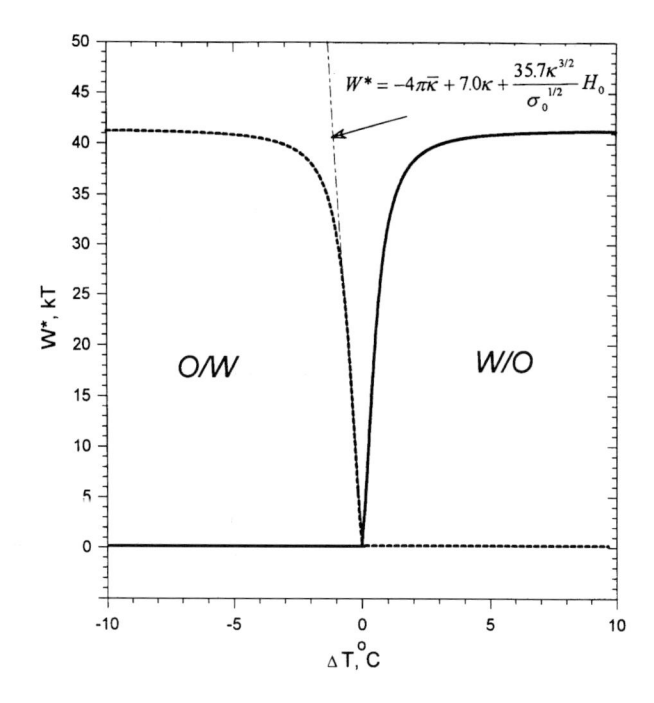

Figure 22 Hole activation barrier, W^*, versus temperature from the balanced point, ΔT, for the n-octane-$C_{12}E_5$-water system ($C_{12}E_5 = C_{12}H_{25}(OCH_2CH_2)_5OH$). Dashed line represents the O/W/O film, while the solid line represents the W/O/W film. The W/O/W film is stable with $W^* = 41$ kT for $\Delta T > 3°C$. The barrier decreases steeply as the balanced point is approached, ultimately leading to film rupture without a barrier for temperatures less than or equal to the balanced point. The mirror image is true for O/W/O films. Adapted, with permission, from Kabalnov and Wennerström (1996).

of H_0. For large positive values of H_0, oil-in-water-in-oil (O/W/O) films are predicted to be stable, with a coalescence barrier given by:

$$W^* = -4\pi\bar{\kappa} + 7.0\kappa + \frac{35.7\kappa^{3/2}}{\sigma_0^{1/2}} H_0 \qquad (5)$$

In contrast, W/O/W films break without a barrier. Conversely, for large negative values of H_0, W/O/W films are stable and O/W/O films break without a barrier. In the vicinity of the balanced state (i.e. $H_0 = 0$), a very steep change in film stability with H_0 is predicted. The predictions of the model are illustrated in Figure 22. The remarkable dependence of emulsion stability in the vicinity of the balanced point has been verified experimentally in the ternary C12E5/n-octane/water system (Kabalnov and Weers, 1996a).

The phospholipid case

Let's now examine the case of phospholipids in more detail. The spontaneous curvature of natural phospholipids (e.g. from egg yolk, EYP) is nearly balanced at

Table 9 Effect of acyl chain saturation on droplet coalescence and flocculation (taken from Pelura et al. (1992), with permission)

EYP	median diameter (μm)	$\omega \times 1000$ (μm^3/month)	η (cps at 1 s^{-1})	free PFOB (vol.%)
E-80-65	0.25	62.1	22.3	4.0
E-80-35	0.24	53.8	27.9	1.0
E-80-3	0.39	155	981.3	0.02
E-100-65	0.22	38.5	21.7	0.04
E-100-35	0.29	34.2	17.9	<0.02
E-100-3	0.30	177.2	1018.3	0.02

the PFC/water interface. Fine adjustment can be achieved by changing the nature of the phospholipid headgroups, the length and degree of saturation of the acyl chains, the composition of the neutral and minor lipid components. Other formulation factors such as electrolyte concentration, fluorocarbon lipophilicity, and temperature also play a role in determining H_0.

As indicated, natural mixtures of EYP contain two principal lipid headgroups, phosphatidylcholine (PC) and phosphatidylethanolamine (PE). PE has a slightly smaller headgroup than PC (headgroup terminus = H_3N^+ vs. $(CH_3)_3N^+$), leading to profound differences in H_0 and equilibrium phase behavior. Whereas PE undergoes a transition from a L_α phase to a reverse hexagonal (H_{II}) phase at high temperatures, PC remains in the L_α phase (Seddon, 1990). Increasing concentrations of PE in PC/PE mixtures adds a negative increment to the spontaneous curvature, thereby destabilizing O/W emulsions (Handa et al., 1990; Ishii, 1992; Pelura et al., 1992; Tarara et al., 1995). Table 9 shows results taken from the study of Pelura et al. (1992), who examined the effect of phospholipid composition and acyl chain saturation on emulsion stability. Large differences in the stability to mechanical stress were noted for the phospholipids (Lipoid KG, Ludigshafen, Germany) containing ca. 20% w/w unsaturated PE (i.e. the E-80 series) relative to the phospholipid containing PC only (i.e. the E-100 series). It is interesting to note that the sample with saturated acyl chains (i.e. E-80-3) also was quite stable to mechanical stress. It appears, therefore, that unsaturation in the PE molecules (i.e. a larger tail volume) is required to effectively destabilize PFC emulsions. This is found in the E-80-35 and E-80-65 phospholipids. The last number in the nomenclature refers to the iodine value, a measure of acyl chain unsaturation. In another study, Tarara et al. (1995) found that PC/PE ratios less than about four dramatically decreased the stability of perflubron emulsions to mechanical stress, ultimately leading to breakage during terminal sterilization for PC/PE = 1. The PC/PE ratio is critical in the formulation of fluorocarbon emulsions since EYP is a natural product whose composition varies between vendors.

The dramatic differences in stabilizing properties between PC and PE has also been observed for submicron triglyceride-in-water emulsions by Ishii (1992) and Handa et al. (1990). These conclusions are, however, not in agreement with earlier studies which had concluded that PC was a poor emulsifier for triglyceride emulsions

(Rydhag and Wilton, 1981; Davis and Hansrani, 1985; Burgess, 1995). These workers hypothesized that minor components (principally charged phospholipids and lysophospholipids) within the natural mixture were responsible for the excellent O/W emulsion stability. Their conclusions were based on studies conducted at planar triglyceride/water interfaces or in crude micron-sized droplets in which the phospholipid was adsorbed from the aqueous phase. Under these conditions the adsorption is exceedingly slow, due in large part to the very low solubility of long-chain phospholipids in water (Kabalnov et al., 1995). The solubility of phospholipids can be approximated from their CMC values, which for dipalmitoylphosphatidylcholine (DPPC) is on the order of 10^{-10} mol L^{-1} (Cevc and Marsh, 1987). Accordingly, the rate of adsorption of DPPC to the triglyceride/water interface can take days. In contrast charged phospholipids and lysophospholipids are readily soluble in water and able to diffuse quickly to the interface. Only in submicron droplets is the diffusion of long-chain phospholipids fast enough to allow accurate conclusions concerning their interfacial properties to be drawn.

For a given phospholipid headgroup, increases in the length and degree of unsaturation of the acyl chains lead to increases in tail volume, thereby decreasing H_0, and destabilizing O/W emulsions with respect to coalescence. Increases in temperature have a similar effect on H_0, increasing the tail volume via increases in the percentage of gauche conformers in the acyl chains.

Minor components within natural phospholipid mixtures can also have a profound effect on H_0. For an extensive review of the effect of various phospholipid types on spontaneous curvature the reader is referred to the excellent review by Seddon (1990). Of particular importance to long term stability of PFC emulsions are the influence of cholesterol and various lipidic oils. In surfactant terms, cholesterol is characterized by a tiny headgroup and a large rigid hydrophobic group (H_0 = negative). The importance of cholesterol levels in phospholipid-stabilized emulsions has been recognized for many years. For example, Corran (1946) found that lecithin (i.e. PC) was an excellent emulsifier for mayonnaise emulsions of the O/W type, while cholesterol favored the stabilization of W/O emulsions. He termed the effect the lecithin/cholesterol antagonism. In PFC emulsions, the addition of cholesterol to EYP at concentrations greater than 10 mol% with respect to EYP, results in breakage during terminal sterilization (Weers and Tarara, unpublished). Similarily, the addition of lipidic oils which penetrate into the phospholipid acyl chains and add a negative increment to the spontaneous curvature dramatically destabilize PFC emulsions. Examples of such oils include medium chainlength triglycerides, diglycerides, monoglycerides, alkanes, and highly lipophilic PFC's. For example, the addition of low concentrations (ca. 10 mol%) of diglycerides leads to phase separation of perflubron emulsions during processing (high pressure homogenization) (Weers and Tarara, 1994, unpublished).

In contrast to the negative increments induced by some minor components, other components provide positive increments to the spontaneous curvature. Included within this group are all single tailed surfactant species (e.g. free fatty acids, lysolecithins), and charged phospholipids (e.g. phosphatidylserine, phosphatidylinositol). Thus, the minor components described by Davis and Hansrani (1981) and Rydhag and Wilton (1981) as being critical for emulsion stability do indeed enhance emulsion stability to coalescence. They are not a prerequisite, however, for emulsion stability. Emulsions stabilized by PC alone are extremely

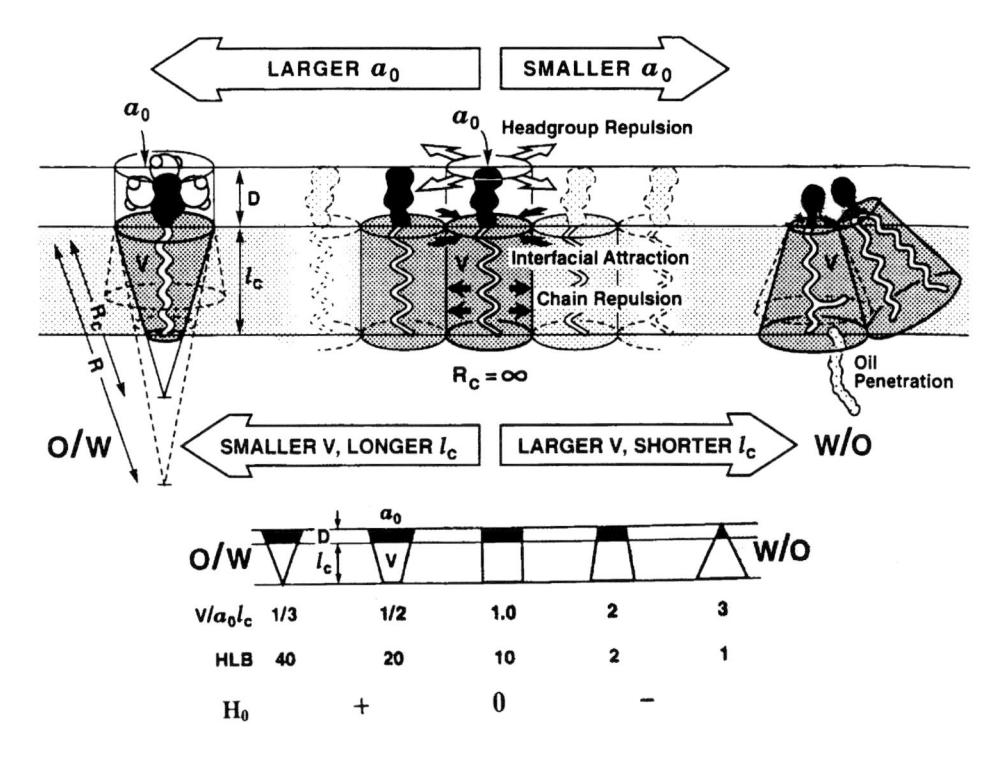

Figure 23 Factors affecting the spontaneous curvature of emulsion films. Adapted from Israelachvili (1994), with permission.

stable with respect to droplet coalescence. The factors affecting the monolayer spontaneous curvature are summarized in Figure 23. The Kabalnov/Wennerström model (1996) provides a quantitative molecular basis for earlier empirical models (i.e. the hydrophilic-lipophilic balance (HLB) method, the oriented wedge theory, Bancroft's rule, and phase-inversion temperature (PIT) concept).

In general, the natural EYP mixture is an excellent emulsifier for PFC emulsions, and coalescence contributes little to irreversible emulsion coarsening on storage. The influence of coalescence is most often observed at elevated temperatures or during product shipping. Care must be taken, however, to ensure that the PC/PE ratio is greater than ca. 4, and that the percentage of cholesterol is low. As well, when formulating highly lipophilic PFC's their stability to terminal sterilization and mechanical stress must be assessed in detail due to potential penetration of these materials between the phospholipid acyl chains.

Steric stabilization with polymeric surfactants

PFC emulsions can also be stabilized with respect to droplet coalescence by the addition of polymeric surfactants which provide a steric barrier preventing droplet contact. This was the approach taken in the first-generation Fluosol formulation (Naito and Yokoyama, 1981; Yokoyama et al., 1982), which contained poloxamer 188.

Table 10 Small angle neutron scattering studies of block copolymers adsorbed to fluorocarbon emulsions (taken from Washington et al. (1996), with permission)

Copolymer	Structure	MW (g/mol)	Bound Fraction	Fraction PO	l (nm)
Poloxamer 188	$(EO)_{76}$-$(PO)_{30}$-$(EO)_{76}$	8,500	0.32	0.16	4.8
+ 0.1 M NaCl			0.22	0.16	8.9
+ 0.2 M NaCl			0.20	0.16	8.7
Poloxamer 407	$(EO)_{98}$-$(PO)_{69}$-$(EO)_{98}$	12,600	0.14	0.26	16.0
Poloxamine 908	$[(EO)_{119}$-$(PO)_{17}]_4 N$	21,000	0.15	0.13	15.2

Washington et al. (1996) used small angle neutron scattering (SANS) to study the adsorption of block copolymers to the surface of PFC emulsion droplets. The emulsions contained 10% v/v FDC, 2% v/v perfluoroperhydrophenanthrene, and 4% w/v polymer. Their results are shown in Table 10. The adsorption of poloxamers at the PFC/water interface is not unlike adsorption onto solid particles since the propylene oxide chains do not effectively penetrate into the dispersed PFC phase. SANS results were consistent with the model that the hydrophobic PO groups adsorb at the particle surface and the EO groups provide a hydrophilic barrier. Differences between different block copolymers were noted, however. A greater fraction of the polymer chain is bound to the particle surface in the case of poloxamer 188 than in the case of either poloxamer 407 or poloxamine 908. The bound fraction for poloxamer 188 is in fact twice as large as the percentage of PO in the polymer, indicating that a significant fraction of the EO groups are also adsorbed to the surface. This also has a large effect on the adsorbed layer thickness, l. In the case of poloxamer 188, l is about three times smaller than in the case of poloxamers 407 and 908, indicating that the hydrophilic brush does not extend nearly as far into solution. The addition of sodium chloride (0.1–0.2 M) was found to significantly reduce the bound fraction of poloxamer 188, leading to a significant increase in the extension of the adsorbed layer. Unfortunately no attempts were made to correlate emulsion stability with l. Crude estimates of the layer thickness in Fluosol 43 emulsions found layer thicknesses for poloxamer 188 on the order of 12 nm (Naito and Yokoyama, 1981). Increased layer thicknesses cannot explain the targeting properties afforded by different polymers. It is likely that there is a complex interplay between structural and biological factors (Davis et al., 1996).

Parfenova et al. (1990) also examined the effect of the nature of the polymer on FDC emulsions. In this case, they examined the force required to achieve droplet coalescence. The results are shown in Table 11. The data show that Proxanol 268 which has the highest molecular mass, has the greatest stabilizing power, while the lower molecular weight Proxanol 226 has the lowest. Proxanols 168 and 456 have practically the same EO group length, but differ considerably in the size of the PO block. These polymers have virtually the same value for the coalescence force. On the other hand, the significantly longer EO chain in Proxanol 268 in comparison with Proxanol 226 results in a significant increase in stability. These results indicate that the length of the EO group or layer thickness is critical in enhancing droplet stabilization to coalescence. Parfenova et al. (1990) found similar trends in surface rheological characteristics.

Table 11 Coalescence forces in FDC emulsions stabilized by block copolymers (taken from Parfenova et al. (1990), with permission)

Copolymer	Structure	MW (g/mol)	$f_c \times 10^6$ (N)
Proxanol 168	$(EO)_{73}$-$(PO)_{28}$-$(EO)_{73}$	8,000	4.3
Proxanol 268	$(EO)_{118}$-$(PO)_{45}$-$(EO)_{118}$	13,000	5.9
Proxanol 226	$(EO)_{38}$-$(PO)_{38}$-$(EO)_{38}$	5,500	3.5
Proxanol 456	$(EO)_{77}$-$(PO)_{77}$-$(EO)_{77}$	11,200	4.9

Although poloxamers significantly improve the stability of PFC emulsions to coalescence at or near room temperature, dramatic destabilization results at high temperatures such as found during terminal sterilization (Johnson et al., 1990). The cloud point of poloxamer 188 is around 110°C, below the normal autoclave temperature of 121°C, preventing terminal sterilization in standard conditions. Johnson et al. (1990) have reported, however, that the addition of 2% soybean oil in a FDC/Pluronic F-68 (20/4 w/v) emulsion raises the cloud point to 128°C, thereby allowing terminal sterilization of poloxamer 188 stabilized FDC emulsions. The role that soybean oil in a FDC/Pluronic F-68 (20/4 w/v) emulsion plays in increasing the polymer's cloud point temperature and emulsion stability is not clearly understood at this time.

Ostwald Ripening

The principal mechanism of irreversible droplet growth in PFC emulsions during storage is Ostwald ripening (Davis et al., 1981; Riess, 1984; Kabalnov et al., 1985; Kabalnov and Shchukin, 1992; Trevino et al., 1993). Ostwald ripening occurs via molecular diffusion of individual PFC molecules through the continuous phase. The driving force for the ripening is the small difference in disperse phase chemical potential which exists between different droplets due to differences in their radii of curvature, i.e. the Kelvin effect (W. Thomson a.k.a. Lord Kelvin, 1870). Smaller, more highly curved droplets have a higher capillary pressure and hence a greater local concentration of disperse phase in their vicinity, viz:

$$C(a) = C(\infty) \exp \frac{2\sigma^i V_m}{RTa} \approx C(\infty) \left(1 + \frac{2\sigma^i V_m}{RTa}\right) \qquad (6)$$

where σ^i is the interfacial tension between the dispersed and continuous phases, V_m is the molar volume of the fluorocarbon, R is the molar gas constant, T is the absolute temperature, $C(a)$ is the solubility surrounding a particle of radius a, and $C(\infty)$ is the bulk phase solubility. Molecular diffusion of fluorocarbon away from the smaller droplets leads to the growth of the larger drops and diminuation in size of the small ones. The differences in chemical potential are substantial only for submicron droplets. Accordingly, Ostwald ripening does not lead to phase separation. Emulsion breakage can occur only by coalescence-mediated droplet growth.

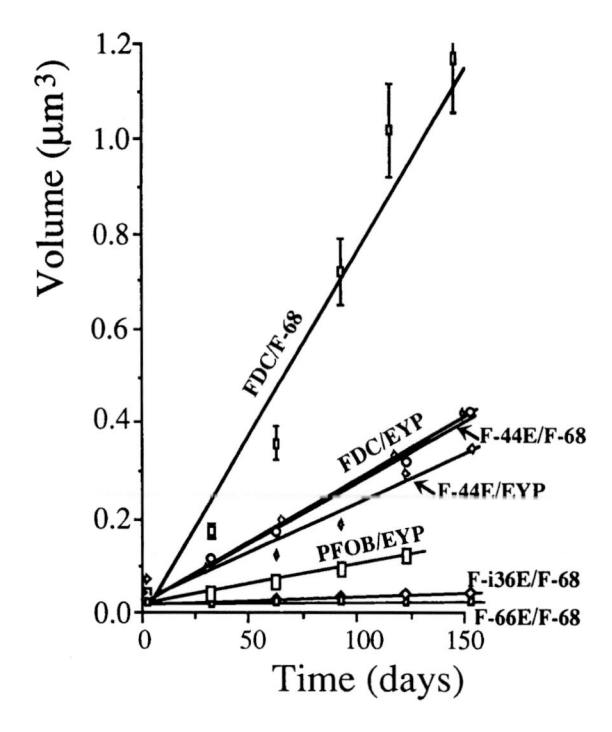

Figure 24 Cubic dependence of emulsion growth rates for diverse fluorocarbons as a function of time illustrating the dramatic dependence of emulsion stability on the nature of the fluorocarbon and surfactant. Taken from Krafft et al. (1992), with permission. FDC: perfluorodecalin (MW 462); F-44E: bis(perfluorobutyl)ethene (MW 464); PFOB: perfluorooctyl bromide (MW 499); F-i36E: (perfluoroisopropyl)(perfluorohexyl)ethene (MW 514); F-66E: bis(perfluorohexyl)ethene (MW = 664); F-68: pluronic F-68; EYP: egg yolk phospholipids.

Lifshitz-Slezov-Wagner (LSW) theory

Particle growth in submicron fluorocarbon emulsions can usually be accurately described in terms of the Lifshitz-Slezov-Wagner (LSW) theory (Lifshitz and Slezov, 1958; Wagner, 1961), which predicts that linear growth rates can be obtained from plots of the cube of the number average droplet radius versus time, viz:

$$\frac{d}{dt}(\bar{a}^3) = \omega = \frac{8\sigma^i DC(\infty) V_m}{9RT} \gamma(\phi) \quad (7)$$

where ω is the Ostwald ripening growth rate, $\bar{a}$ is the mean number droplet radius, D is the diffusion coefficient for the dispersed fluorocarbon phase in the continuous aqueous phase, and the factor $\gamma(\phi)$ reflects the dependence of ω on the dispersed phase volume fraction, ϕ. Figure 24 shows a typical plot of the cubic dependence $\bar{a}$ with time for a few different PFCs. It should be noted, however, that the LSW equation does not take into account the structure of the interfacial film and that it requires the two phases to be isotropic, which may not necessarily be the case, especially near the interface, for example for a multicomponent fluorocarbon phase or surfactant system.

Table 12 Water solubilities of fluorocarbons (adapted from Kabalnov et al. (1990), with permission)

Fluorocarbon	Acronym	S (mol L^{-1})
n-C$_5$F$_{12}$		4.0 × 10^{-6}
n-C$_6$F$_{14}$		2.7 × 10^{-7}
n-C$_7$F$_{16}$		3.1 × 10^{-8}
n-C$_8$F$_{18}$	PFO	3.9 × 10^{-9}
⋏⋏ [a]		5.0 × 10^{-7}
⋏⋏		2.5 × 10^{-9}
◯-		6.7 × 10^{-7}
⋋◯-		2.2 × 10^{-9}
⋋◯-		5.1 × 10^{-10}
◯◯		2.2 × 10^{-6}
◯◯	FDC	9.9 × 10^{-9}
◯N-◯-	FMCP	6.5 × 10^{-10}
N(C$_2$F$_5$)$_3$		1.2 × 10^{-7}
N(C$_3$F$_7$)$_3$	FTPA	2.8 × 10^{-10}
C$_8$F$_{17}$Br	PFOB, perflubron	5.1 × 10^{-9}
C$_{10}$F$_{21}$Br	PFDB	5.0 × 10^{-11}
C$_8$F$_{17}$-C$_2$H$_5$	PFOE, F8H2	7.7 × 10^{-9}
C$_6$F$_{13}$-C$_{10}$H$_{21}$	F6H10	3.4 × 10^{-11}
C$_8$F$_{17}$-C$_8$H$_{17}$	F8H8	5.1 × 10^{-12}

[a]all carbons are perfluorinated in all structures

The effect of the nature of the fluorocarbon

During the early stages of blood substitute research it was recognized that the nature of the PFC played a key role in the resulting emulsion stability (Geyer, 1973; Clark and Moore, 1982; Riess and Le Blanc, 1982). Whereas emulsions of FTBA were found to be stable for periods of years, emulsions of FDC degraded within a matter of days to weeks. It wasn't until Davis et al. (1981) proposed that fluorocarbon emulsions were degraded by Ostwald ripening that the remarkable dependence on fluorocarbon physical properties began to be realized.

Of the parameters in equation 7, only $C(\infty)$ varies significantly between PFCs. The determination of $C(\infty)$ for a range of PFCs is problematic, however, because the values are often below the limits of quantitation of conventional analytical methodologies. Kabalnov et al. (1990) estimated $C(\infty)$ of PFCs from their emulsion growth rates using equation 7 (Table 12). Values range from ca. 10^{-6} mol L^{-1} to

10^{-12} mol L^{-1} depending upon structure. As a general rule of thumb, $C(\infty)$ decreases by a factor of eight with each added CF$_2$ group in a homologous series. The introduction of ether oxygens or tertiary amine nitrogens also decreases $C(\infty)$ by about two-fold, while the introduction of halogens (Br or Cl) leads to only small reductions in solubility. Alternatively, the presence of rings or unsaturation leads, for a given number of carbon atoms, to increases in the water solubility of FCs.

Two-component disperse phases

The instability observed for emulsions containing a moderately water soluble PFC can be corrected by the addition of a small amount of a secondary PFC which has little or no solubility in water (Higuchi and Misra, 1962). In this case, the mass transfer resulting from differences in capillary pressure alters the relative composition of small and large droplets, with the small droplets becoming enriched in the insoluble component and the large droplets being enriched in the faster diffusing soluble component. Eventually the mass transfer stops when the compositional effect compensates for the difference in capillary pressures. This principle was first applied to PFC emulsions by Davis et al. (1981).

A detailed theoretical analysis of Ostwald ripening in two component disperse phase systems was published by Kabalnov et al. (1987). Their predictions have been verified experimentally for perfluorooctyl bromide/perfluorodecyl bromide (PFOB/PFDB) emulsions by Weers and Arlauskas (1995). These authors used sedimentation field-flow fractionation (SdFFF) to separate the polydisperse emulsion droplet population into monodisperse fractions. They then analyzed the fractions for FC content by gas chromatography, showing the predicted component partitioning in different sized droplets. The rate of Ostwald ripening in two-component disperse phases can be approximated by (Kabalnov et al., 1987):

$$\omega_{mix} = (\phi_1/\omega_1 + \phi_2/\omega_2)^{-1} \qquad (8)$$

where ϕ is the volume fraction, and the subscripts 1 and 2 denote the medium soluble component and medium insoluble component, respectively. Equation 8 provides an excellent fit for the decrease in Ostwald ripening rate observed for example in PFOB emulsions stabilized by the addition of PFDB (Figure 25).

The effect of the nature of the surfactant

The nature of the surface active agent also plays an important role in determining the rate of Ostwald ripening. This is illustrated in Figure 25 where the two primary emulsifiers used in PFC emulsions (poloxamer 188 and EYP) are compared (Krafft et al., 1992). For a given PFC, emulsions stabilized by poloxamer 188 grow as much as an order of magnitude faster than those stabilized by EYP (Kabalnov et al., 1995). According to equation 7, the primary manner in which surfactants reduce Ostwald ripening is via reductions in σ^i. The value of σ^i for poloxamer 188 is ca 30 mN m^{-1}, while the value for EYP is a matter of some debate. Burgess and Yoon (1995) reported values of ca. 50 mN m^{-1} for DPPC at F-44E/water interfaces. In contrast, Pelura et al. (1992) when using a spreading solvent (chloroform) to effectively distribute EYP at the PFOB/water interface obtained a value of ca 5 mN m^{-1}. This

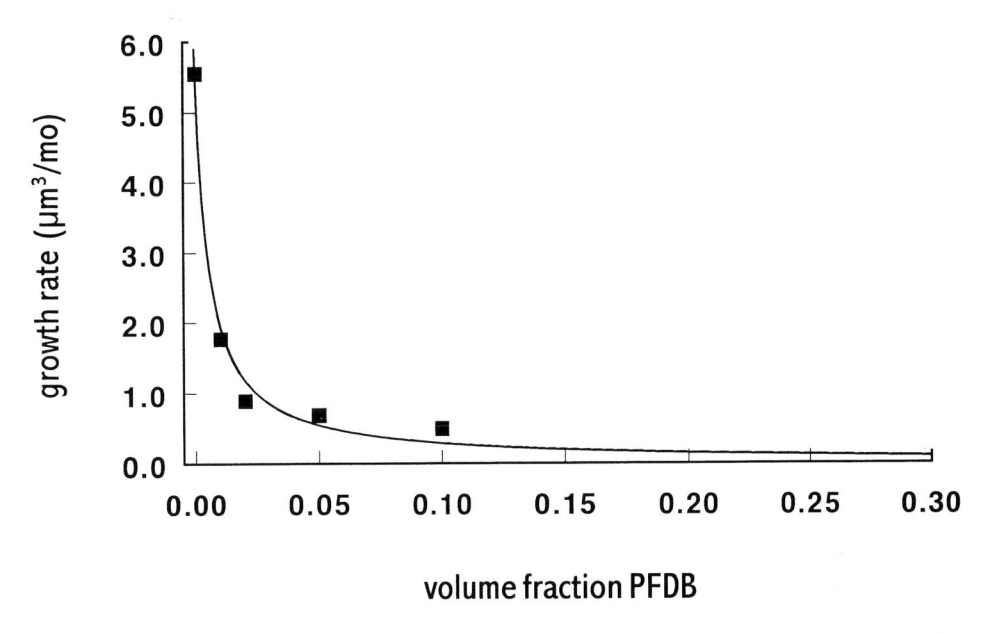

Figure 25 Growth rate vs volume fraction of PFDB in 90% w/v PFOB/PFDB emulsions (T = 40°C). The emulsions are stabilized by 4% w/v EYP. The fit to the experimentally derived points is provided by equation 8. Adapted from Weers et al. (1994), with permission.

value agrees well with studies in which the phospholipid is soluble in the oil phase and able to quickly diffuse to the oil/water interface (see e.g. Li et al., 1996).

The apparent controversy regarding the surface activity of phospholipids is related to the extremely slow kinetics found for phospholipids dispersed in water as they adsorb to planar oil/water interfaces. As discussed previously, Kabalnov et al. (1995) argue that interfacial tension measurements for long-chain phospholipids were usually made under nonequilibrium conditions. These authors estimated the interfacial tension of long-chain phosphatidylcholines via extrapolation of data for short-chain phosphatidylcholines, as shown in Figure 26. Clearly, the equilibrium interfacial tension value is decreasing with increasing chainlength and the value for long-chain phospholipids such as DPPC is likely to be less than 4 mN m^{-1}. The effect of interfacial tension on the rate of Ostwald ripening of perflubron emulsions for a series of water soluble (fast diffusing) surfactants is shown in Figure 27 (Kabalnov et al., 1995). A roughly linear dependence is noted in accordance with LSW theory. Based on the known Ostwald ripening rate for EYP stabilized emulsions, the extrapolated σ value (Figure 27) is on the order of 1 mN m^{-1}.

The relatively low value of the PFC/water interfacial tension found for EYP (1–5 mN m^{-1}) is not surprising in view of the spontaneous curvature of the surfactant film. As discussed previously, solutions of long-chain phospholipids in water result in the formation of a two phase region of lamellar phase in excess water. The lamellar phase consists of planar bilayers of surfactant with low net curvatures. In terms of spontaneous curvature, long chain phospholipids are close to the "balanced state" (i.e. $H_0 = 0$). In the vicinity of the balanced state surfactants show a very steep minimum in the interfacial tension. For microemulsions this minimum can be as

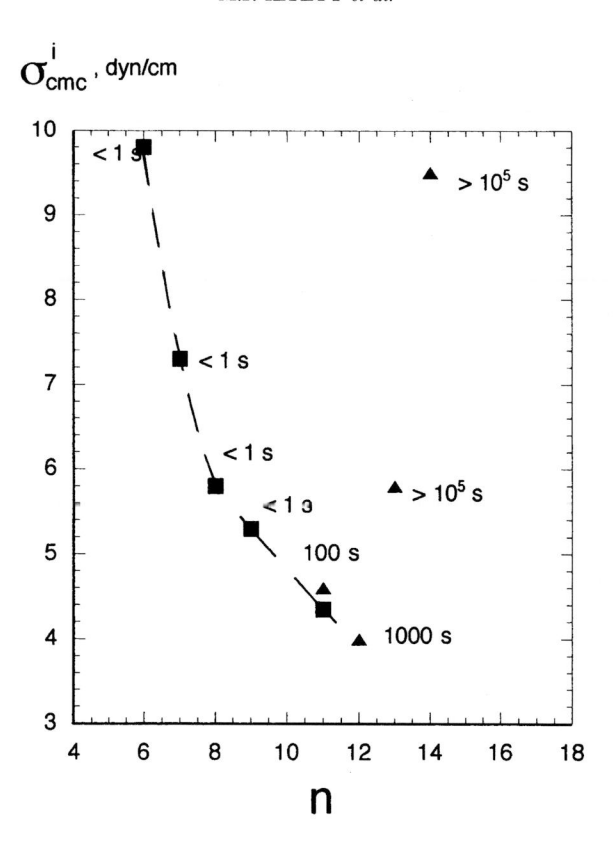

Figure 26 Ultimate interfacial tensions σ^i_{cmc} vs phospholipid chainlength n at the perflubron/water interface (▲: plate; ⊓⊔: ring). The approximate equilibration time is indicated on the plot near the experimental points. From Kabalnov et al. (1995), with permission.

low as 10^{-3} or 10^{-4} mN m^{-1} (Binks, 1993). The minimum in interfacial tension in the balanced state has been attributed to a zeroing of the "frustration bending energy" contribution to the interfacial tension (by frustrated we mean that the curvature of the surfactant monolayer is forced to a value different from the spontaneous curvature) and is given by (de Gennes and Taupin, 1982, Guest and Langevin, 1985, Binks et al., 1989, Strey, 1994):

$$\sigma^i_{cmc} = \frac{2\kappa^2}{\kappa + \bar{\kappa}/2} H_0^2 \tag{9}$$

Assuming that $\kappa \approx \bar{\kappa} \approx 10-100$ kT and $H_0 \approx 0.1$ nm^{-1}, equation 9 yields a value of the interfacial tension on the order of a few mN m^{-1}, in close agreement with experiment.

It has also been hypothesized that changes in the composition of the interfacial layer may alter diffusion of PFC through the interface. Interfacially controlled molecular diffusion would deviate significantly from LSW theory and be characterized by a quadratic scaling of the average radius with time (Kahlweit, 1970). Quadratic scaling has not been observed even with surfactants possessing ultralow CMC values,

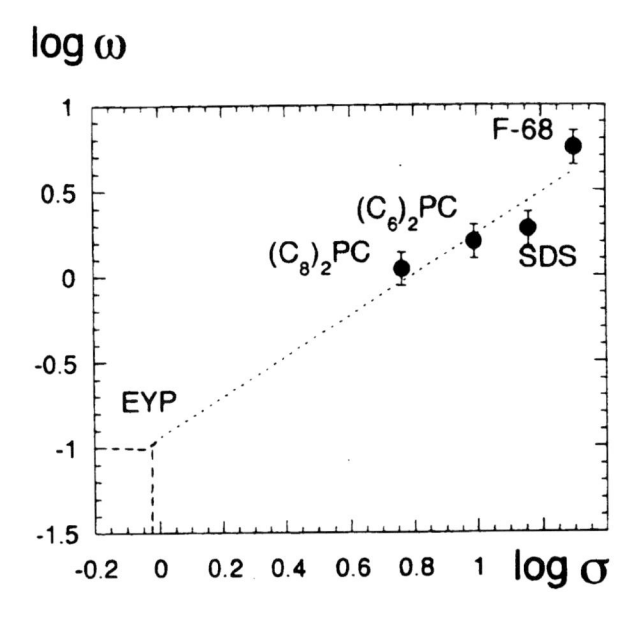

Figure 27 Ostwald ripening rate, w, for PFOB emulsions vs interfacial tension at the PFOB/water interface. Various surfactants were studied including: Pluronic F-68 (F-68), sodium dodecylsulfate (SDS), dihexanoylphosphatidylcholine ((C_6)$_2$PC), dioctanoylphosphatidylcholine ((C_8)$_2$PC), and egg yolk phospholipids (EYP). An estimate of the EYP interfacial tension on the basis of this plot (assuming $\omega = 0.1$ nm^{3}s^{-1}) is 1 mN m^{-1}. From Kabalnov et al. (1995), with permission.

indicating that Ostwald ripening is indeed controlled by the molecular diffusion of the dispersed PFC. For a detailed theoretical description of the requirements for restricted diffusion through the interface the work of Kabalnov et al. (1995) should be consulted.

Fluorinated surfactants

Another means of obtaining highly stable PFC emulsions is to use fluorinated surfactants. XMO-10 provided excellent stabilization of PFC emulsions due to its high surface activity (Clark et al., 1983); however, such emulsions were never developed commercially, probably because of biocompatibility issues.

When used alone, certain fluorinated surfactants are superior stabilizers of PFC emulsions (Figure 28). As compared to poloxamer 188, stability to Ostwald ripening is significantly increased due to strong reduction in interfacial tension. Although excellent emulsion stability can be achieved with some fluorinated surfactants, this is not always the case. For example, recent studies examined the stabilizing properties of three sugar-based perfluoroalkylated surfactants in perflubron emulsions (Riess et al., 1992b). The first two contained nonionic disaccharide moieties (maltose and trehalose) which differed primarily in the point of attachment of the two sugar groups, and consequently in polar headgroup conformation and hydration. The third surfactant was anionic in nature due to the presence of a charged phosphate

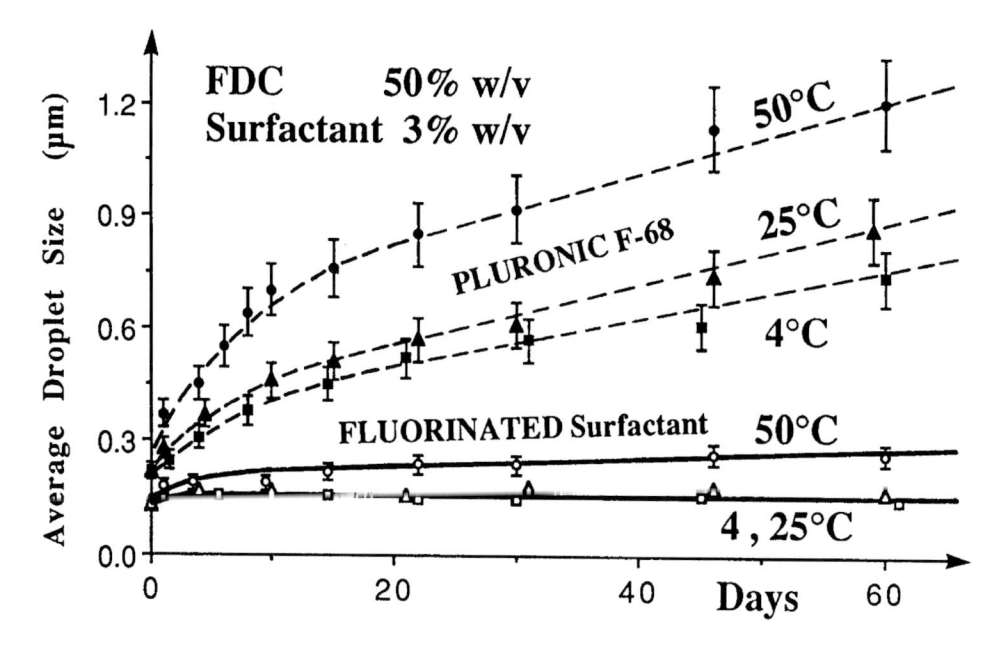

Figure 28 Particle size increase at 4, 25 and 50°C of a 50 w/v% emulsion of perfluorodecalin by a fluorinated surfactant, $C_8F_{17}C_2H_4$-(α,α-trehalose-6), as compared to Pluronic F-68. From Riess et al. (1992b), with permission.

group (glucose phosphate ester). Whereas both the neutral trehalose ester and the negatively charged glucose phosphate ester surfactants were able to very effectively stabilize O/W emulsions, the maltoside surfactant would not even allow for the formation of an emulsion. The observed differences for the three surfactants are likely to be related to the spontaneous curvature of the surfactant monolayer. Due to electrostatic repulsions between the charged headgroups, the glucose phosphate ester is characterized by a large headgroup and small tail (H_0 = positive). Such a geometry favors stabilization of O/W emulsions. The differences between the nonionic surfactants are more curious and difficult to rationalize, but might be related to the geometry of the two sugar groups relative to the fluorinated chain. According to molecular modeling studies the disaccharide moiety is positioned approximately orthogonal to the perfluoroalkyl chain for the trehalose ester, and nearly linear with respect to the perfluoroalkyl chain for the maltose derivative (Weers and Lee, 1996, unpublished). Because these molecules contain rigid cyclic moieties, they are not able to alter their conformation appreciably. As well, it is known that the hydration of isomeric sugars can be significantly different. In terms of surfactant shapes the trehalose ester surfactant is likely to have a wedge-like shape, favorable for stabilization of O/W emulsions, while the maltoside surfactant is nearly cylindrical (i.e. close to balanced), a condition which favors emulsion break. Thus, the observed patterns in emulsion stability found for fluorinated surfactants may also correlate with differences in spontaneous curvature.

Seldom does a single surfactant possess all of the attributes required for emulsion stabilization. Fluosol for example contains three surfactants: poloxamer 188 for effective steric stabilization, EYP for lowering the surface tension and adjusting H_0,

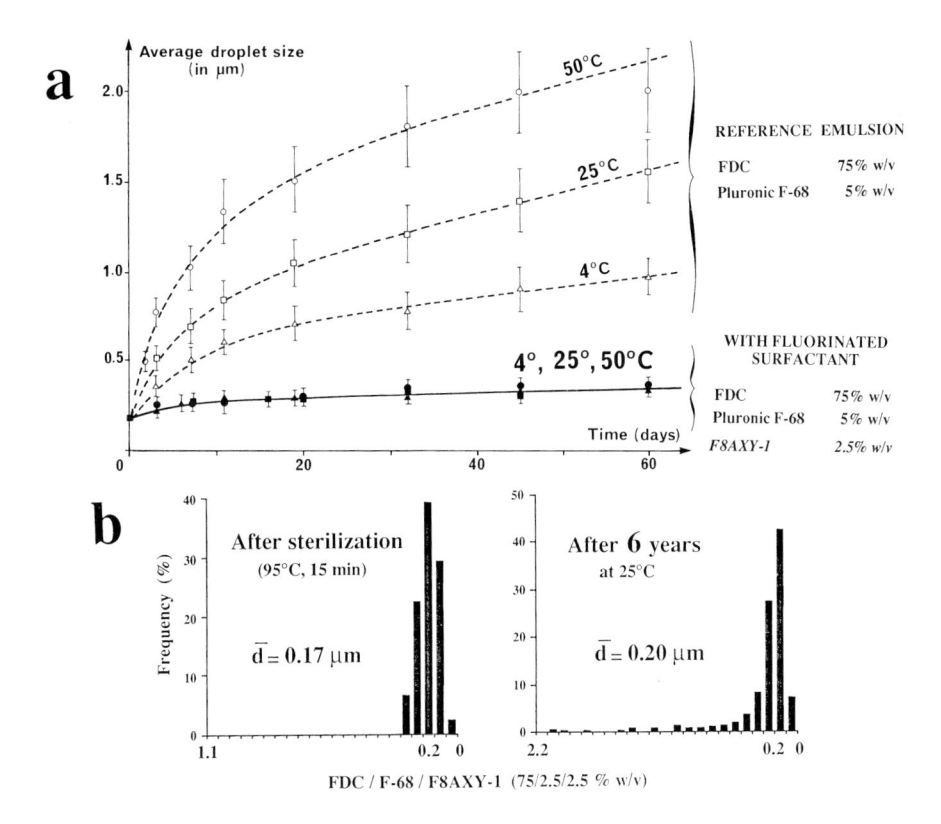

Figure 29 a) Increase in stability of a 75% w/v perfluorodecalin/5% Pluronic F-68 emulsion when one-half of the Pluronic is replaced by a perfluoroalkylated xylitol-derived surfactant, C$_8$F$_{17}$CH$_2$CH=CH-(xylitol-1) (F8AXY-1). b) Particle size histograms measured after sterilization and six years later. From Zarif et al. (1989), with permission.

and potassium oleate for providing electrostatic repulsion between droplets. The nature of the interfacial layer also plays an important role in particle clearance and biocompatibility. Excellent synergistic activity has been noted for mixtures of either EYP (Milius et al., 1992) or poloxamer 188 (Zarif et al., 1989) with fluorinated surfactants (Figure 29).

Mixtures of poloxamer 188 and fluorinated surfactants combine the steric stabilizing power of the poloxamer with the excellent surface activity of the fluorinated surfactant. A synergistic effect was anticipated to occur between the former type of surfactants and fluorinated surfactants with polyhydroxylated headgroups, on the basis that hydrogen bonding would occur between the ether oxygens of the poloxamer and the hydroxyl groups of the fluorinated surfactant. The stabilization achieved with such mixtures is shown in Figure 29. A strong decrease in the interfacial tension of poloxamer 188 at the PFC/water interface can indeed be achieved by the addition of small amounts of a fluorinated surfactant (Riess et al., 1989). A 75% w/v FDC emulsion stabilized with 2.5% poloxamer 188 and 2.5% xylitol-derived perfluoroalkylated surfactant showed only a 20% increase in average particle size over six years at 25°C (Figure 29), whereas the emulsion prepared with poloxamer

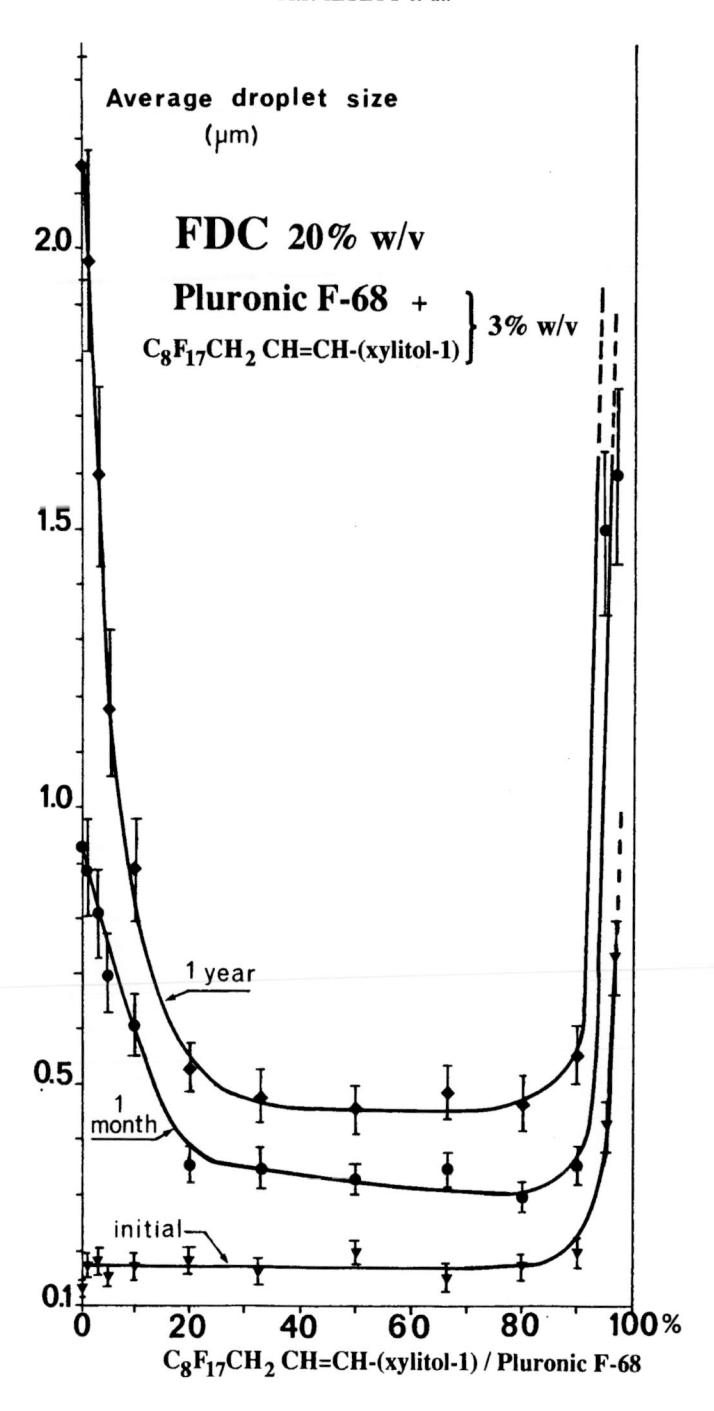

Figure 30 Average particle sizes initially after preparation, at 1 month, and after 1 year at 25°C in a 20% w/v perfluorodecalin emulsion as a function of the ratio of the fluorinated surfactant $C_8F_{17}CH_2CH=CH$-(xylitol-1) to Pluronic F-68 in the surfactant mixture, with the total amount of surfactant being held constant. Note that the fluorinated surfactant alone was unable to produce an emulsion. From Zarif et al. (1989), with permission.

188 alone grew seven-fold in two months. The expected synergistic effect is clearly seen in Figure 30. Significant deviations from LSW theory, as evidenced by nonlinear plots of a^3 vs time, have been observed in some mixtures of fluorinated surfactants with poloxamer 188 (Varescon et al., 1990). Moreover, the magnitude of the stabilization seems, in certain cases, to be greater than the differences in measured interfacial tension values would predict. Such a situation could result from a dependence of σ^i with a resulting from depletion of the fluorinated surfactant solution due to adsorption at the FC/water interface (Kabalnov and Shchukin, 1992).

Other fluorinated surfactants are excellent stabilizers when used in combination with EYP (Milius et al., 1992). One can in principle decrease the interfacial tension to a few tenths of a mN m^{-1}.

Finally, let's examine the degree of stabilization achieved with a typical fluorinated surfactant relative to the current technology of using a secondary PFC for stabilization. EYP is able to provide emulsions with a convenient two-year shelf-life if Ostwald ripening is suppressed by the addition of a secondary PFC component. The advantage of the secondary PFC approach, relative to choosing a fluorinated surfactant is that the stabilizing molecules are completely fluorinated, and not susceptible to metabolic degradation *in-vivo*, as will occur for most fluorinated surfactants. As well, their higher cost and still unknown pharmacology push fluorinated surfactants towards other applications such as drug delivery (Riess, 1994c; Riess and Krafft, 1997, Krafft and Riess, 1998).

The effect of excess surfactant

It has been hypothesized that the presence of excess surfactant in the form of micelles or SUVs may significantly enhance the Ostwald ripening rate (McClements and Dungan, 1993). Kabalnov (1994) and Taylor (1995) found molecular diffusion to be the dominant mechanism of mass transfer for hydrocarbon emulsions stabilized by micelle-forming surfactants. Excess surfactant simply added a small increment (ca. 2–3 fold) to the observed rate. The effect of excess EYP on PFC emulsion stability was examined by Krafft et al. (1991). They found that increases in total surfactant led to significant decreases in emulsion stability. The destabilizing effect observed for EYP/PFC ratios higher than 6% was found to be related to the SUVs and may not be negligible in practice. The importance of micelles/liposomes in the mass transfer process was recently examined theoretically by Kabalnov and Weers (1996b).

The Emulsion Stability/Organ Retention Dilemma

Lipophilic heavier fluorocarbons

Achieving emulsion stability without severely prolonging the half-life of the PFC in the organs of the RES is a problem that has plagued formulators for over 25 years. The dilemma is that an inverse relationship exists between emulsion stability and RES excretion, such that PFCs which possess fast excretion kinetics unfortunately exhibit poor emulsion stability (Riess, 1984). As noted earlier, emulsions of FTBA were found to be stable for long periods of time, but their observed RES half-life is ca 900 days. As discussed previously, PFC excretion depends critically on the solubility of PFC in circulating lipid carriers, and emulsion stability on the solubility of PFC in water. In the case of excretion the solubility in lipids must be maximized, while in the case of emulsion stability the solubility in water must be minimized.

The same problem exists for two-component disperse phase systems. Although less of the higher molecular weight PFC is required for effective stabilization, these components generally still have much longer retention times. Sharma *et al.* (1989) proposed the use of large, sixteen carbon atom polycyclic perfluorocarbons as stabilizers for emulsions of FDC. The physical stability with respect to Ostwald ripening was excellent for these emulsions, unfortunately the organ half-lives of the additives were on the order of hundreds of days, too long to be considered practical.

Based on the mechanisms of emulsion growth and excretion it was proposed to circumvent the emulsion stability/organ retention dilemma by using highly lipophilic PFCs (Weers *et al.*, 1994; Moore *et al.*, 1996). The lipophilicity of PFCs can be increased by the incorporation of polarizable halogen atoms (e.g. Cl or Br), or hydrocarbon blocks (e.g. H or CH_2CH_3) in the terminal position. The profound effect of lipophilic groups on excretion was first noted for perfluorooctyl bromide (PFOB). From plots of organ half-life vs. molecular weight Riess noted that this particular PFC did not fit the general trend: it had a much faster excretion rate than would be predicted for its molecular weight. Later Weers *et al.* (1994) hypothesized that the ten carbon homologue (PFDB) would be an excellent choice for a secondary stabilizing component, combining excellent emulsion stabilizing powers with acceptable excretion characteristics.

Molecular dowels

Fluorocarbon-hydrocarbon diblocks (FmHn) have recently received a great deal of attention due to their excellent stabilizing characteristics and high lipophilicity (Riess and Postel, 1992, Meinert *et al.*, 1992, Riess *et al.*, 1992c). These diblocks may in fact have increased affinity for the PFC/EYP interface and have been termed either molecular dowels (Riess *et al.*, 1992c) or interfacially active compounds (Meinert *et al.*, 1992). The "dowel" concept is illustrated in Figure 31. The hydrocarbon group of the diblock is expected to display good affinity for the acyl chains of the phospholipid monolayer, while the fluorinated group is expected to penetrate the PFC, thus achieving improved adherence of the phospholipid coating to the PFC droplet. The addition of FmHn diblocks to PFC emulsions results in remarkable stabilization for particles ranging in size from 0.13 to 16 μm (Figure 32) (Cornélus *et al.*, 1994a). Riess and coworkers have used the diblocks as additives to the surfactant phase. Their emulsions are processed with the diblock in the initial surfactant dispersion (prior to PFC addition). Because the diblock is thought to act as a molecular dowel, an equimolar concentration (relative to the surfactant) is often used and has proven effective. In support of the dowel hypothesis (i.e. for direct interaction with the surfactant film) is the fact that the addition of diblocks was shown to induce a reduction from 86 to 74 Å^2/molecule of the area occupied by the phospholipids polar headgroups at the interface (Cornélus *et al.*, 1994b). It was also shown (Krafft *et al.*, 1996, unpublished) that differences in stabilization are observed even for very low particle sizes between a diblock (F6H10) and a totally perfluorinated stabilizing additive ($C_{16}F_{34}$) of comparable molecular weight (Figure 31).

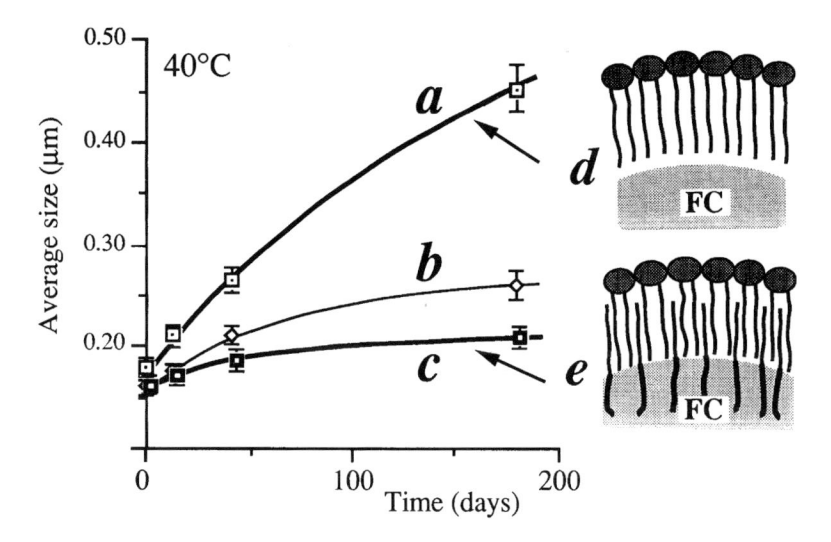

FLUOROCARBON EMULSIONS FOR OXYGEN DELIVERY 305

Figure 31 Particle size increases at 40°C in a fluorocarbon-phospholipid emulsion (90% w/v PFOB, 4% w/v EYP): a) emulsified with EYP alone; b) stabilized with equimolar amounts of EYP and $C_{16}F_{34}$; c) stabilized with equimolar amounts of EYP and $C_6F_{13}C_{10}H_{21}$. $C_{16}F_{34}$ and $C_6F_{13}C_{10}H_{21}$ have close to identical boiling points (242°C) and should have comparable molecular diffusion prevention effects according to the LSW equation. Hypothetical "dowel effect" of a mixed fluorocarbon-hydrocarbon diblock compound at the fluorocarbon-phospholipid film interface: d) without, and e) with $C_6F_{13}C_{10}H_{21}$. From Riess and Weers (1996), with permission.

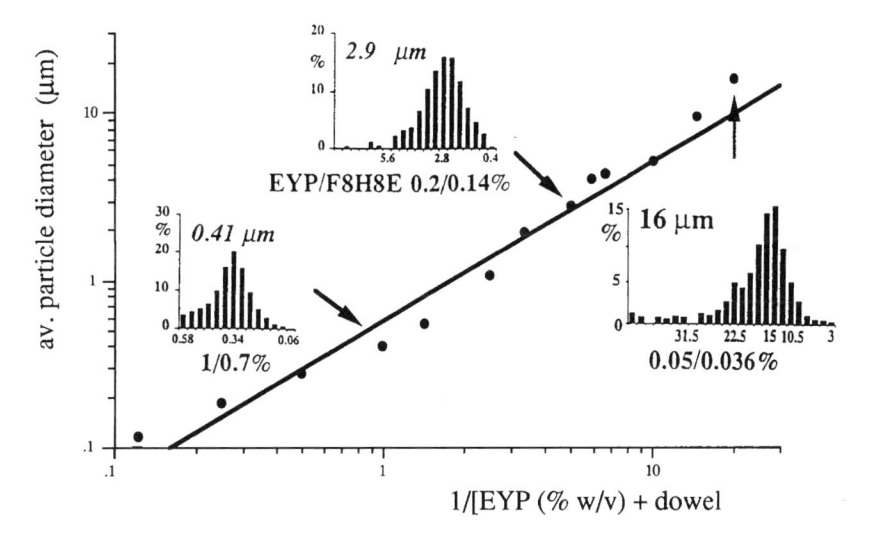

Figure 32 Linear variation of average particle sizes in sterilized 90% w/v perflubron emulsions stabilized by a molecular dowel (C_8F_{17}-CH=CH-C_8H_{17}). Average particle sizes and histograms were measured after a 20 day annealing period. A large range of particle sizes (ca 0.1–16 μm) was obtained by simply varying the EYP + dowel (equimolar) concentration. There was no significant increase in average sizes during the following six-month period. With EYP alone no stable emulsion with particle sizes larger than 4 μm could be obtained. From Cornélus et al. (1994a), with permission.

A dramatic effect on the degree of stabilization is noted depending on the nature of the dispersed PFC phase, such that linear molecules (e.g. PFOB, F-44E, PFOE) are stabilized to a greater extent that cyclics (e.g. FDC) (Cornélus et al., 1994b). The enhanced stabilization is suggested to be due to less favorable arrangement of the diblocks with the rather globular FDC molecules relative to the linear PFCs. Results from Cornélus et al. (1994b) also suggest that diblocks work less efficiently with block copolymers (e.g. poloxamer 188), whose hydrophobic portions are not as well organized in a brush-like fashion at the interface.

As mentioned, increases in droplet stability were noted over a larger range of particle size than attainable with EYP alone (Cornélus et al., 1994a, Cornélus et al., 1994c). Although droplet coarsening in submicron PFC emulsions is controlled by Ostwald ripening, it is likely that the coarsening of droplets greater than 1 μm occurs by coalescence. Cornélus et al. (1994c) noted increases in the stability to droplet coarsening and mechanical stress for the micron-sized droplets containing diblock relative to those containing EYP only, confirming that coalescence is reduced in these larger droplets, and that the diblocks intervene at the level of the surfactant film.

The exact mechanism of stabilization for FnHm diblocks has not been fully elucidated. What is clear is that they provide an excellent solution to the emulsion stability/organ retention dilemma. This is illustrated in Figure 33, where a plot of

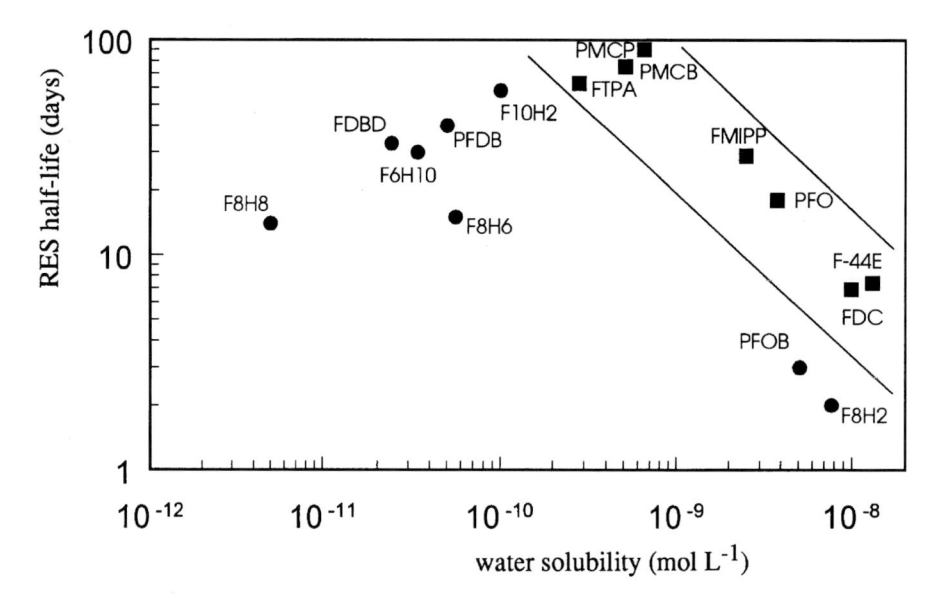

Figure 33 Illustration of the emulsion stability/organ retention dilemma. Emulsion stability increases for nonlipophilic fluorocarbons as water solubility decreases, so too does the organ retention time in the reticuloendothelial system (RES). This dilemma was overcome by the use of highly lipophilic fluorocarbons (●: lipophilic fluorocarbons; ■: non-lipophilic fluorocarbons). Fluorocarbons not defined in Table 1 include: perfluoro-1-methyl-3-isopropylpentane (FMIPP), perfluoro-terbutylcyclohexane (PMCB), perfluorooctane (PFO), (perfluorooctyl)ethane (F8H2), (perfluorodecyl)ethane (F10H2), (perfluorooctyl)hexane (F8H6), (perfluorohexyl)decane (F6H10), (perfluorooctyl)octane (F8H8), perfluorodecyl bromide (PFDB), and α,ω-perfluorodibromodecane (FDBD).

organ half-life vs. PFC water solubility has been made (Weers et al., 1996). The compounds in the upper right hand corner are "true" perfluorocarbons in the sense that they contain only carbon and fluorine in their structure. They clearly illustrate the dilemma in that as the water solubility decreases (and emulsion stability consequently increases) the organ half-life increases dramatically. The lipophilic PFCs do not follow this trend, however. They exhibit significantly lower organ half-lives than would be predicted for their water solubility. For example, (perfluorooctyl)octane (F8H8) has an organ half-life of only 14 days while providing exceedingly efficient emulsion stabilization.

Flocculation

Droplet flocculation has drawn little attention in the blood substitute field, due in part to the generally reversible nature of the process. Although minor components play only a small role in the stability of phospholipid stabilized PFC emulsions with respect to coalescence, they are key in the stability to droplet flocculation. Charged phospholipids increase the zeta potential on the surface of the droplets leading to electrostatic repulsions between droplets. Electrolytes, in particular divalent counterions (e.g. Ca^{2+}) tend to collapse the electrical double layer, leading to flocculation. Johnson et al. (1990) have shown that the zeta potential of 20% w/v FDC emulsions stabilized by 4% w/v PC is on the order of –24 mV. Values close to 0 mV have been reported for a saturated phospholipid (Phospholipon 90H)-stabilized perflubron emulsion (Oleksiak et al., 1994).

The degree of acyl chain saturation plays a key role in droplet flocculation in phospholipid stabilized fluorocarbon emulsions (Pelura et al., 1992). This is illustrated in Table 9 taken from a study by Pelura et al. (1992). Six different types of EYP were studied which differed in the degree of acyl chain saturation and percentage of PC. For example, the E-80-65 sample was derived from egg yolk and composed of ca. 80% PC with an iodine value of 65. The iodine value reflects the degree of acyl chain saturation and is equal to ca. 65–75 for natural EYP, while a value of ca. 3 indicates complete saturation. Perflubron emulsions (90% w/v) stabilized by hydrogenated phospholipids (i.e. E-80-3 and E-100-3) exhibited extensive settling of a viscoelastic gel-like phase upon storage. No such gel-like sediment was observed for the emulsions stabilized by unsaturated phospholipids. The presence of the gel phase is indicated by the relatively high viscosity found for the saturated emulsifiers relative to the unsaturated (ca. 1000 vs. 20 cps). The particle size distributions found for emulsions prepared with saturated phospholipids were broad with a significant tail at large sizes. The median diameters were shifted to larger values and the long term stability was poor. All of these factors point to increased droplet flocculation with the saturated phospholipid emulsifiers.

Oleksiak et al. (1994) also examined flocculation in PFOB emulsions stabilized by Phospholipon 90H using dynamic rheological measurements. Flocculation was prevented by the addition of a negatively charged surfactant (e.g. cholesteryl hemisuccinate), which increased the zeta potential on the droplets, preventing close approach. Fluosol contains added anionic surfactant (i.e. potassium oleate) to increase the zeta potential and decrease the flocculation potential of this formulation.

As noted, other formulation factors, including the concentration of divalent counterions and the presence of chelators (e.g. EDTA) to scavenge counterions, also serve to decrease the potential for emulsion flocculation.

Table 13 Critical depletion flocculation concentrations in proxanol stabilized fluorocarbon emulsions (taken from Amelina et al. (1990), with permission)

Copolymer	Structure	MW (g/mol)	CFC in FDC (wt%)	CFC in FTBA (wt%)
Proxanol 168	$(EO)_{73}$-$(PO)_{28}$-$(EO)_{73}$	8,000	8	>15
Proxanol 268	$(EO)_{118}$-$(PO)_{45}$-$(EO)_{118}$	13,000	8	>15
Proxanol 226	$(EO)_{38}$-$(PO)_{38}$-$(EO)_{38}$	5,500	15	>15
Proxanol 456	$(EO)_{77}$-$(PO)_{77}$-$(EO)_{77}$	11,200	10	>15

Flocculation can also be induced in poloxamer-stabilized PFC emulsions by the presence of free polymer (Kumacheva et al., 1989). Flocculation that is induced by polymer that is free in solution is called depletion flocculation. The attractive force arises when two droplets approach to distances less than the diameter of the polymer molecules. At this point polymer molecules are excluded from the interparticle region, leading to an osmotic pressure difference which causes the droplets to flocculate. Amelina et al. (1990) studied the critical flocculation concentration in 10% v/v FC emulsions stabilized by various levels of Proxanols. The results are illustrated in Table 13.

The concentrations required for depletion flocculation are about a factor of two or more higher than typical concentrations used in blood substitute formulations (e.g. Fluosol), indicating that this form of destabilization poses little practical consideration. Amelina et al. (1990) showed that the critical flocculation concentration (CFC) could be raised dramatically by the addition of small concentrations (0.002 wt%) of an anionic surfactant (e.g. SDS). The increases in initial particle size ascribed to droplet flocculation were irreversible after 7–9 days, due to either irreversible flocculation or droplet coalescence. It is interesting to note that the nature of the PFC phase played a role in the depletion flocculation process. Whereas FDC emulsions readily flocculated at moderate Proxanol concentrations, FTBA emulsions did not. The observed differences possibly result from differences in Proxanol adsorption caused by differences in the lipophilicity of the PFCs.

EMULSION CHARACTERISTICS AND CHARACTERIZATION

In this section two of the most important physico-chemical characteristics relevant to intravascular use of fluorocarbon emulsions, namely particle size and rheology, will be discussed, as well as methods which allow their measurement. Analysis of EYP degradation products and mechanical resistance tests, are also presented.

Emulsion Particle Size

Impact on biocompatibility

Emulsion particle size and distribution play a key role in the biocompatibility, side-effects, and pharmacokinetics of PFC emulsions. A priori the upper limit in terms of particle size must be ca. 7–10 μm (i.e. the size of red blood cells). Although red cells are larger than many capillaries, they are highly deformable and can squeeze

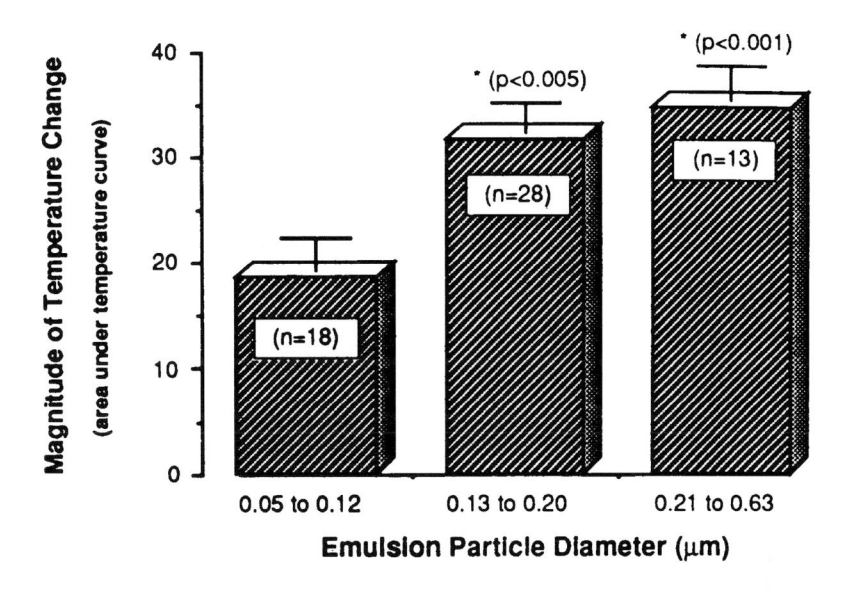

[Figure: Bar chart showing Magnitude of Temperature Change (area under temperature curve) vs Emulsion Particle Diameter (μm). Bars: 0.05 to 0.12 μm ≈ 18 (n=18); 0.13 to 0.20 μm ≈ 32 (n=28, *p<0.005); 0.21 to 0.63 μm ≈ 35 (n=13, *p<0.001).]

Figure 34 Comparison of the magnitude of temperature changes (both duration and intensity, quantified by the area under the temperature curve [AUC]) seen in unrestrained, conscious rats, following injection of perflubron-based emulsions (dose = 2.7 g PFC/kg) having different median particle sizes; * indicates a significant difference compared to the small particle size (0.05–0.12 μm) group. Data shown are means ± SEM for the number of emulsions indicated in each bar. From Keipert et al. (1994), with permission.

through. Emulsion droplets are much less deformable, and so their droplet size must be significantly less than this cutoff. In practice, the upper size limit was defined based on early studies by Green Cross researchers who correlated acute toxicity (lethal dose) with particle size (Fujita et al., 1973, Yokoyama et al., 1982). They observed that emulsion droplets greater than 0.4 μm were considerably more toxic than 0.1 μm droplets, ultimately specifying a median diameter of less than 0.1 μm with no particles greater than 0.6 μm. Coarse emulsions (ca 0.4 μm) were also found by Yokoyama et al. (1975) to intensify RES blockade. Similar claims were made by Russian workers, who promoted that droplets less than 0.1 μm but greater than 0.7 μm (to avoid extravascular leakage or droplets) are preferred (Ivanitsky, 1994).

Keipert et al. (1994b) studied the influence of emulsion particle size on body temperature changes in unrestrained conscious rats. Emulsions with a median particle size between 0.2 and 0.3 μm caused fevers (6 to 8 h duration) which peaked 1–1.5°C above normal. Both the intensity and duration of the febrile response decreased significantly for emulsions with a median particle size of 0.12 μm (Figure 34). Similar results were found in human clinical studies where particle sizes less than 0.2 μm (Oxygent, Formula AF0144) nearly eliminated the febrile response previously observed for PFOB emulsions having a median diameter closer to 0.3 μm (Oxygent, Formula AF0104) (Keipert, 1998).

Smith et al. (1996) examined variations in tumor necrosis factor (TNF-α) of in vitro rat monocytes following incubation with various particle size perflubron emulsions. TNF-α levels increased with particle size for emulsions greater than

0.2 μm, while below 0.2 μm TNF-α levels were similar to saline controls. These results correlate with *in-vivo* TNF-α levels found in humans for 0.3 vs. 0.2 μm sized particles.

Intravascular persistence

Decreases in droplet size also lead to significant increases in intravascular persistence. This has been illustrated in many studies, including early studies by Geyer (1968); see also Yokoyama *et al.*, 1982; Tsuda *et al.*, 1990. The key may be to have a particle size which is smaller than the smallest bacteria (Harashima *et al.*, 1994). The mechanism of particle clearance changes dramatically around 0.2 μm, going from a primarily phagocytosis mediated clearance to that of receptor mediated endocytosis. As the particle size of FC emulsions approaches 0.1 μm, the biological side effects decrease and the avoidance of the RES increases, as noted by increases in intravascular persistence.

Sloviter (1983) showed that intravascular persistence could be dramatically increased by the co-injection of a lipid emulsion. The large number of particles injected effectively blocked uptake by the RES, thereby prolonging the intravascular persistence.

Prolonging the blood half-life is important for indications other than ANH, "bridging" to transfusion, etc. For example, the initial clinical trials for Fluosol targeted patients with chronic anemia. There is no way that current PFC blood substitutes can tackle this problem due to the very short intravascular persistence times ($t_{1/2} \leq 10$ h) of these agents. A continuing need in this area is for the development of agents which have longer blood half-lives. It is only when these half-lives will be on the order of weeks that treatment of chronic anemia will become envisionable (Riess, 1994d). The blood half-life in PFC emulsions depends as we have seen on droplet size. It also depends on the hydrophilicity of the particle surface. Fluosol used a block copolymer to provide a stealthy layer of ethylene oxide groups on the droplet surface. This layer alters the binding of opsonins and slows droplet phagocytosis. Likewise, phagocytic uptake of polystyrene particles by mouse peritoneal macrophages was found to decrease with increased poloxamer or poloxamine layer thickness (Illum *et al.*, 1987). Similar strategies have recently been used to increase the circulation times of liposomes (Lasic and Needham, 1995). Transport of PFC emulsion droplets into the lymphatic vessels (for lymph node imaging) was also reported to depend on particle size (Ikomi *et al.*, 1995).

The effect of Ostwald ripening on initial droplet size

Molecular diffusion has been shown to be the key determinant of initial particle size (hence biological side-effects) in phospholipid-stabilized fluorochemical emulsions (Weers *et al.*, 1994b). These authors showed that attempts to reduce the initial particle size of perflubron emulsions run into a wall at ca. 0.2 μm. At this point increases in total surfactant concentration, homogenization pressure and number of homogenization passes all fail to decrease the droplet size any further. Additional surfactant was found to increase the concentration of phospholipid in free vesicles. The addition of small amounts of a secondary fluorocarbon which reduces Ostwald ripening (i.e. PFDB) allowed dramatic reduction in the initial droplet sizes achievable to less than 0.1 µm, thereby increasing the efficiency of EYP binding to the PFC droplets.

Particle Size Analysis

Modern particle sizing methods can be divided into three categories: those methods which examine individual particles (e.g. microscopy, single-particle sensing), those methods which examine the entire ensemble of particles at one time (e.g. scattering methods), and those methods which fractionate the particles prior to analysis (e.g. field-flow fractionation, photosedimentation).

For submicron emulsion droplets, microscopic analysis requires the use of an electron microscope. Although this technique is excellent for studying the structure of emulsions (e.g. Postel et al., 1991) or for providing subjective information about particle sizes (e.g. the degree of flocculation or presence of multiple emulsion droplets), it is tedious and imprecise for routine analysis. In addition, the technique is expensive, time consuming, and requires skilled operators, a situation not conducive for quality control. Single-particle sensing techniques are also not too useful for the characterization of submicron emulsions since the lower limit of quantitation is ca. 1 µm.

Particle size analysis of submicron emulsions is most frequently done by ensemble techniques, principally quasielastic light scattering (QLS). This technique is preferred because, it is fast, easy, and the equipment is relatively inexpensive. It poses significant problems in the analysis of submicron emulsions, however. Although scattering techniques are excellent for examining monodisperse populations of particles, they are very poor for sizing polydisperse populations of droplets as is most frequently encountered in phospholipid-stabilized PFC emulsions. The problems were pointed out in detail in two recent independent studies with intravenous fat emulsions (Rotenberg et al., 1991; Westesen and Wehler, 1993). QLS was not able to discriminate between emulsion droplets and vesicles. Further, in the polydisperse droplet population QLS was able to account only for the largest population of droplets (Westesen and Wehler, 1993). Although 67% of the droplets had diameters less than 0.14 µm, they were not detected by QLS. Only after the particles had been fractionated by ultracentrifugation was the small droplet population observed. All ensemble techniques (including QLS) must also assume information about the nature of the particle size distribution (e.g. is it log-normal, Gaussian).

Fractionation methods segregate particles due to differences in size and/or density prior to detection. The effective mass of monodisperse fractions of particles are determined via changes in optical density. Among the fractionation methods are the various forms of field-flow fractionation and photosedimentation. Photosedimentation has been used extensively as a quality control tool in sizing submicron PFC emulsions (Klein et al., 1992). Unfortunately, the optical density depends not only on the effective mass of particles in the detector, but also on the scattering properties of the particles. Thus, larger particles, which scatter light to a greater extent are overestimated. This is overcome in commercial photosedimentation instruments by the application of a correction factor (e.g. the Gafford correction) to account for the Mie scattering. Klein et al. (1992) have also shown that photosedimentation devices can be specifically calibrated for PFC emulsions by analyzing the mass distributions obtained after collection of monosized fractions in the sedimentation field-flow fractionation (SdFFF) device. Perhaps the best solution to this problem, however, is to combine the fractionating power of field-flow fractionation (FFF) with the detection power of light scattering. This has been done in a commercial instrument available jointly from FFFractionation Inc. (Salt Lake City, UT)/Wyatt Technology Corporation (Santa Barbara, CA). The new Flow FFF/MALLS technique utilizes a cross-flow to separate particles via differences in particle size. The monodisperse fractions are then detected absolutely (without assumption) using multiangle laser light scattering. A typical fractogram was shown previously in Figure 14.

PFC emulsions for biomedical use generally exhibit a log-normal distribution of droplets, with a "tail" at large sizes. The number of droplets within the tail of the distribution may play a role in the physical characterisitics of the emulsion, and in formulation-related side-effects. Particles greater than ca. 1 μm in size can be quantitatively assessed by single particle counting methods. For example, it is possible to use hemocytometer slides with a known volume to quantitate the total number of particles in a given size range above 1 μm by optical microscopy. Such a procedure is laborius unless an image analysis system is coupled to the method (Jokela et al., 1990). Alternatively, the tail of the distribution can be analyzed by single particle sensing techniques which count individual articles as they pass through a narrow measuring zone. In electrozone (e.g. the Coulter counter), droplets are sized by measuring a small change (pulse) in resistance across a pore between two chambers of partially conducting fluid. As a droplet enters the pore or electrozone it displaces electrolyte. This causes a momentary change in the resistance across the pore, the amplitude of which is dependent on the particle size. By setting pulse-height discriminators, the signal can be accumulated to provide a histogram of particle sizes. Alternatively, the particles can pass through a narrow photozone of uniform illumination (i.e. single particle optical sensing, SPOS). In SPOS, droplets are detected by changes in either light obscuration or light scattering. These methods are excellent for determining the number of particles with droplet size greater than 1 μm. Recently Nicoli et al. (1995) have proposed the marriage of ensemble and single particle counting methods for the analysis of the entire PSD of submicron emulsions. They use quasielastic light scattering to detect the submicron droplet population and SPOS to detect the large particle tail. A commercial instrument combining the two techniques is available from Particle Sizing Systems (Santa Barbara, CA).

The venerable emulsion scientist Paul Becher once said: *"If you want to know if an emulsion has a shelf-life for one year, put it on the shelf for one year."* Sound advice, which is mandated within the pharmaceutical industry by the Food and Drug Administration. For formulation development, however, it is often advantageous to accelerate stability programs. This is generally done by elevating the storage temperature to 40–50°C. Under such conditions the rate of particle growth is dramatically enhanced allowing for rapid stability characterization within a 3 month time-period. Roughly speaking, the degree of particle growth observed each month at 40°C was found to equivalent to 12 months of stability at 5°C (Ni et al., 1994).

Emulsion Rheology

The rheology of FC emulsions depends critically on the volume fraction of dispersed phase, on the degree of droplet flocculation, and to a lesser extent on the particle size and distribution. Increases in viscosity are noted with increases in dispersed phase volume fraction. Below a volume fraction of ca. 0.5, perflubron emulsions behave as Newtonian fluids, with no dependence of viscosity on shear rate (Ni et al., 1992). Above $\phi = 0.5$ dramatic increases in viscosity are noted, and the emulsions become pseudoplastic in nature (Figure 15). The non-Newtonian behavior results from hydrodynamic interactions between the droplets. Difficulties in reproducibly manufacturing emulsions above $\phi = 0.5$ have been noted. These problems were overcome by decreasing the volume fraction slightly to 0.47 (Riess et al., 1992a). The viscosity of the current 60% w/v perflubron emulsions (AF0144) are less than that of human blood (ca. 3 mPas), thereby posing little concern from a hemodynamics perspective (Millard, 1994).

The hydrodynamic interactions depend on the particle size and distance between droplets. In general, the hydrodynamic interactions increase with decreasing particle size. Thus, as particles coarsen during storage slight decreases in PFC emulsion viscosity are noted. For phospholipid emulsifiers, excess EYP leads to an increase in the population of small (ca 0.5 μm) SUV particles (Krafft et al., 1991). This increases the total volume fraction of particles in the formulation leading to concomitant increases in dispersion viscosity.

Emulsion viscosity also depends on the nature of the surfactant. Poloxamers, for example, increase viscosity dramatically. Thus, an attempt to develop a slightly more concentrated Fluosol formulation (Fluosol-DA *35%*) was abandoned, possibly because of increases in viscosity related with the use of a larger concentration of the poloxamer emulsifier.

Flocculated emulsions immobilize continuous phase in the voids between droplets, leading to large increases in viscosity. As discussed in the section on flocculation, PFC emulsions can be flocculated by the addition of divalent counterions, by the use of saturated phospholipid emulsifiers, or by depletion flocculation in emulsions stabilized by poloxamers.

Rheological Analysis

Many commercial instruments are available which can be used for assessing the rheological characteristics of submicron PFC emulsions, and many thorough reviews have been written on this subject (Pal et al., 1992; Sherman, 1983). They range from capillary viscometers, to inexpensive rotating viscometers (e.g. Brookfield, Stoughton, MA) to expensive rheometers which precisely measure shear rates and shear stresses and which are capable of doing dynamic measurements (e.g. Rheometric Scientific, Piscataway, NJ; Bohlin Instruments, Cranbury, NJ). The most widely used of these instruments for quality control purposes is the rotating viscometer available from Brookfield.

Resistance to Mechanical Stress

Measurement of the stability of the emulsion to mechanical stress is generally done in one of two ways. First the emulsion can be shaken at a given frequency (e.g. 250 throws min^{-1}) for a specified period of time (e.g. 1 hr). The application of mechanical stress leads to forced coalescence between droplets, which ultimately leads to phase separation. Thus, instabilities to mechanical stress are generally noted by changes in the percentage of free (i.e. phase separated) PFC, and by measuring changes in the particle size distribution, especially in the large particle tail. Alternatively the emulsion in its bottle and package can be tested using the standard simulated shipping tests available from ASTM or NSTA. Analysis includes mechanical stress tests, drop tests to assess bottle breakage, and tests to assess the stability to repeated freeze/thaw procedures as might be encountered during product shipping.

The Measurement of Egg Yolk Phospholipid Degradation Products

The measurement of EYP oxidative degradation products in PFC emulsions is a daunting task. The oxidation of susceptible lipids leads to literally hundreds of different end-products, including hydroperoxides, endoperoxides, aldehydes, and various condensation products. Some of the possible characterization methods follow. For a more detailed analysis the reader is referred to the excellent review regarding oxidation in emulsions by Corliss and Dugan (1970). The first class of compounds which can be assessed are the peroxides. The evaluation of hydroperoxides can be done by triphenylphosphine oxidation with detection by reverse phase HPLC (Nakamura, 1986; Nakamura and Maeda, 1991). Alternatively, conjugated diene and triene hydroperoxides can be determined by their specific absorbance at 233 nm and 266 nm, with oxidized and nonoxidized species easily distinguished (Borgeat et al., 1990; Klein, 1970).

A number of methods also exist for detection of various aldehydic species (Beckman et al., 1991). Unsaturated aldehydes can be detected by their absorbance at 350 nm following reaction with p-anisidine to form an unsaturated imine. Similarily total aldehydes can be determined by monitoring absorbance at 350–380 nm following reaction with 2,3-dinitrophenylhydrazine (DNPH) to form the hydrazone derivative (Esterbauer, 1982). Direct determination of hydroxyalkenals can be accomplished by HPLC with reverse-phase separation and detection at 220 nm (Esterbauer and Zollner, 1989). Specific measurement of malondialdehydes can be achieved using the thiobarbituric acid method.

Another class of products are condensation products derived from the reaction of malondialdehyde with primary amines (e.g. phosphatidylethanolamine). This reaction produces conjugated Schiff bases which can be detected by fluorescence with excitation at 350 nm and detection at 440 nm (Dillard and Tappel, 1973).

Hydrolysis of EYP leads to the formation of free fatty acids and lysophospholipids. The concentration of free fatty acids is easily determined by a colorimetric assay in which the FFA are reacted with a copper complex to form a deep blue color whose absorbance is detectable at 550 nm (Mahadevan et al., 1969). Lysophospholipids are generally determined via HPLC using an evaporative light scattering detector with reference to calibration curves. Alternatively lysophospholipids can be quantitated by ^{31}P-NMR.

MISCELLANEOUS SUBMICRONIC EMULSIONS WITH A FLUOROCARBON PHASE

A variety of other fluorocarbon preparations have been reported that could find uses as oxygen carriers, contrast agents, protective films, drug delivery systems and in biomedical research (Riess, 1994c,e; Krafft and Riess, 1998).

Microemulsions

Microemulsions, contrary to the usual emulsions (or macroemulsions), form spontaneously and are thermodynamically stable for certain proportions of water, oil and surfactants, i.e. within a certain well-defined, temperature-dependent composition domain. Microemulsions are transparent, or at least translucent, as a result of particle sizes being less than 50 nm, i.e. less than the wave-length of visible light. Transparency, however, is no proof of occurence of a microemulsion, as it can also result from close refractive indexes of the two phases and surfactant film. This can happen with fluorocarbon emulsions, as the refractive indexes of certain fluorocarbons and of water are very close. Being independent of preparation procedure and not needing an input of energy, microemulsions are, for a given composition, highly reproducible. If biocompatibility can be achieved, microemulsions would provide very long-term shelf stability. Tolerance after i.v. injection, however, has never been clearly established. Possible problems can arise from the large amount of surfactant that is usually needed; the biological effects of very small particles are largely unknown (Harashima et al., 1994; Vorobiev, 1992); also unknown is the destiny of the dispersion after mixing with blood when the composition falls out of the often-narrow domain of existence of the microemulsion.

The use of microemulsions of fluorocarbons as a blood substitute for organ preservation was first suggested by Rosano and Gerbacia (1973). Industrial perfluoroalkylated amine oxides and alcohols were mentioned among the suitable surfactants and co-surfactants, but no toxicity data were provided. Another patent claims the use of a mixture of two polydisperse perfluoroalkylated polyoxyethylene surfactants to obtain clear, spontaneously-formed dispersions of fluorocarbons (Chabert et al., 1975). A single neutral perfluoroalkylated polyoxyethylene surfactant was shown to suffice for obtaining fluorocarbon microemulsions (Mathis et al., 1984). Phase diagrams were explored by Mukerjee and Mysels, 1975; Kunieda and Shinoda, 1976; Mathis et al., 1984; Robert and Tondre, 1984; Ravey and Stébé, 1987; Lattes and Rico-Lattes, 1994; Chittofrati et al., 1992. Microemulsions of fluorocarbons could be prepared using mixtures of fluorinated and non-fluorinated surfactants and such mixtures allow control of the temperature of microemulsion formation (Schubert and Kaler, 1994). Lattes et al. prepared microemulsions of mixed fluorocarbon-hydrocarbon diblocks using a non-fluorinated surfactant (Lattes and Rico-Lattes, 1994). The latter preparation was shown to dissolve large amounts of oxygen. Water-in-oil microemulsions have also been reported (Chittofrati et al., 1992; Robert and Tondre, 1984). Further work is clearly needed to evaluate this approach from a biological standpoint.

Gel Emulsions

Gelifying fluorocarbons is, a priori, quite a challenge. Fluorocarbons are indeed extremely fluid and mobile liquids as a consequence of very weak intermolecular cohesive forces, and they do not dissolve the usual gelifying agents. Yet several types of gels have recently been produced. Some are very rich in water and consist of water-in-oil emulsions in which the "continuous phase" is actually a water-in-fluorocarbon microemulsion; the surfactants used were fluorinated ethoxylated alcohols (Ravey and Stébé, 1990).

On the other end of the composition spectrum, stable rigid gels containing up to 99% fluorocarbon and as little as 0.1% of a perfluoroalkylamine oxide could be prepared from a range of compounds, from low boiling-point CFC 113 to high boiling-point polycyclic fluorinated materials (Krafft and Riess, 1994). These gels, or high internal phase ratio emulsions (HIPRE), have a compartmentalized structure consisting of polyhedral fluorocarbon domains (polyaphrons) separated by a reverse hydrated film of surfactant. Other gel formulations with an external aqueous phase were reported that derive from highly concentrated and viscous water-in-fluorocarbon emulsions (Oxynoid et al., 1994) or from fluorocarbon emulsions in the aqueous phase of which collagen was dispersed (Magdassi et al., 1992).

Fluorocarbon gels have been proposed as protective films and for topical drug delivery, in particular for healing of wounds and burns, and for cosmetic uses. A cosmetic fluorocarbon ointment is commercially available that claims to supply oxygen to the skin (Gross et al., 1994).

Low friction gels with a continuous fluorocarbon phase have also been obtained recently (Krafft and Riess, 1995). In this case, gelification was achieved by using a surfactant system consisting of phospholipids and a fluorocarbon-hydrocarbon diblock molecule; this combination is believed, in the presence of water, to form entangled elongated micelles that are dispersed in the fluorocarbon.

Reverse Water-in-Fluorocarbon Emulsions and Microemulsions

Stable reverse, water-in-fluorocarbon emulsions have been obtained, in spite of intrinsically unfavorable solubility and diffusivity parameters, interfacial tension and densities (compared with the direct emulsions) by using a fluorinated surfactant, $C_8F_{17}(CH_2)_{11}OP(O)(N(CH_2CH_2)_2O)_2$ (Sadtler et al., 1996). Fine and fluid, narrowly dispersed reverse emulsions containing from 1 to 30% water could thus be prepared with perfluorooctyl bromide or perfluorooctylethane as the fluorocarbon. A variety of drugs, including antibacterials, vasoactive bronchodilators, a mucolytic agent, a glucocorticoid or an anti-cancer agent were incorporated in such reverse fluorocarbon emulsions without inducing significant loss of stability (Krafft et al., 1995). The inner aqueous compartment can also contain particulates, such as vesicles or other nanostructures. These emulsions have potential for pulmonary drug delivery as they should allow very uniform, reproducible distribution of the drug throughout the lungs, including the dependent areas. Reverse emulsions also give access to multiple emulsions when dispersed in water.

Hydrocarbon-in-Fluorocarbon Emulsions and Microemulsions

Oil-in-fluorocarbon emulsions and microemulsions have recently been obtained. Such preparations are more specifically destined to allow the transport and delivery of lipophilic drugs (Krafft and Riess, 1994, unpubl.). The surfactant consisted, for example, of hydrocarbon/fluorocarbon diblock compounds of the $C_nF_{2m+1}C_mH_{2m+1}$ type or of dimorpholinophosphate derivatives. Oil-in-fluorocarbon-in-water and oil-in-water-in-fluorocarbon triple emulsions, i.e. multiple emulsions with three mutually immiscible phases, have also been produced; the intermediate fluorocarbon phase is expected to allow modulation of drug release from the internal phase into the external aqueous phase.

OUTLOOK

Submicron fluorocarbon-in-water emulsions are being developed as injectable oxygen carrier systems, the so-called blood substitutes. Effective, though temporary delivery of oxygen has been demonstrated in both animals and humans. Maximum effectiveness is reached in hemodiluted patients, i.e. when hemoglobin level is low and cardiac output is high. Low doses of fluorocarbon can then result in significant increase in mixed venous oxygen tension and tissue oxygen consumption.

A new generation of fluorocarbon emulsions is now in advanced clinical trials. Improvements over the earlier, Fluosol-type products include selection of faster-excreted lipophilic fluorocarbons, replacement of the poloxamer emulsifier by the biologically better-accepted egg phospholipids, several-fold increase in fluorocarbon concentration, considerable improvement in shelf stability and ease of use.

Considerable progress has also been achieved where our knowledge and understanding of the structure and physical characteristics, formation and evolution, mechanisms of action and side-effects of fluorocarbons and fluorocarbon emulsions are concerned. This allowed the rational design of strategies that capitalize on the product's advantages, but take into account also its limitations, including principally its short intravascular persistence, so as to maximize benefit for the patient.

One such strategy consists in using the oxygen carrier in conjunction with acute normovolemic hemodilution during surgery. Oxygent, the most advanced of the newer products, has completed phase II clinical trials in Europe and in the US for this application. Infusion of the emulsion to oxygen-breathing hemodiluted patients was seen to result in immediate increase in mixed venous oxygen tension. Oxygent was shown to be more effective than blood in correcting physiological indications for transfusion. Oxygen supplementation to hemodiluted patients is expected to result in increased safety, allowing more profound hemodilution, and enhancement of the potential of ANH to reduce or alleviate the transfusion of donor blood. Such strategies, by offering an effective alternative to red blood cell transfusion, are expected to play a major role in surgery.

Animal and human data indicate that fluorocarbon-based oxygen carriers are safe for use at clinically relevant doses. The flu-like symptoms, frequent with the earlier emulsions, were substantially reduced through formulation and process optimization.

Oxygent is a 60% w/v concentrated emulsion of the somewhat lipophilic perfluorooctyl bromide (perflubron) emulsified with phospholipids. A few percent of perfluorodecyl bromide allow effective reduction of Ostwald ripening without compromising the excretion rate. The present production capacity of perflubron is in the 100-ton/year range and can be upscaled at will. Industrial capacity for producing the emulsion is also in place.

Advantages over hemoglobin-based oxygen carriers include access to virtually unlimited supply, high O_2-extraction by tissues, high O_2-consumption/O_2-delivery ratios, simpler pharmacology, a better understood and controllable side-effect profile, and cost-effectiveness.

Further applications of fluorocarbon-based oxygen delivery systems are being investigated, in particular in the cardiovascular ischemia and cancer treatment area, and for organ preservation.

Future research will undoubtedly aim at prolonging the emulsion's intravascular persistence, which would further extend the range of applications of such products. Achieving circulation half-lifes long enough to allow treatment of persistent anemia represents, however, a formidable challenge for researchers.

Other fluorocarbon emulsion systems that are being investigated comprise reverse and multiple emulsions, microemulsions and gels. Such systems are expected to provide innovative novel drug-delivery systems.

ACKNOWLEDGEMENTS

The authors wish to thank Sarah Brunton and Elizabeth Lepage for help in preparing the manuscript.

REFERENCES

Adams, J.E., Owens, G., Mann, G., Headrick, J.R., Munoz, A., Scott, H.W. (1959) Experimental evaluation of Pluronic F68 (a non-ionic detergent) as a method of diminishing systemic fat emboli resulting from prolonged cardiopulmonary bypass. *Surg. Forum*, **10**, 585–589.

Amelina, E.A., Kumacheva, E.Z., Pertsov, A.V., Shchukin, E.D. (1990) Stability of perfluorocarbon emulsions with respect to Ostwald ripening and flocculation. *Kolloidn. Zh.*, **52**, 216–220.

Amer. Chem. Soc., Symposium on organofluorine compounds in medicine and biology, Amer. Chem. Soc. Natl. Meeting, Las Vegas, March 1982. Abstracts.

American College of Physicians Clinical Guidelines (1992) Practice strategies for elective red blood cell transfusion. *Ann. Intern. Med.*, **116**, 403–406.

Attwood, D., Florence, A.T. (1983) *Surfactant Systems. Their chemistry, pharmacy and biology*. London: Chapman and Hall Ltd.

Banks, R.E. (1982) *Preparation, Properties, and Industrial Applications of Organofluorine Compounds*. Chichester: Ellis Horwood.

Banks, R.E., Tatlow, J.C. (1986) A guide to modern organofluorine chemistry. *J. Fluorine Chem.*, **33**, 227–284.

Banks, R.E., Smart, B.E., Tatlow, J.C. (1994). *Organofluorine Chemistry: Principles and Commercial Applications*. New York: Plenum Press.

Basedow, A., Ebert, K. H. (1977) Ultrasonic degradation of polymers in solution. *Adv. Polymer Sci.*, **22**, 83–148.

Beach, M.C., Morley, J., Spiryda, L., Weinstock, S.B. (1992) Effects of liposome encapsulated hemoglobin on the reticuloendothelial system. *Biomat., Art. Cells, Immob. Biotech.*, **20**, 771–776.

Beckman, J.K., Morley, S.A., Greene, H.L. (1991) Analysis of aldehydic lipid peroxidation products by TLC/densitometry. *Lipids*, **26**, 155–161.

Behan, M., O'Connell, D., Mattrey, R.F., Carney, D.N. (1993) Perfluorooctylbromide as a contrast agent for CT and sonography: preliminary clinical results. *Amer. J. Radiol.*, **160**, 399–405.

Beloyarstev, F.F., Mayevsky, E.I., Islamov, B.I. (1983) *Ftorosan-oxygen Carrying Perfluorochemical Plasma Substitute*. USSR, Pushchino: Acad. Sci.

Bentley, P.K., Davis, S.S., Johnson, O.L., Lowe, K.C., Washington, C. (1989) Purification of Pluronic F-68 for perfluorochemical emulsification. *J. Pharm. Pharmacol.*, **41**, 661–663.

Binks, B.P., Meunier, J., Abillon, O., Langevin, D. (1989) Measurement of film rigidity and interfacial tensions in several ionic surfactant-oil-water microemulsion systems. *Langmuir*, **5**, 415–421.

Binks, B.P. (1993) Emulsion type below and above the cmc in AOT microemulsion systems. *Colloids Surf. A*, **71**, 167–172.

Biro, G.P. (1993) Perfluorocarbon-based red blood cell substitutes. *Transfusion Med. Rev.*, **7**, 84–95.

Bondi, A. (1964) Van der Waals volumes and radii *J. Phys. Chem.*, **58**, 441–451.

Borgeat, P., Picard, S., Vallerand, P., Bourgoin, S., Odelmat, A., Sirois, P., Poubelle, P.E. (1990) Automated on-line extraction and profiling of lipooxygenase products of arachidonic acid by high performance liquid chromatography. *Methods of Enzymology*, **187**, pp. 98–116. San Diego: Academic Press.

Braun, R.D., Goldstick, T.K., Linsenmeier, R.A. (1990) Perfluorocarbon blood substitute enhances retinal oxygenation in cats. *Invest. Ophthalmol. Vis. Sci.*, **31**, 568.

Brasile, L., Clarke, J., Green, E.P., Haisch, C. (1996) The feasability of organ preservation at warmer temperatures. *Transplant. Proceed.*, **28**, 349–351.

Bruneton, J.N., Falewee, M.N., François, E., Cambon, P., Philip, C., Riess, J.G., Balu-Maestro, C., Rogopoulos, A. (1989) Liver, spleen and vessels: Preliminary clinical results of CT with perfluorooctylbromide. *Radiology*, **170**, 179–183.

Bucala, R., Kawakami, M., Cerami, A. (1983) Cytotoxicity of a perfluorocarbon blood substitute to macrophages in vitro. *Science*, **220**, 965–967.

Burgess, D.J., Yoon, J.K. (1995) Influence of interfacial properties on perfluorocarbon/aqueous emulsion stability. *Colloid Surf. B*, **4**, 297–308.

Carr, M.E., Jr., Carr, S.L., High, A.A. (1995) Effects of Poloxamer 407 on the assembly, structure, and dissolution of fibrin clots. *Blood*, **86**, 886A.

Castro, O., Nesbitt, E., Lyles, D. (1984) Effect of a perfluorocarbon emulsion (Fluosol-DA) on reticuloendothelial system clearance function. *Am. J. Hematol.*, **16**, 15–21

Cecutti, C., Rico, I., Lattes, A., Novelli, A., Rico, A., Marion, G., Graciaa, H., Lachaise, J. (1989) New formulation of blood substitutes: optimization of novel fluorinated microemulsions. *Eur J. Med. Chem.*, **24**, 485–492.

Cernaianu, A.C., Spence, R.K., Vassilidze, T.V., Gallucci, J.G., Gaprindashvili, T., Olah, A., Weiss, R.L., Cilley, J.H., Keipert, P.E., Faithfull, N.S., DelRossi, A.J. (1994) Improvement in circulatory and oxygenation status by perflubron emulsion (Oxygent™ HT) in a canine model of surgical hemodilution. *Art. Cells, Blood Subst., Immob. Biotech.*, **22**, 965–977.

Cevc, G. (ed.) (1993) *Phospholipids Handbook*. New York: M. Dekker.

Cevc, G., Marsh, D. (1987) *Phospholipid bilayers: Physical Principles and Models*, p. 39. New York: Wiley.

Chabert, P., Foulletier, L., Lantz, A. (1975) Procédé de préparation de liquides à applications biologiques et transporteurs d'oxygène. *German Offen* 2,452,513.

Chandler, D. (1978) Structures of molecular liquids *Ann. Rev. Phys. Chem.*, **29**, 441–471.

Chang, T.M.S., Riess, J.G., Winslow, R.M. (eds.) (1994) *Proc. Vth Intern. Symp. Blood Substitutes*, vol 1, *Blood Substitutes, General*, published in *Art. Cells, Blood Subst. Immob. Biotech.*, **22**, 123–360.

Chang, T.M.S., Greenburg, G., Tsuchida, E., (eds.) (1997), *Proc. VIth Intern. Symp. Blood Substitutes*, published in *Art. Cells, Blood Subst., Immob. Biotech.*, **25** (in press).

Chang, T.M.S. (ed.) (1998) *Blood Substitutes. Principles, Methods, Products and Clinical Trials*. New York: Karger Landes Systems.

Chapman, K.W., Keipert, P.E., Graham, H.A. (1996) Commercial-scale production of perfluorochemical emulsions. *Art. Cells, Blood Subst., Immob. Biotech.*, **24**, 318 (abstract).

Chen, H.S., Yang, Z.H. (1989) Perfluorocarbon as blood substitute in clinical applications and in war casualties. In *Blood Substitutes*, edited by T.M.S. Chang and R.P. Geyer, pp. 403–410. New York: Dekker.

Chittofrati, A., Sanguineti, A., Visca, M., Kallay, N. (1992) Perfluoropolyether microemulsions: conductivity behavior of three-component W/O systems. *Colloids and Surfaces*, **63**, 219–233.

Clark, L.C., Gollan, F. (1966) Survival of mammals breathing organic liquids equilibrated with oxygen at atmospheric pressure. *Science*, **152**, 1755–1756.

Clark, L. C., Kaplan, S., Becattini, F. (1970) Physiology of synthetic blood. *J. Thorac. Cardiovasc. Surg.*, **60**, 757–772.

Clark, L.C., Becattini, F., Kaplan, S. (1972) The physiological effects of artificial blood made from inert organic oxygen solvents. *Ala. J. Med. Sci.*, **9**, 16–29.

Clark, L.C., Becattini, F., Kaplan, S., Obrock, K. (1973) Perfluorocarbons having a short dwell time in the liver. *Science*, **181**, 680–682.

Clark, L.C., Wesseler, E.P., Miller, M.L., Kaplan, S. (1974) Ring versus straight chain perfluorocarbon emulsions for perfusion media. *Microvasc. Res.*, **8**, 320–340.

Clark, L.C., Wesseler, E.P., Kaplan, S., Miller, M.L., Becker, C., Emory, C., Stanley, L., Becattini, F., Obrock, V. (1975) Emulsions of perfluorinated solvents for intravascular gas transport. *Fed. Proc.*, **34**, 1468–1478.

Clark, L.C., Moore, R.E. (1982) Basic and experimental aspects of oxygen transport by highly fluorinated organic compounds. In *Biomedicinal Aspects of Fluorine Chemistry*, edited by R. Filler, Y. Kobayashi, pp. 213–226. Amsterdam: Elsevier.

Clark, L.C., Clark, E.W., Moore, R.E., Kinnett, D.G., Inscho, E.I. (1983) Room temperature-stable biocompatible fluorocarbon emulsions. *Prog. Clin. Biol. Res.*, **122**, 169–180.

Clark, L.C., Hoffman, R.E., Davis, S.L. (1992) Response of the rabbit lung as a criterion of safety for fluorocarbon breathing and blood substitutes. *Biomat., Art. Cells, Immob. Biotech.*, **20**, 1085–1089.

Colbassani, H.J., Barrow, D.L., Sweeney, K.M., Bakay, R.A.E., Check, I.J., Hunter, R.H. (1989) Modification of acute focal ischemia in rabbits by poloxamer 188. *Stroke*, **20**, 1241–1246.

Collins-Gold, L.C., Lyons, R.T., Bartholow L.C. (1990) Parenteral emulsions for drug delivery. *Adv. Drug Deliv. Rev.*, **5**, 189–208.

Colman, R.W., Chang, L.K., Mukherji, B., Sloviter, H.A. (1980) Effects of a perfluoro erythrocyte substitute on platelets *in vitro* and *in vivo. J. Lab. Clin. Med.*, **95**, 553–562.

Consensus Conference (1988) Perioperative red blood cell transfusion. *JAMA*, **260**, 2700–2703.

Corliss, G.A., Dugan, L.R. (1970) Phospholipid oxidation in emulsions. *Lipids*, **5**, 846–853.

Cornélus, C., Giulieri, F., Krafft, M. P., Riess, J. G. (1993a) Impact of phospholipid dispersions on the stability of fluorocarbon/phospholipid emulsions for biomedical uses. *Colloids Surf.*, **70**, 233–238.

Cornélus, C., Krafft, M.P., Riess, J.G. (1993b) Filtration as an alternative to heat-sterilization for injectable fluorocarbon emulsions. *Proc. 1st World Congress on Emulsions*, Paris, 1993, n°1-12–207.

Cornélus, C., Krafft, M.P., Riess, J.G. (1994a) Improved control over particle sizes and stability of concentrated fluorocarbon emulsions by using mixed fluorocarbon/hydrocarbon dowels. *Art. Cells, Blood Subs., Immob. Biotech.*, **22**, 1183–1191.

Cornélus, C., Krafft, M.P., Riess, J.G. (1994b) About the mechanism of stabilization of fluorocarbon emulsions by mixed fluorocarbon/hydrocarbon additives. *J. Colloid Interface Sci.*, **163**, 391–394.

Cornélus, C., Krafft, M.P., Riess, J.G. (1994c) Mixed fluorocarbon/hydrocarbon molecular dowels help protect concentrated fluorocarbon emulsions with large size droplets against coalescence. *Art. Cells, Blood Subst., Immob. Biotech.*, **22**, 1267–1272.

Corran, J.W. (1946) *Emulsion Technology*, pp. 176. Brooklyn: Chemical Publishing Co.

Dalfors, J.L., Espinosa, C.A. (1992) Terminal sterilization of perfluorocarbon (PFC) emulsions: difficulties and possible solutions. *Biomat., Art. Cells, Immob. Biotech.*, **20**, 869–871.

Davis, S.S., Round, H.P., Purewal, T.S (1981) Ostwald ripening and the stability of emulsion systems: an explanation for the effect of the added third component. *J. Colloid Interface Sci.*, **80**, 508–511.

Davis, S.S., Hansrani, P. (1985) The coalescence behavior of oil droplets stabilized by phospholipid emulsifiers. *J. Colloid Interface Sci.*, **108**, 285–287.

Davis, S.S., Illum, L. (1995) Particulate systems for site specific drug delivery. In *Advances in System Constructs*, edited by G. Gregoriadis, B. McCormack and G. Poste, pp. 183–194. New York: Plenum Press.

Davis, S.S., Illum, L., Stolnik, S. (1996) Polymers in drug delivery. *Curr. Opinion Colloid Interface Sci.*, **1**, 660–666.

de Gennes, P.G., Taupin, C. (1982) Microemulsions and the flexibility of oil/water interfaces. *J. Phys. Chem.*, **86**, 2294–2304.

del Balzo, U., Strnat, C.A., Harrell, R.A., Flaim, S.F. (1997) Effects of perflubron emulsion on cardiac function and oxygenation in the supply-limited isolated, Langendorff perfused heart. *J. Invest. Med.* (in press).

Deschiens (1886). De la transfusion lente, par voie hypodermique, d'un sang artificiel concentré et stérile contenant les principes immédiates du sang naturel. *Disclosure to the French Academy of Science.*

Dillard, C.J., Tappel, A.L. (1973) Fluorescent products from reaction of peroxidizing polyunsaturated fatty acids with phosphatidylethanolamine and phenylalanine. *Lipids*, **8**, 183–189.

Elliott, L.A., Ledgerwood, A.M., Lucas, C.E., McCoy, L.E., McGonigal, M., Sullivan, M.W. (1989) Role of Fluosol-DA 20% in prehospital resuscitation. *Crit. Care Med.*, **17**, 166–172.

Esterbauer, H. (1982) Aldehydic products of lipid peroxidation. In *Free Radicals, Lipid Peroxidation, and Cancer*, edited by D.C.H. McBain, T.F. Slater, pp. 101–172. New York: Academic Press.

Esterbauer, H., Zollner, H. (1989) Methods for determination of aldehydic lipid peroxidation products. *Free Rad. Biol. Med.*, **7**, 197–203.

Evans, R.G., Kimler, B.F., Morantz, R.A., Batnitsky, S. (1993) Lack of complications in long-term survivors after treatment with Fluosol® and oxygen as an adjuvant to radiation therapy for high-grade brain tumors. *Int. J. Rad. Oncol. Biol. Phys.*, **26**, 649–652.

Faithfull, N.S. (1992) Oxygen delivery from fluorocarbon emulsions — aspects of convective and diffusive transport. *Biomat., Art. Cells, Immob. Biotech.*, **20**, 797–804.

Faithfull, N.S. (1994a) The role of perfluorochemicals in surgery and the ITU. In *Yearbook of Intensive Care and Emergency Medicine*, edited by J.L. Vincent, pp. 237–251. Berlin: Springer Verlag.

Faithfull, N.S. (1994b) Mechanisms and efficacy of fluorochemical oxygen transport and delivery. *Art. Cells, Blood Subst., Immob. Biotech.*, **22**, 181–197.

Faithfull, N.S., Rhoades, G.E., Keipert, P.E., Ringle, A.S., Trouwborst, A. (1994). A program to calculate mixed venous oxygen tension — a guide to transfusion? *Adv. Exp. Med. Biol.*, **361**, 139–144.

Fischer, G.W., Hunter, K.W., Wilson, S.R. (1980) Intralipid and reticuloendothelial clearance. *Lancet*, **2**, 1300–1310.

Flaim, S.F. (1994) Pharmacokinetics and side effects of perfluorocarbon-based blood substitutes. *Art. Cells, Blood Subst., Immob. Biotech.*, **22**, 1043–1054.

Flaim, S.F. (1997) Perflubron-based emulsion: efficacy as a temporary oxygen carrier. In *Blood Substitutes: New Frontiers*, edited by R.M. Winslow, K.D. Vandegriff, M. Intaglietta, pp. 91–132. Boston: Birkhauser.

Fluosol 20% intravascular perfluorochemical emulsion (1990) *Product Monograph.* Alpha Therapeutic Corp.

Forman, M.B., Perry, J.M., Wilson, B.H., Verani, M.S., Kaplan, P.R., Shawl, F.A., Friesinger, G.C. (1991) Demonstration of myocardial reperfusion injury in humans: Results of a pilot study utilizing acute coronary angioplasty with perfluorochemical in anterior myocardial infarction. *J. Am. Coll. Cardiol.*, **18**, 911–918.

Friberg, S., Jansson, P.O., Cederberg, E. (1976) Surfactant association structures and emulsion stability. *J. Colloid Interface Sci.*, **55**, 614–623.

Fujita, T., Suyama, T., Yokoyama, K. (1973) Fluorocarbon emulsion as a candidate for artificial blood. *Europ. Surg. Res.*, **3**, 436–453.

Fung, B.M., O'Rear, E.A., Afzal, J., Frech, C.B., Mamrosh, D.L., Gangoda, M. (1989) Perfluorocarbon emulsions with fluorinated surfactants and anticancer drugs. In *Blood Substitutes*, edited by T.M.S. Chang and R.P. Geyer, pp. 439–440. New York: M. Dekker, Inc.

Geyer, R.P., Monroe, R.G., Taylor, K. (1968) Survival of rats having red cells totally replaced with emulsified fluorocarbon (abstract). *Fed. Proc.*, **27**, 384.

Geyer, R.P. (1973) Fluorocarbon-polyol artificial blood substitutes. *New Engl. J. Med.*, **289**, 1077–1082.

Geyer, R.P., Taylor, K., Duffett, E.B., Eccles, R. (1973) Successful complete replacement of the blood of living rats with artificial substitutes. *Fed. Proc.*, **32**, 927.

Geyer, R. P. (1975) "Bloodless" rats through the use of artificial blood substitutes. *Fed. Proc.*, **34**, 1499–1505.

Geyer, R.P. (1979) Perfluorochemical blood replacement preparations. In *Proceed. IVth Intl. Symp. Perfluorochemical Blood Substitutes*, pp. 3–32. Amsterdam: Excerpta Medica.

Ghosh, A., Janic, V., Sloviter, H. (1970) Enzymatic method for measuring dissolved oxygen in nonaqueous materials. *Anal. Biochem.* **38**, 270–276.

Gjaldbaek, J.C.H. (1952) The solubility of hydrogen, oxygen and carbon monoxide in some non-polar solvents *Acta Chem. Scand.* **6**, 623–633.

Gould, S.A., Rosen, L.A., Sehgal, H.L, Langdale, L.A., Krause, L.M., Rice, C.L., Chamberlin, W.H., Moss, G.S. (1986) Fluosol-DA as a red-cell substitute in acute anemia. *New Engl. J. Med.*, **314**, 1653–1656; see also correspondence section *New Engl. J. Med.*, **315**, 1677–1678.

Grec, J.-J., Riess, J.G., Devallez, B. (1985) Etude de solvants perfluoroalkylés à usage biomédical: Températures critiques supérieures de solubilité de bis(F-alkyl)éthènes dans l'hexane et vitesses d'excrétion. Paramètres de solubilité, grandeurs d'excès de mélanges d'acides carboxyliques et de composés perfluoroalkylés. *Nouv. J. Chim.*, **9**, 637–643.

Greiner, J., Riess, J.G., Vierling, P. (1993) Fluorinated surfactants intended for biomedical uses. In *Organofluorine Compounds in Medicinal Chemistry and Biomedical Applications*, edited by R. Filler, Y. Kobayashi and L.M. Yagupolski, pp. 339–380. Amsterdam: Elsevier.

Gross, U., Röding, J., Stanzl, K., Zastrow, L. (1994) Phospholipide enthaldendes Kosmatikum. *German Pat. DE 42 21 255.*

Groves, M.J., Wineberg, M., Brain, A.P.R. (1985) The presence of liposomal material in phosphatide stabilized emulsions. *J. Disp. Sci. Tech.*, **6**, 237–243.

Guest, D., Langevin, D. (1985) Light scattering study of a multiphase microemulsion system. *J. Colloid Interface Sci.*, **112**, 208–220.

Guo, J., White, J.A., Batjer, H.H. (1995). Intravenous Perflubron emulsion administration improves the recovery of auditory evoked potentials after temporary brain stem ischemia in dogs. *Neurosurgery*, **36**, 350–357.

Habif, S.S., Normand, P.E., Oleksiak, C.B., Rosano, H.L. (1992) Perfluorooctyl bromide dispersions in aqueous media for biomedical applications. *Biotechnol. Prog.*, **8**, 454–457.

Habler, O.P., Kleen, M.S., Hutter, J.W., Podtschaske, A.H., Tiede, M., Kemming, G.I., Welte, M.V., Corso, C.O., Batra, S., Keipert, P.E., Faithfull, N.S., Messmer, K.F.W. (1997) Hemodilution and iv. perflubron emulsion as an alternative to blood transfusion: Autologous transfusion versus i.v. administration of perflubron emulsion administration in severe normovolemic anemia: effects on tissue oxygenation. *Transfusion*, **38**, 145–155.

Hammerschmidt, D.E., Vercelotti, G.M. (1989) Limitation of complement activation by fluorocarbon emulsions: superiority of lecithin-emulsified preparations. In *Blood Substitutes*, edited by T.M.S. Chang and R.P. Geyer, pp. 431–440. New York: Marcel Dekker.

Hamza, H., Serratrice, G., Stébé, M.-J., Delpuech, J.-J. (1981) Solute-solvent interactions in perfluorocarbon solutions of oxygen. An NMR study. *J. Am. Chem. Soc.* **103**, 3733–3738.

Handa, T., Saito, H., Miyajima, K. (1990) Phospholipid monolayers at the triolein-saline interface: production of microemulsion particles and conversion of monolayers to bilayers. *Biochemistry*, **29**, 2884–2890.

Hanna, G.K., Ojeda, M.C., Sklenar, T.A. (1992) Application of computer-based experimental design to optimization of processing conditions for perfluorocarbon emulsion. *Biomat., Art. Cells, Immob. Biotech.*, **20**, 849–852.

Harashima, H., Sakata, K., Funato, K., Kiwada, H. (1994) Enhanced hepatic uptake of liposomes through complement activation depending on the size of liposomes. *Pharm. Res.*, **11**, 402–406.

Helfrich, W. (1973) Elastic properties of lipid bilayers: theory and possible experiments. *Z. Naturforsch.*, **28**, 693–703.

Hess, J.R. (1996) Blood substitutes. *Seminars in Hematology*, **33**, 1–11.

Higuchi, W.I., Misra, J. (1962) Physical degradation of emulsions via the molecular diffusion route and the possible prevention thereof. *J. Pharm. Sci.*, **51**, 459–466.

Hildebrand, J.H., Scott, R.L. (1950) *The Solubility of Nonelectrolytes*. New York: Reinhold.

Hogan, M.C., Willford, D.C., Keipert, P.E., Faithfull, N.S., Wagner, P.D. (1992) Increased plasma O_2 solubility improves O_2 uptake of *in situ* dog muscle working maximally. *J. Appl. Physiol.*, **73**, 2470–2475.

Holman, W.L., McGiffin, D.C., Vicente, W.V.A., Spruell, R.D., Pacifico, A.D. (1994) Use of current generation perfluorocarbon emulsions in cardiac surgery. *Art. Cells, Blood Subst., Immob. Biotech.*, **22**, 979–990.

Holman, W.L., Spruell, R.D., Ferguson, E.R., Clymer, J.J., Vicente, W.V.A., Murrah, C.P., Pacifico, A.D. (1995) Tissue oxygenation with graded dissolved oxygen delivery during cardiopulmonary bypass. *J. Thorac. Cardiovasc. Surg.*, **119**, 774–785.

Huang, R., Cooper, D.Y., Sloviter, H.A. (1987) Effects of intravenous emulsified perfluorochemicals on hepatic cytochrome P-450. *Biochem. Pharmac.*, **36**, 4331–4334.

Hunter, R.L., Papadea, C., Gallagher, C.J., Finlayson, D.C., Check, I.J. (1990) Increased whole blood viscosity during coronary artery bypass surgery. *Thrombosis and Haemostasis*, **63**, 6–12.

Ikomi, F., Hanna, G.K., Schmid-Schöenberin, G.W. (1995) Mechanism of colloidal particle uptake into the lymphatic system: basic study with percutaneous lymphography. *Radiology*, **196**, 107–113.

Illum, L., Jacobsen, L.O., Müller, R.H., Mak, E., Davis, S.S. (1987) Surface characteristics and the interaction of colloidal particles with mouse peritoneal macrophages. *Biomaterials*, **8**, 113–117.

Ishii, F. (1992) Phospholipids in emulsion and dispersion systems. *Abura Kagaku*, **41**, 101–106.

Ivanitski, G.R., Vorobiev, S.I. (1993) *Perfluorocarbon emulsions*. Pushchino, Russia: Acad. Sci. Russia.

Ivanitski, G.R. (1994) Int. Symp. "Perfluorocarbon 1994", Pushchino, Russia, June 1994.

Ivanitski, G.R., Vorobiev, S.I. (1996) In blood flow the functional basis of a perfluorocarbon "artificial blood" is structural motility. *Biophysica (Russia)*, **41**, 178–190.

Janco, R.L., Virmani, R., Morris, P.J., Gunter, K. (1985) Perfluorochemical blood substitutes differentially alter human monocyte procoagulant generation and oxidative metabolism. *Transfusion*, **25**, 578–582.

Jeanneaux, F., Le Blanc, M., Riess, J.G., Yokoyama, K. (1984) Fluorocarbons as gas carriers for biomedical applications — 1,2–bis(F-butyl)ethene as a candidate O_2/CO_2 carrier for second-generation blood substitutes. *Nouv. J. Chimie*, **8**, 251–257.

Johnson, O.L., Washington, C., Davis, S.S. (1990) Thermal stability of fluorocarbon emulsions that transport oxygen. *Int. J. Pharm.*, **59**, 131–135.

Jokela, P., Fletcher, P.D.I., Aveyard, R., Lu, J.-R. (1990) The use of computerized microscopic image analysis to determine emulsion droplet size distributions. *J. Colloid Interface Sci.*, **134**, 417–426.

Justicz, A., Lenaerts, V., Raymond, P., Ong, H. (1989) Diffusion of rat atrial natriuretic factor in thermoreversible poloxamer gels. *Biomaterials*, **10**, 265–268.

Kabalnov, A.S., Pertsov, A.V., Aprosin, Yu.D., Shchukin, E.D. (1985) Influence of nature and composition of disperse phase on stability of oil-in-water emulsions against transcondensation. *Kolloidn Zh.*, **47**, 1048–1053.

Kabalnov, A.S., Pertsov, A.V., Shchukin, E.D. (1987) Ostwald ripening in two-component disperse phase systems: application to emulsion stability. *Colloids Surf.*, **24**, 19–32.

Kabalnov, A.S., Makarov, K.N., Shcherbakova, O.V. (1990) Solubility of fluorocarbons in water as a key parameter determining fluorocarbon emulsion stability. *J. Fluorine Chem.*, **50**, 271–284.

Kabalnov, A.S., Makarov, K.N., Shchukin, E.D. (1992) Stability of perfluoroalkyl halide emulsions. *Colloids Surf.*, **62**, 101–104.

Kabalnov, A.S., Shchukin, E.D. (1992) Ostwald ripening theory: applications to fluorocarbon emulsion stability. *Adv. Colloid Interface Sci.*, **38**, 69–97.

Kabalnov, A.S. (1994) Can micelles mediate a mass transfer between oil droplets? *Langmuir*, **10**, 680–684.

Kabalnov, A., Weers, J., Arlauskas, R., Tarara, T. (1995) Phospholipids as emulsion stabilizers. 1. Interfacial tensions. *Langmuir*, **11**, 2966–2974.

Kabalnov, A., Tarara, T., Arlauskas, R., Weers, J. (1996) Phospholipids as emulsion stabilizers. 2. Phase behavior versus emulsion stability. *J. Colloid Interface Sci.*, **184**, 227–235.

Kabalnov, A., Weers, J. (1996a) Macroemulsion stability within the Winsor III region: theory versus experiment. *Langmuir*, **12**, 1931–1935.

Kabalnov, A., Weers, J. (1996b) Kinetics of mass transfer in micellar systems: surfactant adsorption, solubilization kinetics, and ripening. *Langmuir*, **12**, 3442–3448.

Kabalnov, A., Wennerström, H. (1996) Macroemulsion stability: the oriented wedge theory revisited. *Langmuir*, **12**, 276–292.

Kahlweit, M. (1970) Precipitation and aging. In *Physical Chemistry: An Advanced Treatise*, edited by H. Eyring, D. Henderson, W. Jost, Volume X, pp. 719–759. New York: Academic Press.

Kaufman, R.J. (1994) The results of a Phase I clinical trial of a 40v/v% emulsion of HM351 (Oxyfluor) in healthy volunteers. *IBC Conf. on Blood Substitutes and Related Products*, Washington.

Kaufman, R.J. (1995) Clinical development of perfluorocarbon-based emulsions as red cell substitutes. In *Blood Substitutes: Physiological Basis of Efficacy*, edited by R.M. Winslow, K.D. Vandegriff, M. Intaglietta, pp. 53–75. Boston: Birkhäuser.

Kaufman, R.J., Richard, T.J. (1995) Red blood cell substitute emulsions containing alkyl- or alkylglycerophosphoryl choline surfactants and methods of use. *United States Patent No.* 5,439,944.

Keipert, P.E., Faithfull, N.S., Bradley, J.D., Hazard, D.Y., Hogan, J., Levisetti, M.S., Peters, R.M. (1994a) Oxygen delivery augmentation by low-dose perfluorochemical emulsion during profound normovolemic hemodilution. *Adv. Exp. Med. Biol.*, **345**, 194–204.

Keipert, P.E., Otto, S., Flaim, S.F., Weers, J.G., Schutt, E.A., Pelura, T.J., Klein, D.H., Yaksh, T.L. (1994b) Influence of perflubron emulsion particle size on blood half-life and febrile response in rats. *Art. Cells, Blood Subst., Immob. Biotech.*, **22**, 1169–1174.

Keipert, P.E. (1995) Use of Oxygent™, a perfluorochemical-based oxygen carrier, as an alternative to intraoperative blood transfusion. *Art. Cells, Blood Subst., Immob. Biotech.*, **23**, 381–394.

Keipert, P.E., Conlan, M.G. (1996) Advances in perflubron emulsion development: potential use during surgery and cardiopulmonary bypass to avoid donor blood transfusion and prevent tissue hypoxia. *Art. Cells, Blood Subst., Immob. Biotech.*, **24**, 359 (abstract).

Keipert, P.E., Faithfull, N.S., Roth, D.J., Bradley, J.D., Batra, S., Jochelson, P., Flaim, K.E. (1996) Supporting tissue oxygenation during acute surgical bleeding using a perfluorochemical-based oxygen carrier. In *Oxygen Transport to Tissue XVII*, edited by C. Ince, J. Kesecioglu, L. Telci, K. Akpir, pp. 603–609. New York: Plenum Press.

Keipert, P.E. (1998) Perflurochemical emulsions: future alternatives to transfusion. In *Blood Substitutes*, edited by T.M.S. Chang, pp. 127–156. New York: Karger Landes Systems.

Kennan, R.P., Pollack, G.L. (1988) Solubility of xenon in perfluoroalkanes: Temperature dependence and thermodynamics. *J. Chem. Phys.*, **89**, 517–521;

Kent, K.M., Cleman, M.W., Cowley, M.J., Forman, M.B., Jaffe, C.C., Kaplan, M., King, S.P. III, Krucoff, M.W., Lasser, T., McAuley, B., Smith, R., Wisdom, C., Wohlgelernter, D. (1990) Reduction of myocardial ischemia during percutaneous transluminal coronary angioplasty with oxygenated Fluosol. *Am. J. Cardiol.*, **66**, 279–284.

Kerins, D.M. (1994) Role of perfluorocarbon Fluosol-DA in coronary angioplasty. *Am. J. Med. Sci.*, **307**, 218–221.

Kitazawa, M., Ohnishi, Y. (1982) Long-term experiment of perfluorochemicals using rabbits. *Virchows Arch. Pathol. Anat.*, **398**, 1–10.

Klein, D.H., Burtner, D.B., Trevino, L.A., Arlauskas, R.A. (1992) Particle size distribution of concentrated perfluorocarbon emulsions by sedimentation field-flow fractionation. *Biomat., Art. Cells, Immob. Biotech.*, **20**, 859–864.

Klein, D.H., Jones, R.C., Keipert, P.E., Luena, G.A., Otto, S., Weers, J.G. (1994) Intravascular behavior of perflubron emulsions. *Colloids Surf.*, **84**, 98–95.

Klein, H.G. (1994) Oxygen carriers and transfusion medicine. *Art. Cells, Blood Subst., Immob. Biotech.*, **22**, 123–135.

Klein, R.A. (1970) The detection of oxidation in liposome preparations. *Biochim. Biophys. Acta*, **210**, 486–489.

Kloner, R.A., Hale, S. (1994) Cardiovascular applications of fluorocarbons in regional ischemia/reperfusion. *Art. Cells, Blood Subst., Immob. Biotech.*, **22**, 1069–1081.

Kong, C.F., Fung, B.M., O'Rear, E.A. (1985) Interaction between perfluoro chemicals and phosphatidylcholine vesicles. *J. Phys. Chem.*, **89**, 4386–4390.

Korstvedt, H., Nikopoulos, G., Chandounet, S., Siciliano, A. (1985) Microfluidization for making fine emulsions and dispersions. *American Paints and Coating Journal*, **22**, 38–39.

Krafft, M.P., Rolland, J.-P., Riess, J.G. (1991) Detrimental effect of excess lecithin on the stability of fluorocarbon/lecithin emulsions. *J. Phys. Chem.*, **95**, 5673–5676.

Krafft, M.P., Postel, M., Riess J.G., Ni, Y., Pelura, T.J., Hanna, G.K., Song, D. (1992) Drop size stability assessment of fluorocarbon emulsions. *Biomat., Art. Cells, Immob. Biotech.*, **20**, 865–868.

Krafft, M.P., Riess J.G. (1994). Stable highly concentrated fluorocarbon gels. *Angew. Chem. Int. Ed. Engl.*, **33**, 1100–1101.

Krafft, M.P., Sadtler, V., Riess, J.G. (1995) Water-in-fluorocarbon emulsions for pulmonary drug delivery. *Proceed. Int. Symp. Control. Rel. Bioact. Mater.*, **22**, 464–465.

Krafft, M.P., Riess, J.G. (1995) Gels inverses avec une phase fluorocarbure continue. Fr. Patent 2,737,135.

Krafft, M.P., Riess, J.G. (1998) Highly fluorinated amphiphiles and colloidal systems, and their applications in the biomedical field – A contribution. *Biochimie*.

Kumacheva, E.E., Amelina, E.A., Pertsov, A.V., Shchukin, E.D. (1989) Effect of a lipid on reverse distillation in aqueous emulsions of perfluorocarbons. *Kolloidn Zh.*, **51**, 1214–1216.

Kunieda, H., Shinoda, K. (1976) Krafft points, critical micelle concentrations, surface tensions and solubilizing power of aqueous solutions of fluorinated surfactants. *J. Phys. Chem.*, **80**, 2468–2470.

Lane, T.A., Lampkin, G. (1984) Paralysis of phagocyte migration due to an artificial blood substitute. *Blood*, **64**, 400–405.

Lane, T.A., Lampkin, G. (1986) Increased infection mortality and decreased neutrophil migration due to a component of an artificial blood substitute. *Blood*, **68**, 351–354.

Lane, T.A., Krukonis, V. (1988) Reduction in the toxicity of a component of an artificial blood substitute by supercritical fluid fractionation. *Transfusion*, **28**, 375–378.

Lasic, D.D., Needham, D. (1995) The stealth liposome: a prototypical biomaterial. *Chem. Rev.*, **95**, 2601–2628.

Lattes, A., Rico-Lattes, I. (1994) Microemulsions of perfluorinated and semi-fluorinated compounds. *Art. cells, Blood Subst., Immob. Biotech.*, **22**, 1007–1018.

Lawson, D.D., Moacanin, J., Scherer, K.V., Terranova, T.F., Ingham, J.D. (1978) Methods for the estimation of vapor pressures and oxygen solubilities of fluorochemicals for possible application in artificial blood formulations. *J. Fluorine Chem.*, **12**, 221–236.

Le, T.D., Arlauskas, R.A., Weers, J.G. (1996) Characterization of the lipophilicity of fluorocarbon derivatives containing halogens or hydrocarbon blocks. *J. Fluorine Chem.*, **78**, 155–163.

Leach, C.L., Greenspan, J.S., Rubenstein, S.D., Shaffer, T.H., Wolfson, M.R., Jackson, J.C., DeLemos, R., Fuhrman, B.P. (1996) Partial liquid ventilation with perflubron in premature infants with severe respiratory distress syndrome. *New Engl. J. Med.*, **335**, 761–767.

Leakakos, T., Schutt, E.G., Cavin, J.C., Smith, D., Bradley, J.D., Strnat, C.A., de Balzo, U., Hazard, D.Y., Otto, S., Fields, T.K., Keipert, P.E., Klein, D.H., Flaim, S.F. (1994) Pulmonary gas trapping differences among animal species in response to intravenous infusion of perfluorocarbon emulsions. *Art. Cells, Blood Subst., Immob. Biotech.*, **22**, 1199–1204.

Le Blanc, M., Riess, J.G. (1982) A strategy for the synthesis of pure, inert perfluoroalkylated derivatives designed for blood substitution. *Oxygen-carrying Colloidal Blood Substitutes*, pp. 43–49. Munich: W. Zuckschwerdt Verlag.

Le Blanc, M., Riess, J.G., Poggi, D., Follana, R. (1985) Use of lymphoblastoid Namalva cell cultures in a toxicity test. Application to the monitoring of detoxification procedures for fluorocarbons to be used as intravascular oxygen-carriers. *Pharm. Res.*, 245–248.

Li, J., Miller, R., Möhwald, H. (1996) Characterization of phospholipid layers at liquid interfaces. 1. Dynamics of adsorbed phospholipid at the chloroform/water interface. *Colloids Surf. A*, **114**, 113–121.

Lidgate, D.M., Fu, R.C., Fleitman, J.S. (1989) Using a microfluidizer to manufacture parenteral emulsions. *BioPharm*, October 1989, 28–34.

Lifshitz, I.M., Slezov, V.V. (1959) Kinetics of diffusive decomposition of supersaturated solid solutions. *Sov. Phys. JETP*, **35**, 331–339.
Long, D.M., Liu, M., Szanto, P.S., Alrenga, D.P., Patel, M.M., Rios, M.V., Nyhus, L.M. (1972) Efficacy and toxicity studies with radiopaque perfluorocarbon. *Radiology*, **105**, 323–332.
Long, D.M., Higgins, C.B., Mattrey, R.F., Mitten, R.M., Multer, F.K. (1988) Is there a time and place for radiopaque fluorocarbons? In *Preparation, Properties and Industrial Applications of Organofluorine Compounds*, edited by R.E. Banks, pp. 139–156. UK: Ellis Horwood Ltd., Chichester.
Long, D.C., Long, D.M., Riess, J.G., Follana, R., Burgan, A., Mattrey, R.F. (1989) Preparation and application of highly concentrated perfluorooctyl bromide fluorocarbon emulsions. In *Blood Substitutes*, edited by T.M.S. Chang and R.P. Geyer, pp. 441–443. New York: M. Dekker.
Lowe, K.C. (1994a) Properties and biomedical applications of perfluorochemicals and their emulsions. In *Organofluorine Chemistry, Principles and Commercial Applications*, edited by R.E. Banks, B.E. Smart and J.C. Tatlow, pp. 555–577. New York: Plenum Press.
Lowe, K.C. (1994b) Perfluorochemicals in medicine and cell biotechnology. In *Fluorine in Medicine in the 21st Century*, edited by R.E. Banks and K.C. Lowe, Chapter 19. Shawbury, UK: Rapra Technol. Ltd.
Lutz, J. (1985) Effect of perfluorochemicals on host defense, especially on the reticuloendothelial system. *Int. Anesth. Clin.*, **23**, 63–93.
Lutz, J., Stark, M. (1987) Half-life and changes in the composition of a perfluorochemical emulsion within the vascular system of rats. *Plügers Arch.*, **410**, 181–184.
Magdassi, S., Royz, M., Shoshan, S. (1992). Interactions between collagen and perfluorocarbon emulsions. *Int. J. Pharm.*, **88**, 171–176.
Mahadevan, S., Dillard, C.J., Tappel, A.L. (1969) A modified colorimetric micro method for long-chain fatty acids and its application for assay of lipolytic enzymes. *Anal. Biochem.*, **27**, 387–396.
Makowski, H. (1978) The properties of Fluosol-DA infusion in the treatment of hemorrhagic shock. In *Proc. IVth Intern. Symp. on Perfluorochemical Blood Substitutes*, Kyoto, Japan, Oct. 1978, pp. 439–448. Amsterdam: Excerpta Medica.
Malet-Martino, M.C., Betbeder, D., Lattes, A., Lopez, A., Martino, R., Francois, G., Cros, S. (1984) Fluosol 43 intravascular persistence in mice measured by ^{19}F nmr. *J. Pharm. Pharmacol.*, **36**, 556–559.
Marchbank, A. (1995) Fluorocarbon emulsions. *Perfusion*, **10**, 67–88.
Marsh, D. (1987) *CRC Handbook of lipid bilayers*. Boca Raton: CRC Press.
Mathis, G.P., Leempoel, P., Ravey, J-C., Selve, C., Delpuech, J.-J. (1984) A novel class of nonionic microemulsions: fluorocarbons in aqueous solutions of fluorinated poly(oxyethylene) surfactants. *J. Am. Chem. Soc.*, **106**, 6162–6171.
Mathy-Hartert, M., Krafft, M.P., Deby, C., Deby-Dupont, G., Meurisse, M., Lamy, M., Riess, J.G. (1997) Effects of perfluorocarbon emulsions on cultured human endothelial cells. *Art. Cells, Blood Subst., Immob. Biotech.*, **25**, 563–575.
Mattrey, R.F., Scheible, F.W., Gosink, B.B., Leopold, G.R., Long, D.M., Higgins, C.B. (1982) Perfluorooctyl bromide, a liver/spleen specific and a tumor imaging ultra-sound contrast material. *Radiology*, **145**, 759–762.
Mattrey, R.F. (1994) The potential role of perfluorochemicals (PFCs) in diagnostic imaging. *Art. Cells, Blood Subst., Immob. Biotech.*, **22**, 295–313.
Mayer, D.C., Strada, S.J., Hoff, C., Hunter, R.L., Artman, M. (1994) Effects of poloxamer 188 in a rabbit model of hemorrhagic shock. *Ann. Clin. Lab. Sci.* **24**, 302–311.
McClements, D.J., Dungan, S.R. (1993) Factors that affect the rate of oil exchange between oil-in-water emulsion droplets stabilized by a nonionic surfactant: droplet size, surfactant concentration, and ionic strength. *J. Phys. Chem.*, **97**, 7304–7308.
Meinert, H., Fackler, R., Knoblich, A., Mader, J., Reuter, P., Röhlke, W. (1992) On the perfluorocarbon emulsions of second generation. *Biomat., Art. Cells, Immob. Biotech.*, **20**, 805–818.
Meinert, H., Reuter, P., Röhlke, W., Cambon, A., Szönyi, S., Gaysinski, M. (1994) Liposomes and liposome-like vesicles in perfluorocarbon emulsions. *J. Fluorine Chem.*, **66**, 203–207.
Menasché, P., Fleury, J.P., Piwnica, A. (1992) Fluorocarbons: a potential treatment of cerebral air embolism in open-heart surgery, 1992 update. *Ann. Thorac. Surg.* **54**, 392–393.
Milius, A., Greiner, J., Riess, J.G. (1992) Improvement in emulsification ease, particle size reduction, and stabilization of concentrated fluorocarbon emulsions by small amounts of (d-glucosyl)[2-(perfluoroalkyl)ethyl]phosphate as surfactants. *Colloids Surf.*, **63**, 281–289.
Millard, R.W. (1994) Oxygen solubility, rheology, and hemodynamics of perfluorocarbon emulsion blood substitutes. *Art. Cells, Blood Subst., Immob. Biotech.*, **22**, 235–244.

Miller, M.L., Wesseler, E.P., Jones, S.C., Clark, L.C. (1976) Some morphologic effects of "inert" particulate loading on hemopoietic elements in mice. *J. Reticuloendothelial. Soc.*, **20**, 385–398.

Mitsuno, T., Ohyanagi, H., Naito, R. (1982a) Clinical studies of perfluorochemical whole blood substitute (Fluosol-DA): summary of 186 cases. *Ann. Surg.*, **195**, 60–69.

Mitsuno, T., Ohyanagi, H. Naito, R. (1982b) Clinical studies of a perfluorochemical whole blood substitute (Fluosol-DA). In *Oxygen Carrying Colloidal Blood Substitutes*, edited by R. Frey, H. Beisbarth, K. Stosseck, pp. 30–40. Munich: W. Zuckschwerdt Verlag.

Mitten, R.M., Burgan, A.R., Hamblin, A., Yee, G., Long, D.C., Long, D.M., Mattrey, R.F. (1989) Dose related biodistribution and elimination of 100% PFOB emulsion. In *Blood Substitutes*, edited by T.M.S. Chang and R.P. Geyer, pp. 683–684. New York: M. Dekker, Inc.

Miyauchi, Y., Inoue, J., Paton, B.C. (1966) Adjunctive use of surface active agent in extracorporeal circulation. *Circulation*, **33**, 171.

Moghimi, S.M., Muir, I.S., Illum, L., Davis, S.S., Kolb-Bachofen, V. (1993) Coating particles with a block co-polymer (poloxamin-908) suppresses opsonization but permits the activity of dysopsonins in the serum. *Biochim. Biophys. Acta*, **1179**, 157–165.

Moore, G.G.I., Flynn, R.M., Guerra, M.A. (1996) Physiologically acceptable emulsions containing perfluorocarbon ether hydrides and methods of use. *US Patent 5,567,765*.

Moore, R.E., Clark, L.C. (1982) Synthesis and physical properties of perfluorocompounds useful as synthetic blood candidates. In *Oxygen-carrying Colloidal Blood Substitutes*, edited by R. Frey, H. Beisbarth and K. Stosseck, pp. 50–60. Munich: W. Zuckschwerdt Verlag.

Moore, R.E., Clark, L.C. (1985) Chemistry of fluorocarbons in biomedical use. *Int. Anesth. Clin.*, **23**, 11–24.

Moore, R.E. (1989) Physical properties of a new synthetic oxygen carrier. In *Blood Substitutes*, edited by T.M.S. Chang and R.P. Geyer, pp. 443–445. New York: M. Dekker, Inc.

Mukerjee, P., Mysels, K. J. (1975) Anomalies of partially fluorinated surfactant micelles. *ACS Symp. Ser. 9. Am. Chem. Soc.*, pp. 239–252. Washington, DC.

Mukherji, B.M., Sloviter, H.A. (1991) A stable perfluorochemical blood substitute. *Transfusion*, **31**, 324–326.

Naito, R., Yokoyama, K. (1975) On the perfluorodecalin/phospholipid emulsion as a red cell substitute. *Proc. Xth Inter. Cong. Nutrition — Symp. on Perfluorochemical Artificial Blood*, Kyoto, pp. 55–72. Osaka: Igakushodo Medical Publ.

Naito, R., Yokoyama, K. (1978) An improved perfluorodecalin emulsion. In *Blood Substitutes and Plasma Expanders*, pp. 81–84. New York: Alan Liss.

Naito, R., Yokoyama, K. (1981) *Perfluorochemical blood substitutes. Technical Information Ser. n° 5*. Osaka, Japan: The Green Cross Corp.

Nakamura, T. (1986) Prostaglandin-like substances formed during autooxidation of methyl linoleate. *Lipids*, **21**, 553–557.

Nakamura, T., Maeda, H. (1991) A simple assay for lipid hydroperoxides based on triphenylphosphine oxidation and high-performance liquid chromatography. *Lipids*, **26**, 765–767.

Nakashima, K., Anzai, T., Fujimoto, Y. (1994) Fluorescence studies on the properties of a Pluronic® F68 micelle. *Langmuir*, **10**, 658–661.

Navari, R.M., Rosenblum, W.I., Kontos, H.A., Patterson, J.L. (1977) Mass transfer properties of gases in fluorocarbons. *Res. Exp. Med.*, **170**, 169–180.

Newman, R.J., Podolsky, D., Loeb, P. (1994) Bad Blood. *U.S. News*, June, pp. 68–78.

Ni, Y., Klein, D. H., Pelura, T. J. (1992) Rheology of concentrated perfluorocarbon emulsions. *Biomat., Art. Cells, Immob. Biotech.*, **20**, 869–871.

Ni, Y., Pelura, T. J., Sklenar, T. A., Kinner, R. A., Song, D. (1994) Effects of formulation, processing and sorage parameters on the characteristics and stability of perflubron emulsion. *Art. Cells, Blood Subs., Immob. Biotech.*, **22**, 1307–1315.

Ni, Y., Klein, D., Song, D. (1996) Recent developments in pharmacokinetic modeling of perfluorocarbon emulsions. *Art. Cells, Blood Subst., Immob. Biotech.*, **24**, 81–90.

Nicoli, D.F., Wu, J.S., Chang, Y.J., McKenzie, D.C., Hasapidis, K. (1995) Wide dynamic range particle size analysis by DLS-SPOS. *American Laboratory*, April.

Obraztsov, V.V., Kabalnov, A.S., Sklifas, A.N., Makarov, K.N. (1992) A new model describing the elimination of fluorocarbons from the body: dissolution of fluorocarbons in the lipid components of the blood. *Biophysics*, **37**, 298–302.

Obraztsov, V.V. (1994) Fluorocarbon blood substitutes in Russia. *Art. Cells, Blood Subst., Immob. Biotech.*, **22**, 1019–1027.

Ogilby, J.D., Noma, S., DiLoretto, G., Stets, G. (1992) Preservation of myocardial function during ischemia with intracoronary perfluorooctylbromide (Oxygent™). *Biomat., Art. Cells, Immob. Biotech.*, **20**, 973–977.

Ogilby, J.D. (1994) Cardiovascular applications of fluorocarbons: current status and future direction — a critical clinical appraisal. *Art. Cells, Blood Subst., Immob. Biotech.*, **22**, 1083–1096.

Ohyanagi, H., Mitsuno, T. (1975) Biophysiological effects of perfluorochemicals as artificial blood. *Proc. Xth Intern. Cong. of Nutrition — Symp. on Perfluorochemical Artificial Blood*, pp. 21–54. Kyoto, Japan.

Ohyanagi, H., Itoh, T., Sekita, M., Okamoto, M., Mitsuno, T. (1977) Kinetic studies of oxygen and carbon dioxide transport into or from perfluorochemical particles. *Art. Organs*, **2** (Suppl.), 90–92.

Ohyanagi, H., Saitoh, Y., Mitsuno, T., Watanabe, M., Yamanouchi, K., Yokoyama, K. (1990) A new perfluorochemical emulsion: An Overview. *Art. Organs*, **14**, 199–200.

Okada, K., Kosugi, I., Kawashima, Y., Yamagushi, Y., Yoshikawa, H., Yamamura, H. (1975) Effect of Fluosol-DC on tissue pO_2 and pCO_2 in treatment of hemorrhagic hypotension. *Proc. Xth Intern. Cong. of Nutrition — Symp. on Perfluorochemical Artificial Blood*, pp. 215–224. Kyoto, Japan.

Okamoto, H., Yamanouchi, K., Imagawa, T., Murashima, R., Yokoyama, K., Watanabe, R., Naito, R. (1973) Persistence of fluorocarbons in circulating blood and organs. *Proc. IInd Intercompany Conf.*, Osaka.

Okamoto, H., Yamanouchi, K., Yokoyama, (1975) Retention of perfluorochemicals in circulating blood and organs of animals after intravenous injection of their emulsions. *Chem. Pharm. Bull. Jap.*, **23**, 1452–1457.

Oleksiak, C.B., Habif, S.S., Rosano, H.L. (1994) Flocculation of perfluorocarbon emulsions. *Colloids Surf. A*, **84**, 71–79.

Oxynoid, O.E., Sydliarov, D.P., Aprosin, Yu. D., Obraztsov, V.V. (1994). Application of fluorocarbon emulsions as components of cosmetics and medical ointments. In *Art. Cells, Blood Subst., Immob. Biotech.*, **22**, 1331–1336.

Pal, R., Yan, Y., Masliyah, J. (1992) Rheology of emulsions. In *Emulsions: Fundamentals and Applications in the Petroleum Industry*, edited by L. Schramm, pp. 131–170. Washington: American Chemical Society.

Pandolfe, W.D. (1983) Recent developments in the understanding of homogenization parameters. Summer Nat. Meeting, Am. Inst. Chem. Engineers, Denver, August 1983.

Parfenova, A.M., Amelina, E.A., Vitvitskii, V.M., Makarov, K.N., Gervits, L.L., Shchukin, E.D. (1990) Influence of different proxanols on the coalescence resistance of perfluorodecalin droplets. *Kolloidn Zh.*, **52**, 801–803.

Patrick, C.R. (1982) Mixing and solution properties of organofluorine compounds. In *Preparation, Properties and Applications of Selected Organofluorine Compounds*, edited by R.E. Banks, pp. 323–342. Chichester, UK: Ellis Horwood.

Peczeli, C.F. (1975) Fluid shear device. *US Pat 1 520 482*.

Pelura, T.J., Johnson, C.S., Tarara, T.E., Weers, J.G. (1992) Stabilization of perflubron emulsions with egg-yolk phospholipid. *Biomat., Art. Cells, Immob. Biotech.*, **20**, 845–848.

Pierotti, R.A. (1976) A scaled particle theory of aqueous and nonaqueous solutions *Chem. Rev.*, **76**, 717–726.

Pollack, G.L., Kennan, R.P., Himm, J.F. (1989) Solubility of xenon in 45 organic solvents including cycloalkanes, acids, and alkanals: Experiment and theory. *J. Chem. Phys.*, **90**, 6569–6579.

Pollack, G.L., Kennan, R.P., Holm, G.T. (1992) Solubility of inert gases in PFC blood substitutes, blood plasma, and mixtures. *Biomat., Art. Cells, Immob. Biotech.*, **20**, 1101–1104.

Porter, C.J.H., Moghimi, S.M., Illum, L., Davis, S.S. (1992) The polyoxyethylene/polyoxypropylene block co-polymer Poloxamer-407 selectively redirects intravenously injected microspheres to sinusoidal endothelium cells of rabbit bone marrow. *FEBS Letters*, **305**, 62–66.

Postel, M., Chang, P., Rolland, J.P., Krafft, M.P., Riess, J.G. (1991) Fluorocarbon/lecithin emulsions: identification of EYP-coated fluorocarbon droplets and fluorocarbon-empty vesicles by freeze-fracture electron microscopy. *Biochim. Biophys. Acta*, **1086**, 95–98.

Postel, M., Riess, J.G., Weers, J.G. (1994) Fluorocarbon emulsions — the stability issue. *Art. Cells, Blood Subst., Immob. Biotech.*, **22**, 991–1005.

Putyatina, T.K., Aprosin, U.D., Afonin, N.I. (1994) The elimination peculiarities of perfluorocarbon emulsions stabilized with egg yolk phospholipid. *Art. Cells, Blood Subst., Immob. Biotech.*, **22**, 1281–1285.

Ravey, J.C., Stébé, M.J. (1987). Phase and structure behavior of fluorinated nonionic surfactant systems. *Prog. Colloid. Polym. Sci.*, **73**, 127–133.

Ravey, J.C., Stébé, M.J. (1990). Structure of inverse micelles and emulsion-gels with fluorinated nonionic surfactants. A small-angle neutron scattering study. *Prog. Colloid. Polym. Sci.*, **82**, 218–228.

Ravis, W.R., Hoke, J.F., Parsons, D.L. (1991) Perfluorochemical erythrocyte substitutes: disposition and effects on drug distribution and elimination. *Drug. Metabol. Rev.*, **23**, 375–411.

Reeve, L.E. (1997) The poloxamers: their chemistry and medical applications. In *Handbook of Biodegradable Polymers*, edited by A. Domb, J. Kost and D. Wiseman. Amsterdam: Harwood Academic Publ.

Riess, J.G., Le Blanc, M. (1978) Perfluoro compounds as blood substitutes. *Angew. Chem. Intl. Ed. Engl.*, **17**, 621–634.

Riess, J.G., Le Blanc, M. (1982) Solubility and transport phenomena in perfluorochemicals relevant to blood substitution and other biomedical applications. *Pure Appl. Chem.* **54**, 2383–2406.

Riess, J.G. (1984). Reassessment of criteria for the selection of perfluorochemicals for second generation blood substitutes. Analysis of structure/property relationships. *Artif. Organs*, **8**, 44–56.

Riess, J.G. (1987) Post-Fluosol progress in fluorocarbon emulsions for *in vivo* oxygen delivery. *La Trasf. del Sangue*, **32**, 316–334.

Riess, J.G., Le Blanc, M. (1988) Preparation of perfluorochemical emulsions for biomedical use: principles, materials and methods. In *Blood Substitutes: Preparation, Physiology and Medical Applications*, edited by K.C. Lowe, pp. 94–129. Chichester, UK: Ellis Horwood.

Riess, J.G., Arlen, C., Greiner, J., LeBlanc, M., Manfredi, A., Pace, S., Varescon, C., Zarif, L. (1989) Design, synthesis and evaluation of fluorocarbons and surfactants for *in vivo* applications: new perfluoroalkylated polyhydroxylated surfactants. In *Blood Substitutes*, edited by T.M.S. Chang and R.P. Geyer, pp. 421–430. New York: Marcel Dekker.

Riess, J.G. (1990) Hemocompatible fluorocarbon emulsions. In *Blood compatible materials and devices: prospectives towards the 21st century*, edited by C.P. Sharma and M. Szycher, pp. 237–270. Lancaster: Technomics.

Riess, J.G. (1992) Overview of progress in the fluorocarbon approach to in vivo oxygen delivery. *Biomat., Art. Cells, Immob. Biotech.*, **20**, 183–202.

Riess, J.G., Krafft, M.P. (1992) Elaboration of fluorocarbon emulsions with improved oxygen-carrying capacity. *Adv. Exp. Med. Biol.*, **317**, 465–472.

Riess, J.G., Postel, M. (1992) Stability and stabilization of fluorocarbon emulsions destined to injection. *Biomat., Art. Cells, Immob. Biotech.*, **20**, 819–829.

Riess, J.G., Dalfors, J.L., Hanna, G.K., Klein, D.H., Krafft, M.P., Pelura, T.J., Schutt, E.G. (1992a) Development of highly fluid, concentrated and stable fluorocarbon emulsions for diagnosis and therapy. *Biomat., Art. Cells, Immob. Biotech.*, **20**, 839–842.

Riess, J.G., Greiner, J., Abouhilale, Milius, A. (1992b) Stabilization of fluorocarbon emulsions by sugar-derived perfluoroalkylated surfactants and co-surfactants. *Prog. Colloid Polym Sci.*, **88**, 123–130.

Riess, J.R., Sole-Violan, L., Postel, M. (1992c) A new concept in the stabilization of injectable fluorocarbon emulsions: the use of mixed fluorocarbon-hydrocarbon dowels. *J. Disp. Sci. Technol.*, **13**, 349–355.

Riess, J.G. (ed.) (1994a). *Proc. Vth Intern. Symp. on Blood Substitutes*, vol. 3, *Blood Substitutes, the Fluorocarbon Approach.*, published in *Art. Cells, Blood Subst., Immob. Biotech.*, **22**, 945–1543.

Riess, J.G. (1994b) Perfluorochemical emulsions for intravascular use. In *Fluorine in Medicine in the 21st Century*, edited by R.E. Banks and K.C. Lowe, Chap. 20. Shawbury, UK: Rapra Technol. Ltd.

Riess, J.G. (1994c) Highly fluorinated systems for oxygen transport, diagnosis and drug delivery. *Colloids Surf.*, **84**, 33–48.

Riess, J.G. (1994d) The design and development of improved fluorocarbon-based products for use in medicine and biology. *Art. Cells, Blood Subst., Immob. Biotech.*, **22**, 215–234.

Riess, J.G. (1994e) Fluorinated vesicles. *J. Drug Target.*, **2**, 455–468.

Riess, J.G., Cornélus, C., Follana, R., Krafft, M.P., Mahé, A.M., Postel, M., Zarif, L. (1994) Novel fluorocarbon-based injectable oxygen-carrying formulations with long-term room-temperature storage stability. *Adv. Exp. Med. Biol.*, **345**, 227–234.

Riess, J.G., Frézard, F., Greiner, J., Krafft, M.P., Santaella, C., Vierling, P., Zarif, L. (1996). In *Handbook of Nonmedical Applications of Liposomes, Volume III*, edited by Y. Barenholz and D.D. Lasic, Chap. 8, pp. 98–141. Boca Raton, Florida: CRC Press Inc.

Riess, J.G., Weers, J.G. (1996) Emulsions for biomedical uses. *Curr. Opinion Colloid Interface Sci.*, **1**, 652–659.

Riess, J.G., Krafft, M.P. (1997) Advanced fluorocarbon-based systems for oxygen and drug delivery, and diagnosis. *Art. Cells, Blood Subst., Immob. Biotech.*, **25**, 43–52.

Riess, J.G., Krafft, M.P. (1998) Fluorinated materials for *in vivo* oxygen transport (blood substitutes), diagnosis and drug delivery. *Biomaterials*, **31**, xx.

Riess, J.G. (1998) Fluorocarbon-based oxygen delivery: basic principles and product development. In *Blood Substitutes*, edited by T.M.S. Chang, p. 101–126. New York: Karger Landes Systems.

Riess, J.G., Keipert, P.E. (1998) Update on perfluorocarbon-based oxygen delivery systems. In *Present and Future Perspectives of Blood Substitutes*, edited by E. Tsuchida. Lausanne: Elsevier Science.

Robert, A., Tondre, C. (1984) Solubilization of water in binary mixtures of fluorocarbons and nonionic fluorinated surfactants: existence domains of reverse emulsions. *J. Colloid. Interface Sci.*, **98**, 515–522.

Rockwell, S. (1994) Perfluorochemical emulsions and radiation therapy. *Art. Cells, Blood Subst., Immob. Biotech.*, **22**, 1097–1108.

Rosano, H.L., Gerbacia, W.E. (1973) Fluorocarbon microemulsions. U.S. Patent 3,778,381.

Rosenberg, M.D. (1971) Discrimination among dispersion forces at the aqueous-fluorocarbon interface. *Fed. Proc.*, **30**, 1623–1630.

Rotenberg, M., Rubin, M., Boc, A., Meynhas, D., Talmon, Y., Lichtenberg, D. (1991) Physico-chemical characterization of Intralipid™ emulsion. *Biochim. Biophys. Acta*, **1086**, 265–272.

Rudolph, A.S. (1994) Encapsulated hemoglobin: current issues and future goals. *Art. Cells, Blood Subst., Immob. Biotech.*, **22**, 347–360.

Rydhag, L. (1979) The importance of the phase behavior of phospholipids from emulsion stability. *Fette Seifen Anstrichmitt.*, **81**, 168–173.

Rydhag, L., Wilton, I. (1981) The function of phospholipids of soybean lecithin in emulsions. *J. Am. Oil Chem. Soc.*, **58**, 830–837.

Sadtler, V., Krafft, M.P., Riess, J.G. (1996). Achieving stable reverse water-in-fluorocarbon emulsions. *Angew. Chem. Intl. Ed. Engl.*, **35**, 1976–1978.

Sanchez, V., Zarif, L., Greiner, J., Riess, J.G., Cippolini, S., Bruneton, J.N. (1994) Novel injectable fluorinated contrast agents with enhanced radiopacity. *Art. Cells, Blood Subst., Immob. Biotech.*, **22**, 1421–1439.

Schaer, G.L., Hursey, T.L., Abrahams, S.L., Buddemeier, K., Ennis, B., Rodriguez, E.R., Hubbell, J.P., Moy, J., Parrillo, J.E. (1994) Reduction of reperfusion-induced myocardial necrosis in dogs by RheothRx injection (poloxamer 188 N.F.), a hemorheological agent that alters neutrophil function. *Circulation*, **90**, 2964–2975.

Schmolka, I.R. (1977) A review of block polymer surfactants. *J. Am. Oil Chem. Soc.*, **54**, 110.

Schmolka, I.R. (1992) Applications of the poloxamer surfactants in the medical and pharmaceutical industries. Proceed. 3rd World Surfactant Congress, London, June 1992, pp. 186–194.

Schmolka, I.R. (1994) Physical basis for poloxamer interactions. *Annals of New York Academy of Science*, **720**, 92–97.

Schubert, O., Wretlind, A. (1961) Intravenous infusion of fat emulsions, phosphatides and emulsifiers. *Acta Chir. Scand.*, **278 Suppl.**, 3–21.

Schubert, K.-V., Kaler, E.W. (1994) Microemulsifying fluorinated oils with mixtures of fluorinated and hydrogenated surfactants. *Colloids Surf. A: Physicochem. Engin. Aspects*, **84**, 97–106.

Schutt, E., Barber, P., Fields, T., Flaim, S., Horodniak, J., Keipert, P., Kinner, R., Kornbrust, L., Leakakos, T., Pelura, T., Weers, J., Houmes, R., Lachmann, B. (1994) Proposed mechanism of pulmonary gas trapping (PGT) following intravenous perfluorocarbon emulsion administration. *Art. Cells, Blood Subst., Immob. Biotech.*, **22**, 1205–1214.

Seddon, J.M. (1990) Structure of the inverted hexagonal (H_{II}) phase, and non-lamellar phase transitions of lipids. *Biochim. Biophys. Acta*, **1031**, 1–69.

Sellards, A.W., Minot, G.R. (1916) Injection of haemoglobin in man and its relation to blood destruction, with special reference to the anemias. *J. Med. Res.*, **34**, 469–494.

Selve, C., Castro, B., Leempoel, P., Mathis, G., Gartiser, T., Delpuech, J.J. (1983) Synthesis of homogenous polyoxyethylene perfluoroalkyl surfactants. *Tetrahedron*, **39**, 1313–1316.

Serratrice, G., Delpuech, J.J., Diguet, R. (1982) Compressibilités isothermes des fluorocarbures. Relation avec la solubilité des gaz. *Nouv. J. Chim.*, **6**, 489–493.

Shakir, K.M.M., Williams, T.J. (1982) Inhibition of phospholipase A_2 activity by Fluosol®, an artificial blood substitute. *Prostaglandins*, **23**, 919–920.

Sharma, S.K., Lowe, K.C., Davis, S.S. (1988) Emulsification methods for perfluorochemicals. *Drug Develop. Ind. Pharm.*, **14**, 2371–2376.

Sharma, S.K., Lowe, K.C., Davis, S.S. (1989) Novel compositions of emulsified perfluorochemicals for biological uses. In *Blood Substitutes*, edited by T.M.S. Chang and R.P. Geyer, pp. 447–450. New York: Marcel Dekker.

Sharts, C.M., Reese, H.R., Ginsberg, K.A., Multer, F.K., Nielson, M.D., Greenburg, A.G., Peskin, G.W., Long, D.M. (1978) The solubility of oxygen in aqueous fluorocarbon emulsions. *J. Fluorine Chem.*, **11**, 637–641.

Sherman, P. (1983) Rheological properties of emulsions. In *Encyclopedia of Emulsion Technology: Basic Theory*, edited by P. Becher, volume 1, pp. 405–438. New York: Marcel Dekker.

Sjölund, M., Lindblom, G., Rilfors, L., Arvidson, G. (1987) Hydrophobic molecules in lecithin-water systems I. Formation of reversed hexagonal phases at high and low water contents. *Biophys. J.*, **52**, 145–153.

Sloviter, H, Kamimoto, T. (1967) Erythrocyte substitute for perfusion of brain. *Nature*, **216**, 458–460.

Sloviter, H.A., Mukherji, B. (1983) Prolonged retention in the circulation of emulsified lipid-coated perfluorochemicals. *Progr. Clin. Biol. Res.*, **122**, 181–187.

Sloviter, H. A. (1985) Process for preparing perfluorochemical emulsion artificial blood. *US Pat.* 4,497,829.

Smart, B.E. (1983) Fluorocarbons. In *The Chemistry of Halides, Pseudo Halides and Azides*, edited by S. Patai and Z. Rappoport, Part 2, pp. 603–655. Chichester, UK: Wiley-Interscience.

Smith, D., Obraztsov, V., Neslund, G., Arlauskas, R., Weers, J. (1996) Influence of particle size distribution of perflubron-based emulsions on tumor necrosis factor (TNF) release from rat monocytes *in-vitro*. *Art. Cells, Blood Subst., Immob. Biotech.*, **24**, 432.

Song, D., Pelura, T.J., Liu, J., Ni, Y. (1994) Effects of buffer pH and phosphate concentration on the droplet size and EYP hydrolysis of perflubron/EYP emulsions. *Art. Cells, Blood Subst., Immob. Biotech.*, **22**, 1299–1305.

Spence, R.K., McCoy, S., Costabelle, J., Norcross, E.D., Pello, M.J., Alexander, J.B., Wisdom, R.C. (1990) Fluosol DA-20 in the treatment of severe anemia: randomized controlled study of 46 patients. *Crit. Care Med.*, **18**, 1227–1230.

Spence, R.K. (1995) Perfluorocarbons in the twenty-first century: clinical applications as transfusion alternatives. *Art. Cells, Blood Subst., Immob. Biotech.*, **23**, 367–380.

Spiess, B.D., Braverman, B., Woronowicz, A.W., Ivankovich, A.D. (1986) Protection from cerebral air emboli with perfluorocarbons in rabbits. *Stroke*, **17**, 1146–1149.

Spiess, B.D. (1995) Perfluorocarbon emulsions: one approach to intravenous artificial respiratory gas transport. *Int. Anesth. Clin.*, **33**, 103–113.

Stern, S., Guichard, M. (1996) Efficacy of agents counteracting hypoxia in fractionated radiation regimes. *Radiother. Oncol.*, **41**, 143–149.

Stolnik, S., Illum, L., Davis, S.S. (1995) Long circulating microparticulate drug carriers. *Adv. Drug Delivery Rev.*, **16**, 195–214.

Storm, G., Oussoren, C., Peeters, P.A.M., Barenholz, Y. (1993) Tolerability of liposomes *in vivo*. In *Liposome Technology*, edited by G. Gregoriadis, Vol. III, pp. 345–383.

Strey, R. (1994) Microemulsion microstructure and interfacial curvature. *Colloid Polym. Sci.*, **272**, 1005–1019.

Tadros, T.F., Vincent, G. (1983) Emulsion stability. In *Encyclopedia of Emulsion Technology*, edited by P. Becher, pp. 129–285. New York: M. Dekker.

Tarara, T.E., Malinoff, S.H., Pelura, T.J. (1994) Oxidative assessment of phospholipid-stabilized perfluorocarbon-based blood substitutes. *Art. Cells, Blood Subst., Immob. Biotech.*, **22**, 1287–1293.

Tarara, T.E., Dellamary, L.A., Kabalnov, A., Trevino, L.A., Weers, J.G. (1995) The role of spontaneous curvature in emulsions and its effect on stability to coalescence. Presented at the 210th American Chemical Society National Meeting, Chicago, IL.

Taylor, P. (1995) Ostwald ripening in emulsions. *Colloids Surf. A.*, **99**, 175–185.

Teelmann, K., Schläppi, B., Schüpbach, M., Kistler, A. (1984) Preclinical safety evaluation of intravenously administered mixed micelles. *Arzneim. Forsch./Drug Res.*, **34**, 1517–1523.

Teicher, B. A. (1995) An overview on oxygen carriers in cancer therapy. *Art. Cells, Blood Subst., Immob. Biotech.*, **23**, 395–405.

Thomas, T.G. (1878) The intravenous injection of milk as a substitute for the transfusion of blood. Illustrated by seven operations. *New York Med. J.*, **27**, 449–65.

Thomson, W. (Lord Kelvin) (1870) On the equilibrium of vapour at a curved surface of liquid. *Proc. Royal Soc. Edinburgh*, 63–68.

Tremper, K., Friedman, A., Levine, E.M., Lapin, R., Camarillo, D. (1982) The preoperative treatment of severely anemic patients with a perfluorochemical oxygen-carrying fluid, Fluosol-DA. *New Engl. J. Med.*, **307**, 277–283.

Tremper, K., Vercelotti, G.M., Hammerschmidt, E.D. (1984) Hemodynamic profile of adverse clinical reactions to Fluosol-DA 20%. *Crit. Care Med.*, **12**, 428–431.

Tremper, K., Wahr, J.A. (1995) Blood use and non-use: designing blood substitutes. In *Critical Care, State of the Art, Soc. Crit. Care Med.*, edited by M.M. Parker, M.J. Shapiro, Porembra, pp. 143–162.

Trevino, L., Sole-Violan, L., Daumur, P., Devallez, B., Postel, M., Riess, J.G. (1993) Molecular diffusion in concentrated fluorocarbon emulsions and its effect on emulsion stability. *New J Chem*, **17**, 275–278.

Tsuda, Y., Yamanouchi, K., Yokoyama, K., Suyama, T., Watanabe, M., Ohyanagi, H., Saitoh, Y. (1988) Discussion and considerations for the excretion mechanism of perfluorochemical emulsion. *Biomat., Art. Cells, Art. Org.*, **16**, 473–483.

Tsuda, Y., Nakura, K., Yamanouchi, K., Yokoyama, K., Watanabe, M., Ohyanagi, H., Saitoh, Y. (1989) Study of the excretion mechanism of a perfluorochemical emulsion. *Art. Organs*, **13**, 197–203.

Tsuda, Y., Yamanouchi, K., Okamoto, H., Yokoyama, K., Heldebrandt, C. (1990) Intravascular behavior of a perfluorochemical emulsion. *J. Pharmacobio-Dyn.*, **13**, 165–171.

U.S. Naval Research Advisory Committee Report (1992) Delivery of artificial blood to the military.

Vamvaskas, E.C., Taswell, H.F. (1994) Epidemiology of blood transfusion. *Transfusion*, **34**, 464–479.

Varescon, C., Arlen, C., LeBlanc, M., Riess, J.G. (1989) An easy convenient way of describing the stability of fluorocarbon emulsions. *J. Chim. Phys.*, **86**, 2111–2117.

Varescon, C., Le Blanc, M., Riess, J.G. (1990) Deviation from molecular diffusion ageing model in fluorocarbon emulsions stabilized by perfluoroalkylated surfactants. *J. Colloid Interface Sci.*, **137**, 373–379.

Vaslef, S.N., Goldstick, T.K (1994). Enhanced oxygen delivery induced by perfluorocarbon emulsions in capillary tube oxygenators. *ASAIO J.*, **40**, M643–648.

Virmani, R., Warren, D., Rees, R., Fink, L., English, D. (1983) Effect of perfluorochemical blood substitutes on phagocytic function of leukocytes. *Transfusion*, **23**, 512–515.

Virmani, R., Fink, L.M., Gunter, K., English, D. (1984b) Effect of perfluorochemical blood substitutes on human neutrophil function. *Transfusion*, **24**, 343–347.

Voiglio, E.J., Zarif, L., Gorry, F., Krafft, M.P., Margonari, J., Dubernard, J.M, Riess, J.G. (1996) Aerobic preservation of organs using a new perflubron/lecithin emulsion stabilized by molecular dowels. *J. Surg. Res.*, **63**, 439–446.

Vorobyev, S.I., Ivanitsky, G.R. (1994). *Perfluorocarbon Emulsion Stabilized by Proxanol*. Pushchino, Russia: Russian Acad. of Sciences.

Wagner, C. (1961) Theorie der alterung von niederschlagen durch umlosen (Ostwald-reifung). *Z. Electrochem*, **35**, 581.

Wahr, J.A., Trouwborst, A., Spence, R.K., Henny, C.P., Cernaianu, A.C., Graziano, G.P., Tremper, K.K., Flaim, K.E., Keipert, P.E., Faithfull, S., Clymer, J.J. (1996) A pilot study of the effects of a Perflubron emulsion, AF0104, on mixed venous oxygen tension in anesthetized surgical patients. *Anesth. Analg.*, **82**, 103–10

Wake, E.J., Studzinski, G.P. Bhandal, A. (1985) Changes in human cultured cells exposed to a perfluorocarbon emulsion. *Transfusion*, **25**, 73–77.

Wallace, E.L., Churchill, W.H., Surgenor, D.M., An, J., Cho, G., McGurk, S., Murphy, L. (1995) Collection and transfusion of blood and blood components in the United States 1992. *Transfusion*, **35**, 802–812.

Walstra, P. (1983) Formation of emulsions. In *Encyclopedia of Emulsion Technology*, edited by P. Becher, pp. 57–127. New York: M. Dekker.

Wanka, G., Hoffmann, H., Ulbricht, W. (1990) Polymer science: the aggregation behavior of poly-(oxyethylene)-poly-(oxypropylene)-poly-(oxyethylene) block copolymers in aqueous solution. *Colloid Polymer Sci.*, **268**, 101–117.

Waschke, K.F., Riedel, M., Albrecht, D.M., van Ackern, K., Kuschinsky, W. (1994) Effects of a perfluorocarbon emulsion on regional cerebral blood flow and metabolism after fluid resuscitation from hemorrhage in conscious rats. *Anesth. Analg.*, **79**, 874–882.

Washington, C. (1996) Stability of lipid emulsions for drug delivery. *Adv. Drug Delivery Rev.*, **20**, 131–145.

Washington, C., King, S.M., Heenan, R.K. (1996) Structure of block copolymers adsorbed to perfluorocarbon emulsions. *J. Phys. Chem.*, **100**, 7603–7609.

Watanabe, R., Inahara, H., Motoyama, Y. (1975) Oxygen carrying capacity of perfluorochemical emulsion mixed with blood *in vitro. Proc. Intern. Cong. Nutrition — Symp. Perfluorochemical Artificial Blood*, p. 113–119. Osaka: Kyoto. Igakushobo Medical Pub.

Weers, J.G. (1993) A physicochemical evaluation of perfluorochemicals for oxygen transport applications. *J. Fluorine Chem.*, **64**, 73–93.

Weers, J.G., Liu, J., Resch, P., Cavin, J., Arlauskas, R.A. (1994a) Room temperature stable perfluorocarbon emulsions with acceptable half-lives in the reticuloendothelial system. *Art. Cells, Blood Subst., Immob. Biotech.*, **22**, 1175–1182.

Weers, J.G., Ni, Y., Tarara, T.E., Pelura ,T.J., Arlauskas, R.A. (1994b) The effect of molecular diffusion on initial particle size distributions in phospholipid-stabilized fluorocarbon emulsions. *Colloids Surf. A*, **84**, 81–87.

Weers, J.G., Arlauskas, R.A. (1995) Sedimentation field-flow fractionation studies of Ostwald ripening in fluorocarbon emulsions containing two disperse phase components. *Langmuir*, **11**, 474–477.

Weers, J.G., Arlanskas, R.A., Harris, M., Otto, S. (1996) The use of lipophilic secondary fluorocarbons to solve the emulsion stability/organ retention dilemma in blood substitutes. *Art. Cells, Blood Subst., Immob. Biotech.*, **24**, 458 (abstract)

Wendel, A. (1995) *Lecithin Encyclopedia of Chemical Technology*, IVth edition, **15**, 192–209.

Wesseler, E.P., Iltis, R., Clark, L.C. (1977) The solubility of oxygen in highly fluorinated liquids. *J. Fluorine Chem.* **9**, 137– 146.

Westesen, L., Wehler, T. (1993) Particle size determination of a submicron-sized emulsion. *Colloids Surf. A*, **78**, 125–132.

Williams, J.H., Chen, M., Drew, J., Panigan, E., Hosseini, S. (1988) Modulation of rat granulocyte traffic by a surface active agent *in vitro* and bleomycin injury. *Proceed. Soc. Exp. Biol. Med.*, **188**, 461–470.

Winslow, R.M. (1992) *Hemoglobin-based Red Cell Substitutes*. Baltimore: The John Hopkins University Press.

Winslow, R.M. (ed.) (1994) *Proc. Vth Intern. Symp. Blood Substitutes*, vol 2, *Blood Substitutes: Modified Hemoglobin*, published in *Art. Cells, Blood Subst. Immob. Biotech.*, **22**, 361–944.

Winslow, R.M., Vandegriff, K.D., Intaglietta, M. (eds.) (1995) *Blood Substitutes: Physiological Basis for Efficacy*. Boston: Birkhäuser.

Wretlind, A. (1977) Lipid emulsions and technique of peripheral administration in parenteral nutrition. In *Current Concepts of Parenteral Nutrition*, edited by J.M. Greep, P.B. Socters, R.I.C. Wisdrop, C.W.R. Phaf and J.E. Fisher. The Hague: Nartinus Hijhoff Medical Division.

Wretlind, A. (1987) The when and why of parenteral nutrition. *Med. Corps Int.*, **3**, 39–47.

Yamanouchi, K., Tanaka, M., Tsuda, Y., Yokoyama, K., Awazu, S. Kobayashi, Y. (1985) Quantitative structure *in vivo* half-life relationships of perfluorochemicals for use as oxygen transporters. *Chem. Pharm. Bull*, **33**, 1221–1231.

Yokoyama, K., Yamanouchi, K., Watanabe, M., Matsumoto, T., Murashima, R., Daimoto, T., Hamano, T., Okamoto, H., Suyama, T., Watanabe, R., Naito, R. (1975) Preparation of perfluorodecalin emulsion, an approach to the red cells substitute. *Fed. Proc.*, **34**, 1478–1483.

Yokoyama, K., Yamanouchi, K., Ohyanagi, H., Mitsuno, T. (1978) Fate of perfluorochemicals in animals after intravenous injection or hemodilution with their emulsions. *Chem. Pharm. Bull. Jap.*, **26**, 956–966.

Yokoyama, K., Watanabe, M., Naito, R. (1981) Retention of perfluorochemicals (PFCs) in blood of human recipients after infusion of Fluosol-DA 20%. *Oxygen-carrying Colloidal Blood Substitutes:* 5th Int. Symp. Perfluorochemical Blood Substitutes, Mainz, Germany, 1981, pp. 214–219. Munich: W. Zuckschwerdt Verlag.

Yokoyama, K., Suyama, T., Naito, R. (1982) Development of perfluorochemical (PFC) emulsion as an artificial blood substitute. In *Biomedicinal Aspects of Fluorine Chemistry*, edited by R. Filler and Y. Kobayashi, pp. 191–212. Amsterdam: Elsevier.

Yokoyama, K., Naito, R. (1983) Selection of 53 PFC substances for better stability of emulsion and improved artificial blood substitutes. *Prog. Clin. Biol. Res.*, **122**, 189–196.

Yokoyama, K., Yamanouchi, K., Suyama, T. (1983) Recent advances in a perfluorochemical blood substitute and its biomedical application. *Life Chem. Reports*, **2**, 35–93.

Yokoyama, K., Suyama, T., Okamoto, H., Watanabe, M., Ohyanagi, H., Saitoh, Y. (1984) A perfluorochemical emulsion as an oxygen carrier. *Artif. Org.*, **8**, 34–40.

Yoon, J.K., Burgess, D.J. (1996) Interfacial properties as stability predictors of lecithin-stabilized fluorocarbon emulsions. *Pharm. Dev. Technol.*, **1**, 333–341.

Zander, R. (1974) O_2-Löslichkeit in Fluorcarbonen. *Res. Exp. Med.*, **164**, 97–109

Zarif, L., Greiner, J., Pace, S., Riess, J.G. (1990) Synthesis and evaluation of perfluoroalkylxylitol ethers and esters: new surfactants for biomedical uses. *J. Med. Chem.*, **33**, 1262–1269.

Zarif, L., Manfredi, A., Le Blanc, M., Riess, J.G. (1989) Synergistic stabilization of fluorocarbon emulsions by Pluronic F-68 and a perfluoroalkylated polyhydroxylated surfactant derived from xylitol or maltose. *J. Am. Oil Chem. Soc.*, **66**, 1515–1523.

Zaritskii, A.R., Kuznetsova, I.N., Perevedentseva, E.V., Fok, M.V. (1993) Effect of perfluorochemical emulsions on the rate of blood oxygenation-deoxygenation. *Russian J. Phys. Chem.*, **67**, 533–536.

Zuck, T.F., Riess, J.G. (1994) Current status of injectable oxygen carriers. *Crit. Rev. Clin. Lab. Sci.*, **31**, 295–324.

Zweier, J.L., Chzhan, M., Ewert, U., Schneider, G., Kuppusamy, P. (1994) Development of a highly sensitive probe for measuring oxygen in biological tissues. *J. Mag. Reson.*, **105**, 52–57.

INDEX

Acute normovolemic hemodilution (ANH) 236, 243, 317
Amorphous drug clusters 227
Amphotericin B 137
Antiinflammatory activity
　bethamethasone 167
　diclofenac 159
　Indomethacin 162
　jojoba oil 162
　lidocaine 168
　naproxen 162
　NSAID 159
　piroxicam 162
　tetracaine 168
　ubiquinone 169
Apoliprotein C 100
Apoliprotein E 101
Artificial blood 237
Autocorrelation function 32

Beta (β) 40
Bioavailability 188
Blood substitutes 235, 317
Burst release 224

Capillary hydrodynamic fractionation (CDHF) 78
Capillary zone electrophoresis (CZE) 79
Carnitine 9
Cavitation 223
Centrifugal ultrafiltration technique 130
Cetylpalmitate 230
Classical light scattering (CLS) 43
Coalescence 287
Coalescence monitoring 57, 89
Coenzyme Q_{10} 189
Coincidence counting 62
Coincidence events 62
Cold homogenization technique 220
Colloidal suspension 205
Compritol 229
CONTIN 42
Co-surfactant
　Highly mobile 216
　Micelle-forming 216

Coulter counter 79
Critical crystallization temperature 185
Cryo-electron microscopy 192, 210
Crystal face 209
Crystallization 182, 186
Cumulants 41
Cyclosporine A 146
Cytotoxicity 229

De Weir equation 15
Dexamethasone palmitate 135
Diazemuls® 131
Diazepam-lipuro® 131
Dielectric spectroscopy 77
Differential Scanning Calorimetry (DSC) 182, 193
Diffusion 35
Diprivan® 134
Direct counting methods 30
Disc centrifuge 78
Dissolution rate 188
Drug release profile 224
Drug retention 110
Dyalisis sac diffusion technique 128
Dynamic light scattering (DLS) 32

Egg lecithin 229
Egg yolk phospholipids 266, 314
Electrolyte displacement 79
Electron microscopy 67
Electrozone 79
Electrical field-flow fractionation (EFFF) 74
Emulsifier 262, 296
　excess 213
　mobility 216
Emulsion stability 286, 302
Emulsions for parenteral nutrition 228
Emulsions of supercooled melts 176, 181
Energy expenditure 15
Ensemble sizing methods 30
Entrapment efficiency 223
Epirubicin 145
Epitaxical effect 214

INDEX

Etomidat® 135
Exponential sampling 42

Fiber optics 36
Field flow fractionation (FFF) 69
Fish oil 11
Flocculation 307
   monitoring 57, 89
Flow field-flow fractionation (FFFF) 69, 74
Fluorinated surfactants 299
Fluorocarbons 235, 302
   excretion 252, 253
   organ retention 256, 302
   oxygen dissolving capacity 241, 248
   synthesis 247
   toxicity 258
Fluorocarbon/hydrocarbon diblocks 276, 304
Fluorocarbon-in-water emulsions 235
   clinical trials 239, 245, 317
   efficacy 239, 243
   particle size 308, 311
   pharmacokinetics 252
   processing 278, 283
   production flow chart 280
   rheology 275, 312
   side-effects 277, 308
   stability 286, 302
   sterilization 285
fluorocarbons 315
Fluorosurfactants 299
Fluosol 239, 255, 272
Flurbiprofen axetil 135
FO-QELS 37
Fraunhofer diffraction 49
Fractogram 71
Freeze-fracture microscopy 69

Gap homogenizer 220
Gel
   Formation 208, 213
   Network 212
GRAS status 229
Gel 208, 212, 215
Gel-emulsions 315

Halothane 142
Hard fat 186
Heterodyne 36

HIAC 62
High pressure homogenization 280, 220
Homodyne 36
Hot homogenization technique 220
Hydrocarbon-in-fluorocarbon emulsions 316
Hydrodynamic chromatography (HDC) 78
Hydrodynamic size 74
Hydrophilization 188

Indomethacin 162
Intensity fluctuation spectroscopy (IFS) 32
Intensity light scattering (ILS) 50
Interaction of emulsion with plasma 84
Intravascular persistance 252, 310
In vitro toxicity 229
In vivo toxicity 229

jojoba oil 162
   lidocaine 168

Laser diffraction 32
LCT emulsion 7
Lecithin 206
Lifshitz-Slezov-Wagner theory 294
Light blockage 60
Light scattering 61
Limethason® 134
Lipid emulsion
   effect on immune function 8
   oxidation rate 15
Lipid matrix 208
Lipid microspheres 219
Lipid nanopellets 219
Lipid suspension
   Colloidal 205
   Differences to lipid emulsions 206
Lipiodol 145
Liple® 132
Lipolysis 99
Lipo-NSAID® 135
Lipopearls® 220
Lipophilic fluorocarbons 258, 302
Lipophilicity 99, 111
Lipoprotein 100
Lipoprotein lipase 100
Liposomes 219, 230

INDEX

Lipospheres 219
Long chain triglycerides emulsion 7
Long term stability 228
Lusk equation 15

Medium chain triglycerides (MCT) 121
   Emulsion 9
Mean size 25
Melt-homogenization 175, 182, 207
Miconazole 140
Microemulsions 219
Microfluidization 280
Mie scattering 46
Mobility 206, 215
Monolayer spontaneous curvature 287
Mononuclear phagocyte system 102, 105
Multilamellar vesicles 215
Multiple exponential 42
Multiple light scattering (MLS) 36

Nanocrystal 209, 216
Nanoparticles
   Lipid nanoparticles 175
   Solid lipid nanoparticles 175, 187
   Ubidecarenone nanoparticles 189, 192
NMR spectroscopy 77, 182
Nitrosourea 145
Nucleation 176
   Heterogenous nucleation 177, 199
   Homogenous nucleation 176
   Nucleation rate 177, 199

Obscuration-SPOS 59
Oil-in-water emulsion 220
Omega-3 (Ω-3) fatty acids 11
Omega-6 (Ω-6) fatty acids 11
Organ distribution clearance 106
Ostwald ripening 293, 310
Oxygen carrier 235
Oxygen delivery 236, 241
Oxygent® 240, 274, 317

Paclitaxel 143
Parenteral administration 181
Particle size 103, 181, 198
Particle size distribution 22
Paw edema model 160
Pay load 223
Penclomedine 144

Penetration enhancers 153, 170
Perflubron 240, 260
Perfluorocarbons 245, 260
Perfluorochemicals 245
Perfluorodecalin 238
Perfluorooctylbromide 240, 258
PGI$_2$ 146
Phospholipids 121, 181, 215, 266, 284, 314
Photon correlation spectroscopy (PCS) 32
Physical state 188
Pluronic 264
Polarization intensity differential scattering (PIDS) 43
Polarized light microscopy 214
Poloxamers 263
Poloxamer 188 229
Polymeric nanoparticles 229
Polysorbate 80 229
Poorly water-soluble drugs 187
Pregnanolone 142
Prodrug 112
Propofol 134
Prostacyclin 146
Pulmonary embolism 23, 84

Quasielastic light scattering (QELS) 32

Rayleigh scattering 44
Rayleigh-Gans-Debye (RGD) scattering 45
Recrystallization 214
Release kinetics 127
Resting energy expenditure (REE) 13
Reticuloendothelial system (RES) 12
Reverse emulsions 316
Reverse sac diffusion technique 128
Rhizoxin 143
Ropion® 135

Scanning electron microscopy (SEM) 67
Scattering-SPOS 60
Sedimentation field-flow fractionation 69, 71
Semisolid 207
Separation methods 31
Single particle optical sensing (SPOS) 57
Size exclusion chromatography (SEC) 78
SLN® 219
Small unilamellar vesicles 210

SME topical cream 154
Sodium cholate 229
Solid lipid nanoparticles 207, 219
   Gel formation 208
   Long-term stability 213
   Phospholipid-stabilized 210
Solid triglycerides 187
Soybean oil 120
Spingomyelin 101, 108
Stability 199
Static light scattering (SLS) 43
Steric stabilization 292
Steric field-flow fractionation (SFFF) 72
Strokes-Einstein equation 35
Structured triglycerides 9
Structure 213
Supercooling 175, 198
   Supercooled drugs 187
   Supercooled melts 183, 189, 199
Surface charge 125
Surfactant availability 216
Systemic toxicity 229

Targeting 99, 113
Taxol® 143
Topical drug carrier 154
Total parenteral nutrition (TPN) 7
Transfusion reduction 235
Transmission electron microscopy (TEM) 67, 181, 192, 209

Tricaprin 187
Triglycerides 180, 186
Trilaurin 176
Trimyristin 182
Tripalmitate
   β-modification 209
   dispersion 209, 214
   gel 208, 212, 215
   nanocrystal 209dicl
   suspension 205, 215
Tumorigenesis 11
Turbidimetry 52

Ubidecarenone 189, 193
Ultrafiltration technique at low pressure 130
Ultrasound spectroscopy 55

Viability 229
Viscosity 181, 185
Vitalipid® 134
Volume weighting 26

Water-in-fluorocarbon emulsions 316
Wettability 188

X-ray diffraction 181, 193

z-average 25
Zeta Potential 105, 125